Imaging for Medicine

Volume 1

NUCLEAR MEDICINE, ULTRASONICS, and THERMOGRAPHY

Imaging for Medicine

Volume 1 Nuclear Medicine, Ultrasonics, and Thermography
Volume 2 Diagnostic Radiology
Volume 3 From the Ultraviolet to the Near Infrared

Imaging for Medicine

Volume 1

NUCLEAR MEDICINE, ULTRASONICS, and THERMOGRAPHY

Edited by

SOL NUDELMAN
DENNIS D. PATTON

University of Arizona School of Medicine
Tucson, Arizona

PLENUM PRESS · NEW YORK AND LONDON

Library of Congress Cataloging in Publication Data

Main entry under title:

Imaging for medicine.

Includes index.

CONTENTS: v. 1. Nuclear Medicine, ultrasonics, and thermography.

1. Diagnosis, Radioscopic, 2. Radiology, Medical. 3. Imaging systems in medicine. I. Nudelman, Sol. II. Patton, Dennis D. [DNLM: 1. Ultrasonics–Diagnostic use. 2. Thermography. 3. Diagnosis–Instrumentation. 4. Radionuclide imaging. WB141.3 I31]

RC78.I45 616.07'57 79-25680

ISBN 978-1-4684-3673-0 ISBN 978-1-4684-3671-6 (eBook)
DOI 10.1007/978-1-4684-3671-6

Softcover reprint of the hardcover 1st edition 1980
A Division of Plenum Publishing Corporation
227 West 17th Street, New York, N.Y. 10011

Contributors

H. H. Barrett, Optical Sciences Center, University of Arizona, Tucson, Arizona 85721

Theodore Bowen, Department of Physics, University of Arizona, Tucson, Arizona 85721

Eustace L. Dereniak, Optical Sciences Center, University of Arizona, Tucson, Arizona 85721

Irwin M. Freundlich, Department of Radiology, Health Sciences Center, University of Arizona, Tucson, Arizona 85724

Kai Haber, Department of Radiology, Health Sciences Center, University of Arizona, Tucson, Arizona 85724

Ronald E. McKeighen, Searle Diagnostics, Inc., 2000 Nuclear Drive, Des Plaines, Illinois 60018. *Present address:* K. B. Aerotech, P.O. Box 350, Lewistown, Pennsylvania 17044

G. Muehllehner, Searle Diagnostics, Inc., 2000 Nuclear Drive, Des Plaines, Illinois 60018. *Present address:* Hospital of the University of Pennsylvania, 3400 Spruce Street, Philadelphia, Pennsylvania 19104

Dennis D. Patton, Division of Nuclear Medicine, Health Sciences Center, University of Arizona, Tucson, Arizona 85724

J.A. Patton, Department of Radiology, Vanderbilt University, Nashville, Tennessee 37232

Götz Rassow, Siemens Aktiengesellschaft, Medical Engineering Group, Postfach 3260, D-8520 Erlangen, West Germany

R.G. Simpson, Optical Sciences Center, University of Arizona, Tucson, Arizona 85721

F. R. Whitehead, Searle Diagnostics, Inc., 2000 Nuclear Drive, Des Plaines, Illinois 60018. *Present address:* General Electric Medical Systems Division, 11505 Douglas Road, Rancho Cordova, California 95670

William L. Wolfe, Optical Sciences Center, University of Arizona, Tucson, Arizona 85721

Preface

The material in this volume was prepared and collected over the past four years with the growing realization that a technical revolution was in progress for diagnostic medicine. It became clear that for the wide variety of imaging instruments and methods finding their way into applications for research and clinical medicine, there was a scarcity of reference and text books for the scientist and engineer beginning in the field. Thus what began as a relatively small project for a single volume has grown into certainly two and probably three volumes to adequately cover the field. This first volume is expected to be followed within a few months by a second volume, dealing with diagnostic radiology, and within a year by a third volume, covering most other aspects of medicine that utilize spectra from the ultraviolet through the visible into the near-infrared.

The chapters in this book are divided into three groups. The first group deals with nuclear medicine and includes Chapters 1–8. These chapters are arranged to begin with a broad introduction to the subject (Chapter 1) followed by a sequence of four chapters (Chapters 2–5) that provide an in-depth review of the imaging instrumentation developed for the field. Chapter 6 deals with "evaluation" of imaging device performance, while Chapters 7 and 8 discuss two areas of considerable research activity.

The second group of chapters, Chapters 9 and 10, covers ultrasonic imaging. Chapter 9 provides a tutorial treatment of the physician's approach to ultrasonic examination, and Chapter 10 provides a theoretical analysis of the various aspects important in ultrasonic imaging. The third group of chapters, Chapters 11–13, spans the field of thermography. Chapter 11 again introduces the subject from the physician's point of view, Chapter 12 reviews instrumentation available as well as under development, and Chapter 13 presents a detailed theoretical treatment of the subject.

It is hoped that by mixing chapters covering the physician's diagnostic approach with the technical chapters, a more practical understanding of the strengths and weaknesses of the different modalities will be possible, and that it might even inspire new directions of research and development.

We are indebted to and thank Professor M. Paul Capp for his continuous encouragement and assistance, in addition to Ms. Beverly Bindes, Ms. Betty Porter, and Ms. Georgie May Quinn for their secretarial assistance.

University of Arizona
College of Medicine

Sol Nudelman, Ph.D.
Dennis D. Patton, M.D.

Contents

1. Basic Information on Routine Diagnosis in Nuclear Medicine

Götz Rassow

2. Scintillation Camera Collimators

G. Muehllehner

3. Rectilinear Scanners
Dennis D. Patton

4. A Review of Gamma Camera Technology for Medical Imaging
Ronald E. McKeighen

5. Tomography

J.A. Patton

6. Quantitative Analysis of Minimum Detectable Uptake Ratios for Nuclear Medicine Imaging Systems

F.R. Whitehead

7. X-Ray Fluorescence Imaging

J.A. Patton

8. Coded-Aperture Imaging

R.G. Simpson and H.H. Barrett

9. Diagnostic Uses of Ultrasonic Imaging

Kai Haber

10. Ultrasonic Imaging: Basic Principles

Theodore Bowen

11. Medical Aspects of Thermography

Irwin M. Freundlich

12. Thermographic Instrumentation

Eustace L. Dereniak

13. General Infrared System Analysis

William L. Wolfe and Eustace L. Dereniak

CHAPTER 1

Basic Information on Routine Diagnosis in Nuclear Medicine*

GÖTZ RASSOW

1.1. INTRODUCTION

The application of radionuclides in medicine has proved to be so fruitful that a separate scientific branch has developed: nuclear medicine.

Radionuclides are radioactive isotopes of the chemical elements and have the same chemical behavior as the stable (nonradioactive) isotopes. Radionuclides differ from them in their ability to undergo spontaneous nuclear disintegration. Nuclear medicine makes use of the effect of the radiation produced by the nuclear disintegration.

Nuclear medicine is divided into diagnostic and therapeutic procedures.

* *Note from editor*. This chapter was originally published as a booklet by Siemens Aktiengesellschaft, Berlin/Munich, 1970. We are indebted for their kind permission to use it as an introduction for our discussion on the "state of the art" in diagnosis with nuclear medicine. Although newer radiotracers are now used, the principles remain the same.

GÖTZ RASSOW • Siemens Aktiengesellschaft, Medical Engineering Group, Postfach 3260, D-8520 Erlangen, West Germany.

1.1.1. Nuclear Therapy

Therapy makes use of the radiation effect of incorporated radionuclides for selective cell and tissue destruction.

1.1.2. Nuclear Diagnosis

Diagnosis makes use of the radiation effect of incorporated and non-incorporated radionuclides for information.

With the aid of radionuclides, medical research has made considerable advances, which have given rise to many routine methods of diagnosis. Since physics and engineering play a considerable role in this development, nuclear-medical diagnosis represents a complex scientific field. This chapter is intended to give the newcomer to nuclear medicine an insight into this field and to explain the physical and engineering terms required for an understanding of this subject.

1.2. NUCLEAR DIAGNOSIS

1.2.1. Indicator Method

Nuclear-medical diagnosis is based on the indicator method. The indicator method with radionuclides has the characteristic that the information carried by them does not flow continuously as is the case of the indicator method with dyes. While individual color particles can be recognized as an indicator at any time through their color effect, radionuclides reveal their indicator effect only at the moment of nuclear disintegration.

On account of the spontaneity of nuclear disintegration, however, the disintegrations are statistically distributed with respect to time. Consequently, a large number of radionuclides have the effect of an indicator with continuously flowing information, when the information is conceived as disintegration rate, i.e., as the number of disintegrations per time interval.

Since nuclear disintegration manifests itself by the emission of radiation and the effect of the radiation is measured as an electric voltage pulse, the count rate is the measured quantity of the indicator method, i.e., as the number of pulses per time interval (Fig. 1-1). In practice, in most cases it is not necessary to distinguish between disintegration rate and count rate as absolute values are not measured. It is sufficient to know that under the measuring conditions used in nuclear medicine the count rate is proportional to the disintegration rate. The disintegration rate is referred to as activity A (cf. Section 1.4.2).

The simplest information that can be obtained from the indicator method consists of the comparison between various activities (finding the

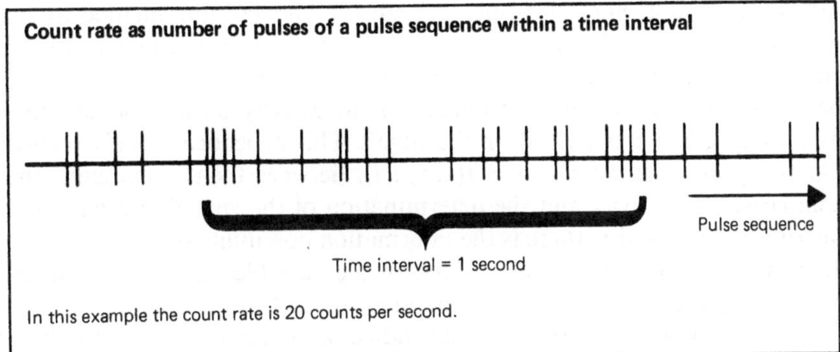

Count rate as number of pulses of a pulse sequence within a time interval
Pulse sequence
Time interval = 1 second
In this example the count rate is 20 counts per second.

Fig. 1-1

Graphic displays as example of basic technique 2

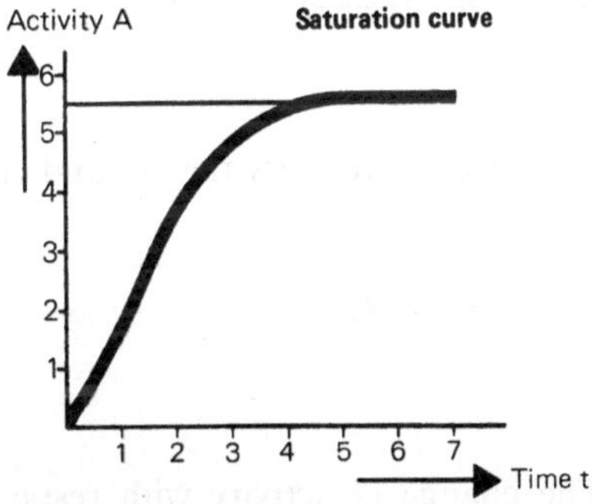

Activity A

Saturation curve

1 2 3 4 5 6 7

Time t

Typical curve obtained when a certain quantity of indicator finally ends up at the site of measurement.

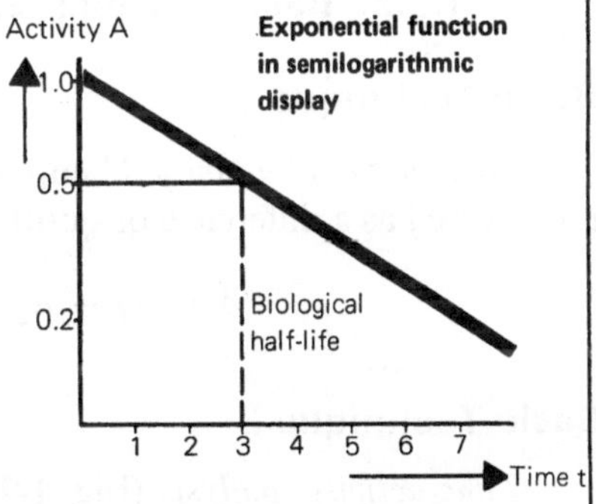

Activity A

Exponential function in semilogarithmic display

1.0

0.5

0.2

Biological half-life

1 2 3 4 5 6 7

Time t

Typical curve obtained when a certain quantity of indicator is transported from the measuring site at a speed proportional to the quantity still present.

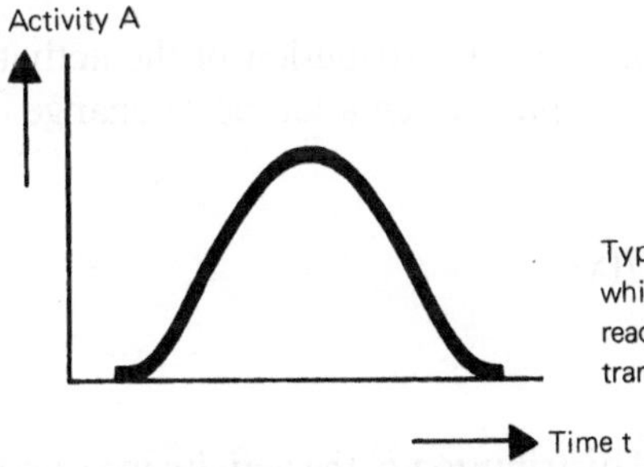

Activity A

Typical functional measuring curve, which indicates how fast the indicator reaches the site and how fast it is transported away.

Time t

Fig. 1-2

difference or quotient of the values A_1 and A_2). The indicator method would be fully exploited if information were given on the spatial and temporal change of the activity distribution in the organism. In this ideal case it would be necessary to know the dependence of the activity on the spatial coordinates x, y, and z as well as on the time t. This dependence is also called function f and it is written $A = f(x, y, z, t)$. Between the two extremes, the comparison of activity and the determination of the spatial and temporal distribution of activity, there is the information possibility of measuring the activity as a function of one or more of the variables x, y, z, or t, while neglecting the dependence of the remaining variables.

The analytical approach to the indicator method as described here forms a supporting frame into which the manifold nuclear-medical applications can be clearly arranged. The supporting frame is built up of five basic techniques of obtaining information now to be discussed.

1.2.2. Basic Techniques of the Indicator Method

Basic Technique 1

Comparison of activity. Comparison between two activities A_1 and A_2 is expressed as a difference or quotient, i.e.,

$$A = A_1 - A_2 \quad \text{or} \quad A = A_1/A_2$$

Basic Technique 2

Time-activity analysis (Fig. 1-2). The change of activity with respect to time at given site is given as

$$A = f(t)$$

Basic Technique 3

Profile Scintigraphy (Fig. 1-3). The spatial distribution of the activity measured as activity distribution along a path when a temporal change of activity can be neglected:

$$A = f(x)$$

Basic Technique 4

Scintigraphy (Fig. 1-4). The spatial distribution of the activity measured as activity distribution in a plane when a temporal change of activity can

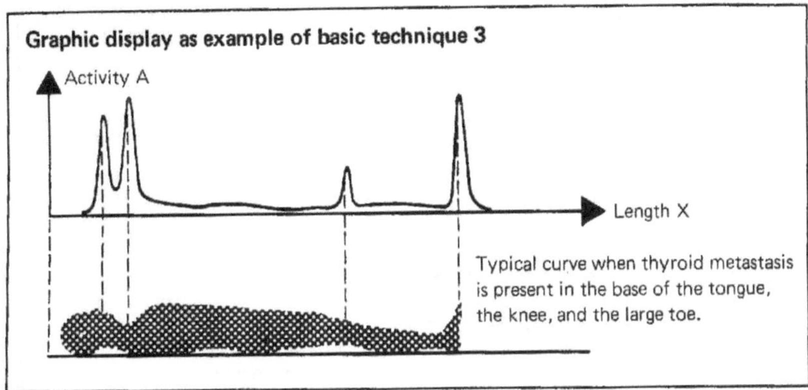

Fig. 1-3

be neglected:

$$A = f(x, y)$$

Photoscan (Fig. 1-5). If a photorecorder is used for displaying the data, the change in the activity appears as a variation in the film blackening. In this case graphical display in a plane is possible.

Color Dot Scan (Fig. 1-6). If a color dot printer is used for displaying the data, the change in the activity appears as colored regions. In this case graphic display in a plane is possible.

Basic Technique 5

Camera Scintigraphy. The spatial distribution of the activity measured as activity distribution in a plane at various times is given as

$$A = f(x, y, t)$$

Serial Scintigraphy (Fig. 1-7). The graphical representation of a quantity as the function of three variables is unclear. Since with scintigraphic camera exposures a change of activity results in a step between light and dark, graphic representation in space is possible.

With serial scintigraphy the principle of cinematography is realized in scintigraphy. In this representation the information obtained reproduces very clearly the spatial changes of activity within the camera field of vision if the pictures "shot" at various times are compared with each other.

Function Scintigraphy (Fig. 1-8). Another representation of the information obtained with camera pictures is possible with special technical means, which only allow small regions of the field of vision of the camera, i.e., picture elements, to be evaluated. The evaluation of the change of activity

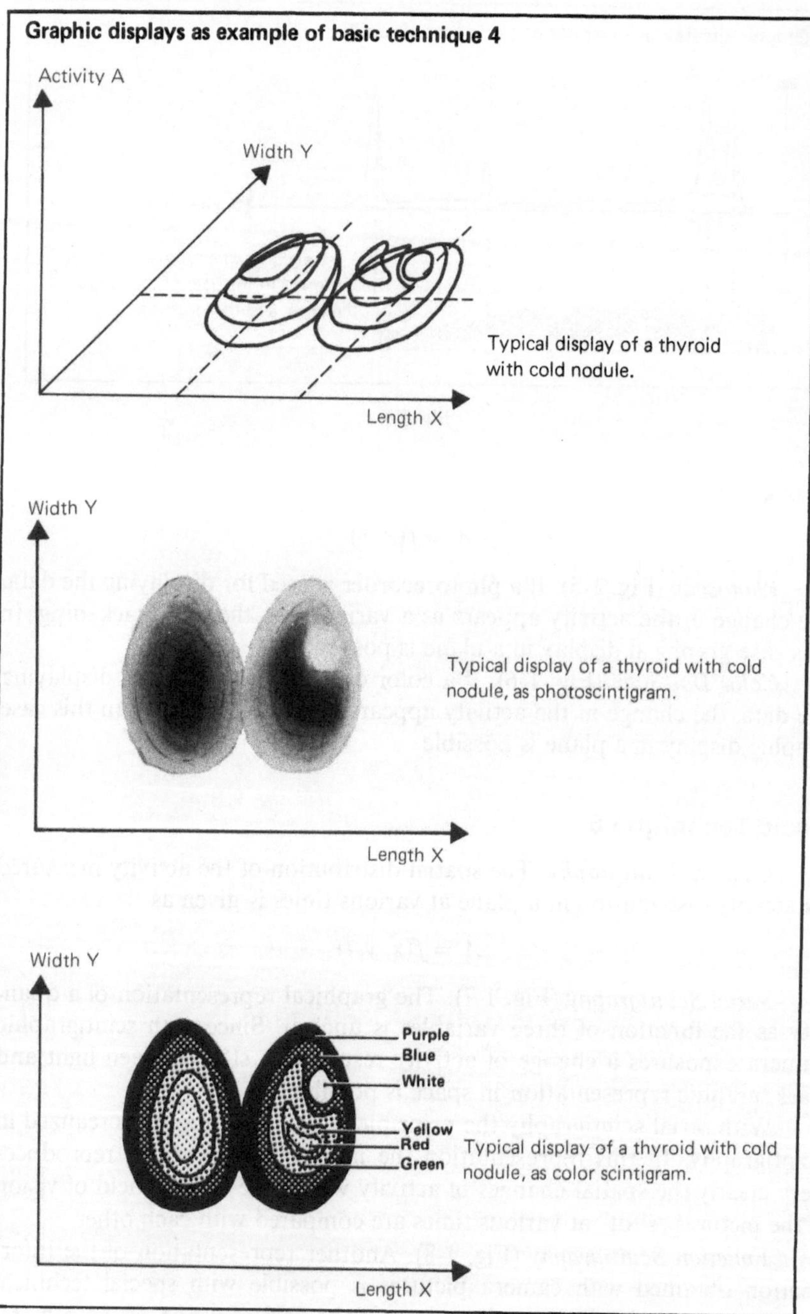

Fig. 1-4 (top), Fig. 1-5 (middle), and Fig. 1-6 (bottom)

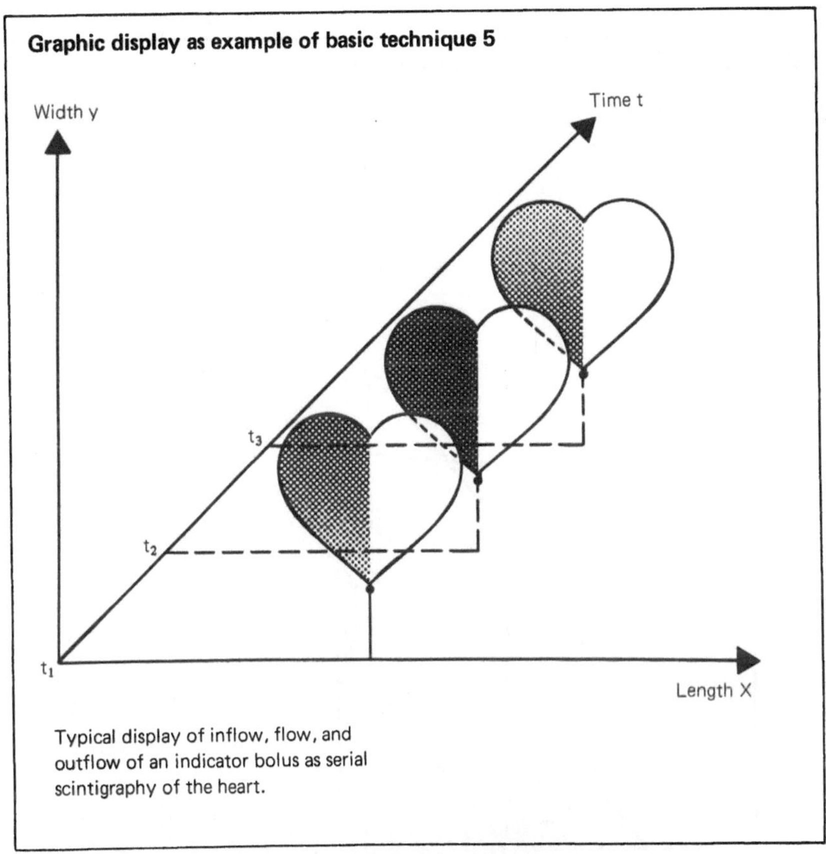

Fig. 1-7

in certain definite picture elements of various pictures results in time–activity information about an organ region as in function studies. However, here we are not dealing with continuous function measurements, but individual values are measured at various times.

Although the medical applications of the indicator method emanate from these basic informations, they are alone not sufficient for the physician. For instance, if information is required on the blood volume and an indicator is used that can leave the vascular compartment, then determining the activity of the blood would lead to false results. For this reason the results of all nuclear-medical methods are based on combinations of information obtained from the indicator method with a special knowledge of medicine, biochemistry, and physics. It is these combinations that account for the diversity of nuclear-medical methods. Starting from the basic informations as a supporting frame, well-proven methods—the routine methods—will now be dealt with.

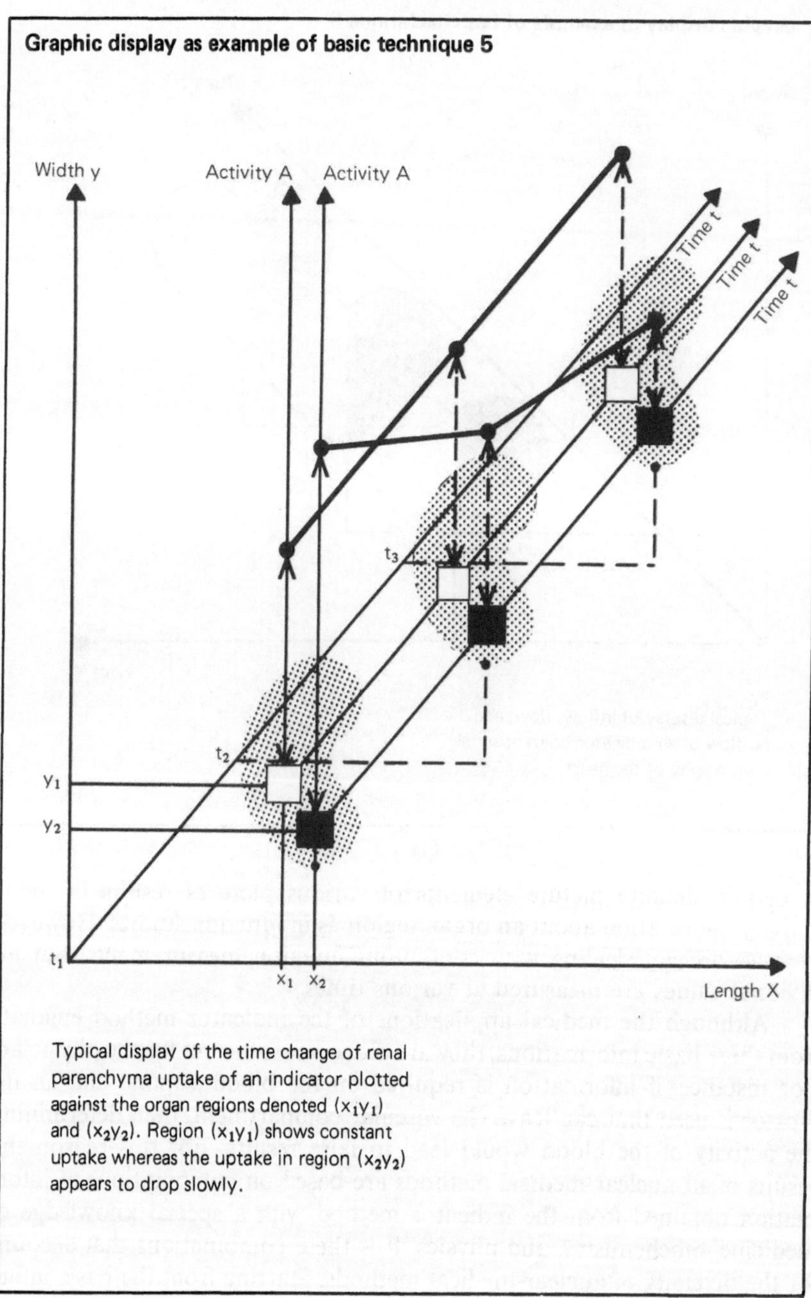
Graphic display as example of basic technique 5
Width y
Activity A
Activity A
Time t
Time t
Time t
t₃
t₂
y₁
y₂
t₁
x₁ x₂
Length X
Typical display of the time change of renal parenchyma uptake of an indicator plotted against the organ regions denoted (x₁y₁) and (x₂y₂). Region (x₁y₁) shows constant uptake whereas the uptake in region (x₂y₂) appears to drop slowly.

Fig. 1-8

1.2.3. Routine Methods

1.2.3.1. Comparison of Activity

The methods that are based on the comparison of activity can be divided into three groups: methods with which dilution analysis is carried out, methods with which saturation analysis is carried out, and methods with which transport analysis is carried out.

1.2.3.1.1. Dilution Analysis. Dilution analysis makes use of the fact that the indicator concentration (K), e.g., as activity per milliliter (A/ml), of a liquid is reduced by the factor $1/F$ after dilution. F is the dilution factor and characterizes the volume ratio of the diluted liquid ($V + v$) to the diluting liquid (v):

$$F = \frac{V + v}{v}$$

If K_1 is the concentration before dilution and K_2 the concentration after dilution, then

$$K_2 = \frac{1}{F} K_1 \quad \text{or} \quad \frac{K_1}{K_2} = F = \frac{V + v}{v}$$

Consequently, the volume of the dilution liquid can be calculated when K_1, K_2, and v have been measured. Since v is very small compared with V, for the calculation $V + v \approx V$ is used (Fig. 1-9).

Dilution analysis is suitable for determining the blood volume and body water.

Measurement of Blood Volume. If 1 ml radioactive liquid of activity A_1 is injected intravenously into a patient and after a reasonable mixing time the activity A_2 of a 1-ml blood sample taken from the patient is measured, then the volume of the vascular compartment, which the radioactive substance cannot leave, is

$$V = \frac{A_1}{A_2} v$$

If Cr-51-labeled erythrocytes are used as an indicator, then V indicates the volume in which the erythrocytes are distributed. In order to calculate the blood volume from the erythrocyte volume, the haematocrit value must be allowed for. In a similar way the plasma volume can be determined with iodine-labeled serum albumin.

The blood volume is not measured directly, as are the erythrocyte or plasma volume. This is due to the fact that dilution analysis applies only to the compartment in which the indicator has become uniformly distributed.

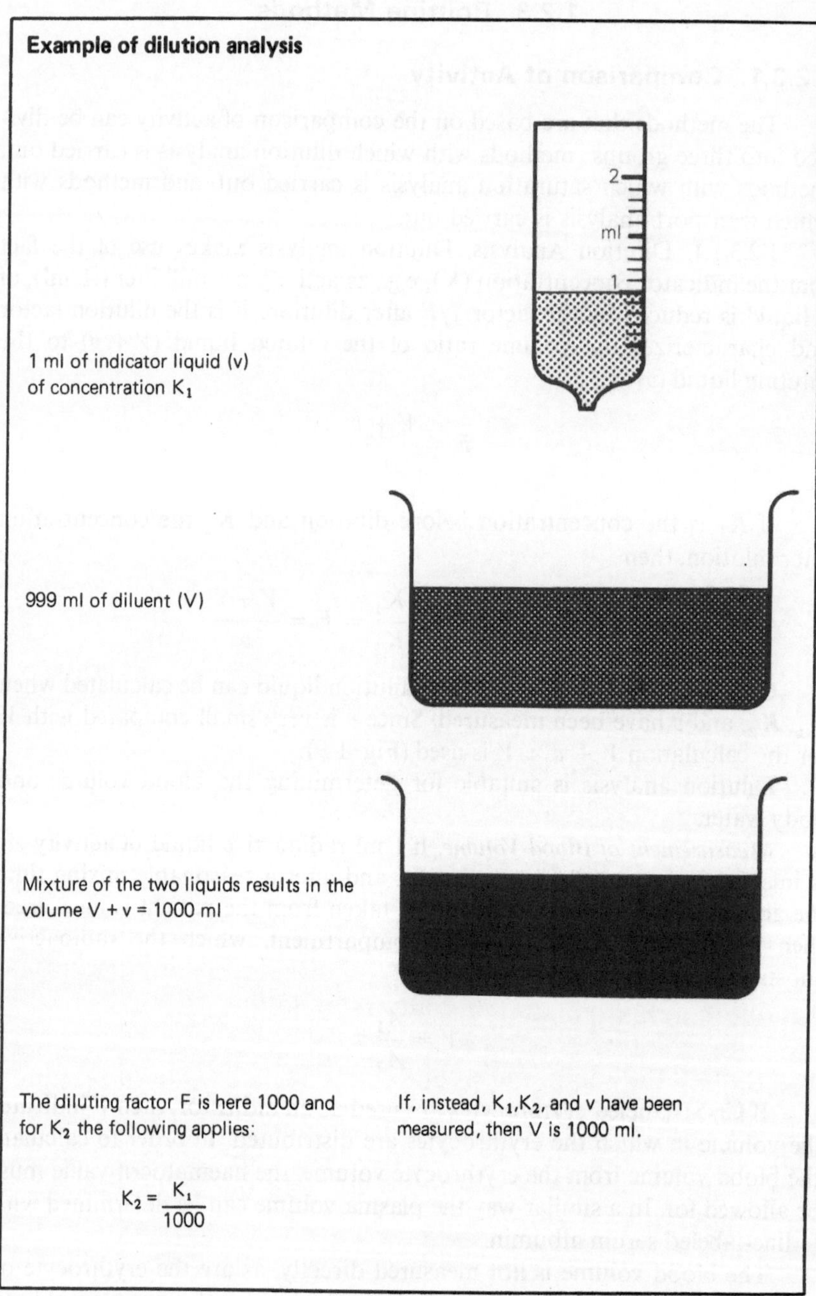
Example of dilution analysis
2
ml
1
1 ml of indicator liquid (v)
of concentration K_1
999 ml of diluent (V)
Mixture of the two liquids results in the
volume V + v = 1000 ml
The diluting factor F is here 1000 and
for K_2 the following applies:
$K_2 = \frac{K_1}{1000}$
If, instead, K_1,K_2, and v have been
measured, then V is 1000 ml.

Fig. 1-9

1.2.3.1.2. Saturation Analysis. Saturation analysis makes use of the fact that when molecules bind to a molecule carrier, the nonsaturated binding capacity of the carrier represents an inverse measure of the quantity of bound molecules. With radionuclides the free binding capacity is relatively easy to assay. All that is needed is a quantity of this molecule in a radioactively labeled form and a separating method in order to be able to measure either the activity of the carrier or the activity of the free radioactive molecules remaining after the saturation process. Figure 1-10 shows the principle of saturation analysis.

In essence a solution of the carrier with the quantity of molecules under investigation is mixed with a solution of the molecules in radioactive form. This mixed solution gives the activity A (total). If, after a reasonable period for saturation of the carrier with radioactive molecules, the total quantity of the carrier is separated from the mixture, then measurement of this carrier fraction gives the activity A (bound). This value represents the quantity of bound radioactive molecules. The result

$$A_1 = \frac{A\,(\text{bound})}{A\,(\text{total})}$$

is a relative measure of the free binding capacity. If, on the other hand, the mixture is measured after removal of the carrier, then the activity (free) is obtained. This represents the quantity of radioactive molecules that are still free after the saturation has been completed. The result

$$A_2 = \frac{A\,(\text{free})}{A\,(\text{total})}$$

is a relative measure of the occupied binding capacity and thus of the quantity of molecules under investigation.

When the quantity of molecules to be determined is available in an unbound form and a suitable carrier is available, then the saturation analysis is capable of calibration and gives absolute values after preparation of a calibration curve with known quantities of molecules.

Saturation analysis is suitable for measuring protein-bound thyroid hormone and iron in the blood.

Thyroid Hormone Determination. It is well known that the hormone passing from the thyroid into the blood is bound to protein carriers. A depot form of the hormone is involved since the binding is reversible and on an average the carriers only bind or release the quantity of hormone required to maintain a certain free hormone level in the blood.

The method of estimating the binding capacity of the hormone-occupied carrier from the relative values of the saturation analysis is called the T3 test (T3 = triiodothyronine). The T4 test (T4 = tetraiodothyronine =

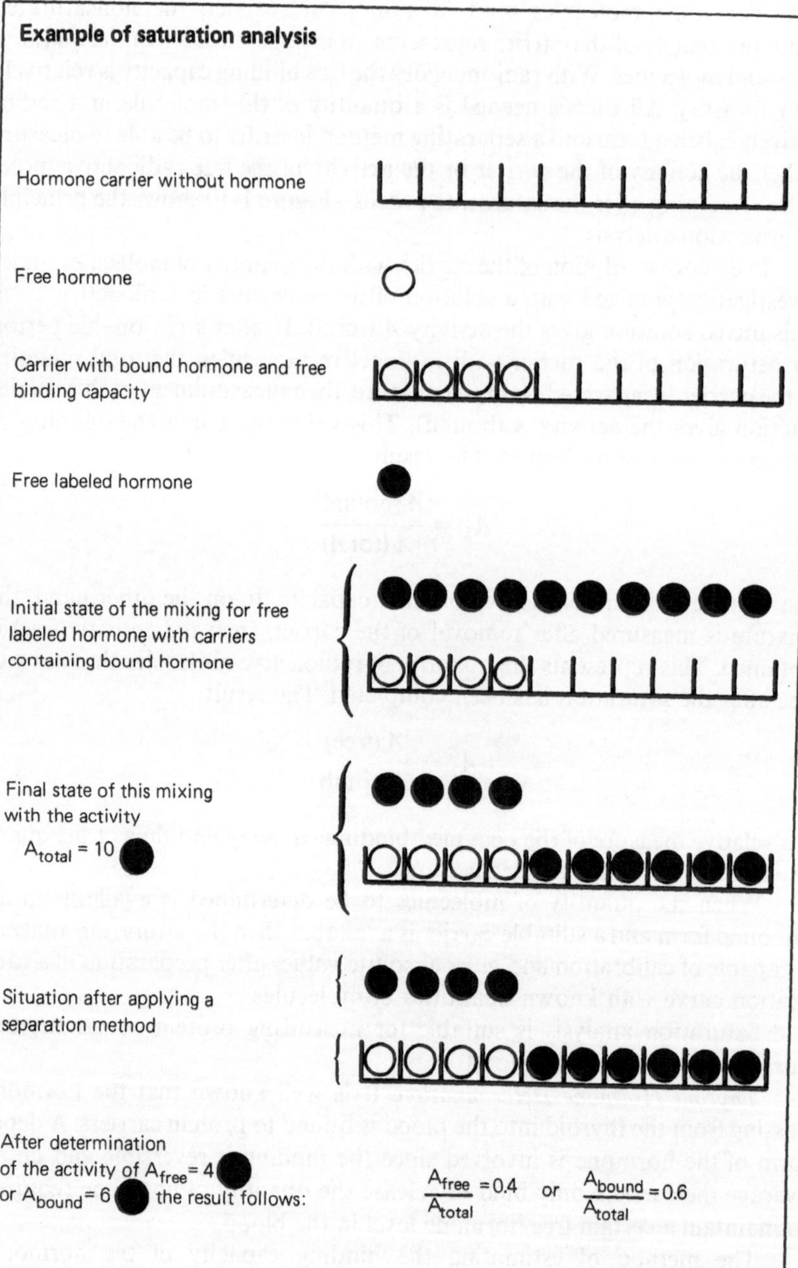
Example of saturation analysis
Hormone carrier without hormone
Free hormone
Carrier with bound hormone and free binding capacity
Free labeled hormone
Initial state of the mixing for free labeled hormone with carriers containing bound hormone
Final state of this mixing with the activity
A total = 10
Situation after applying a separation method
After determination of the activity of A free = 4
or A bound = 6 the result follows:
A free / A total = 0.4 or A bound / A total = 0.6

Fig. 1-10

thyroxine), on the other hand, describes a method in which the hormone is extracted from the binding protein by means of alcohol before the start of the saturation analysis.* For the analysis a normal serum is used as carrier, a mixture from persons with normal thyroids. A large quantity of normal serum is calibrated with known quantities of thyroxine. As long as this stock lasts absolute determination of hormone quantities extracted from the serum of patients can be carried out.

The diagnostically important value, however, is not so much the quantity of depot hormone, which is shown relatively by the T3 test, or the total hormone concentration of the serum, as revealed by the T4 test, but the fraction of all thyroid hormones made up by the non-protein-bound hormones, i.e., the hormone level of the blood available to the tissue. Consequently, by combining the results of the T3 test and the T4 test an endeavour is made to estimate the concentration of the hormones available to the tissues. The difficulty of direct measurement is understandable when we bear in mind that the concentration of the hormones available to the tissue is only about one-thousandth of the depot concentration.

1.2.3.1.3. Transport Analysis. Transport analysis makes use of the fact that the activity of the administered radionuclide is—after deduction of the reduction in activity in accordance with the physical half-life—equal to the sum of the activities distributed in and excreted from the organism. Therefore, if the administered radionuclides travel along a defined path, it is possible to determine the percentage of activity transported by measuring the capacity at the beginning and at the end.

In this way it is possible to check whether the transport of a substance along a certain path is blocked for pathological reasons or whether a new path has opened up as a result of pathological changes. If an orally administered substance usually passes into the blood through the intestinal wall, an absorption test can be carried out by comparing the activities of samples of the blood and of the substance administered. It is also possible to detect any intestinal protein loss by intravenous injection of a labeled protein fraction. Here we speak of excretion tests.

A further example is given by the measurement of the activity of C-14-labeled exhaled carbon dioxide. If a substance is labeled with C-14 at a structural site, of which it is known that its C-14 is used in the course of metabolism for the formation of carbon dioxide, then by measuring the activity of the exhaled air it is possible to determine how much of the original substance has been involved in the metabolic process.

Since the labeled forms of a substance have the same chemical behavior as the inactive form, only small quantities of the labeled form are required

* The designations T3 test and T4 test are based on the radioactive hormone used. Both test results, however, refer to the hormone content, which embraces both T3 and T4.

for mixing with the inactive substance. This follows because in this case the percentage of transported labeled substance is the same as the percentage of transported inactive substance.

1.2.3.1.3.1. Absorption Test (Schilling Test). The cobalt-containing substance vitamin B12 is easily labeled with Co-57. The absorption test checks whether the labeled vitamin can pass through the intestinal wall into the blood and from there into the urine (Fig. 1-11). The value of the activity determined in the urine and that of the test substance gives as quotient the percentage absorption of the vitamin. In order to ensure that a small dose of the radioactive substance is adequate, the patient is given a high intramuscular dose of the unlabeled vitamin 2 hr after oral administration of the labeled vitamin. Without this precaution the labeled vitamin would largely wander to binding sites and get "lost" inside the organism so that the activity in the urine would remain unnecessarily low. Now, however, the labeled vitamin passing through the intestinal wall is displaced from its binding sites in the organism particularly into the liver and onto the plasma protein of the blood and the main portion appears in the urine.

If the outcome of this test is abnormal, intrinsic factor is administered in order to establish whether a lack of this substance is responsible for the blockage of the vitamin absorption in the intestinal wall or whether the faulty absorption is due to an intestinal disease.

1.2.3.1.3.2. Excretion Test (Gordon Test). The Gordon test tries to estimate the extent of the intestinal protein loss in various diseases. When an intravenous injection of labeled serum albumin is given, a certain amount of the albumin enters the intestine in pathological cases. By measuring the activity of the feces as a percentage of the applied activity it is possible to estimate the intestinal protein loss.

As a rule there are a number of enzymes in the intestines that split up the plasma protein when it passes into the GI tract. Some products of splitting, however, are able to reenter the vascular compartment through reabsorption. Such products of splitting must not be the carrier of the indicator as otherwise measurement of the feces would lead to false results.

In routine work the use of iodine-131- or iodine-125-labeled polyvinylpyrrolidone (PVP) has proved satisfactory. It is a plastic particle fraction, whose particles—in the event of intestinal albumin loss—pass through the intestinal wall in the same way as the serum albumin, but are not subjected to catabolism.

As the binding of the radioactive iodine to the PVP particles is partly broken in the blood and in the intestines, a certain error must be reckoned with. A splitting off of the iodine in the blood causes a reduction of the measuring effect. Splitting off of the iodine in the intestines has a similar effect since the iodine is largely reabsorbed. In order to overcome this disadvantage Cr-51-labeled serum albumin has been used with success.

Example of transport analysis

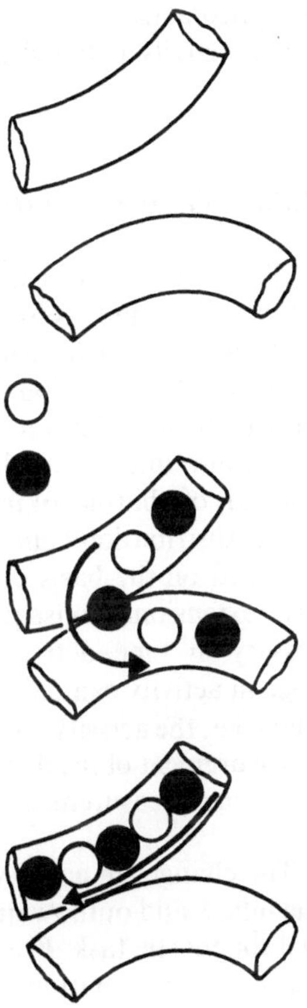

Intestinal lumen

Vascular spaces

Vitamin

Labeled vitamin

Path of the vitamin and of the labeled vitamin in the normal case

Path of the vitamin and of the labeled vitamin in the case of blockage

The labeled vitamin travels along the same paths as the unlabeled vitamin. At the instant when all orally administered vitamins can normally be found in the vascular spaces, the following applies:

$$\frac{\text{Labeled vitamin in vascular spaces}}{\text{Orally administered labeled vitamin}} = \frac{\text{Vitamin in vascular spaces}}{\text{Orally administered vitamin}}$$

Thus the ratio of the blood activity to the orally administered activity is a measure of vitamin transport. The fact that in practice the urine activity and not the blood activity is measured, makes no difference to the principle.

Fig. 1-11

Chromium is also split off in the intestines, but it is reabsorbed only slightly.

The results of the excretion test are a comparison of activity between the applied activity and the activity of the feces. Normally about 1% of the injected activity is found in the feces, which have been collected for a few days.

1.2.3.2. Time–Activity Measurements

Time–activity measurements reveal the rate of accumulation or clearance of activity in a volume of the organism.

If the volume concerns an organ or an anatomically important region, then we speak of function analysis or function measurements. If the volume concerns the distribution compartment of a radionuclide, as is defined for instance in a dilution analysis, then we speak of indicator kinetics and, in particular, of pharmacokinetics when the indicator is a pharmaceutical.

The distribution compartment is often an abstract quantity, i.e., its size is assumed on the basis of measurements without information on its geometric extension. Consequently, establishment of a measuring site as is necessary in time–activity measurements is futile. Measurement of the change in activity can only be made by determining the activity per volume element, i.e., the activity concentration, which is assumed to be representative for measurement of the distribution compartment. Therefore, we are dealing with *in vitro* measurement of liquids or excretory products taken from the patient.

The changes in activity of the volume under study are due to changes in the inflow and outflow quantities. Recognition of the causes for this is the actual diagnostic task. Frequently, the volume under study is not identical to the overall distribution compartment. For instance, the distribution compartment of iodide also includes the salivary glands and the gastric mucosa, but in thyroid function studies only the rate of uptake in this gland is evaluated. Limitation of the volume under study to this region of the distribution compartment is due to the characteristic iodine accumulation in this particular gland. A further example is iron utilization. After intravenous injection of radioactive iron, the iron is first distributed in the vascular compartment. Soon, however, the distribution compartment is extended since the iron spreads to the blood-forming centers in bone marrow. The rate of accumulation in the blood-forming centers, which is of diagnostic interest, can be measured both as clearance rate from the blood and as uptake rate by functional measurements via the sacrum. In both cases different sections of the distribution compartment are covered, and in the case of functional measurement via the sacrum even a part of the vascular compartment.

As the results of a method are the more accurate the smaller the number of variable influences during the measurement, an endeavor is always made to restrict the measurement to that part of the distribution compartment that is relevant to the diagnosis. This is possible when one part can be macroscopically delimited from another, as with the study of the absorption kinetics from the intestinal lumen into the blood. In the renal parenchyma it is not possible to measure the activity of the vascular system independently from the urinal system by external measurement, since the two systems can only be microscopically separated from each other. The time–activity curve of a radioactive kidney-seeking substance, obtained as function measurement over the kidney, therefore represents superimpositioning.

One tries to eliminate the basic difficulties mentioned here by obtaining additional information on the time–activity behavior of the regions involved in the distribution compartment. In effect the most suitable method would be the catheterization of the various regions in order to analyze the time–activity behaviors independently of each other. However, this would mean forgoing the advantage of the indicator method with radionuclides, i.e., that measurement can be carried out remotely from the site of measurement; operation of the organism would thus be necessary. The better way is to try to measure additionally the time–activity behavior of an involved region at a different, more representative site and to use the measured value as a correction. In many cases, however, evaluation of the uncorrected, superimposed time–activity curves, together with the nonnuclear medical data and case history, supplies sufficient information for making a diagnosis.

1.2.3.2.1. Iron Utilization. Investigation of iron utilization, also known as ferrokinetics, comprises the testing of the reabsorption of orally administered iron by means of transport analysis as well as the clearance rate from the blood into the blood-forming centers and the rate at which iron returns to the blood as a cell component. Usually function measurements over the heart, liver, spleen, and sacrum follow, which can give information on any possible blood-forming centers outside the bone marrow.

As radionuclide Fe-59 is used, which has a half-life of 47 days (cf. Section 1.3.5). The clearance of the iron from the blood is in accordance with an exponential function (Fig. 1-2). The clearance rate is therefore given as a biologic half-life. The normal values of the biologic half-life lie between 1 to 2 hr. Lower values point to lack of iron, hyperplastic anemia, or polycythemia, and increased values to hypoplastic anemia.

It takes several days before the iron returns to the circulation as a cell constituent. The time–activity measurement of the blood yields in this case a saturation curve (Fig. 1-2), whose maximum value is normally reached after 10–12 days. Hypoferric anemia results in higher maximum values, which are attained more quickly. Hypoplastic anemia gives much reduced maximum values that are only reached after a long time.

1.2.3.2.2. Red Cell Survival. Red blood cells can be labeled *in vitro* by incubation with Cr-51 sodium chromate. After disappearance of the labeled red blood cells, the Cr-51 is not further utilized by the organism but is excreted. If labeled red blood cells are injected they do not age any quicker than other cells of the same patient. Consequently, the time–activity curve indicates the disappearance rate of the red blood cells. Since the decrease in activity, measured as a change in concentration of the blood in samples, follows an exponential function, semilogarithmic display results in a straight line. From this curve it is possible to read the biological half-life, which is given as the measuring quantity for the red cell survival. Normally red cells disappear from the circulation in approximately 30 days and in pathological cases (hemolytic anemia) in a few days. This quantity is only proportional to the mean life of the red cells (normally about 120 days).

Since red cells also disappear in the liver and spleen, it is also of diagnostic interest to check the disappearance over each organ by function measurement. These time–activity curves are usually grouped together by finding the ratio, so that each point of the curve corresponds to a ratio of the measured spleen and liver activity. Normally a slightly domed curve is obtained having a maximum at 15–20 days. It is characteristic that all the ratios are slightly greater than one, i.e., only slightly more cells disappear in the spleen than in the liver. In the case of hemolytic anemia, however, the values of the ratios increase considerably with respect to time, since the red cells disappear almost exclusively in the spleen.

The red cell survival and the spleen–liver ratio permit coordination to pathological changes of the red cells. By means of a trick it is possible to obtain information on pathological changes to the spleen from measurement of the elimination of red cells. The healthy spleen has such narrow capillaries that normal red cells can just about slip through. Red cells that are no longer elastic and have become spherocytes block the capillaries and are prematurely eliminated. Spherocytes can be obtained either by heat treatment (thermally aged red cells) or by chemical treatment with bromomercurihydroxypropane (BMHP). In the case of treatment with Hg-197-labeled BMHP the labeling simultaneously forms a union with the spherocytes so that extra marking is not necessary.

Within a few minutes after the injection of labeled spherocytes, almost all of them are filtered out of the blood by a healthy spleen. Certain pathological changes rob the spleen of this ability, so that the spherocytes can be used to diagnose changes in the spleen.

1.2.3.2.3. Thyroid Function Analysis. Since the thyroid takes up iodide, uses the stored iodide for incorporation in the hormone, and releases the iodine-containing hormone into the blood—20% triiodothyronine (T3) and 80% thyroxine (T4)—function measurement over the thyroid gives information on the uptake rate from the blood and on the hormone secretion. The increase of the time–activity curve shows the iodide phase and the decrease the hormone phase. This function analysis is therefore also known as the two-phase study. Since the curve covers a time period of several days and the specific deviations of the curve shape for the various clinical pictures occur particularly after 2, 24, and 48 hr, samples are taken at these times. The values measured are recorded as a percentage of the orally administered activity.

Since the immediate cause for the clinical pictures of hyper- and hypothyroidism is due to an increased or decreased supply of the tissue-disposable hormone, it is clear that the function analysis of the thyroid only checks one of many conditions for the occurrence of hyper- or hypothyroidism. Consequently, the two-phase study is employed together with scintigraphy and other diagnostic methods.

1.2.3.2.4. Renal Function Analysis. If a urine-seeking, labeled substance such as Hippuran, which is quickly excreted, is intravenously injected, then a time–activity curve consisting of the superpositioning of three time-related processes is obtained (Fig. 1-12). Normally the curve increases rapidly within a few seconds, a sign that the radioactive blood has reached the kidney (initial phase). While the kidney is filling with radioactive blood, the Hippuran is glomerularly filtered and tubularly secreted and finally accumulates in the renal calyces (secretion phase). The curve climbs further as, on the one hand, Hippuran is coming in with the blood and, on the other hand, the first Hippuran molecules have not yet left the renal calyces. Finally the curve forms a maximum and gradually drops as the excretion of the Hippuran into the ureters starts (excretory phase).

The exact breakdown of the time–activity curve into the components vascular phase, secretory phase, and excretory phase is so problematic that in routine diagnosis the curve is only evaluated qualitatively and other diagnostic measures are needed. Comparison of the behavior of the two kidneys plays a considerable role. Experience has revealed a number of correlations of typical curve forms to specific diagnostic findings so that renal function analysis is widely used (Fig. 1-13).

1.2.3.2.5. Liver Function Analysis. As an excretory organ, the liver continuously handles substances from the blood in order to pass them on to the intestines via the bile ducts. The liver function can be tested by intravenous injection of a labeled substance that is treated by the liver in exactly the same way as the natural breakdown products of the organism.

Function measurement of the liver with I-131 rose bengal gives a time–activity curve, which is made up of two exponential functions. The biological half-lives corresponding to them can be determined from the semilogarithmic display and give a measure of the uptake and excretion rate of rose bengal.

Normally the biological half-life is about 10 min for the uptake and

Renal functional analysis
Activity A
Initial phase
Secretion phase
Excretory phase

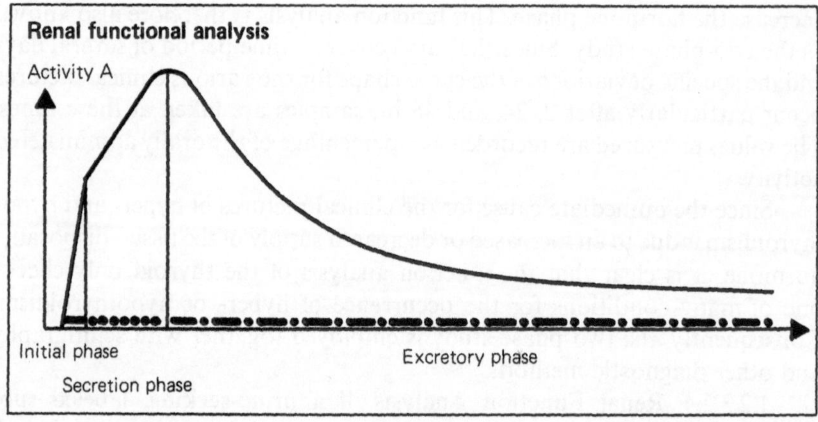

Fig. 1-12

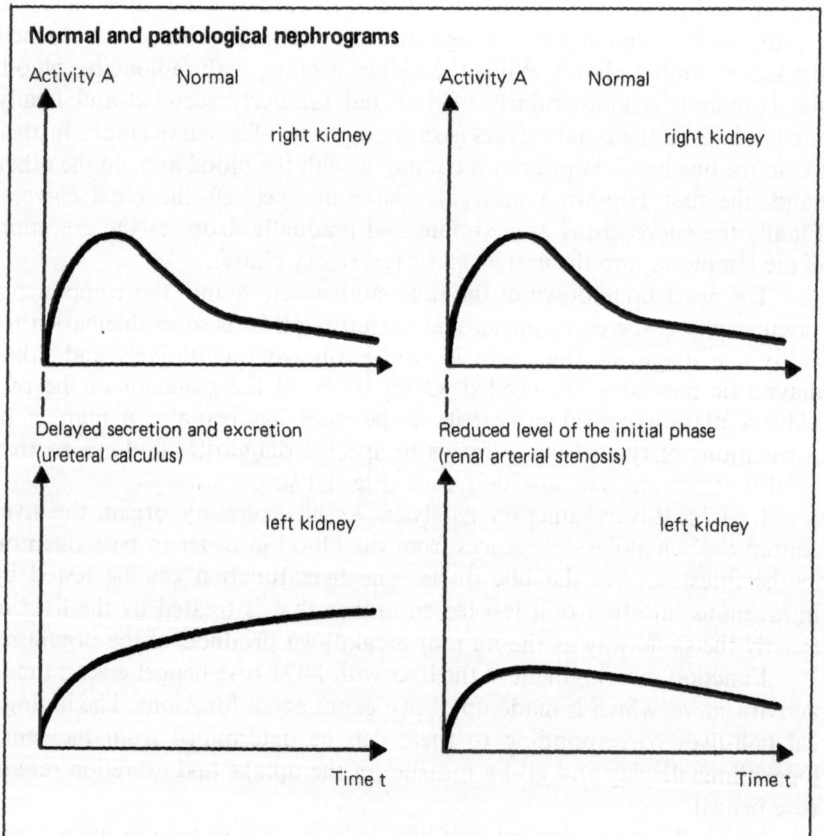

Normal and pathological nephrograms
Activity A
Normal
right kidney
Activity A
Normal
right kidney
Delayed secretion and excretion
(ureteral calculus)
left kidney
Time t
Reduced level of the initial phase
(renal arterial stenosis)
left kidney
Time t

Fig. 1-13

100 min for the excretion. Hepatitis and cirrhosis delay the uptake, gall-bladder diseases and obstructive jaundice delay the excretion.

1.2.3.2.6. Blood Flow through Organs. To obtain an answer to the diagnostically important question about the blood flow through the organs, it appears at first sight that function measurement over the organ is the ideal method. Blood is relatively easy to mark with labeled red blood cells or other indicators and it is possible to measure the time–activity curve over the organ under examination. However, the administered activity is distributed over the entire volume of the blood so that it is not known what quantity of activity A_{in} flows to the organ whose time–activity curve is being measured. In this form the measurement is nonspecific with respect to the flow of blood through the organ since there can be many reasons why the quantity of activity flowing to the organ is large or small. The same applies when the quantity of activity A_{out} flowing from the organ is unknown since it cannot be excluded that the indicator may take a path other than that of the blood. This state of affairs is regulated by the Fick principle and it relates dA/dt, an expression of the slope of the time–activity curve, to the blood flow F in ml/min:

$$F = \frac{dA/dt}{A_{in} - A_{out}}$$

Exact knowledge of A_{in} and A_{out} can be obtained by catheterization, but this is not conducive to making the method routine. Therefore, various tricks have been conceived in order to obtain a representative value for the blood circulation without having to measure A_{in} and A_{out} directly.

Since nuclear medicine is by no means the only source of diagnostic information, it is often sufficient for the physician to know that A_{in} is constant without having knowledge of the absolute value. This can be found out by making a massive single injection. If a radioactive indicator is administered as a massive single injection, the blood carries the indicator as a "spherical mass," also known as a bolus, away from the site of injection without the indicator mixing with the blood. Injected at a suitable site, the indicator bolus reaches the organ by a direct path so that when making the function measurement of the organ a definite value A_{in} can be used as a basis.

That is the method used in the determination of the cardiac time volume (CTV). The function measurement over the heart gives a time–activity curve, which momentarily increases to a maximum as the bolus enters the inside of the heart and then slowly drops to the activity value corresponding to the blood activity after complete mixing of the bolus activity (Fig. 1-14). If the stroke volume is large, then most of the activity brought in by the bolus will be quickly washed out of the volume covered by the measure-

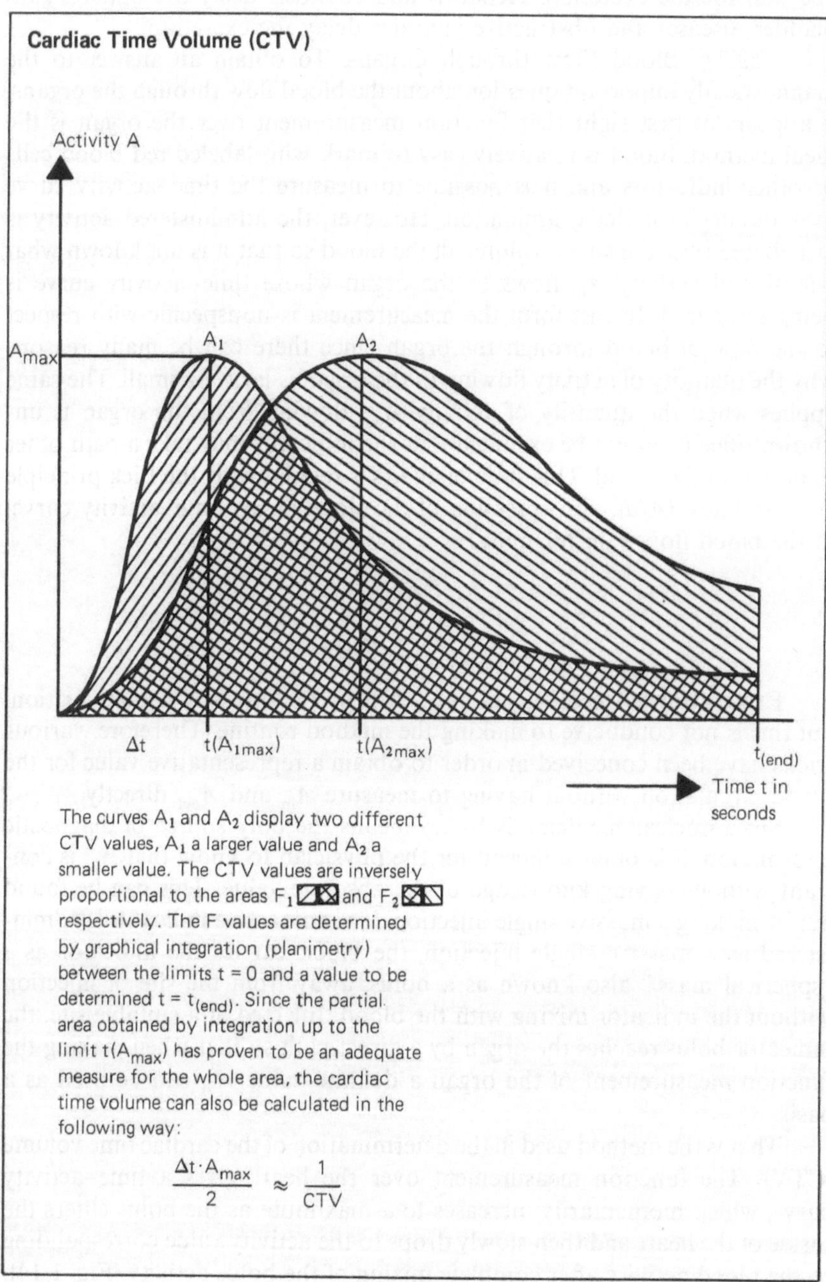
Cardiac Time Volume (CTV)
Activity A
A_max
A₁
A₂
Δt
t(A_1max)
t(A_2max)
t_(end)
Time t in seconds
The curves A_1 and A_2 display two different CTV values, A_1 a larger value and A_2 a smaller value. The CTV values are inversely proportional to the areas F_1 and F_2 respectively. The F values are determined by graphical integration (planimetry) between the limits t = 0 and a value to be determined $t = t_{(end)}$. Since the partial area obtained by integration up to the limit $t(A_{max})$ has proven to be an adequate measure for the whole area, the cardiac time volume can also be calculated in the following way:
$$\frac{\Delta t \cdot A_{max}}{2} \approx \frac{1}{CTV}$$

Fig. 1-14

ment; if the stroke volume is small, the washing out procedure will take more time. If the end of the measuring time is taken to be the time before completion of the activity mixing in the blood volume, then the time–activity curve together with the time axis encloses an area, whose size is inversely proportional to the cardiac time volume. As shown by experience, when the area is determined, the quantity A_{out} is also allowed for without it being accessible to the measurement. This method is routinely used, since adequate diagnostic information is obtained with little effort.

A massive single injection is also used for determining the cerebral circulation. Xe-133, a radioactive gas, which is dissolved in physiological saline, is injected into the internal carotid artery. Most of the Xe-133 is quickly taken up from the cerebral capillaries by the grey and white matter and the rest is almost completely eliminated by the lungs. The xenon-free blood following the bolus is now enriched by the xenon diffusing out of the grey and white matter owing to the reversed concentration gradient, a process that is known as washing out. The time–activity curve measured over the brain first reveals a maximum, a sign that the bolus is distributed over the capillaries. The drop in activity following shows essentially the process of washing out. The evaluation of the time–activity curve is made in the same manner as that of the cardiac time volume determination. It has been established, however, that the time–activity curve in the region of the washing out represents superpositioning of two exponential functions, whose biological half-lives are to be evaluated as measure of a greater and a lesser blood flow. Apparently this reflects the difference in blood circulation in the grey and white matter. Each hemisphere of the brain should be examined separately. Usually several detectors are located over selected regions of the head so that information over the local cerebral circulation can be obtained. On the other hand, the regional cerebral circulation is an example for the application of serial and functional scintigraphy (cf. Section 1.2.3.3).

Considerable success has been obtained with the labeling of artificially produced macroaggregated albumin (MAA). After injection of MAA at a suitable site of the circulation, temporary microemboli are produced on a scale giving indirect information on the circulation. With the aid of this method measurement of the circulation is transposed to the field of localization.

1.2.3.3. Localization Analysis

Localization analysis gives information on the location of activities in the organism. The localization measurement calls for two basic measures:

1. Collimation, i.e., suitable shielding of the detector, so that the de-

tector receives gamma radiation primarily from a limited volume at a certain distance (cf. Section 1.4.5.2.6).

2. A position finder, which not only records the activity values of the volumes selected by the collimation but also establishes the relative position of the volumes to each other.

Two different position finders are used. In one case a relatively small detector is moved over the organism. For activity measurement at each site the entire detector is employed and the spatial relationship of the activity values results from the position of the moving detector. With the other position-finding system a large detector is selected, which stands still during the measurement and is positioned over the region of interest. For activity measurement at each site only part of the detector is used, namely, the part nearest to the volume to be located, and the spatial relationship of the activity values results from the relative position of the gamma absorption events to each other in the detector.

Since localization analysis almost exclusively employs measurement of gamma radiation and the detectors used are scintillation detectors, this nuclear-medical field is known as scintigraphy. Imaging systems with moving detectors are called scanners and those with stationary detectors are known as gamma cameras, as localization is made with them in a similar manner to that used in a photographic camera.

Scintigraphy gives rise to pictures, whose image points appear in succession line by line with moving systems or, in the case of stationary systems, simultaneously during the exposure time. Such a picture is called a scintigram and if the mode is to be emphasized we speak of a scan or a scintiphoto.

The result of scintigraphy is the representation of either an accumulation *effect* or an accumulation *defect*. For this reason a distinction is made between positive and negative scintigraphy. Positive scintigraphy is based on the affinity an indicator has for selected regions of the organism (Fig. 1-15). Negative scintigraphy is based on the loss of affinity in those regions (Fig. 1-16).

Positive scintigraphy includes organ representation, which gives information on the size, form, and position of the organ and can supply the basis for determining the weight. It also includes visualization of lesions in which conditions have arisen which respond to the affinity of indicators. In this way brain lesions can be localized that have destroyed the blood–brain barrier and have thus created a path for intravenously injected indicators. Another example is the increased transformation rate in bone lesions, which can be made visible by injecting radioactive fluorine or strontium. The search for metastasis is also an important application of positive scintigraphy. Finally, there is scintigraphy as therapy control, for which examples of negative scintigraphy can also be mentioned.

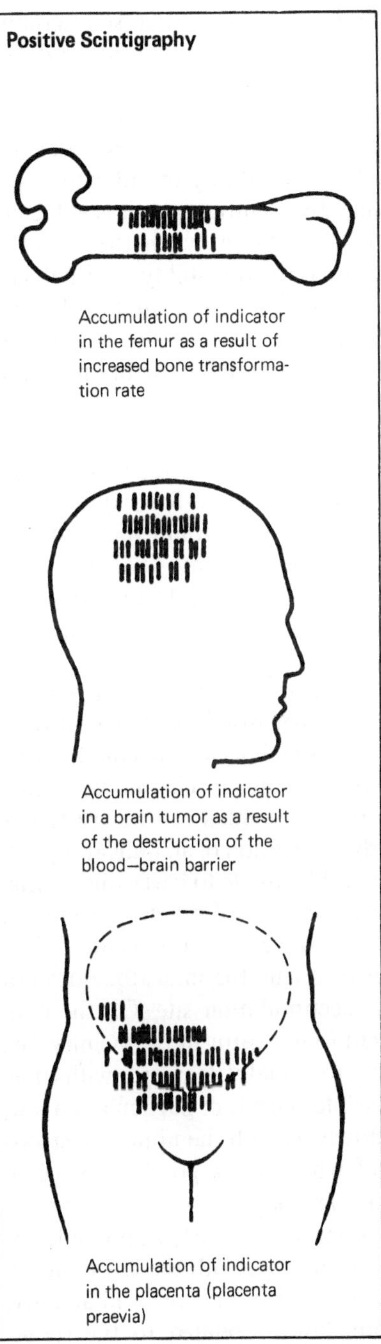

Positive Scintigraphy
Accumulation of indicator in the femur as a result of increased bone transformation rate
Accumulation of indicator in a brain tumor as a result of the destruction of the blood–brain barrier
Accumulation of indicator in the placenta (placenta praevia)

Fig. 1-15

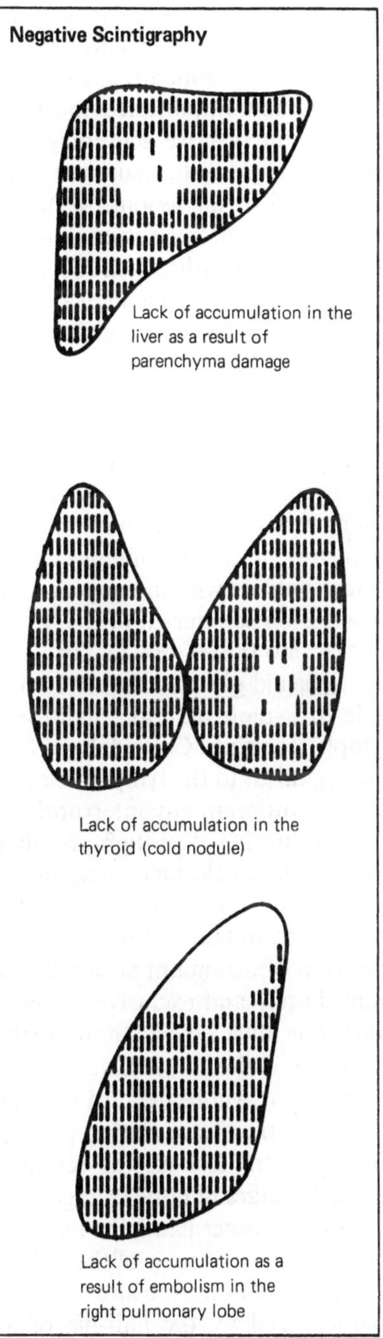

Lack of accumulation as a result of embolism in the right pulmonary lobe

Fig. 1-16

In principle, negative scintigraphy is inferior to positive scintigraphy since an accumulation effect can be more sensitively recorded than a defect within an accumulation effect. Nevertheless, negative scintigraphy is of considerable importance and it is more widely used at present in routine work than positive scintigraphy. This has the following reason. Positive scintigraphy has to make use of the biochemical affinity of indicators that is dictated by the lesions. In the case of negative scintigraphy it is sufficient that any indicator is accumulated in normal organs or moves in the organism along normal paths. Consequently, here there is the possibility of visualizing an organ with various indicators or various organs with a single indicator. For instance, parenchyma defects of the thyroid can be recorded with iodide or with pertechnetate. Or, with a mercury compound both brain lesions and parenchyma defects of the kidneys can be established.

The fact that mechanical fixation of the indicators can be used for scintigraphy is shown by perfusion scintigraphy of the lungs with labeled macroaggregates (MA). The macroaggregates occlude a few capillaries of lungs with normal circulation after injection into the cubital vein and consequently in the case of lungs with poor circulation they are fixed to a slight extent only or with missing circulation (emboli) not at all. In the same way a perfusion scintigram of the lower extremities can be made after injection of MA into the femoral artery.

The aid given to negative scintigraphy through the possibility of being able to exploit natural conditions of the normal organ is shown also by lymph scanning. Colloidal gold, subcutaneously injected, is conveyed by the organism to the lymphatic system as an inorganic foreign body, so that in the scintigram any interruption of the lymph channel can be visualized.

The timing of scintigraphy after the administration of an indicator plays an important role. Of course, an endeavor will be made to carry out scintigraphy during maximum accumulation at the region of diagnostic interest in order to obtain a scan of high contrast. However, contrast is not only a question of maximum accumulation since as a rule the indicator does not immediately and exclusively seek out the accumulation site. On the contrary, one must expect a noteworthy content of indicator in the vicinity, i.e., especially in the blood. Since the blood activity usually decreases with time, scintigraphy will be delayed as long as possible. This is of particular advantage when the accumulation takes place slowly as with the uptake of strontium by bone lesions, the scintigraphy of which gives good evidence of the early stages of bone changes even after a few days.

On the other hand, the reasons for scintigraphy as early as possible are the decrease in activity of the indicator in accordance with the law of decay and the radiation exposure to the patient. The natural decrease in activity, characterized by the half-life of a radionuclide, is related to the radiation exposure in the sense that the activity administered to maintain a permissible radiation burden may be the higher, the shorter the half-life is. For instance, the half-life of 65 days of Sr-85 is unnecessarily high for bone scintigraphy since an indicator with a half-life of a few days would be adequate for the method. Furthermore, with a shorter half-life a higher activity could be administered, which can be more accurately measured. With respect to radiation burden, Tc-99m with its half-life of 2.7 hr permits the administration of particularly high activities, an advantage that can outweigh the disadvantages of early scintigraphy, i.e., high blood activity and too early timing for maximum accumulation. This example shows that the maximum accumulation as time effect of indicator kinetics does not have to be identical to optimum accumulation, as can be achieved by selection of suitable radionuclides.

The time effect of indicator accumulation is also of importance from another aspect. Although biochemists have been trying for a long time to discover the reasons for degenerative tissue and cell changes, only in a few cases has it been possible to develop indicator preparations that, on account of their molecular properties, seek out the site of a specific change. Such molecule indicators will certainly become very important since they offer an ideal method of differential diagnosis. The special role which an indicator plays in changed tissue of the organism can also find its expression in the time effect of the accumulation, a fact that can be used as a basis for differential diagnosis. In cerebral scintigraphy with iodine-labeled serum albumin it is largely possible to distinguish between durosarcoma, gliosarcoma, and metastasis owing to the lesion-caused time effect of the accumulation.

The considerations on the impact of the time effect of the accumulation apply to scintigraphy with both moving and stationary detectors. Since scintigraphy with a stationary detector makes possible scintigraphic times of the order of magnitude of minutes or seconds, whereas a scan even of a small organ cannot be made under 10 min, it is possible with the gamma camera to carry out serial scintigraphy. Serial scintigraphy (Fig. 1-7) means the exposure of scintiphotos in rapid succession with the aim of capturing spatial changes in the activity accumulation in the region covered by the scintiphoto. A variation of serial scintigraphy is functional scintigraphy. This views only partial regions of the serial scintiphoto (Fig. 1-8). By evaluating congruent partial regions of various scintiphotos of a series, a time–activity curve is obtained, which gives additional important diagnostic information. For reasons of radiation burden alone, an effort is made to obtain as much information as possible from the single administration of an indicator.

Within the field of nuclear-medical diagnosis, the greatest activities are administered in scintigraphy. Nevertheless, the radiation burden is often less than that of individual roentgenological examinations. However, while in radiology the radiation exposure is restricted to the transirradiated volume, in scintigraphy the radiation exposure can also occur at a part of the organism remote from the area under investigation. This is a result of the transport of the indicator and the excretion of the indicator, which can take many paths. Frequently, while traveling along these paths the indicator may stop for a considerable time so that the radiation exposure there is higher than at the site of diagnostic interest. In addition to information on the radiation burden of the organ under examination and general information on whole-body radiation exposure, in such cases further information will be necessary on the radiation burden of the so-called critical organs and occasionally also on the gonadal exposure.

The radiation exposure is, unfortunately, not only a question of gamma radiation, whose disadvantages must be accepted along with the advantages of nuclear-medical diagnosis, but also of the beta radiation, which does not contribute to scintigraphic diagnosis at all. This only applies to a limited extent to positive beta radiation, the positrons, since they give rise to the diagnostically valuable annihilation radiation, a gamma radiation.

However, we are not free in the selection of radionuclides as we are governed by their biochemical suitability as an indicator or their suitability for labeling biochemical indicators. The gamma energy must also be borne in mind. Too low a gamma energy means difficult localization in deep-seated layers of the organism, and too high an energy creates problems with respect to collimation. Roughly speaking gamma energies suitable for scanning lie in the range between 0.08 MeV (Xe-133; Hg-197) and 0.51 MeV (annihilation radiation). For the gamma camera, energies at the bottom end of this range are preferred.

The following paragraphs will now deal with the most important routine scintigraphic examinations.

1.2.3.3.1 Scintigraphy in the Head Region. In the head region scintigraphy is used for examining the brain, the fluid spaces, the cerebral circulation, the thyroid, the parathyroid, and the salivary glands. Of these examinations brain scintigraphy and thyroid scintigraphy have the greatest importance. These will be dealt with later.

The fluid spaces are visualized positively some time after intrathecal injection of I-131-labeled serum albumin. If, in addition, the region of the spinal column is scintigraphed, then possible interruption of the indicator transport to the intracranial fluid spaces or displacement or constriction of the vertebral fluid space can be detected. The circulation can be checked after injection of I-131- or Tc-99m-labeled macroaggregates (MA) into the carotid artery. Pertechnetate is taken up by the salivary glands so that scintigraphy can reveal organ enlargement or changes to the parenchyma. For scintigraphy of the parathyroid in the case of hyperfunction, a labeled amino acid (Se-75 methionine) is used as an indicator, which is required by the gland for hormone synthesis. The uptake of the indicator by the normal gland is too poor for it to result in visualization of the organ. In this way regions of increased hormone synthesis can be located (adenoma).

1.2.3.3.1.1. Brain Scintigraphy. Scintigraphy of the brain does not image the healthy organ since the blood–brain barrier does not allow much indicator from the blood to diffuse into the brain. In most cases, however, brain diseases destroy this barrier so that the path is free for the indicators. Consequently, lesions can be positively visualized (Fig. 1-15).

The indicator of preference is Tc-99m since it gives excellent results with either a scanner or camera and with low radiation exposure. Deeper-seated lesions are not so easy to locate as the gamma energy of Tc-99m with 0.14 MeV is relatively low. In this respect I-131 (0.36 MeV) and Hg-203 (0.28 MeV) are suitable. As human I-131 serum albumin (HSA) and Hg-203 neohydrin they are taken up by brain lesions. In contrast to Tc-99m, both radionuclides also emit beta radiation and thus cause a higher radiation burden. For I-131 HSA blood is the critical organ. The uptake in lesions is somewhat stronger than with Tc-99m and owing to the time effect of the accumulation, differential diagnosis is possible. For Hg-203 the kidney is the critical organ since it stays there longer than in the brain lesion. Unfortunately the radiation exposure for the kidney is extremely high, and Hg-203 is being used less and less.

Recently introduced into brain scintigraphy is In-113m (0.39 MeV), which with a half-life of 1.7 hr can be applied in a similar manner to Tc-99m and it can also be located easily in deeper-lying lesions. Furthermore, it has the advantage that, bound to a chelate (DTPA or EDTA), it accumulates in brain lesions but not in the salivary glands, as is unfortunately the case with pertechnetate. Consequently, lesions close to the base can be better located.

Another localization method should be mentioned here that does not make use of the scanner or camera, namely, gamma encephalography, a method in which a large number of detectors are applied to selected sites of the skull. The measured results of the right and left halves of the skull are compared with each other. Here the position of the individual detectors is used to locate the lesions.

1.2.3.3.1.2. Thyroid Scintigraphy. Since the thyroid takes up iodine selectively and incorporates it in the hormone, a suitable indicator is sought amongst the radionuclides of iodine. Of the more than 20 known radionuclides of iodine, many can be excluded because they are too short lived. From the remaining isotopes, only a few are available to the physician owing to production reasons. I-131 with a gamma energy of 0.36 MeV is of primary importance and well suited to scintigraphy, but it also emits beta radiation.

The most favorable time for the scan is the first or second day after intravenous or oral administration so that the half-life of eight days of I-131 is quite suitable. Since the diagnostic value of thyroid scintigraphy is increased if the evaluation is made together with that of function diagnosis, it is usual during function studies to administer sufficient I-131 for scintigraphy as well.

Tc-99m also accumulates in the thyroid as pertechnetate, but as a result of the half-life of 6 hr a completely different situation arises. Scintigraphy after a few days is not possible, but the short half-life makes it possible to use high activities with low radiation exposure so that scintigraphy can be carried out 30–60 min after intravenous injection.

There are reasons to state that in conjunction with scintigraphic findings, evaluation of function studies 2 hr after the injection permits adequate diagnosis to be made in many cases. For such cases a short test has been developed, which combines Tc-99m scintigraphy with I-132 function analysis. Tc-99m cannot be used alone since it is not incorporated into the thyroid hormone. With a half-life of 2.4 hr, I-132 does not contribute very much to radiation exposure. Evaluation of this short test can be concluded in about 6 hr. The short half-lives of these two radionuclides permit repetition of the examination after about one day, a fact that is of advantage when carrying out the stimulation and suppression tests (discussed below).

Scintigraphy with pertechnetate or iodide images the normal gland so that accumulation defects reveal changes (Fig. 1-16). However, there are also parenchymal changes which lead to excessive accumulation (hot nodules). In most cases an adenoma is involved, which is autonomously producing thyroid hormone (toxic adenoma). In its hormone production, it is independent of the hormone secretion of the diencephalon and the pituitary gland. On the other hand, since strong hormone production of the toxic adenoma reduces the hormone excretion of the diencephalon and the pituitary gland, the remaining thyroid parenchyma receives only little or no stimulation by the pituitary hormone thyrotrophin. The automatic control system (thyroid hormone content of the blood—diencephalon—pituitary gland—thyroid hormone production) is ineffective for the toxic adenoma and blocked for the rest of the thyroid.

Depending upon whether, in addition to the toxic adenoma, the thyroid can be imaged slightly or not all in the scintigram, we speak of a compensated or decompensated adenoma. In the case of the compensated adenoma the automatic control system is intact but blocked. In the other case the automatic control system in not intact.

In order to detect a compensated adenoma, there is the suppression test. Before renewed scintigraphy, thyroid hormone is administered to the patient for several days. This reduces the thyrotrophin excretion even more and the thyroid is no longer visualized in the scintigram along with the adenoma.

In order to detect a decompensated adenoma, there is the stimulation test. Before renewed scintigraphy, the patient is given an intramuscular injection of thyrotrophin. Any thyroid parenchyma still present is then visualized in the scintigram along with the decompensated adenoma.

1.2.3.3.2. Scintigraphy in the Trunk and Extremity Region

1.2.3.3.2.1. Cardiac Scintigraphy. For scintigraphic imaging of the myocardium the radioactive alkalies such as cesium and rubidium are suitable. Infarcted tissue is revealed in the scan as an accumulation defect. For positive scintigraphy of the infarct Tc-99m pyrophosphate has been used. Furthermore, it is possible to image scintigraphically the chambers of the heart. For this purpose serum albumin is labeled with Tc-99m or In-113m and reinjected. These indicators have, on the one hand, a short half-life and, on the other hand, stay sufficiently long in the vascular system to obtain good results with a scanner without overexposure to the patient. After injection of an activity bolus the dynamics of the filling of the heart can be recorded by means of a scintigraphic series made with the gamma camera.

1.2.3.3.2.2. Lung Scintigraphy. For the examination of the lungs two different techniques have been adopted, perfusion scintigraphy and ventilation scintigraphy. Thus far perfusion scintigraphy has been used in routine work. Ventilation scintigraphy is more complicated and has not always proved necessary from the diagnostic aspect since ventilation disorders are usually manifest as perfusion disorders (Euler–Liljestrand mechanism). Xe-133 gas is used.

Perfusion scintigraphy makes use of macroaggregates (MA), which are labeled with I-131, Tc-99m, or In-113m. In-133m has the advantage of a very short half-life of 1.7 hr, but also means that the MA must be rapidly prepared just before the injection. Perfusion scintigraphy is of particular importance since it permits segmental or lobar failure of the pulmonary circulation to be detected earlier than is possible with roentgenologic means (Fig. 1-16).

1.2.3.3.2.3. Liver Scintigraphy. Since colloidal gold is taken up by the liver and conveyed to the hepatic reticuloendothelial system (RES), the liver can be imaged by injecting intravenously Au-198 colloid. Cysts, abscesses, hematomas, and tumors can be detected as accumulation defects (Fig. 1-16). In the case of serious liver damage, the spleen takes over the elimination of the colloid to an increasing extent so that spleen scintigraphy is often resorted to in order to evaluate the damage. Tc-99m-labeled colloids have also been introduced in order to exploit the well-known advantages of this radionuclide. Whilst Au-198 can be located even at deep regions of the liver owing to its gamma energy of 0.41 MeV, the application of Tc-99m is restricted to the discovery of more superficial lesions of the liver.

The excretion of the colloid taken up in the RES occurs relatively slowly so that serial scintigraphy brings no additional advantage. I-131-labeled rose bengal, however, is well suited to serial scintigraphic function testing of the excretory passages between liver, gallbladder, and intestines (cf. Section 1.2.3.2.5).

1.2.3.3.2.4. Scintigraphy of the Pancreas. Thus far the pancreas can only be visualized scintigraphically with Se-75-labeled methionine, which is a constituent of the pancreatic enzyme. The suitability of this indicator is based on accumulation in regions of increased protein synthesis, for which this amino acid is required. The accumulation effect of Se-75 methionine is, however, relatively nonspecific as the organism incorporates the methionine in proteins at many sites, especially in the liver. Consequently, a number of measures have been evolved to reduce as much as possible the influence of the adjacent liver on the scintigram. These include special positioning of the patient to prevent overlapping of the liver and dietary measures to stimulate the enzyme production. Good results can also be obtained by making a separate liver scintigram with Au-198 and comparing it with the Se-75 methionine scintigram. The evaluation of the accumulation defects can be carried out by the subtraction method used in radiology or by electronic means.

1.2.3.3.2.5. Spleen Scintigraphy. The spherocytes used for function analysis of the spleen, i.e., both thermally and chemically treated red blood cells (cf. Section 1.2.3.2.2), are equally good indicators for scintigraphy of the spleen. Cr-51-labeled red blood cells must be aged at just about 50°C. In the case of chemical treatment with Hg-197 bromomercurihydroxypropane (BMHP) the labeling with Hg-197 is done at the same time. In contrast to storage of colloid in the RES, sequestration of the spherocytes is a special property of the spleen. Consequently, the spleen exhibits a good accumulation effect, which permits relatively exact determination of the size and weight when scans of the supine and lateral positions are evaluated. Since the Hg-197 is released in the spleen during the breakdown of red blood cells and accumulates in the tubules of the kidneys, renal scintigraphy is possible after several hours.

1.2.3.2.6. Renal Scintigraphy. For visualizing the kidneys mercury compounds are suitable indicators since they are kept in the renal parenchyma for a relatively long time. Accumulation defects give evidence of cysts, infarction, and tumors. Owing to the high renal affinity of mercury a lower activity is required than in cerebral scanning. Nevertheless, even in renal scintigraphy Hg-203 is avoided if possible. Frequently, Hg-197 is used as the radiation dose to the patient is only about one-third. The disadvantage of its lower gamma energy (0.08 MeV) is not so important as the kidneys are close to the surface of the body.

Good results have been obtained with Tc-99m-labeled iron–ascorbic-acid complex as indicator. With this indicator the radiation exposure to the kidneys is reduced to about 1/20 of that of Hg-203. Furthermore, compared with Hg-197 (half-life 65 days) this indicator has the advantage of a shorter half-life of 6 hr and a higher gamma energy of 0.14 MeV.

For use with the scanner, kidney-seeking substances are usually not suitable as their excretion from the kidney takes place too quickly. For I-131 Hippuran a method has been developed, whereby the injection is made to a small extent intravenously and to a large extent intramuscularly. With the intramuscular injection in the thigh a depot effect is achieved. In this way the kidneys receive a relatively constant supply of Hippuran.

But it is this rapid excretion of intravenously administered Hippuran that supplies the basis for serial scintigraphy. The serial scans reveal the momentary position of the indicator in the kidney so accurately that evaluation with respect to time in the individual picture regions is possible (functional scintigraphy, Fig. 1-8). In this way the functional values for the renal cortex, renal medulla, and urinary tract can be obtained separately.

1.2.3.3.2.7. Placental Scintigraphy. For determining the position of the placenta various indicators have been used with success (Fig. 1-15). Since we have been able to label patient plasma with In-113m, this indicator is given preference as the radiation exposure caused by it is much lower than that of abdominal radiography. Furthermore, the dose to the fetus is low since the indicator hardly passes through the placenta to the fetus. Essentially all placental localization is now done with ultrasound.

1.2.3.3.2.8. Bone Scintigraphy. Bone scintigraphy belongs to positive scintigraphy. Of the bone-seeking substances strontium and fluorine are available as radionuclides with good physical properties. F-18 has the disadvantage that it has to be produced in a cyclotron or nuclear reactor. Consequently, with a half-life of 112 min this indicator is not available to all doctors. The advantage of F-18 is that the fluorine disappears from the blood more quickly than strontium does, and a lower blood activity shows the lesion more clearly in the scan (Fig. 1-15).

The use of short-lived indicators in bone scintigraphy means a compromise because the accumulation effect in bone lesions is a relatively slow procedure. With Sr-85 this state of affairs is better as the half-life of 65 days makes it possible to carry out scanning even after a few days. The problem of radiation exposure in the case of long half-lives can be avoided with Sr-87m, but its half-life of 2.8 hr is only about twice as long as that of F-18. Compared with F-18, however, Sr-87m has the advantage that it is a daughter nuclide of Y-87, a radionuclide with a half-life of 3.3 days. With Y-87 a generator system is available, which can be used as a source of Sr-87m in clinical application. Also of interest is Ba-131, which with a half-life of 11 days lies between the extremes of Sr-87m and Sr-85. Most bone scans now are done with Tc-99m phosphate complexes; Tc-99m has a 6-hr half-life, no beta radiation, and good imaging characteristics. It is cheap and chemically versatile.

Bone scintigraphy is of particular importance since it reveals lesions at an earlier stage than is possible with radiography.

1.2.3.3.2.9. Isotopic Lymphography. Isotopic lymphography is carried out with colloidal Au-198. The colloid must be injected into the appropriate lymphatic collecting area whose lymphatic system is to be visualized. The advantage over radiographic lymphangiography is that only a subcutaneous injection is necessary and not exposure of the lymphatic vessel. After interdigital injection between the first and second toe, the radioactive gold first accumulates in the lymphatic system of the extremities and later in the pertaining iliac and para-aortic lymph nodes so that the lymphatic pathways into the lower abdominal cavity can be followed scintigraphically. For various pathological reasons these pathways may become partially or completely blocked. This is revealed by reduced or absent accumulation of Au-198. Other parts of the lymphatic system can also be checked by choosing a suitable injection site.

1.3. PHYSICAL TERMS

1.3.1. Chemical Elements, Isotopes, Nuclides

Chemists regard the chemical elements as the building blocks of matter (Fig. 1-17). From the physical aspect they are atoms, i.e., they consist of an atomic nucleus and an electron shell (Fig. 1-18). Chemical compounds and chemical reactions derive from the structure of the electron shell. Since this structure is determined by the protons in the nucleus, the number of protons in the nucleus is the physical characteristic of a chemical element. It is the atomic number. It indicates the position of the chemical element in the periodic system. Since the proton carries the positive electrical elementary charge, this principle of order is based on the nuclear charge of the atoms (Fig. 1-19).

Apart from the hydrogen nucleus, the nuclei of the chemical elements also contain neutrons. These are uncharged particles with almost the same mass as the proton. Owing to their lack of charge, they influence the structure of the electron shell to such a small extent that atoms of the same number of protons but a different number of neutrons cannot be distinguished from each other by chemical means. Such atoms are called isotopes (Fig. 1-20). This principle of order is based on the mass of the atomic nucleus (Fig. 1-21).

All the chemical elements with their isotopes make up the wide variety of atoms. They are called nuclides and are clearly determined by the number of protons and the number of neutrons in their nuclei.

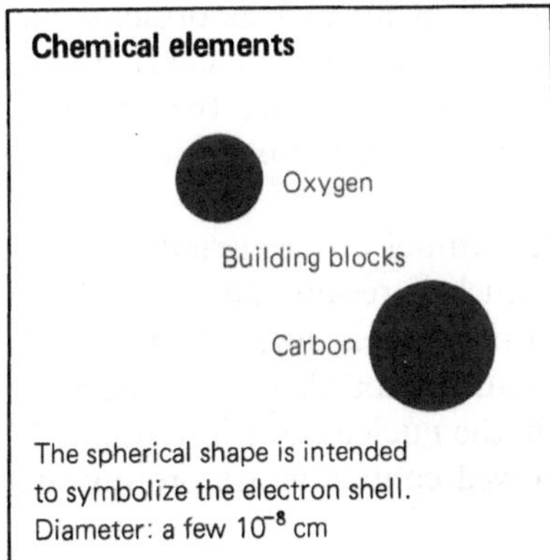

Chemical elements
Oxygen
Building blocks
Carbon
The spherical shape is intended to symbolize the electron shell.
Diameter: a few 10^{-8} cm

Fig. 1-17

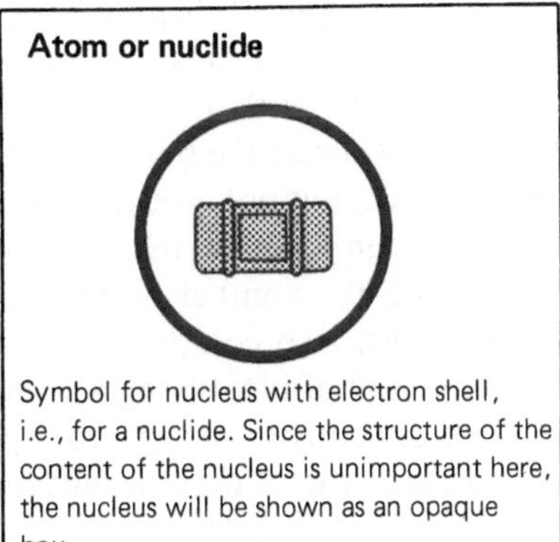

Atom or nuclide
Symbol for nucleus with electron shell, i.e., for a nuclide. Since the structure of the content of the nucleus is unimportant here, the nucleus will be shown as an opaque box.

Fig. 1-18

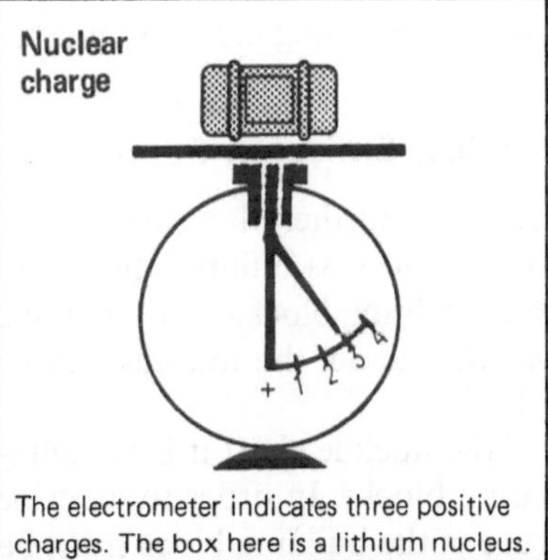

Nuclear charge
+ 1 2 3 4
The electrometer indicates three positive charges. The box here is a lithium nucleus.

Fig. 1-19

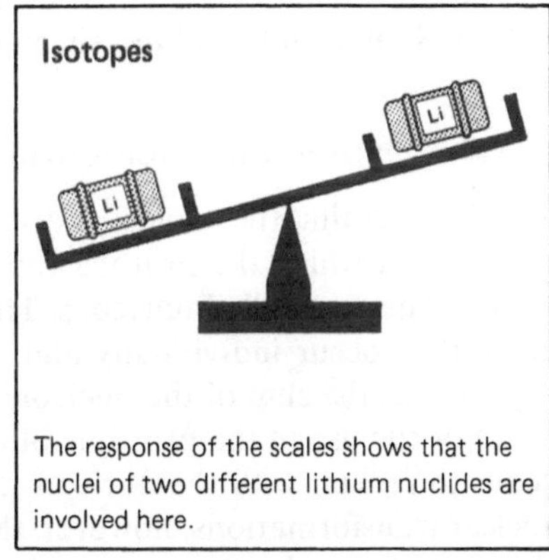

Isotopes
Li
Li
The response of the scales shows that the nuclei of two different lithium nuclides are involved here.

Fig. 1-20

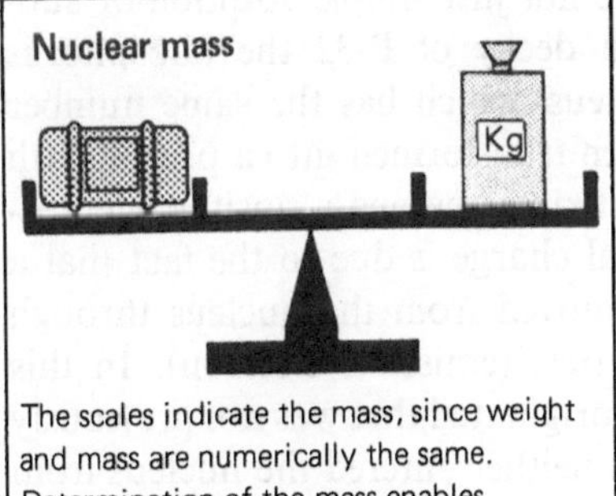

Nuclear mass
Kg
The scales indicate the mass, since weight and mass are numerically the same. Determination of the mass enables conclusions to be drawn about the number of nucleons in the nucleus.

Fig. 1-21

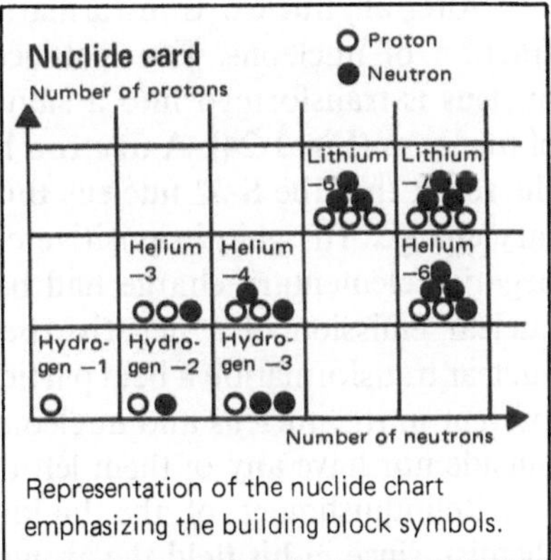

Fig. 1-22

Their graphical display with the number of protons as ordinate and the number of neutrons as abscissa is known as the nuclide chart. Such a chart displays both principles of order, the physical and the chemical. Figure 1-22 shows the beginning of the nuclide chart. A box corresponds to each nuclide, but not a nuclide to each box.

The sign for a chemical element is its symbol in the periodic system, from which the number of protons of the nucleus results. The symbol of a nuclide must also contain information on the nuclear mass. A simple but exact method of identifying a nuclide is to add to the chemical symbol the number of neutrons and protons present in the nucleus. For instance, C-12 would mean that a carbon nucleus is involved containing six protons and six neutrons (Fig. 1-23).

Chemically pure substances of a chemical element consist of a mixture of their isotopes. Consequently, determination of the atomic mass results in a mean atomic mass, which deviates from the mass of the isotopes involved. Seen from this plane, the nuclides are the building blocks of matter.

1.3.2. Nucleons, Elementary Particles, Emission Particles

The fact that the nucleus is divisible leads to a further plane of observation, within which the protons and neutrons appear as building blocks of matter. They are called nucleons. They act as building blocks as, on the one hand, they occur individually and, on the other hand, the nucleus can be regarded as the sum of the nucleons (Fig. 1-23).

For the use of the principle of order of the nuclide chart it is advantageous to reckon with the nucleons as building blocks. In order to describe nuclear transformations, however, the picture of the building block must be abandoned, as shown in the following example, and consequently the nucleons are usually referred to as elementary particles.

After all, nuclear transformations are not just simple addition or subtraction of nucleons. For instance, with decay of P-32 the phosphorus nucleus is transformed into a sulfur nucleus, which has the same number of nucleons (Fig. 1-24). A neutron has been transformed into a proton with the result that the S-32 nucleus thus created has gained a positive elementary charge. The gain in positive electrical charge is due to the fact that a negative elementary charge had been removed from the nucleus through nuclear emission of a negative beta particle (emission electron). In this nuclear transformation a beta particle has originated that was not previously existent in the nucleus and nucleons have neither entered the nucleus from outside nor have any of them left the nucleus by emission.

Relinquishment of the building block concept is unusual for the chemist, since in his field the atoms can always be individually detected in the molecule and crystal forms (Fig. 1-25) and chemical synthesis and con-

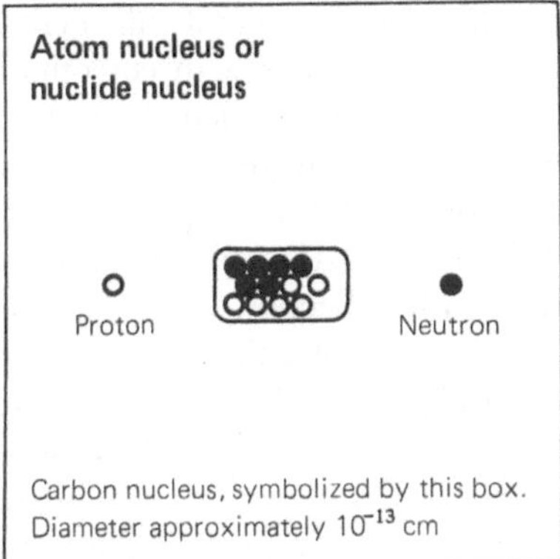

Atom nucleus or nuclide nucleus
Proton
Neutron
Carbon nucleus, symbolized by this box. Diameter approximately 10^{-13} cm

Fig. 1-23

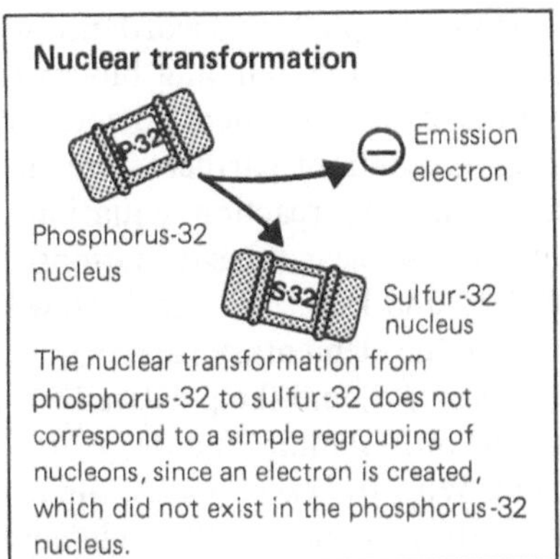

Nuclear transformation
P-32
Emission electron
Phosphorus-32 nucleus
S32
Sulfur-32 nucleus
The nuclear transformation from phosphorus-32 to sulfur-32 does not correspond to a simple regrouping of nucleons, since an electron is created, which did not exist in the phosphorus-32 nucleus.

Fig. 1-24

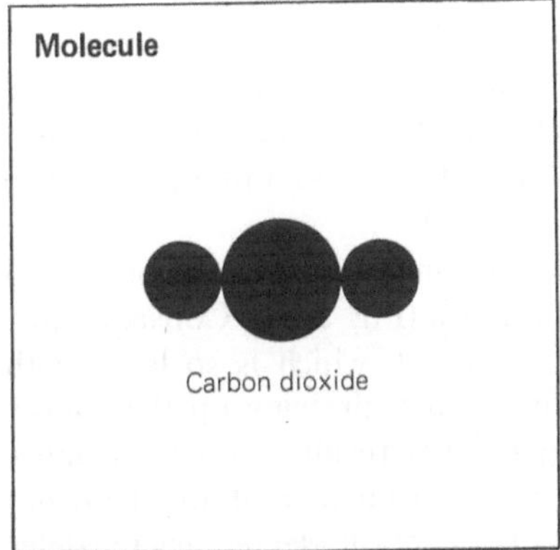

Fig. 1-25

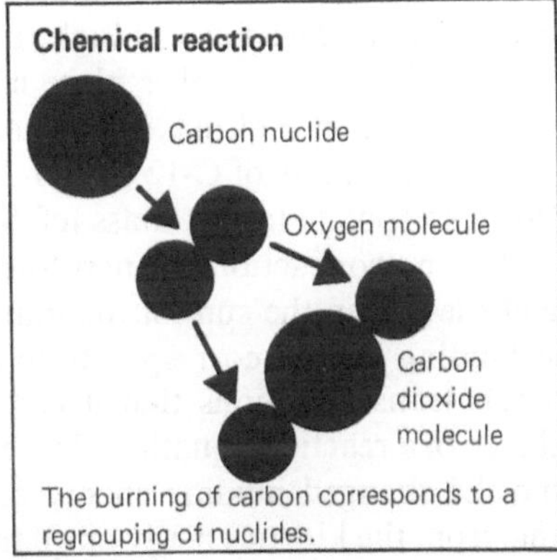

Fig. 1-26

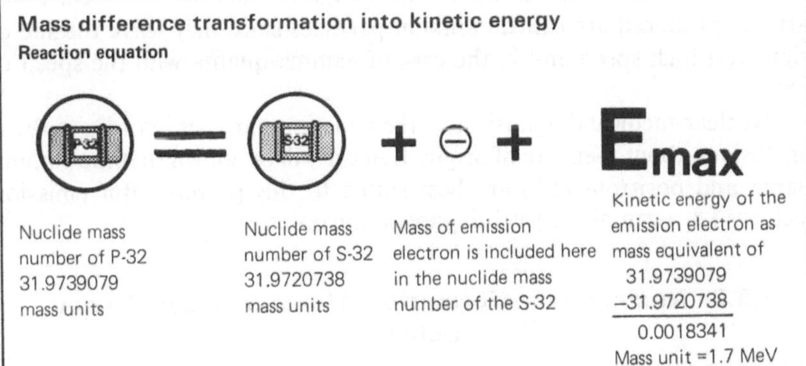

Fig. 1-27

version take place in accordance with the rules of addition and subtraction of unconvertible building blocks (Fig. 1-26). All conflicts with customary notions can be avoided, however, by simply regarding the elementary particles as reactions partners in nuclear transformations. In this way they can be defined in reaction equations, which correspond to experimentally observed nuclear transformations (Fig. 1-27). The neutrino, which has been neglected in Figs. 1-24 and 1-27, will be dealt with in Section 1.3.8.

Of the elementary particles, apart from the nucleons, the negative beta particles (β^-) and the positive beta particles (β^+), also called positrons, are important. Gamma quanta, which are electrically neutral, also belong to them. With the exception of the proton, which when alone corresponds to the hydrogen nucleus, these elementary particles do not represent a nucleus since they are incapable of forming an electron shell around themselves.

A comparison between nuclear transformations and chemical reactions brings to light a further difference. When dealing with nuclear forces, the energies involved are so high that measurable conversion of mass into energy and vice versa takes place in accordance with the Einstein relation on the equivalence of mass and energy. The unit of mass has been defined as 1/12 of the mass of C-12 (Fig. 1-28). An energy of 931.4 million electron volts corresponds to this mass (cf. Section 1.3.8).

When two reaction partners form a compound, the resulting compound weighs less than the sum of the individual parts (Fig. 1-29). Consequently, the binding energy corresponds to a mass defect, which is so large with nuclear transformations that it can be used when drawing up the energy balance of a reaction equation. The energy balance results, on the one hand, from the changed binding energy of the reacting nuclei and, on the other hand, from the kinetic energy or quantum energy of the elementary particles involved.

The nucleus that undergoes conversion is called the starting nucleus; the resulting nucleus is known as the daughter nucleus. The elementary particles produced are called emission particles since they leave the site of origin at a high speed and in the case of gamma quanta with the speed of light.

Nuclear-medical diagnosis uses the emission particles in order to draw conclusions about their site of origin. Later it will be shown that the gamma quanta and positrons (β^+) are best suited to this purpose. But emission electrons (β^-) can also serve diagnostic purposes.

1.3.3. Nuclear Transformation, Nuclear Decay, Decay Scheme

A change in the mass or charge of the nuclide nucleus is called a nuclear transformation. The starting nucleus gives rise to a daughter nucleus, to

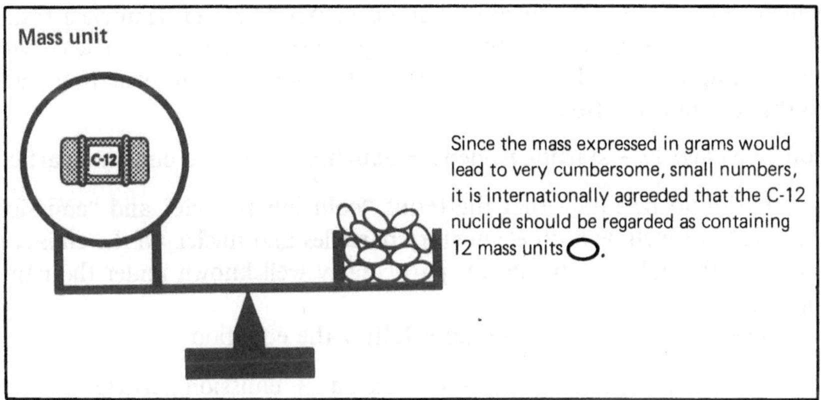

Mass unit
C-12
Since the mass expressed in grams would lead to very cumbersome, small numbers, it is internationally agreeded that the C-12 nuclide should be regarded as containing 12 mass units.

Fig. 1-28

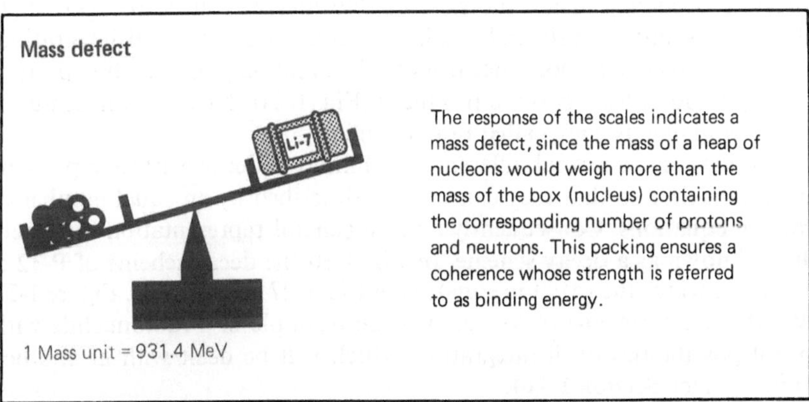

Mass defect
Li-7
The response of the scales indicates a mass defect, since the mass of a heap of nucleons would weigh more than the mass of the box (nucleus) containing the corresponding number of protons and neutrons. This packing ensures a coherence whose strength is referred to as binding energy.
1 Mass unit = 931.4 MeV

Fig. 1-29

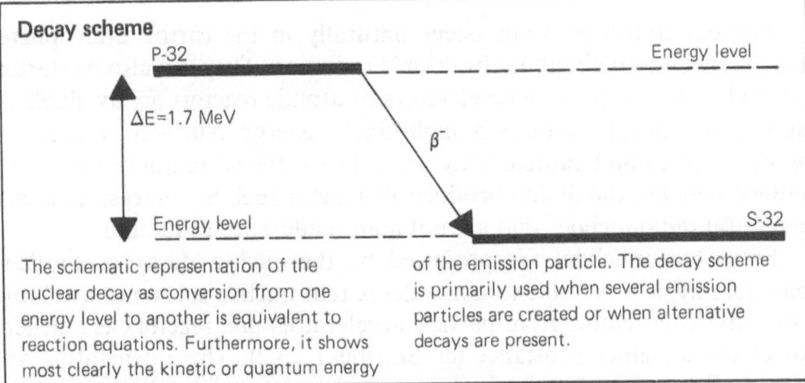

Decay scheme
P-32
Energy level
ΔE=1.7 MeV
β⁻
Energy level
S-32
The schematic representation of the nuclear decay as conversion from one energy level to another is equivalent to reaction equations. Furthermore, it shows most clearly the kinetic or quantum energy of the emission particle. The decay scheme is primarily used when several emission particles are created or when alternative decays are present.

Fig. 1-30

which a new place in the nuclide chart corresponds. As a rule nuclear transformations are started by collision of high-speed elementary particles with the starting nucleus. The general form of the nuclear transformation leads to the reaction equation

collision particle + starting nucleus = daughter nucleus + emission particle

It should be noted that the terms "collision particle" and "emission particle" can include both elementary particles and nuclei. Of the emission particles, the helium-4 nucleus is particularly well known under the name alpha particle.

Special nuclear transformations follow the equation

starting nucleus = daughter nucleus + emission particle

The reason for this special nuclear transformation is to be found in processes occurring inside the nucleus. No motive can be recognized. It takes place spontaneously and is called spontaneous nuclear disintegration. We speak of disintegration since prior to the event only one reaction partner is present and at least two are produced (Fig. 1-24). Nuclides whose nuclei decay spontaneously are called radionuclides.

In many cases several different possibilities of decay exist for a particular radionuclide so that they can only be described by an equal number of reaction equations. Consequently a more general representation is chosen. This is known as a decay scheme. In Fig. 1-30 the decay scheme of P-32 is shown, for which the reaction equation in Fig. 1-27 is illustrated. Figure 1-32 gives the decay scheme of Mo-99. It is an example of a radionuclide with several possibilities of disintegration, which will be dealt with in another connection (cf. Section 1.3.6).

1.3.4. Artificial and Natural Radionuclides

Nuclear transformations occur naturally in the earth's atmosphere, where they are brought about by cosmic radiation. They can also be started in the laboratory if particle accelerators or atomic reactors are available as a source of collision particles of high kinetic energy. Nuclides obtained in this way that exhibit radioactivity are called artificial radionuclides. Also included here are the fission products of reactor fuel. In contrast there are the natural radionuclides that are not man-made, such as radium.

Some radionuclides are produced by the nuclear decay of another. Consequently, it is possible to make the parent nuclide substance available to the physician remote from particle accelerators and reactors as a generator of the daughter substance (cf. Section 1.2.3.2). These generators are not only important for producing special radionuclides but also offer advantages when the daughter nuclide has a short half-life and the parent nuclide a long half-life.

1.3.5. Stability, Half-Life

The stability of a nucleus depends upon the ratio of neutrons to protons. It requires for a given number of protons an equal or almost equal number of neutrons. For this reason stable nuclides are found at the approximate center of a nuclide chart line. For nuclides at either side of the center there is the tendency to correct the nucleon ratio of the nucleus by spontaneous nuclear decay, i.e., the nucleus is unstable.

This tendency of unstable nuclides is stronger the further the nuclides are away from the center of the nuclide chart line. The strength of the tendency finds its expression in the life of a nuclide nucleus. On account of the phenomenon of spontaneous nuclear decay, it is not possible to determine the life of an individual nucleus. Statistics on the nuclear decay of large quantities of a radionuclide show (decay law) that the time interval during which half the nuclei disintegrate is independent of the number of nuclei present at the beginning (Fig. 1-31). This time interval is a characteristic of the pure radionuclide substance and is called the physical half-life. It is a statement of probability on the life of a radionuclide and consequently belongs to the data printed on the nuclide chart.

All processes that can be formulated mathematically as an exponential function result in a straight line when plotted semilogarithmically, which can be clearly established by the half-value. The notion of half-value is found not only in the law of decay. Further examples of half-value are the biological half-life (cf. Section 1.2.3.2.1) and the half-value layer of radiation shielding (cf. Section 1.4.5.2.6).

1.3.6. Metastability

The daughter nucleus formed during nuclear decay is either stable or is itself a radionuclide. There are radionuclides, however, in the case of which the decay process in the daughter nucleus leaves behind an excited state, which can be compensated not only by a change in the nucleon ratio but also by emission of a gamma quantum.

Such daughter nuclei are radionuclides, because they are radioactive, but they do not disintegrate into a new daughter nucleus differing in mass and charge. Instead they undergo a quantum transition to a state of lower energy. This change of state occurs spontaneously and occasions a half-life of the pure nuclide substance just like spontaneous nuclear decay.

The reverse process, transition to a state of higher energy, is called nuclear excitation, and the state of such nuclei is referred to as metastable. Actually, the excitation of any nucleus is possible by means of energy-supplying processes. As a rule, however, the excitation is instantly reversed by emission of a gamma quantum so that cause and effect are to be regarded as a common process. To distinguish from this process, the term "meta-

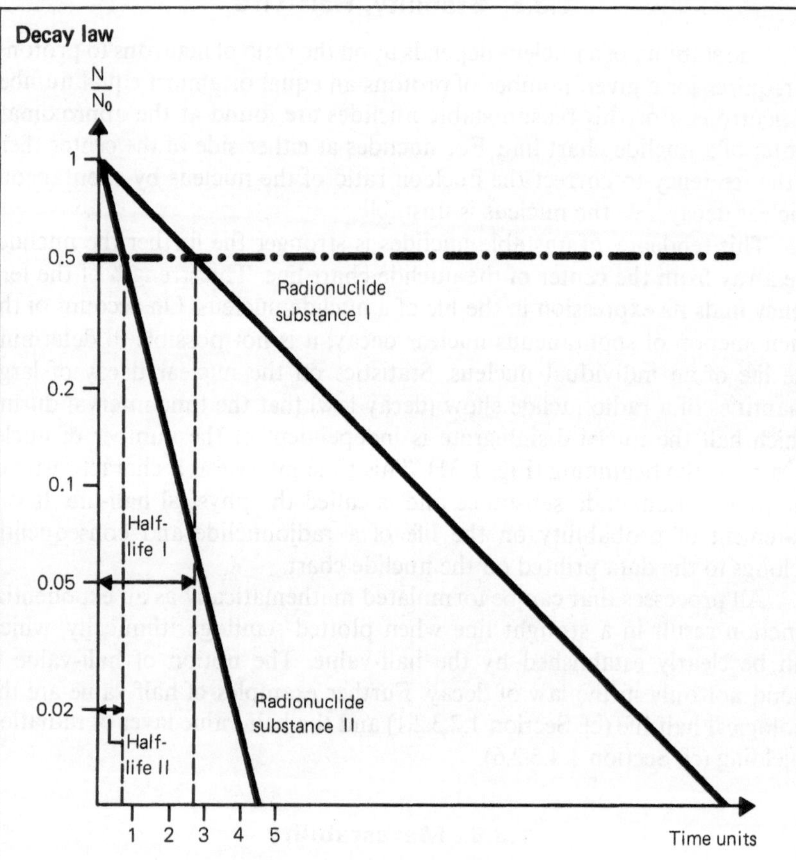

Processes that can be described as a change of quantity and in the case of which the change of this quantity is proportional to the unchanged quantity at the beginning, can be formulated mathematically as exponential functions. This applies to the decrease in the quantity N of a radionuclide with respect to time as a result of nuclear decay, and the following applies:

$dN/dt = -\lambda N$ or $N = N_0 \cdot e^{-\lambda t}$

and applying logarithms

$\ln (N/N_0) = -\lambda t$

In semilogarithmic representation of N/N_0 with respect to t we obtain a straight line with the gradient $-\lambda$.

The proportionality factor λ is called the decay constant and is a measure of the rate of decrease of the nondisintegrated nuclei. The same purpose is met by the half-life

$$\text{half-life} = \frac{\ln 2}{\lambda}$$

Fig. 1-31

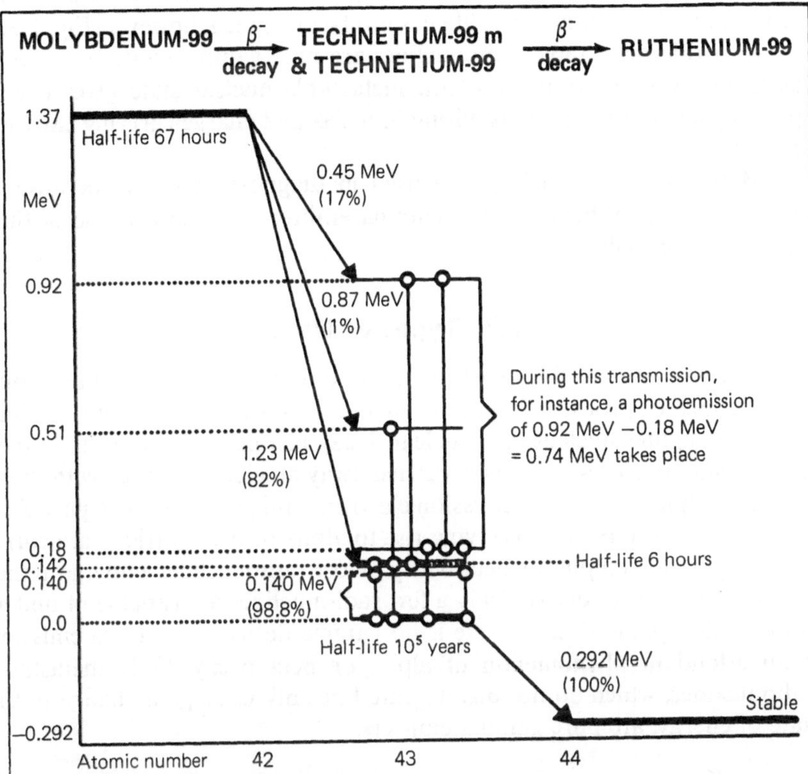

The decay scheme is a two-dimensional representation of the nuclear disintegration. The horizontal axis contains the atomic number of the chemical element and the vertical axis an energy scale. The energy levels indicated by heavy lines signify the positions of nonexcited nuclide nuclei and the energy levels indicated by thin lines the positions of the excited nuclear states. The arrows show which energy levels can be attained by beta decay. If several arrows start from the same level, these indicate that various types of beta decay are involved. The percentage figures in brackets state the frequency with which the individual decay types occur when a radionuclide substance is assayed. The vertical lines between the energy levels refer to gamma energies. If several such lines start from the same level, alternative types of gamma emission are involved. The decay scheme is similar to a timetable. A reaction equation, i.e., a decay type, corresponds to each train between two nonexcited nuclide nuclei. The time of changing over to the energy level and the travel time are negligibly short. Some nuclide nuclei, however, have a special energy level (marked by the heavy dashed line) at which the changing over involves such a long waiting time that it will be possible to isolate nuclei in this excited state as a substance with a certain definite half-life. They are the metastable radionuclides.

Fig. 1-32

stable" is applied only to those excited nuclear states having lifetimes that are measurable. A "limit" half-life has not been defined, however (Fig. 1-32).

As a rule metastable radionuclides are pure gamma emitters. In some cases, however, the transition to a metastable nuclear state gives rise to spontaneous nuclear decay resulting in mass- and charge-carrying emission particles.

Metastable radionuclides are used in diagnosis not only because of their advantage of being a pure gamma emitter but also because of their relatively short half-life.

1.3.7. Types of Decay

Nuclides of a nuclide chart line differ only in the number of neutrons. The number of protons changes from line to line. If the starting nucleus and the daughter nucleus of a nuclear decay belong to different lines, then the emission particles must have carried away an electric charge with them, i.e., either alpha particles or emission electrons and positrons (beta particles).

Nuclear disintegrations giving rise to alpha or beta particles are correspondingly called alpha or beta decay. Most radionuclides undergo either alpha decay or beta decay. Only a few radionuclides are capable of undergoing both types of decay. There is no gamma decay, i.e., gamma emission is an attendant phenomenon of alpha or beta decay. Only metastable radionuclides, which do not disintegrate but only undergo a change in the state of energy, are pure gamma emitters.

1.3.8. Energy of Emission Particles

The energy of the emission particles originates from the transformation of the mass difference between the starting nucleus and the daughter nucleus into energy. The distribution of the energy amongst the emission particles formed is made in a specific way for the type of decay of a particular radionuclide. Since the type of decay goes back to the properties of the starting nucleus, the energy of the emission particles formed is given in the nuclide chart.

While alpha particles and gamma quanta receive a characteristic energy amount for the nuclear decay, the beta particle only receives a characteristic energy together with another simultaneously produced elementary particle, the neutrino. Consequently, the energies of the beta particle and of the neutrino supplement each other with respect to this characteristic amount, whereas the energy distribution between the two appears to be arbitrary.

Since the neutrino—an elementary particle without a charge and with an extremely small mass compared with the beta particle—can only be detected by nuclear research means, its energy portion remains in the dark.

Therefore, as a characteristic quantity of the beta energy, the maximum beta energy occurring is given in the nuclide chart.

The practical result of the energy distribution between a beta particle and a neutrino is that measurement of a radionuclide substance yields an extensive spectrum of beta energy (Fig. 1-33). In diagnosis the beta energy only plays a role in the evaluation of the emission electron, since the evaluation of the positron is based exclusively on annihilation radiation, which is produced when positrons and electrons combine (cf. Section 1.3.9).

The energies of the emission particles are measured in electron volts (eV). The energies of interest here, however, are expressed in millions of electron volts (MeV). The energy of an electron is increased by 1 eV when it is accelerated in a vacuum through a potential difference of 1 V.

1.3.9. Absorption of Emission Particles

On account of their mass, charge, kinetic energy, or quantum energy, emission particles interact with matter. The complete or partial loss of their energy is known as absorption.

As a result of the aforementioned definition of elementary particles that gamma quanta, which carry neither mass nor charge but only energy, also belong to the elementary particles, it is customary to regard the absorption not only of alpha and beta particles but also that of the gamma quanta as a collision process. Complete absorption means that the energy of an emission particle has been completely used up by one or more collisions.

The collision partners of emission particles after nuclear decay are largely the shell electrons of the nuclides in the vicinity of the decayed radionuclide, since, on account of their large number, they are the most likely an obstacle for the emission particles. Nuclei are less likely to be collision partners.

Since shell electrons have discrete energy states in accordance with their binding energy, collision with shell electrons leads either to a state of higher energy or to complete liberation from their bond with the nucleus (cf. Section 1.3.10). In the first case an electrically neutral nuclide in the state of excitation remains, in the second case a positively charged nuclide (ion). The second case occurs when the impact emission particle is carrying at least the ionization energy, the first case is possible with less energy.

Emission particles have such high energy when they are formed that up to their complete absorption they undergo almost exclusively ionizing collision processes (Fig. 1-34). The number of ion pairs produced in air per beta particle of 1 MeV is in the order of magnitude of 30,000 and the number of pairs produced per alpha particle of 1 MeV goes into the hundreds of thousands.

As long as it is of high kinetic energy, the positron behaves like an

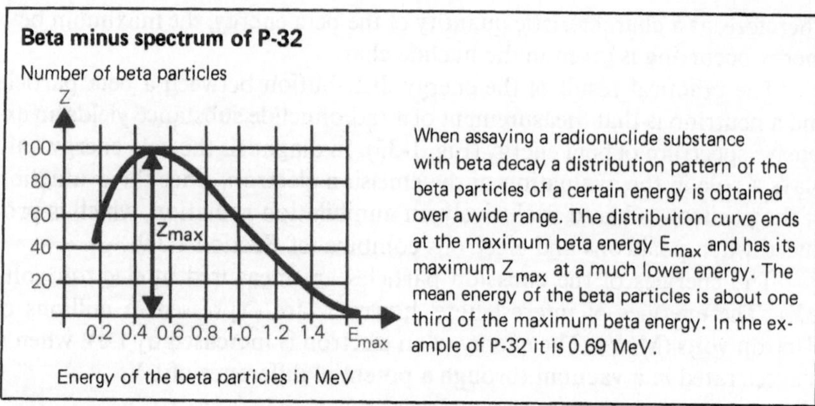

Fig. 1-33

Ionization as absorption process of alpha and beta particles

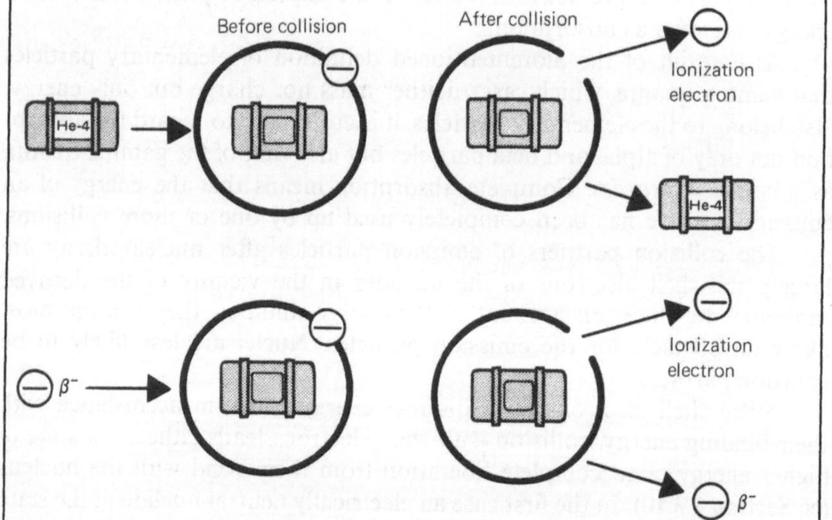

Before collision

After collision

He-4

Ionization electron

He-4

β^-

Ionization electron

β^-

β^+

Ionization electron

β^+

Fig. 1-34

emission electron, i.e., has an ionizing effect. But as soon as the kinetic energy is almost exhausted through a number of absorption processes, the next collision with an electron leads to annihilation of both collision partners and two gamma quanta are produced, which are emitted in opposite directions (Fig. 1-35). These gamma quanta are called annihilation radiation and both possess a quantum energy of 0.51 MeV. Since, in the body, this positron absorption process occurs within a few millimeters of the site of the nuclear decay producing annihilation radiation, positron decay can be located by gamma measurement. To distinguish from other radiation the angular relation of the annihilation radiation can be made use of.

Collision processes of gamma quanta with shell electrons leads, depending upon the quantum energy, to two different results. A collision process, in which the gamma quantum releases its energy completely, is known as photoeffect in analogy to light absorption (Fig. 1-36). A collision process in which the gamma quantum loses only part of its energy to a shell electron and the remaining energy appears in the form of a correspondingly low-energy quantum is called the Compton effect (Fig. 1-37).

As a rule, like the absorption of alpha and beta particles, both collision processes create an accelerated electron. Such electrons are called secondary electrons. They contain in the case of the photoeffect the entire gamma energy minus the ionization energy, and in the case of the Compton effect the difference in energy between the colliding gamma quantum and created Compton quantum minus the ionization energy.

1.3.10. Effects of Nuclear Decay

On the one hand, nuclear decay results in the creation of a new nuclide with different chemical properties in place of the decaying nuclide. Consequently, at this site changed chemical conditions are suddenly created, which can result in chemical reactions. However, since diagnosis with radionuclides employs quantities between 10^{-10} and 10^{-14} g, poisoning by these new nuclides is not to be feared.

On the other hand, nuclear decay results in the released energy being distributed over the surrounding area. The distribution is not continuous, but to discrete sites, the sites of absorption. If we imagine all the absorption sites over which the entire energy of an emission particle has been distributed to be connected by lines in the direction of the energy transport whose thickness designates the amount of the energy transported, then a picture of a branch is obtained with many short and long twigs.

This is shown schematically in Fig. 1-38 for the case where a gamma quantum emitted from the nucleus gives rise to a photoeffect. The energy of this emission particle has the energy E, of which the fraction E_1 is released at the first absorption site O_1. The remaining energy E_2 is carried further

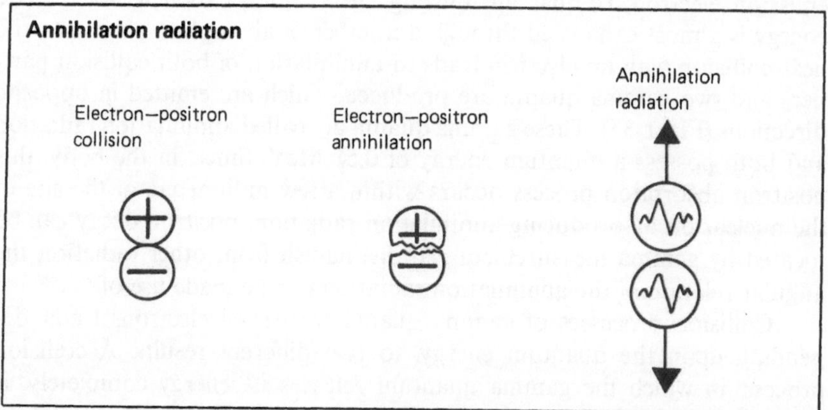

Fig. 1-35

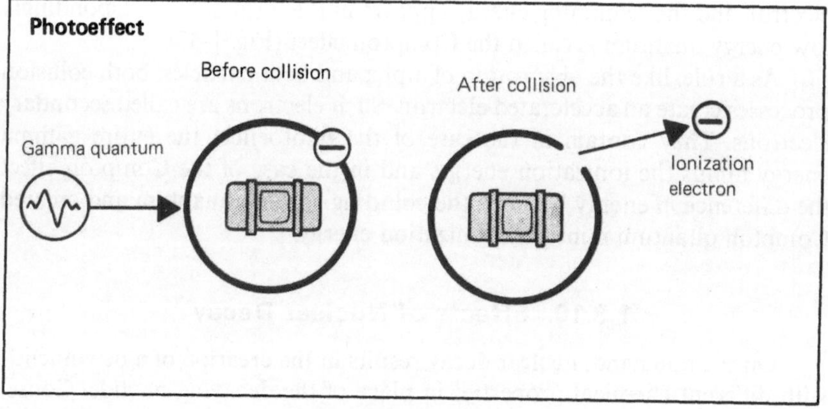

Fig. 1-36

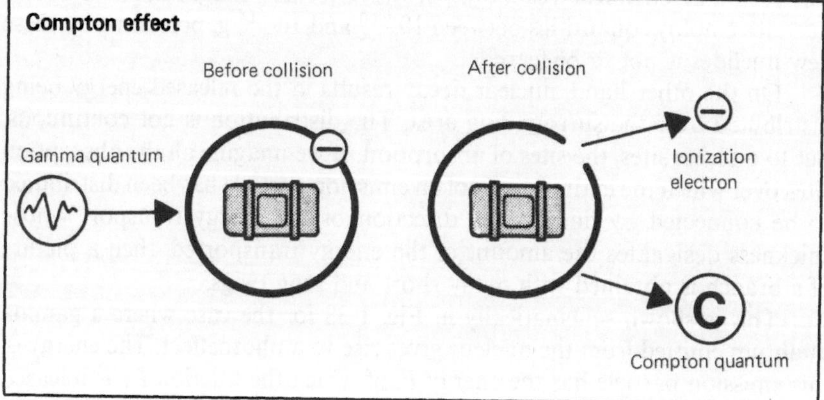

Fig. 1-37

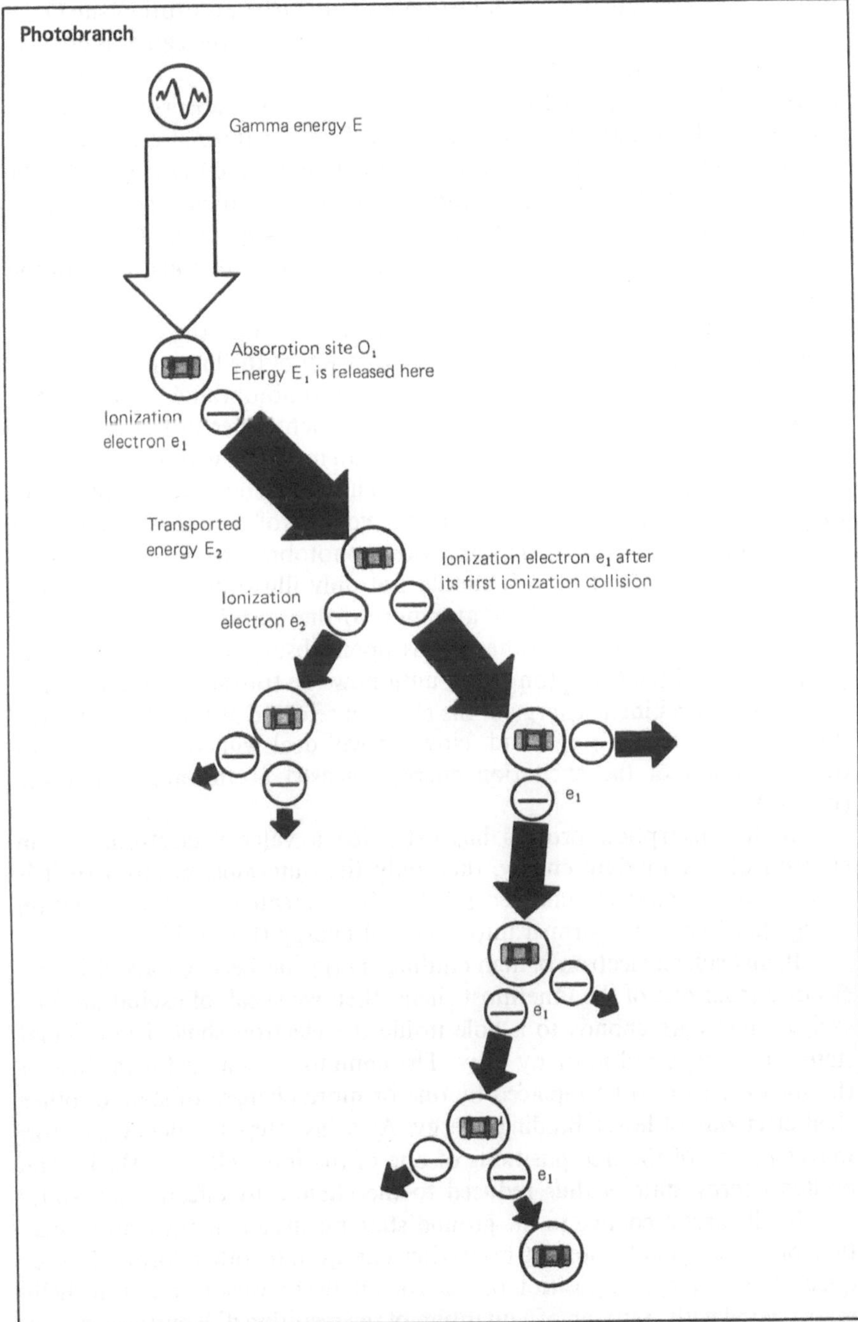
Photobranch
Gamma energy E
Absorption site O_1
Energy E_1 is released here
Ionization electron e_1
Transported energy E_2
Ionization electron e_1 after its first ionization collision
Ionization electron e_2
e_1
e_1
e_1

Fig. 1-38

by the electron e_1 created by ionization up to the next absorption site O_2. If the energy E_2 of e_1 is adequate to give rise to ionization then an e_2 is created. In the course of this a fraction E_3 of E_2 is released at O_2. The remaining energy will be transported by e_1 and e_2 up to further absorption sites O_3 and O_4, etc. In this way the energy E is transferred to the matter.

In contrast to the photoeffect, with the Compton effect (Fig. 1-39) the energy transport branches off already at the first site of absorption O_1. In addition to the ionization electron e_1 the Compton quantum C is created, whose energy is finally absorbed by ionization processes just as with the photoeffect.

Each emission particle forms its own branch and the amount of its energy is roughly related to the spatial extension of the branch. The spatial extension of branches created by the photoeffect (photobranch) and branches created by the Compton effect (Compton branch) differ in that Compton quanta on an average cover a much longer path in matter without absorption than ionization electrons of equal energy. The Compton branch looks more like a double branch and a much larger volume of matter is required to observe this branch than is the case with a photobranch (cf. Section 1.4.1).

The picture of the branch should not only illustrate the paths of the energy transport, but also draw attention to the branch points as sites of transfer of the energy into other forms upon absorption. In studying the photoeffect and the Compton effect, until now the transformation of quantum energy into kinetic energy of the electron released at the site of absorption has been in the foreground. Now we will deal with the possibility of transformation of the excitation energy released at the absorption site (Fig. 1-40).

If the absorption process has extracted a valency electron, i.e., an electron of low binding energy, then only the outermost electron shell is concerned. A positively charged ion has been created. i.e., the excitation energy has been transformed into chemical energy (Fig. 1-40, example 3).

If, instead, an electron of high binding energy has been extracted, i.e., an electron from one of the innermost shells, then we speak of excitation. The excited state corresponds to a hole inside the electron shell. The original state can be regained in many ways. The commonest way is for the loss of the shell electron to be replaced by one or more changes of state of other shell electrons of lesser binding energy. As a last step, a valency electron moves to one of the free positions of one of the inner electron shells. The excited energy state is thus reduced to the chemically effective ion state.

In all cases a change to the ground state means an energy transformation of the originally present excitation energy into other forms. Consequently, the change of position of electrons between various electron shells is associated with emission of a quantum of the resulting difference in energy. In accordance with their nature of origin these quanta are X-rays (Fig. 1-40,

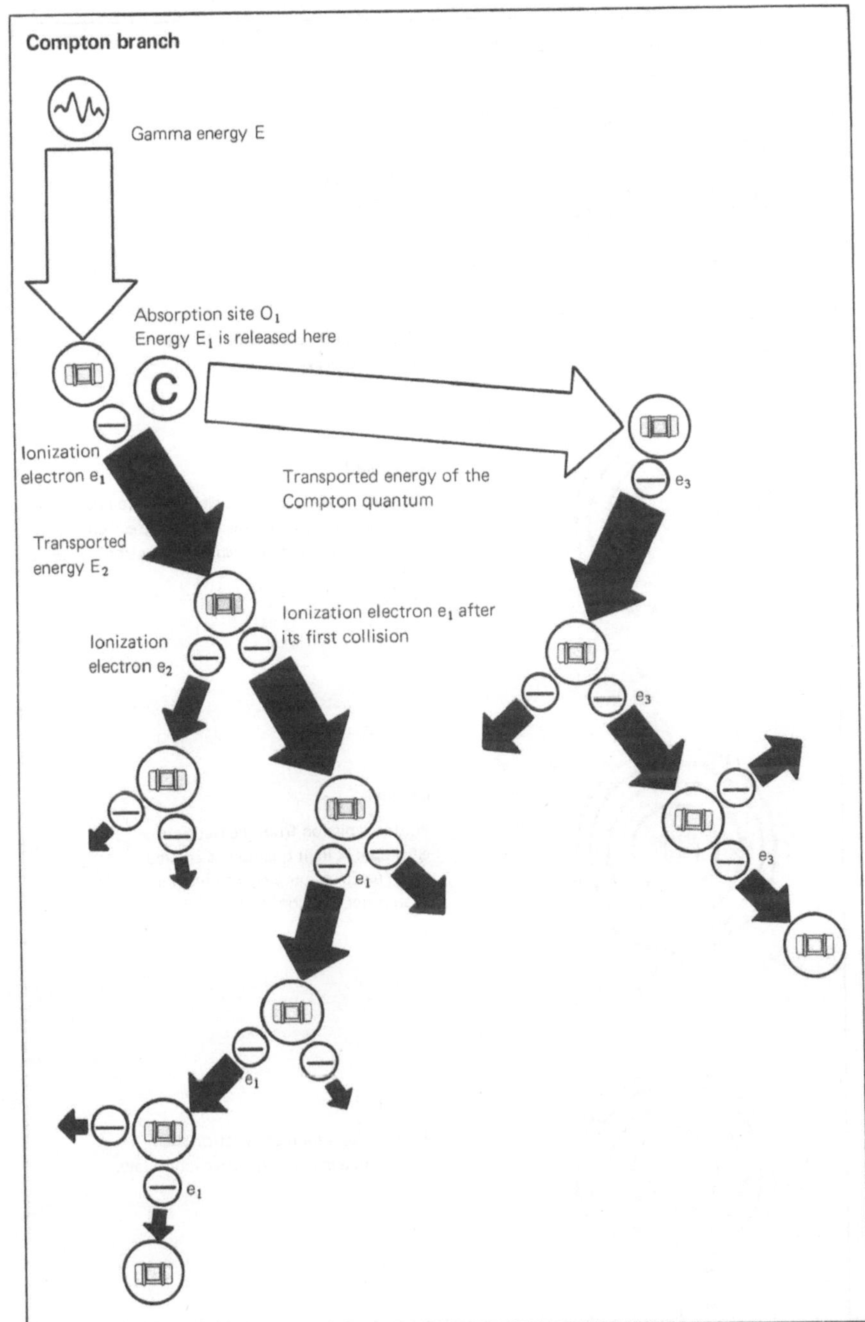
Compton branch
Gamma energy E
Absorption site O_1
Energy E_1 is released here
C
Ionization electron e_1
Transported energy of the Compton quantum
e_3
Transported energy E_2
Ionization electron e_1 after its first collision
Ionization electron e_2
e_3
e_3
e_1
e_1
e_1

Fig. 1-39

Transformation of the released energy

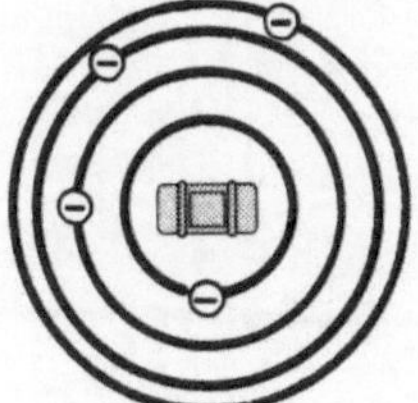

Symbolic electron envelope with several electron shells

Electron shells disarranged by the released energy

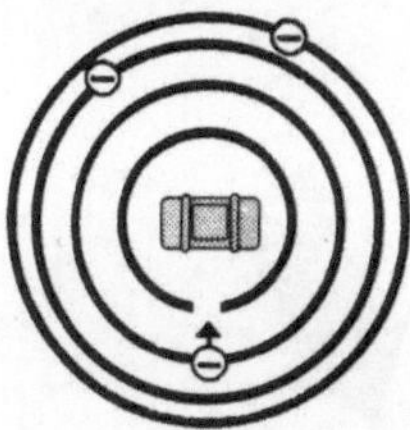

Example 1

Photon emission from the electron envelope: An X-ray quantum is created by an electron jumping into the hole in an inner electron shell.

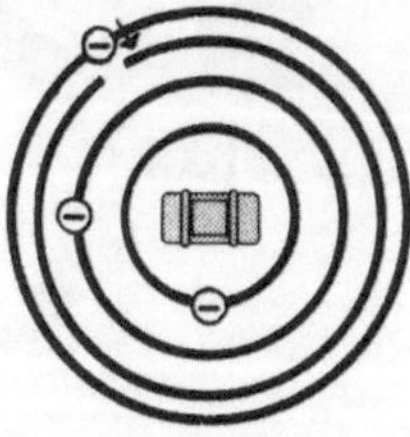

Example 2

Photon emission from the electron envelope: A light quantum is created by an electron jumping into the hole in an outer electron shell.

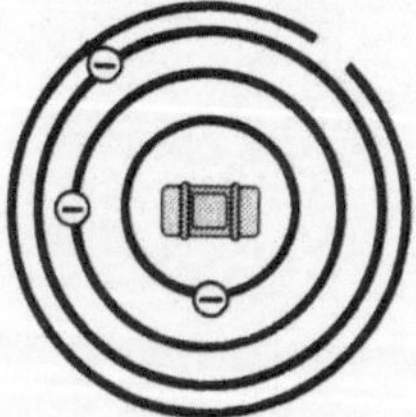

Example 3

Holes in the outermost electron shell give rise to a chemically active ionic state.

Fig. 1-40

example 1). Quanta of lower energy of the order of magnitude of a few electron volts can also be created. This process is known as scintillation (Fig. 1-40, example 2). Quanta of such low energy appear as ultraviolet or visible light. In extension of the term "light", which originally referred only to the visible part of the spectrum, it is now customary to include radiation of the adjacent spectral ranges so that we speak of ultraviolet light.

The most prominent feature of nuclear radiation in biology and medicine is the ionization effect, since, on the one hand, the yield of ions per emission particle is great and, on the other hand, ionization means a transformation of energy into a form that is chemically very effective. Nevertheless, the reason why the transformation of energy into scintillation light is preferred in diagnosis for measuring nuclear radiation will be dealt with in the next section.

1.4. INSTRUMENTATION

Nuclear-medical diagnosis requires counting and localization of the nuclear decay events. Of course nuclear decay cannot be detected by simply observing the event. Consequently, the effect of the nuclear radiation is measured. The fact that nuclear decay events at a remote site can be detected by the effects of the nuclear decay makes the indicator method with radionuclides very valuable in diagnosis. Consequently, we must measure the effect in order to draw conclusions about the cause. For this conclusion it is necessary to check whether the measuring effect as effect clearly corresponds to the nuclear decay as cause.

The measuring effect is firstly the absorption effect of the emission particles in the detector. As a rule, the end result does not follow directly from this measuring effect but from other effects caused by it. If the emission particle absorption is measured as scintillation light, then this measuring effect is converted in the secondary electron multiplier into an electronic measuring effect, which is in turn subjected to a further change by a selection principle in the discriminator. It is important to bear this stepwise change of the measuring effect in mind since the value of the final results depends upon the accuracy of the relation of the measuring effects of the various stages to each other.

The question as to the relation and thus also the measuring accuracy is a problem of a special kind, since we do not wish to measure only a single nuclear decay, but the total activity of a radionuclide substance, i.e., a statistical quantity. Consequently, counting of nuclear decay events only leads to a decay rate, i.e., as nuclear decay number per time interval, for establishing an activity value. Also the resulting measuring effects are statistical quantities with inherent inaccuracies—the statistical errors (cf. Section 1.4.4).

A result of the statistical nature of the nuclear decay rate is that a high decay rate can be measured more accurately than a low one. For various reasons, however, it is extremely difficult to determine the actual number of nuclear decays occurring in a certain period of time. Since for the emission of particles there is no preferential direction, the object under study must be completely surrounded by detector material, a measure that is not even suitable for some aims in diagnosis. Therefore, in practice, only a fraction of the decaying nuclei is detected.

The task of measuring nuclear-medical radiation is the determination of a quantity proportional to the nuclear decay rate. Generally speaking this quantity is based on the summation of absorption effects of nuclear radiation. Refinement of results of a radiation measurement occurs when the absorption effects can be counted. The best results are obtained when only the absorption effects are counted that in all probability have resulted from a single emission particle.

In accordance with practical importance, in the following pages radiation measurement with scintillation detectors will be in the foreground. Measuring equipment based on the ionization effect of radiation will be dealt with only in passing.

1.4.1. Detection and Energy Determination of Individual Emission Particles

An emission particle can be detected by measuring one of its effects. As a rule for measurement either the ionization or the scintillation is brought into play. Thus the detection is based on either electrical conductivity produced by ionization or scintillation light yield in a substance, in which the absorption process of the emission particle has taken place. The substance used for the measurement is called detector.

Detection of an emission particle gives no information about its energy. However, the sum of all ionization or scintillation processes has proved to be a sufficiently reproducible measure of the emission particle energy. Consequently, the measuring effects of the conductivity change or light yield of the emission particle energy are proportional as long as the measurement covers all ionizations or scintillations of an emission particle (Fig. 1-41). If we imagine a branch to picture the absorption processes started by an emission particle (cf. Section 1.3.10), then it is clear that we can only draw conclusions about the emission particle energy from the magnitude of the measuring effect when the branch is completely encompassed by the detector volume (Fig. 1-42).

If only part of the branch is encompassed by the detector volume, then

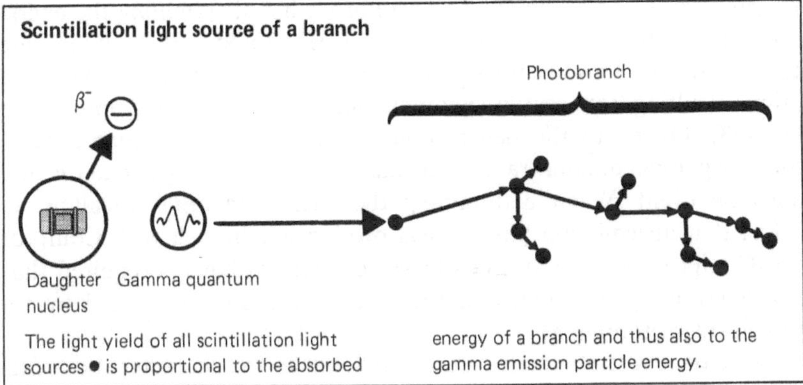

Fig. 1-41

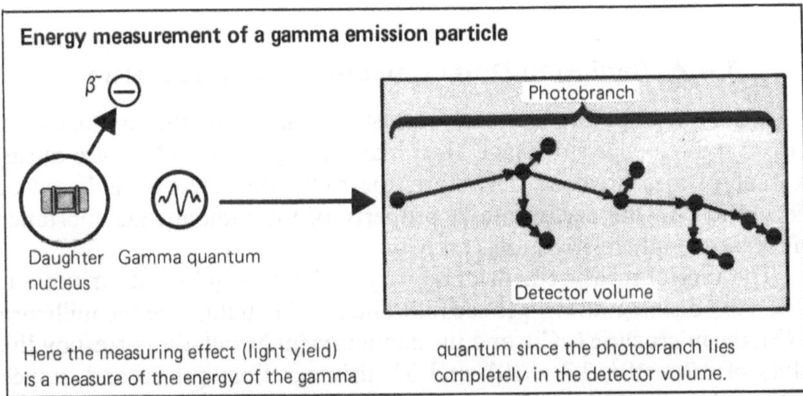

Fig. 1-42

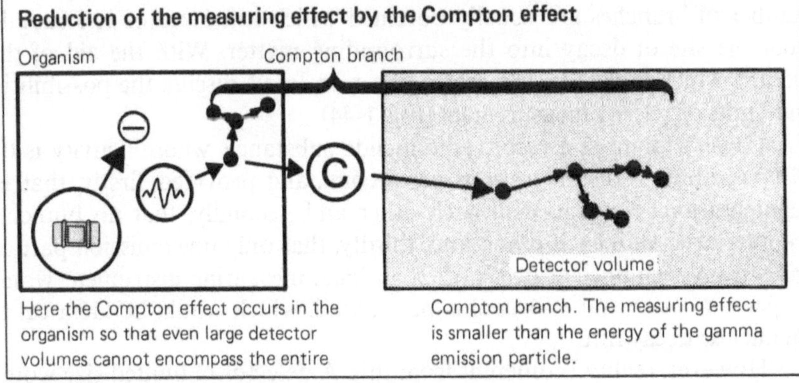

Reduction of the measuring effect by the Compton effect
Organism
Compton branch
C
Detector volume
Here the Compton effect occurs in the organism so that even large detector volumes cannot encompass the entire Compton branch. The measuring effect is smaller than the energy of the gamma emission particle.

Fig. 1-43

the energy measured is too small. Therefore, when determining the energy the detector with its substance volume must be tailored to the volume effect of the absorption. This becomes a problem when the branch contains ramifications resulting from scattered gamma quanta as with the Compton effect (Fig. 1-43). Owing to the penetration capacity of gamma quanta, these secondary gamma quanta travel some distance before giving rise to the next absorption event. When determining the energy, in order to allow for this fact that an emission particle has produced a branch with Compton effect (Compton branch), a much larger detector volume is required than when determining the energy in the case of a branch produced by the photoeffect (photobranch).

Since the emission particle energy belongs to the characteristics of the radionuclide and is always known in nuclear medicine, determination of the energy forms the basis for unequivocal coordination of measuring effect and decay event.

1.4.2. Radiation Detection and Energy Spectrum

If the object of measurement consists of a large number of nuclei, i.e., if it is a radionuclide substance, then many decay events take place during the time of measurement. Therefore, the radiation detection is based on information on the decay rate, a property of the radionuclide substance, which is generally referred to as activity.

The unit of measurement of activity is the curie (Ci) and amounts to 3.7×10^{10} disintegrations per second. The usual subunits are the millicurie (mCi), the microcurie (μCi), and the nanocurie (nCi) with the corresponding values of 3.7×10^7, 3.7×10^4, and 37 disintegrations per second, respectively. A Becquerel (Bq) equals one disintegration per second (1 dps).

Since the decay events follow each other in a random manner, when illustrating the absorption of emission particles even over a short period a number of branches are usually obtained which run more or less radially from the site of decay into the surrounding matter. With the aid of this picture, which looks like the crown of a tree, let us discuss the possibilities and limits of activity measurement (Fig. 1-44).

Given a point source of radionuclide substance, whose activity is 0.1 nCi, i.e., about 4 disintegrations per second, and provided, firstly, that no disintegrations coincide with each other and, secondly, that no branches are interlaced with each other, and, thirdly, that only one emission particle arises from each nuclear decay, then an ideal measuring instrument would measure a count rate of 4 counts per second, which would be identical to the nuclear decay rate.

However, reality is different from this. A detector of limited size would prevent all the branches from being measured, especially when it does not

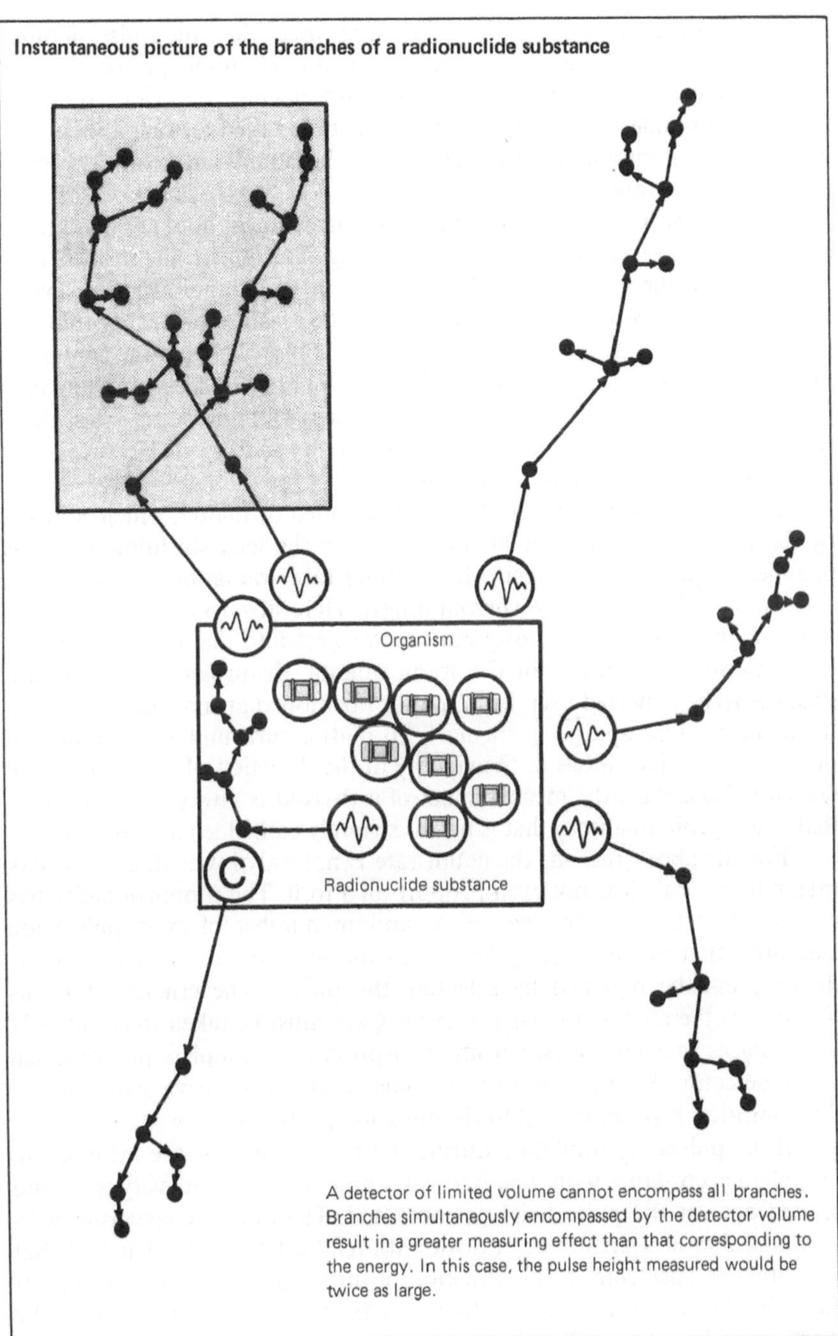
Instantaneous picture of the branches of a radionuclide substance
Organism
C
Radionuclide substance
A detector of limited volume cannot encompass all branches. Branches simultaneously encompassed by the detector volume result in a greater measuring effect than that corresponding to the energy. In this case, the pulse height measured would be twice as large.

Fig. 1-44

completely encompass the radionuclide substance. Since the emission directions are statistically distributed, the count rate will no longer be identical to the decay rate. For the same reason interlacing of various branches cannot be excluded so that two branches can be taken for one if they have been produced simultaneously. Therefore, the count rate is always lower than the decay rate.

Furthermore, since an ideal measuring instrument does not exist, there are additional reservations. Each measuring instrument has a dead time during which the system is unable to respond to another signal or event. With scintillation-measuring instruments the dead time lies within the range of 10^{-6} sec so that after reception of a pulse the next one cannot be measured for some microseconds. Since the pulse sequence is a statistical process, in all probability there will be cases even with low count rates where the pulses follow each other too quickly to be measured. However, this only plays a role with high count rates.

Moreover, the detector is always surrounded by matter, which is struck by the radiation. Of particular importance is the lead shielding, which is intended to protect the detector from undesirable radiation (cosmic radiation, radioactivity from the surroundings). Here absorption will also give rise to Compton effects, whose branches project into the detector volume. On account of the range of Compton quanta, disturbance by Compton effects is to be expected even from matter positioned at some distance from the detector. This applies particularly to matter surrounding the object of measurement, since it lies in the vicinity of the direction of reception of the detector. Consequently, measurement of a thyroid is always different from that of a thyroid phantom that is not so strongly embedded in material.

For the above reasons the count rate is not only lower than the decay rate, but as a rule it is not even proportional to it. The proportionality has only been lost, however, because a random number of extra pulses are measured that do not clearly belong to the nuclear decays. The proportionality can be regained by selecting the pulses. The criterion for this selection is the emission particle energy. Care must be taken to count only those pulses that have arisen from absorption of a complete photobranch in the detector. For the selection the pulse height is decisive, which under this condition is proportional to the emission particle energy.

If the pulses accumulating during the measuring time are arranged in a graph in accordance with their frequency and height, an intensity spectrum plotted against the pulse height is obtained. The intensity spectrum with beta emission has already been dealt with (cf. Section 1.3.8). The fact that this intensity spectrum in the direction of increasing pulse heights ends at the pulse height corresponding to the maximum beta energy allows the spectrum to be calibrated so that an energy spectrum is obtained (Fig. 1-33).

The emission spectrum with gamma radiation can also be calibrated.

However, the energy spectrum obtained is not to be interpreted as a spectrum of emission particles with different energies as with the beta emission. The gamma emission spectrum has discrete energies, and measurement of the emission spectrum cannot lead to a continuous spectrum as with measurement of the beta emission spectrum. The fact that over wide energy ranges a continuous spectrum is nevertheless found plotted against the energy is due both to the Compton effect and the various influences of spectral-line broadening.

If there were no Compton effect, only a photoeffect, then measurement of a radionuclide substance with gamma emission would give rise to an intensity spectrum with a photopeak at a certain pulse height (Fig. 1-45). This means that pulses of a certain height are measured very frequently. Since in all probability the same pulse height only arises when a complete photobranch is in the detector, the pulse height at which most of the pulses are found must correspond to the gamma emission particle energy. With this correlation of the pulse height of the intensity maximum to the emission particle energy, calibration of the intensity spectrum plotted against the energy is achieved. If a radionuclide substance emits several emission particles of differing gamma energy, the intensity spectrum will have the corresponding number of maxima. In this case the term energy spectrum for the intensity spectrum is exactly right. Each of these maxima is a photopeak.

The photopeak ranks above a pulse height interval. The edges of the photopeak are partially due, on the one hand, to the fact that individual photobranches are not completely in the detector and, on the other hand, to the fact that several photobranches are in the detector at the same time. If this were the only criterion, the edges would be steeper than they actually are. The chief reason for flattening of the edges is the inaccuracies of the measuring instrument.

Through the occurrence of the Compton effect additional pulses are to be found in the intensity spectrum. If the improbable case of the Compton branch being completely in the detector is disregarded, then the pulses involved must have a height lower than that corresponding to the gamma energy of the emission particle, since with the Compton effect the emission particle energy is split up and only part of it is transported away by the scattered gamma quantum. Since the energy distribution between the scattered gamma quantum and the ionization electron is random, just like the energy distribution in the nucleus between the beta emission particle and the neutrino, the pulses created in the detector by the scattered gamma quanta give rise to a continuous intensity spectrum plotted against an extensive pulse height range (Fig. 1-46). This part of the intensity spectrum is therefore called the Compton continuum.

The typical position of the Compton continuum relative to the photo-

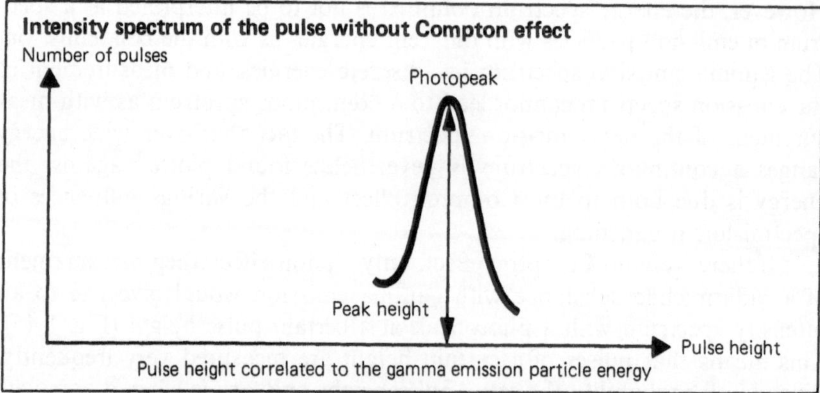

Fig. 1-45

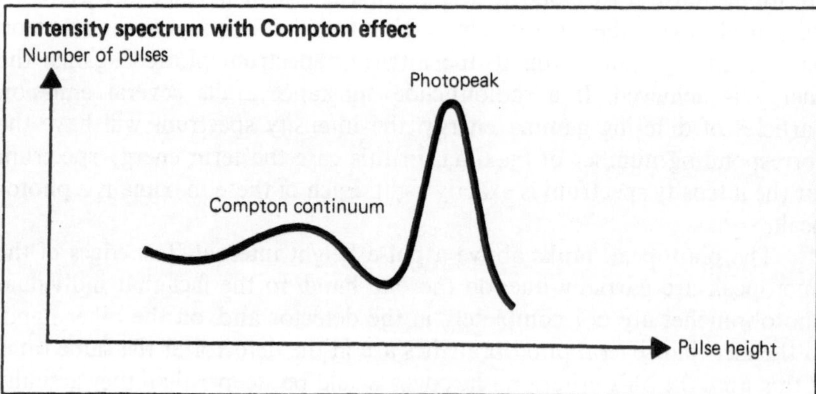

Fig. 1-46

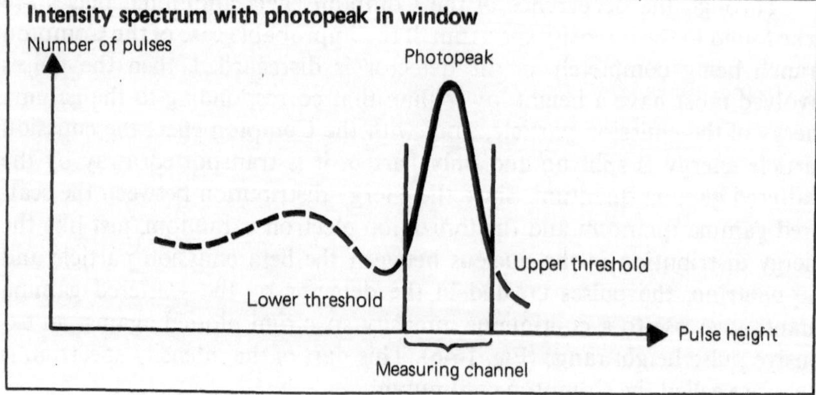

Fig. 1-47

peak makes it easy to distinguish the two parts of the intensity spectrum. If selection in accordance with the pulse height is not intended, then the measuring effect consists of a count rate that is made up of all the pulses of the intensity spectrum accumulating during the measuring time. If selection in accordance with the pulse height is possible, as with a discriminator in the radiation measuring system, then parts of the intensity spectrum can be suppressed (Fig. 1-47). If only the lower part of the intensity spectrum is suppressed, we speak of *integral count rate* measurement. The threshold can be set at a pulse height between the Compton continuum and the photopeak so that all pulses created by absorption of scattered gamma quanta in the detector are eliminated.

Technically, it is also possible to provide a second threshold, which eliminates all pulses of the intensity spectrum exceeding it in pulse height. If both thresholds are employed at the same time, then a "window" (measuring channel) is produced, which only allows those pulses to pass whose height falls between the upper and lower thresholds of the intensity spectrum. This is called *differential count rate* measurement. The thresholds of the measuring channel can be set so that the window straddles the photopeak. It is that part of the intensity spectrum in which the pulses fall that have been created by absorption of entire photobranches in the detector.

The straddling of the photopeak is the technical solution of forming a count rate that meets the proportionality condition with respect to the nuclear decay rate. Each narrowing of the measuring channel reduces the resulting count rate so that in practice a compromise must be made between the magnitude of the measuring effect and the width of the window straddling the photopeak.

For radiation detection the integral measuring mode is adequate. If numerical information is required on the nuclear decay rate, then the differential measuring mode is to be preferred over the integral one.

1.4.3. Radiation Detector Types

For *in vivo* examinations nuclear-medical diagnosis relies mainly on gamma measurements, and for *in vitro* examinations beta and gamma measurements. Since both types of radiation are detected by measuring the absorption energy, in principle any detector substance that is suitable for measuring beta radiation is also suitable for measuring gamma radiation and vice versa. The counter efficiency of a detector substance for beta and gamma radiation varies as much as the volume effect of the beta and gamma absorption. Since the volume effect is a function of the density of the detector substance, with gamma radiation a detector substance of greater density is selected instead of increasing the detector volume. Therefore, the usual types of detector differ in the detector substance. Further differences result from the state of aggregation of the detector material, since solid, liquid, and gaseous materials are used. Finally, the detectors differ in their construction, depending upon whether light produced by the absorption or the electric charge is to be measured.

By selection of suitable detector substances, detector types have been created that are tailored to the special tasks of beta and gamma radiation measurement, as required by the counting and locating of nuclear decay events.

1.4.3.1. Scintillation Detectors

It has already been mentioned that the absorbed radiation energy leads to a rearrangement in the electron shell of the nuclide in question. If an energy transformation into ultraviolet or visible light takes place, we speak of scintillation.

If a detector substance is brought into optical contact with a photoelectric meter, photons having an energy falling within the response range of the instrument will be registered. For measuring scintillation light the secondary electron multiplier is used (cf. Section 1.4.5.2.1). It is known as a photomultiplier or just multiplier. The photomultiplier supplies electric voltage pulses whose heights are proportional to the light yield. It is important that the detector substance be transparent for the scintillation light. Furthermore, the detector substance should have a density as high as possible if it is intended for measuring gamma radiation.

All these requirements with respect to gamma radiation are met by the following detector:

The detector substance is sodium iodide (NaI), which has been activated with a trace of thallium. The substance is produced as a single crystal, i.e., the crystalline structure is regular from face to face. Therefore the propagation of the scintillation light inside the crystal is not interfered with by inhomogeneity. The transparency for the scintillation light is so good that even crystal cylinders of several inches height and diameter can be employed with good light yield. The maximum of the scintillation light spectrum lies at about 410 nm corresponding to a photon energy of about 3 eV and is thus in the ultraviolet spectral range. The measuring instrument is a photomultiplier, whose maximum spectral sensitivity lies at about 400 nm. The density of the sodium iodide crystal (3.67 g/cm^3) is sufficiently high so that in diagnosis, which chiefly has to do with gamma energies up to 0.51 MeV, crystals thicker than 2 in in the direction of reception of the radiation are seldom used. A further favorable property of NaI crystals is the short decay time of the light pulses (about 10^{-7} sec).

Since crystalline NaI is hygroscopic, the crystal is supplied in a thin-walled aluminium case with a glass window at one end. Of course the aluminium walls also protect the crystal against beta radiation so that in this form it cannot be used for beta measurements. There are a number of nonhygroscopic crystals such as cesium iodide or anthracene, which can be used unprotected and are well suited to beta measurement. As gamma detectors, however, they are inferior to NaI so that they are primarily used for beta measurement. Since the depth of penetration of beta radiation is in the order of magnitude of millimeters, crystal disks of only 5 mm thickness are chiefly employed.

Since in diagnosis the measuring tasks involving beta radiation chiefly occur in laboratory examinations, where small quantities of a radionuclide-containing substance have to be measured, which can be brought into the immediate vicinity of the detector, the conditions are ideal for embedding the substance to be measured in the detector substance. This idea has been realized with liquid scintillation substances. For this purpose organic substances are used that are soluble in aromatic solvents such as xylene or toluene. For beta measurements a few milliliters of the scintillation solution are mixed with the radionuclide-containing sample and the light yield is measured with a photomultiplier.

In practice, however, a number of difficulties crop up. For instance, the compatibility of the scintillation substance and the sample, i.e., mixing them can cause turbidity and discoloration of the solution as well as disturbance of the scintillation by chemical reactions. Poor compatibility means a reduction in the light yield, which, however, is frequently outweighed by the extreme sensitivity in detecting even low-energy beta radiation.

1.4.3.2. Ionization Detectors

Ionization means the separation of charges of opposite sign, which were united in a previously electrically neutral atom. This separation produces in a substance positive and negative charges, whose movement under the influence of an electric potential can be measured as an electric current. The more mobile the charge carriers are in the voltage field and the longer it takes before they recombine through random collision, the more sensitive the current measurement is for the ionization events. It is clear that such conditions are best met by gaseous detector substances.

In principle, gas-filled ionization detectors consist of a gas-tight vessel provided with two electrodes, with which the detector is connected to an electric potential via a resistor. Ionization events in the detector substance give rise to an electric current, which in turn results in a voltage drop across the resistor, which can be amplified by electrical means.

When the electrode voltage exceeds a certain value, the height of the pulses ceases to depend alone upon the charge produced by the ionizing radiation. This is because high voltages are able to accelerate charge carriers to such an extent that they themselves give rise to ionization events. Since a primary event usually produces many secondary events, higher-voltage pulses are also formed across the resistor, an advantage that is known as gas amplification. Gas-filled detectors that make use of gas amplification are called counter tubes, whereas tubes that are operated at a potential too low for gas amplification are called ionization chambers. Counter tubes of moderate operating potential are called proportional counter tubes since just like ionization chambers they supply voltage pulses whose heights are proportional to the number of primary ionization events.

The proportionality between pulse height and particle energy is lost when the voltage applied to the gas-filled detector is higher than that for operating proportional counter tubes. In this case a primary ionization event gives rise to so many secondary ionizations that the detector gas is completely ionized and further primary events have no effect on the height of the voltage pulse. This type of detector tube is the Geiger–Müller counter. With it emission particles can be counted but their energy cannot be determined.

The low density of gaseous detector substances results in the fact that the counter efficiency is very poor for gamma radiation. Consequently, gas-filled detectors play a subordinate role in diagnosis. They are chiefly used in radiation monitors, which are only used for detecting radiation.

Furthermore, the case wall necessary for gaseous detector substances has an attenuating effect on beta radiation. Consequently, for measuring low-energy beta radiation a detector type has been developed in which the sample to be measured is placed in the gas volume. The problem of loss of gas while changing the sample has been overcome by allowing a suitable gas to flow through the volume. This type of detector is known as a gas flow counter.

Included amongst the ionization detectors are the semiconductor detectors. In semiconductor crystals the absorption causes separation of a shell electron from the shell of a nuclide in the same way as in gaseous detector substances. However, in the semiconductor no ions are formed, which wander under the influence of an electric potential, since all the atoms are firmly established in the crystal lattice. The positive charges produced by the absorption are instead transported by movement of adjacent shell electrons to the vacant "holes" in the electron shell under the influence of the electric potential.

Consequently, ionization in semiconductors produces electron-hole pairs. For this process only about one tenth of the energy is required as for the production of electron-ion pairs in gases. This means that the measuring effect of a certain amount of absorbed energy is one order of magnitude greater than with an ionization chamber, since ten times as many charges are available for the measurement. The measuring effect, which can be measured as a voltage drop across a resistor connected to the circuit, is proportional to the charge produced, so that semiconductor detectors can be used for both counting and measuring the energy of emission particles.

This and other superior features of the semiconductor detector seldom outweigh in diagnosis the disadvantage resulting from its small volume. Semiconductor detectors are effective only in a layer scarcely thicker than one half of a millimeter without a loss of detector quality. Their field of application is to be found in methods requiring the use of small probes.

1.4.4. Statistical Error

As a rule, under constant measuring conditions the same results are to be expected when the same object of measurement is measured if the properties of the object have also remained the same. However, the nuclear decay rate of a radionuclide substance is by no means a quantity that remains constant with repeated measurements, even when the physical half-life is extremely long. This is due to the randomness of nuclear decay. It is not possible to predict the time when a decay event will take place.

This also applies to the count rates of radiation measurements (Fig. 1-48). If count rates are measured in immediate succession, it appears to be a mere chance whether a pulse is measured with the first count rate or with the next. By chance one count rate is then higher than the other.

On the other hand, if a radionuclide substance with an extremely long half-life is measured frequently in rapid sequence, then some values of the count rate are measured more often than others. This accumulation effect becomes the more evident, the higher the activity, i.e., the greater the mean count rate.

If the count rates measured are now distributed in accordance with their values as balls in glass tubes, which are arranged in ascending order, and the filling height of the tubes is marked, then a distribution curve is obtained (Fig. 1-49). If the mean count rate is not too small, a bell-shaped curve, known as a Gaussian distribution curve, is obtained and here the mean count rate is the most frequent count rate. The most frequent count rate is the closest value to the quantity of the nuclear decay of a radionuclide substance and is thus the best measured value of the activity (statistical expected value).

In practice it is not always possible to carry out a large number of measurements in order to determine the activity, particularly when the determination calls for rapidly changing activities. This results in errors since with a few or even only a single measurement it is not known to what extent the count rate deviates from the most frequent value. Therefore limits are drawn in the bell-shaped curve, which mark a symmetric interval $\pm x$ around the most frequent value of the count rate on the abscissa, and

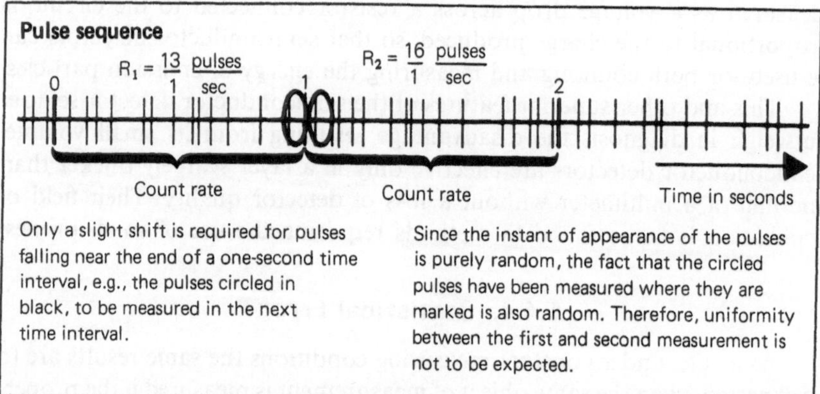

Pulse sequence
$R_1 = \frac{13}{1} \frac{\text{pulses}}{\text{sec}}$
$R_2 = \frac{16}{1} \frac{\text{pulses}}{\text{sec}}$
0
1
2
Count rate
Count rate
Time in seconds
Only a slight shift is required for pulses falling near the end of a one-second time interval, e.g., the pulses circled in black, to be measured in the next time interval.
Since the instant of appearance of the pulses is purely random, the fact that the circled pulses have been measured where they are marked is also random. Therefore, uniformity between the first and second measurement is not to be expected.

Fig. 1-48

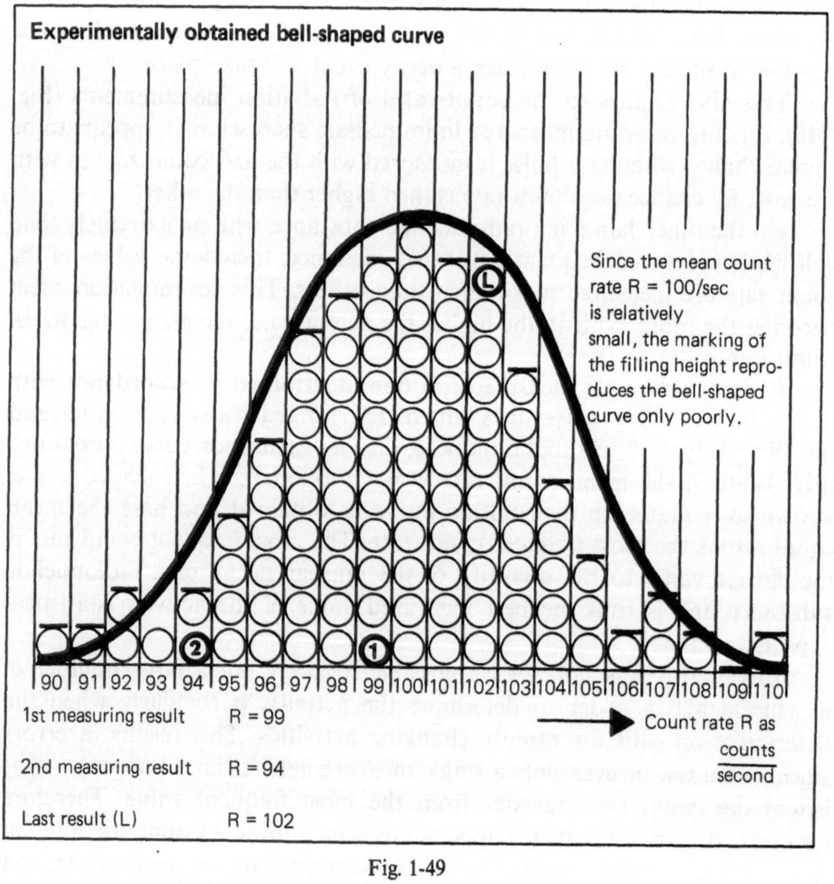

Experimentally obtained bell-shaped curve

Since the mean count rate R = 100/sec is relatively small, the marking of the filling height reproduces the bell-shaped curve only poorly.

90 91 92 93 94 95 96 97 98 99 100 101 102 103 104 105 106 107 108 109 110

Count rate R as $\frac{\text{counts}}{\text{second}}$

1st measuring result R = 99

2nd measuring result R = 94

Last result (L) R = 102

Fig. 1-49

the probability P as to whether the count rate measured is within these limits is determined.

This probability P is evaluated as a percentage of the count rates distributed within the limits and is given as a percentage of the area enclosed by the bell-shaped curve and the limits compared with the total area enclosed by the curve.

Let the count rate R of a single measurement result in the value $R = N/t$, where N is the count during the time t. If we now hypothetically assume that this value R belongs to the most frequent count rate, then a bell-shaped curve can be calculated since each most frequent count rate has its own bell-shaped curve. One property of all Gaussian distribution curves is, however, that the limits of the interval with $x = \pm N^{1/2} \equiv \sigma$ enclose, together with the bell-shaped curve, an area of 68.3%. Consequently, with a probability of $P = 68.3\%$ count rates in the value range between $R = (N - N^{1/2})/t$ and $R = (N + N^{1/2})/t$ can be expected.

Forgetting the hypothetical assumption that the individual measurement R is the most frequent count rate of this radiation measurement, then it is obvious that the most frequent count must be greater or smaller than R. However, with the same interval $\sigma = \pm N^{1/2}$ it is possible to calculate how much greater or smaller the most frequent count rate can be at the most with a probability of $P = 68.3\%$. If the calculation is based on 2σ, then $P = 95\%$; if 3σ is selected, then P increases to 99.7%.

Therefore, extraction of the square root of the count of a count rate offers, within the range of validity of the Gaussian distribution, a means of determining the maximum possible deviation with respect to the most frequent count rate, of course under the proviso of a certain probability P. This maximum possible deviation is called the statistical error.

When measuring low activities, long measuring times will be selected in order to keep the statistical error small. For instance, if 98 pulses per minute are counted, then $\sigma = \pm 9.9$. With 10,000 pulses per minute $\sigma = \pm 100$.

In the first case the result is as follows: The most frequent count rate lies in a count rate range between 88.1 and 107.9 counts per minute with a probability $P = 68.3\%$. In the second case the result is as follows: The most frequent count rate lies in a count range between 9,900 and 10,100 counts per minute with a probability $P = 68.3\%$.

The result can be formulated more simply by expressing σ as a percentage of the measured count N, i.e., by giving the percentage statistical error

$$\frac{\sigma \times 100}{N}\,\%$$

In the present example, in the first case the result has a statistical error of 9.8% and in the second case an error of 1%.

In other words, generally speaking, the smaller the percentage statistical error is, the greater the count is. The count can be increased either by prolonging the measuring time or by increasing the activity.

1.4.5. Radiation-Measuring Instruments

1.4.5.1. Instruments for Radiation Detection

The pen dosimeter, which is worn like a fountain pen, consists of an electrically charged capacitor, which is enclosed in a gas-filled chamber, and a charge indicator. Each ionization process in the gas chamber promotes the discharge and after complete discharge it is known that the chamber and thus the person wearing the pen dosimeter has received a radiation dose that can be established by calibration. No fixed reference is given to time, since if, for instance, the capacitor has become discharged after one day, there is nothing to indicate whether the dose has been evenly distributed over this period.

In contrast, dose-rate meters indicate the dose per time unit. They are provided with a gas chamber and a voltage source (battery or power pack), which is connected to the gas chamber via a current measuring instrument (ammeter). When many ionization events are taking place in the chamber, a high current flows owing to the high electrical conductivity. When no ionization events are taking place, a minimum current flows. From the above it follows that the scale of a pen dosimeter indicates the dose in Roentgens and that of a dose-rate meter the dose rate in Roentgens per hour.

Radiation warning devices are called monitors. Some monitors use a scintillation detector instead of an ionization detector.

1.4.5.2. Radiation-Measuring Instruments with a Scintillation Crystal

On account of the high sensitivity of scintillation detectors with respect to gamma radiation and the most frequent demand for directional radiation measurement, such detectors are provided with a relatively thick lead shield against gamma radiation not coming from the object being measured. The heavy weight makes it necessary to use a stand, which must be so constructed that it permits adjustment in various directions.

To keep the weight within reasonable limits, only the most essential technical components are mechanically coupled to the detector. These include the photomultiplier and a preamplifier, which ensures that the electric pulses of the photomultiplier are not deformed on their way through the connecting cable to the electronic system. Detector crystal, photomultiplier, preamplifier, and lead shielding are together called the measuring head.

Apart from the measuring head, the following are required for the radiation measurement: a pulse amplifier (linear amplifier), an electronic selection of pulses in accordance with their height (discriminator), a pulse counter, and a measuring value display.

1.4.5.2.1. Measuring Head. The important elements for understanding the function of the measuring head are the scintillation crystal and the photomultiplier. The task and functioning of the scintillation crystal have already been described.

The photomultiplier converts the scintillation light into electrical voltage pulses. The conversion takes place in a photoelectric layer, in which electrons are ejected from the layer substance by light absorption. The layer is applied to the inner surface of an evacuated glass vessel and is held at a high potential with respect to other electrodes protruding into the vessel. Through this means expelled electrons are accelerated towards the next electrode.

In principle, this conversion can be carried out by means of a layer as cathode and a positively biased electrode as anode. However, by suitable arrangement of several electrodes in sequence, which are called dynodes, an amplification effect can be achieved by maintaining the dynodes at successively higher positive potentials with respect to the cathode. This is explained by the fact that from a certain acceleration the expelled layer electrons are able to expel several secondary electrons from the first dynode, which are then accelerated toward the next dynode owing to the potential difference. Consequently there is an avalanche-like increase of secondary electrons from dynode to dynode so that there is a considerable flow of electrons at the anode.

The gain factor is about 10^5–10^6. It depends upon the potential applied. Therefore, the value of the potential applied must be strictly stable. Adjustment of this value permits regulation of the gain of the photomultiplier.

Since the scintillation, which is produced by absorption of a gamma quantum in the crystal, comprises many light quanta, the pulse height that is measured at the anode of the photomultiplier is made up of the sum of many secondary electron avalanches. Through the reflection of light it occurs that some light quanta do not reach the cathode of the photomultiplier, particularly when optical contact between the crystal and cathode is poor. As a result less avalanches are started per gamma quantum absorbed. Since the event of light reflection for a light quantum depends upon the random emission direction, this influence represents a statistical quantity, which gives rise to line broadening in the energy spectrum, i.e., here a broadening of the photopeak. The transit-time effects of the avalanche electrons in the photomultiplier have a similar action.

1.4.5.2.2. Linear Amplifier. The measuring head supplies pulses of varying height, which follow each other statistically. The amplification of this measuring effect has the aim of increasing the height of each pulse. An amplifier that increases the height of each pulse in proportion to its original height is known as a linear amplifier. This fact is expressed in the intensity spectrum in the following manner: the pulse height gain spreads the spectrum over a bigger pulse height range of the abscissa (Fig. 1-50). During the spreading the curve points of the intensity spectrum retain their ordinate values.

The amplification has the task of matching the magnitude of the measuring effect to the electrical conditions, whose maintenance is essential for the function of the discriminator. The use of a linear amplifier facilitates the determination of the position of the intensity spectrum with respect to the pulse height scale. If the gain is doubled, one maximum of a photopeak, which previously lay over a pulse height of 5 V, now lies over a pulse height of 10 V. Conversely, by reducing the gain by 50% we can now say that the maximum of the photopeak is over the pulse height of 2.5 V.

1.4.5.2.3. Discriminator. The pulse train, which leaves the linear amplifier, is conveyed to the discriminator, which selects and passes voltage pulses of a certain amplitude. Each pulse of the pulse train is compared with a given electric potential. The decision is then made whether the pulse is to be passed on or suppressed.

In integral radiation measurement only *one* reference potential is selected. Only voltage pulses that have a lower amplitude than this reference potential are suppressed. In differential radiation measurement *two* reference potentials are set. The discriminator ensures that only pulses of an amplitude greater than the first reference potential but smaller than the second reference potential are passed. The two reference potentials are referred to as the lower and upper thresholds, respectively, and the voltage range between them is called the window (Fig. 1-47).

Usually discriminators are so constructed that the voltage range of the window can be set relative to the voltage of the lower threshold. The lower threshold is therefore called the base. First of all the base potential is set and with the upper threshold a window width is set in volts. As the window width selected does not change when the base is adjusted, it is sufficient to shift the base over the entire voltage range in order to obtain the spectrum.

1.4.5.2.4. Pulse Spectroscope. A survey of the pulse spectrum can be obtained immediately with the pulse spectroscope. The spectroscope is provided with a cathode-ray tube with horizontal and vertical beam deflection. The pulse train from the linear amplifier is conveyed to the horizontal beam deflection electrodes so that the electron beam and thus the light spot are deflected horizontally to an extent depending upon the pulse height (Fig. 1-51).

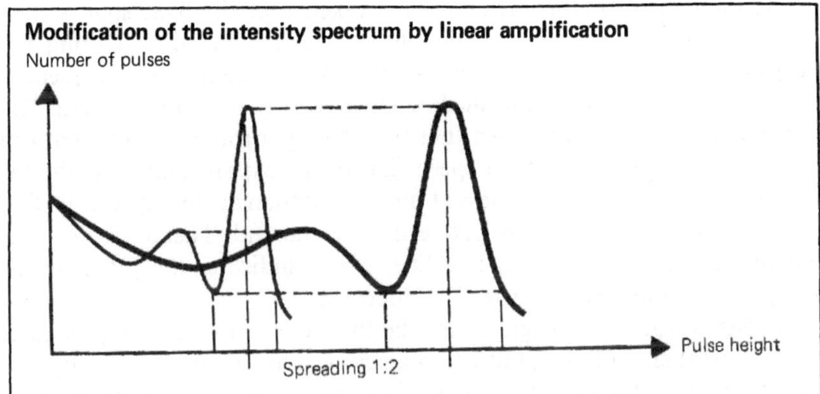

Fig. 1-50

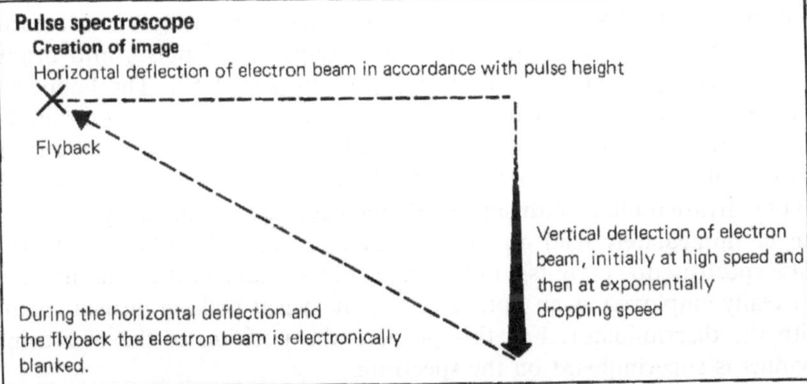

Fig. 1-51

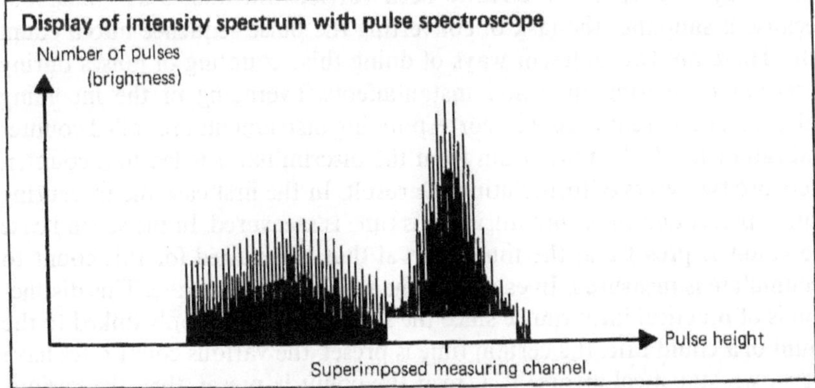

Fig. 1-52

At the end of the deflection care is taken that the light spot is then deflected vertically before returning to its starting position. During the sweep and flyback the electron beam is electronically blanked. Consequently, for each pulse only a line is formed on the screen from top to bottom. The vertical deflection is so arranged that the light spot traces its line from top to bottom starting with a high speed that drops exponentially. As the luminous intensity of the spot is less at high speed than at slow speed, the line produced by a single pulse is not seen until the end. Therefore, for each incoming pulse there is a vertical line, which indicates the pulse height through its position in the horizontal direction.

Pulses of the same height cause the lines to be traced on top of each other. Thus, at sites of great pulse frequency such as the site of a photopeak, not only are great line densities obtained but also lines of extreme brightness. Enhancement of the brightness by superpositioning is, however, also effective in those cases where the electron beam does not visualize the line owing to its high vertical sweep speed, so that the visible line length is increased.

The pulse spectroscope transforms a sequence of pulses into bright lines of varying length on a dark background (Fig. 1-52). The boundary between light and dark represents the curve of the intensity spectrum. In contrast to spectra which have been picked up with the aid of the discriminator point for point by forming the pulse rates, the spectrum here is built up of individual lines. With sufficiently high activity, the intensity spectrum can be immediately read on the luminescent screen. In other words, the pulse spectroscope permits a rapid survey of the shape of the spectrum and is usually employed as an optical setting aid when making measurements with the discriminator. For this purpose the position of the measuring channel is superimposed on the spectrum.

1.4.5.2.5. Counter and Ratemeter. The discriminator supplies a pulse sequence consisting of pulses of uniform height. This is possible since the pulse height analysis has already been carried out and is advantageous because it simplifies the task of converting the pulse sequence into a count rate. There are two different ways of doing this: counting of pulses during a certain measuring time and instantaneous averaging of the incoming pulses of a pulse sequence. The corresponding instruments are called counter and ratemeter. If the pulse train from the discriminator is fed to a counter, there are two ways of formulating the result. In the first case the measuring time is preset and the count during this time is measured. In the second case the count is preset and the time interval that is required for this count to accumulate is measured. In each case the result is a count rate. This distinction is of practical importance since the statistical error is only linked to the count of a count rate. If a certain time is preset, the various count rates have their own statistical errors; if instead the count is preset, then the various count rates have the same statistical error.

For time measurement the counter is provided with a frequency generator. If preset counting is intended, then an additional device is required for interrupting the counting after the preset count has accumulated. In any case, the counter is provided with a digital display. It consists of a number of glow lamps, each of which contains ten glow electrodes, whose form is that of the ten figures. If a potential is applied to a glow electrode, the figure concerned lights up. A glow lamp is required for each digit of the number to be displayed. As a rule the number display consists of six glow lamps, so that figures up to 999,999 can be displayed either as accumulated count or expired time units. These values can also be conveyed as an electric signal to a digital printer for documentation. The use of a digital printer not only brings the advantage of permanent recording, but also that of automation. For instance, activity measurements of a sample changer can be kept going through the night without surveillance.

Apart from digital display, there is also analog display. While in digital display the results appear as a sequence of individual measurements, which can be expressed in figures, the analog display reproduces the results of a continuous measurement so that they can be displayed as curves of, for instance, a time function.

Based on this principle is the ratemeter, an instrument that gives a higher reading with a quick sequence of pulses than with a slow sequence. This can be done by the incoming pulses charging a capacitor, which can only be discharged across a constant electrical resistance. Consequently, at the capacitor an electric potential can be measured, which at any given moment corresponds to the average rate of the pulse sequence.

The display instrument of a ratemeter is a voltmeter whose reading corresponds to the mean count rate. Usually, the measuring instrument has a linear scale, i.e., a twice as large pointer deflection corresponds to a twice as large count rate. However, ratemeters with a logarithmic scale are also used. Logarithmic scales cover several decades so that switching over of the measuring range is not necessary. Linear ratemeters in contrast have a range switch.

Furthermore, linear ratemeters are provided with a switch for selecting the time constant T. The time constant T is a characteristic of the ratemeter and has an influence on the setting time of the pointer of the instrument. The time taken for the pointer to settle down to the actual reading is about three times the time T. If T is extremely short, the pointer follows each pulse with a movement. If T is long, the pointer movement results from many pulses. Since averaging of a large number of pulses results in a smaller statistical error, increasing of T leads to more exact results. However, this advantage is obtained at the expense of the setting time, which becomes longer, a limitation that can have a detrimental effect on the measurement of quickly changing activities. These facts make a compromise necessary and the ratemeter is provided with a variable time constant so that it can be matched to the conditions on hand.

The electric potentials displayed by the ratemeter can also be conveyed to a strip-chart recorder. Such a recorder writes a time–activity curve on a uniformly moving strip chart.

1.4.5.2.6. Collimators. Usually, detectors are provided with lead shielding to prevent background radiation from influencing the measuring result. They also have a directional effect since only a certain spatial angle is now open for picking up the radiation. Since lead has a high density, it is excellent for shielding against gamma radiation. The shielding effect obeys an almost exponential function so that a half-value layer can be defined. The half-value layer is the thickness of any material that absorbs 50% of the incident emission particles. It is dependent upon the emission particle energy and amounts to 5 mm of lead with a gamma energy of 0.51 MeV. To increase the shielding effect to 99.9%, layer thickness of ten half-value layers are required. For gamma quanta of 0.51 MeV the thickness of the lead shielding must be 5 cm.

It has been shown that special directional characteristics of radiation pickup can be achieved by using special forms of lead shielding. In order not to limit the use of the measuring heads, the protective lead shielding has been kept separate from the shielding with directional characteristics, called collimators. This makes it possible to use various collimators on a single measuring head.

The simplest form of collimator is the hollow cylinder. It is used in functional analysis and has the task of delimiting a definite field size on the skin surface. The definition of the field size is related to a plane, which lies in front of the collimator at the skin distance to be selected, as it can be easily checked experimentally in this way. Naturally, the actual measuring volume lies under the skin embedded in tissue, and as Compton scatter occurs in it, a definition of the field size there is not easily possible.

Collimators of scanners have a different task. They should accept as much radiation as possible from a small volume at a certain distance from the measuring head. Such collimators are provided with a large number of conical bores, whose axes meet at a certain distance from the collimator. In analogy to the conditions in optics, where radiation is focused, we also speak of a focus distance of the collimator although radiation is not focused here but selection of radiation takes place, which is emitted as a divergent beam from the volume to be located. Also in conjunction with this analogy we speak of this volume as a focus volume.

The bores of a camera collimator, in contrast, run parallel to each other. While with the scanner the whole detector serves for production of an image element, in gamma scintigraphy an image element is produced by gamma absorption in only one part of the detector. Since from the relative position of the absorption of various gamma quanta in the detector, the camera electronics determines at which site of the camera image a received image element must be placed. Consequently, the collimator must only accept parallel gamma radiation rays that strike the detector perpendicularly. Only in this way is it possible to ensure that the locating system of the camera is not confused by oblique gamma radiation rays emanating from the object to be imaged.

CHAPTER 2

Scintillation Camera Collimators

G. MUEHLLEHNER

2.1. INTRODUCTION

A collimator is essentially a block of lead larger than the detector, containing an arrangement of holes which allows gamma rays to pass through from a specified direction and form the image. The lead thickness is sufficient to absorb unwanted radiation, so that the radiation reaching the detector face must have originated from a known direction. This is determined by the orientation of the hole in the lead. A typical collimator is shown in Fig. 2-1. There are broadly four types of collimators: parallel hole, converging, diverging, and pinhole. They are described below, with particular attention paid to the principle governing the performance of the parallel hole collimator.

The standard collimator in use with the scintillation camera is the parallel hole collimator, the performance of which is measured by the

G. MUEHLLEHNER • Searle Diagnostics, Inc., 2000 Nuclear Drive, Des Plaines, Illinois 60018. *Present address*: Hospital of the University of Pennsylvania, 3400 Spruce Street, Philadelphia, Pennsylvania 19104.

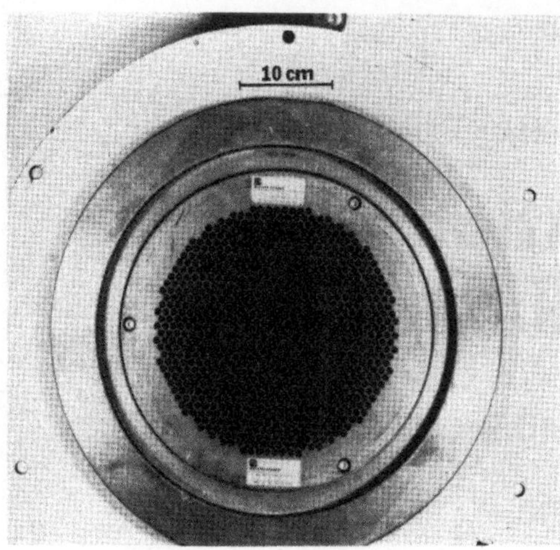

Fig. 2-1. Typical multihole collimator for gamma camera (diverging collimator). Bottom plate has been removed. The array of holes is 28 cm in diameter and 8 cm deep.

three quantities resolution, efficiency, and septum penetration, which in turn are determined by the three collimator dimensions height, hole diameter, and septum thickness. The only additional variable is hole shape such as round, hexagonal, square, triangular, and straight or tapered. Other secondary factors which do not affect performance must nevertheless be considered in the design of collimators, notably manufacturing technique, which becomes of overriding importance in the design of low-energy collimators where hole diameters of the order of 1 mm and septum thickness less than 0.2 mm are optimum; at the higher energies, especially at 511 keV, hole separation must be chosen such as to avoid noticeable image artifacts.

It is, however, not sufficient to relate the three physical collimator dimensions to the three performance quantities, but a formulation must be found to choose such collimator dimensions as to optimize efficiency for a stated resolution or equivalently to optimize resolution for a stated efficiency, as has been described by Keller (1968). Beyond this it becomes necessary to develop a criterion useful in selecting a desired resolution or efficiency as a function of the clinical imaging conditions. This criterion may be related to the information density in the scintiphoto or it may be related more directly to lesion detectability.

Only if these three separate problems are solved is it possible to arrive at that collimator best suited for a particular investigation. From a practical point of view it becomes necessary to group types of investigations such that a limited number of collimators may serve all types of studies. These clinical considerations, however, shall not be discussed here.

2.2. RESOLUTION

Resolution is the quantity most directly related to the amount of detail visible in the image. For this reason it is often measured using closely spaced line sources or lead bars of various width separated by a distance equal to their width, placed over a sheet source. In either case, it is sometimes difficult to judge whether a pattern is visible or not and the only firm statement one can make is that resolution is better than a certain value but worse than another. It has therefore become accepted practice to measure the line source response function (LSRF). It is then possible to compare the full width at half-maximum (FWHM) of various collimator LSRFs as long as their shape is nearly identical, or preferably to compare the modulation transfer functions (MTF) derived directly from the LSRFs by a Fourier transformation.

The only theoretical formulation of parallel hole collimator resolution in closed form is that given by Anger (1964). He derives the shape and FWHM of the point source response function (PSRF). Two assumptions in the derivation are particularly noteworthy. With the collimator stationary, the shape of the PSRF is highly irregular and is dependent upon the exact location of the point source with respect to the centerline of the nearest collimator hole. The value which is usually desired, however, is an average value independent of the exact location. It is therefore assumed in the derivation that the collimator moves much like a Bucky filter used in radiology. Because of this assumption the septum thickness does not enter in the formula for resolution. This is quite acceptable as long as the intrinsic resolution of the camera device is inferior to the hole-to-hole separation of the collimator so that individual holes are not visible in the final image. This assumption is only partially satisfied at medium energies (360–410 keV) where collimator structures become visible if images are obtained of phantoms with regular holes in the collimator (Bonte, 1971). This can be remedied by moving the collimator during an exposure (Wilks, 1969).

The second assumption which affects the accuracy and usefulness of the formula is the generalization of the solution from one dimension to two dimensions. The formula as derived is valid only for square holes with the response measured parallel to one of the sides of the hole; for round holes the shape of the response curve as well as the FWHM would be different. Kibby (1969) has calculated the response function using a computer and has noted that Anger's formula gives values roughly 15% higher than the values obtained by her for round holes.

While these assumptions have to be kept in mind in judging the accuracy and applicability of the results obtained, the formula is nevertheless very useful in optimizing collimator dimensions. According to Anger, the index

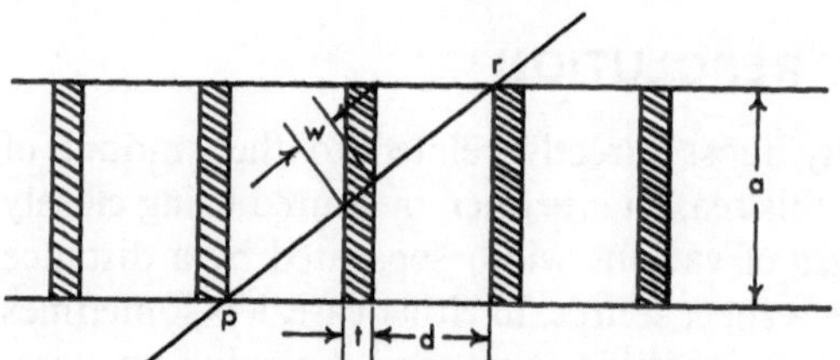

Fig. 2-2. Sketch showing collimator dimensions.

of resolution (FWHM) is given by

$$R = \frac{a + b + c}{a} d \tag{2-1}$$

where all dimensions are shown in Fig. 2-2 (*a* is collimator height, *b* is the distance from the object to the collimator, *c* is the distance from the collimator to the scintillation crystal, and *d* is hole diameter). This formula has been used to design many collimators, and measurements have shown good agreement between measured and calculated values (Walker, 1969). The formula predicts a monotonic decrease in resolution as a function of collimator to object distance (*b*), the slope of which is a function of collimator height (*a*). Thus the longer the collimator, the smaller the variation of resolution as a function of distance from the collimator.

One important question in collimator design is the resolution as a function of hole shape. In general, the hole shape was dictated in the past by the construction technique used, rather than by any consideration of relative performance. It is reasonable to assume that the difference in performance would be small, yet any gain made in resolution by proper selection of hole shape would have to be made without making some sacrifice in another area. Different hole shapes can only be compared if the shape of the PSRF or LSRF is known accurately. The response function most useful for a comparison of hole shape would be one obtained as an average over different locations of the source relative to the central axis of the hole and as an average over the different rotational angles. The PSRF may be obtained analytically by a ray-tracing technique (Muehllehner and Luig, 1973). Use of this technique shows that the influence of specific hole shape is quite small (Muehllehner *et al.*, 1976).

2.3. EFFICIENCY

Important concepts in evaluating an imaging system are sensitivity and efficiency. Sensitivity is the measure of the overall response or counting efficiency of a system and includes the detector efficiency as well as the collimator geometric efficiency. Further, the efficiency defined for a collimator depends on whether the source distribution it is viewing is a point source, line source, area source, or volume source. The efficiency for a point source, for instance, depends upon the relative position of the source to the collimator. One of the more practical measures of collimator efficiency is the area efficiency, ε_a, which is the response to a sheet source distribution of activity larger than the field of view of the collimator (MacIntyre *et al.*, 1969). Its value is independent of how far away the sheet source is from the collimator face, and indeed can be measured with the source right on the collimator. Area efficiency then is the ratio of the number of photons per second passing through the collimator to the number of photons per second per square centimeter emitted by the plane source. Area efficiency, ε_a, has the dimensions of the area, and thus is bigger the larger the size of the collimator–detector. In the past it has been of interest to compare the performance of various imaging systems such as moving detector scanners vs. stationary cameras. For this, it is useful to talk about the efficiency normalized for the field of view. So we have

$$E = \frac{\varepsilon_a}{A_{\text{tot}}} \tag{2-2}$$

which is dimensionless and is the effective geometric efficiency of the collimator. Note though that a system with the higher geometric efficiency does not necessarily give statistically reliable images in the shortest time, since counting rate depends on the size of the detector.

The geometric efficiency of any collimator can be derived from the generic relationship

$$E = \frac{A_{\text{hole}}}{4\pi a^2} \frac{A_{\text{open}}}{A_{\text{total}}} \tag{2-3}$$

where the first term is the fractional solid angle subtended by a single collimator hole having size A_{hole} at the detector side, and the second term represents the fractional transparent area of the entrance side of the collimator.

For a collimator having square straight holes in a square array, Eq. (2-3) becomes

$$E = \frac{d^4}{4\pi a^2 (d + t)^2} = \left[\frac{0.282 d^2}{a(d + t)} \right]^2 \tag{2-4}$$

For a collimator having round straight holes in a hexagonal array, Eq. (2-3) becomes

$$E = \frac{\pi d^4 \cos 30^\circ}{48 a^2 (d + t)^2} = \left[\frac{0.238 d^2}{a(d + t)} \right]^2 \tag{2-5}$$

The formulas for other hole shapes or tapered holes can readily be derived from Eq. (2-3).

Mather (1957) has shown that due to penetration of the edges of the holes by the gamma rays, the efficiency of the hole is increased by an amount which is equivalent to shortening the collimator hole by two times the linear attenuation coefficient. Thus, in Eq. (2-3), (2-4), and (2-5) the collimator height a should be replaced by an effective thickness a_e, where

$$a_e = a - 2\mu^{-1} \tag{2-6}$$

It should be noted that this correction factor only includes penetration of the edges of the holes for gamma rays traveling down that particular hole, which has the effect of only slightly widening the response curve but does not include penetration of the septa where the gamma ray originates in one hole but leaves the collimator via a neighboring hole or one that is even more distant, which is responsible for the long tail in the response curve.

2.4. SEPTUM PENETRATION

Anger (1966) has described a method of choosing septum thickness by calculating the minimum path length W which a gamma ray must traverse in the collimator material (Fig. 2-2). He states the following:

> From experimental studies it has been determined that acceptable images result when total (Compton + photoelectric) attenuation of gamma rays taking the path **pr** is 95% or more. This is achieved when $\mu^{-1} \times W = 3$, where μ is the total linear absorption coefficient. Septum thickness t is given to a good approximation by
>
> $$t = \frac{2dW}{a - W} \qquad [(2\text{-}7)]$$
>
> where all dimensions are shown in [Fig. 2-2].

The use of much thicker septa has been proposed (Kibby, 1969) by simply setting $\mu^{-1} \times W = 5$. However, the lower efficiency associated with thicker septa was not discussed. Since the above criterion only considers attenuation along the minimum path in the collimator material it does not provide useful answers to detailed questions regarding the penetration fraction. Unfortunately, the problem of septum penetration is so complicated that it would be quite difficult to solve in closed form. One method of obtaining an answer to the above mentioned problem is to use an expanded version of the ray-tracing method described in Section 2.2 on resolution. This has been discussed in detail (Muehllehner and Luig, 1973).

Experience has shown that Anger's formulas can be used to design useful collimators having resolution and sensitivity as predicted and septum penetration which is tolerable but generally a little too high. However, to answer detailed questions about hole shape and the connection between septum thickness and the distribution of the penetrated gamma rays a more accurate formulation must be used which has not been provided so far in closed form.

2.5. SYSTEM RESOLUTION

When the whole imaging system is considered the collimator resolution (R_c) must be combined with the intrinsic detector resolution (R_I) to calculate the system performance. Since the line spread function for both the camera and the collimator is nearly Gaussian—except for collimators with unacceptable septum penetration—system resolution (R_s) is given by

$$R_s = (R_I^2 + R_c^2)^{1/2} \tag{2-8}$$

The performance of Anger scintillation cameras has been improved by a continued improvement in intrinsic resolution first through the introduction of photomultipliers with bialkali photocathodes (intrinsic resolution $R_I = 11$ mm for 120 keV), then through the use of threshold preamplifiers ($R_I = 8.5$ mm), and recently through the use of 2-in.- instead of 3-in.-diameter photomultipliers ($R_I = 5$ mm). The effect of these changes on system resolution for a particular collimator is shown in Fig. 2-3. The figure also shows how the system would improve if the intrinsic resolution were reduced to 2 mm (FWHM) instead of 4–6 mm currently achieved with 2-in. photomultipliers and nonlinear preamplifiers. As the intrinsic resolution is improved the system resolution is determined to an ever increasing amount by the collimator resolution.

Improvements in collimators have received less attention than improvements in camera resolution but have nevertheless been significant for low-energy collimators. Since we now understand the nature of collimation and can calculate and fabricate the optimum parallel hole collimator for any given set of design parameters we can expect only small improvements to be made in the future. This leaves us only free to sacrifice sensitivity for better resolution or vice versa. As smaller and smaller structures need to be resolved the number of resolution elements increases, the count density per resolution element must stay constant to preserve the statistical accuracy of the data, and the count density per unit area must therefore increase. Any improvement in resolution gained at the expense of collimator sensitivity is therefore doubly painful: a 40% improvement in collimator resolution decreases the collimator sensitivity by a factor of 2 (Vetter and Pizer, 1971), thus requiring an increase in flux by a factor of 4. Since imaging time cannot reasonably be lengthened substantially nor is it appropriate

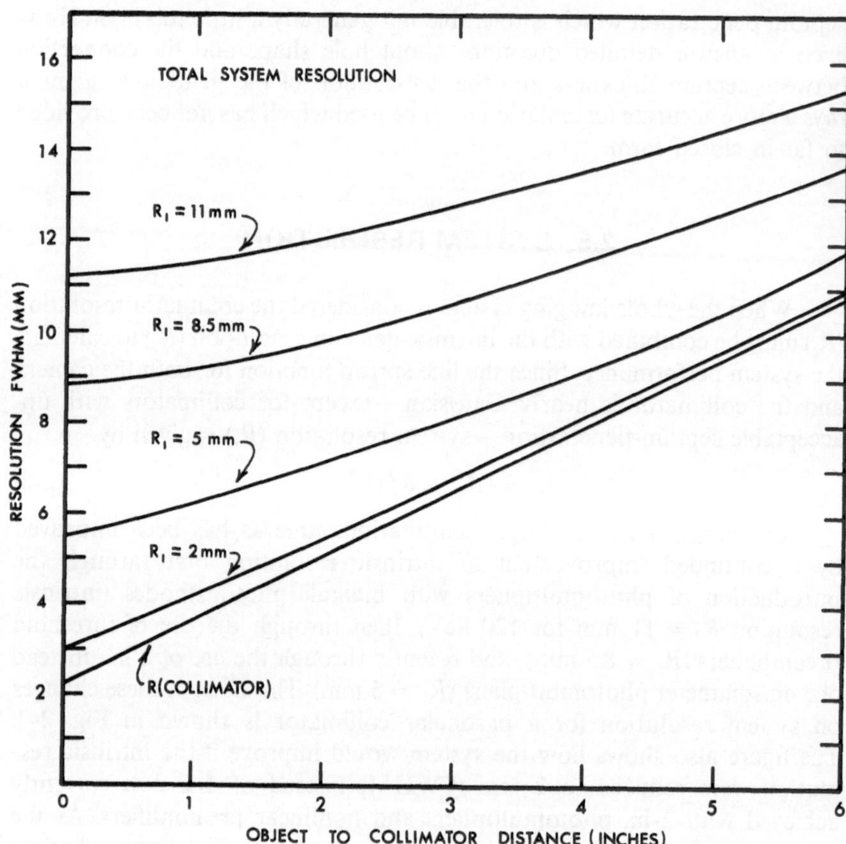

Fig. 2-3. System resolution (R_s) as a function of object distance for various values of intrinsic resolution (R_I) and for a particular collimator [$R_s = (R_I^2 + R_c^2)^{1/2}$].

to inject significantly larger amounts of activity we cannot greatly improve image quality by improving collimator resolution at the expense of sensitivity and must therefore look elsewhere for significant improvements in instrumentation.

2.6. CONVERGING COLLIMATORS

A converging collimator is one with its holes directed towards a focal point some distance (about 30 cm) away from the collimator face. On the detector side the holes cover the detector face; on the patient side the holes are closer together. The general design of the converging collimator is not basically different from that of the focusing collimator used on the rectilinear scanner, though on the gamma camera there is no focusing effect; the design matches a smaller radiation source to a larger imaging instrument. It is useful in imaging pediatric patients.

The concept of converging collimators allows improvements in efficiency and/or resolution at the expense of the field of view of the camera (Moyer, 1974; Dowdey and Bonte, 1972; Rudin *et al.*, 1971). Deficiency in field of view may then be remedied by using an enlarged camera. Significant improvements can be made by the use of a large-diameter camera—useful field diameter approximately 38.5 cm—using 37 3-in.-diameter photomultiplier tubes in conjunction with a converging collimator giving a 25-cm field of view at 10 cm from the collimator. The improvement in performance is due to a combination of two effects: since twice the scintillation crystal area is used to look at the same object area when compared to a 25-cm-diameter camera using a parallel hole collimator the efficiency increases roughly by a factor of 2; furthermore, since the object is enlarged onto the crystal, the intrinsic camera resolution is effectively improved by a factor equal to the magnification, which at 10 cm from the collimator is 1.52.

An important difference between parallel and converging collimators is the variation of sensitivity as a function of depth; while parallel hole collimators have a sensitivity in air which is virtually constant as a function of distance from the collimator, the sensitivity of a converging collimator *increases* with distance, up to its focal point, in the absence of any attenuating

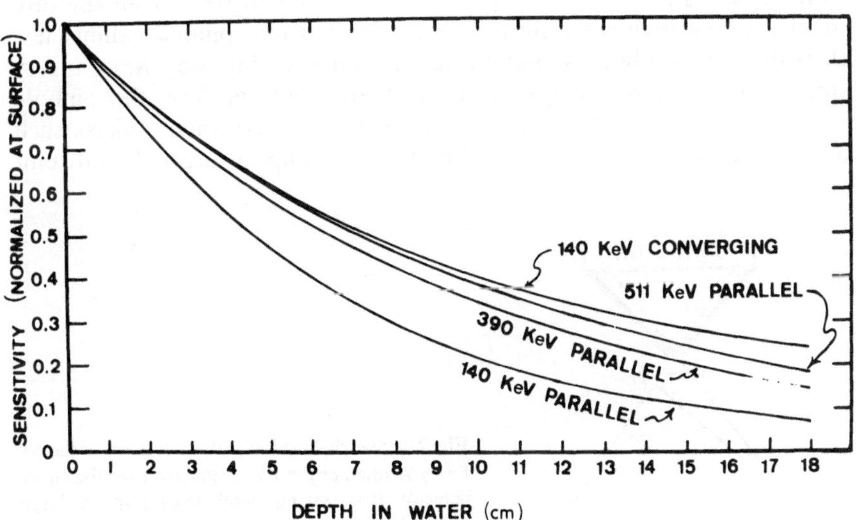

Fig. 2-4. Collimator sensitivity as a function of depth in absorbing material (water) for various energies and both parallel and converging collimators.

material. Fig. 2-4 compares the sensitivity of a parallel hole collimator for various gamma ray energies in water as attenuating material to the sensitivity of a converging collimator at 140 keV which is comparable to that of a parallel hole collimator at 511 keV. This improved depth response should be helpful in many situations, notably the imaging of areas of decreased activity deep in the liver where overlying activity tends to mask the area of decreased uptake.

2.7. DIVERGING COLLIMATORS

It is possible to image a source larger than the detector by using a collimator whose holes are directed outwards. A diverging collimator can by made by reversing a converging collimator, i.e., upside-down, and in fact such dual-purpose collimators are commercially available. The diverging collimator is used to image the entire lung field in one view, and to image large body areas (liver and spleen; kidneys and bladder).

2.8. PINHOLE COLLIMATORS

The pinhole collimator is a large cone of lead (apex outwards—toward the patient) with a small hole through which all radiation must pass to reach the detector as shown in Fig. 2-5. As with most other collimators there is an inverse trade-off between sensitivity and resolution, not only with respect to the size of the aperture but with the distance from aperture to object. Sensitivity is typically very low; a 3-mm pinhole admits less than 10^{-4} of the photons emitted from a source 10 cm away. Since a very small object can be imaged over the entire detector face, the pinhole collimator allows the best available resolution of very small objects such as the thyroid, small bones, etc. Closer objects appear larger than distant

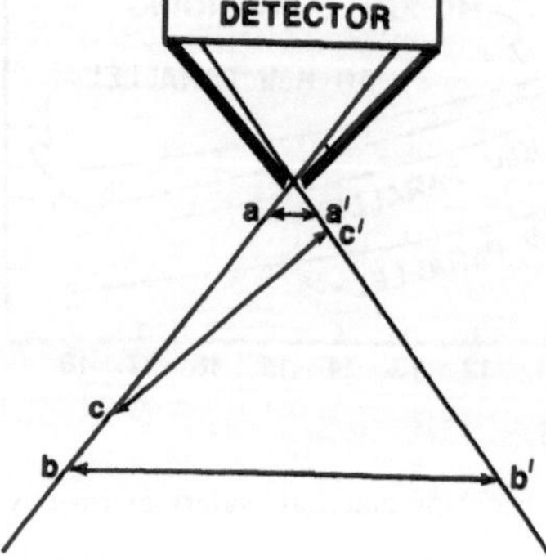

Fig. 2-5. Sketch showing pinhole collimator (heavy lines). A small object (*aa'*) is imaged over the entire detector face, giving good resolution. A large object (*bb'*) is imaged over the same area. Distortion is seen in angled object *cc'*, where the closer portion *c'* appears larger than the distant portion.

objects, and this geometric distortion sometimes makes it difficult to interpret medical images made this way, as the closer parts of the organ being imaged will appear to be magnified.

REFERENCES

Anger, H.O. (1964), Scintillation camera with multichannel collimators, *J. Nucl. Med.* **5**: 515–531.

Anger, H.O. (1966), Survey of radioisotope cameras, *ISA Trans.* **5**:311–334.

Bonte, F.J., Graham, K.D., Dowdey, J.E. (1971), Image aberrations produced by multichannel collimators for a scintillation camera, *Radiology* **98**:329–334.

Dowdy, J.E., and Bonte, F.J. (1972), Principles of scintillation camera image magnification with multichannel converging collimators, *Radiology* **104**:89–96.

Keller, E.L. (1968), Optimum dimensions of parallel-hole, multi-aperture collimators for gamma-ray cameras, *J. Nucl. Med.* **9**:233–235.

Kibby, P.M. (1969), The design of multichannel collimators for radioisotope cameras, *Br. J. Radiol.* **42**:91–101.

MacIntyre, W.J., Fedoruk, S.O., Harris, C.C., *et al.* (1969), Sensitivity and resolution in radioisotope scanning, in *Medical Radioisotope Scintigraphy*, Vol 1, IAEA, Vienna, pp. 391–435.

Mather, R.L. (1957), Gamma ray collimator penetration and scattering effects, *J. Appl. Phys.* **28**:1200.

Moyer, R.A. (1974), A low-energy multi-hole converging collimator compared with a pinhole collimator, *J. Nucl. Med.* **15**:59–64.

Muehllehner, G., and Luig, H. (1973), Septal penetration in scintillation camera collimators, *Phys. Med. Biol.* **18**:855–862.

Muehllehner, G., Dudek, J., and Moyer, R. (1976), Influence of hole shape on collimator performance, *Phys. Med. Biol.* **21**:242–250.

Rudin, S., Bardfeld, P.A., and Hart, H. (1971), Use of magnifying multi-hole collimators in the gamma-ray system, *J. Nucl. Med.* **12**:831–834.

Vetter, H.G., and Pizer, S.M. (1971), A measure for radioisotope scan image quality, *J. Nucl. Med.* **12**:526–529.

Walker, W.G. (1969), The design and analysis of scintillation camera lead collimators using a digital computer, in *Medical Radioisotope Scintigraphy*, Vol. 1, IAEA, Vienna, pp. 545–560.

Wilks, R.J., Mallard, J.R., and Taylor, C.G. (1969), The collywobber—A moving collimator image-processing device for stationary detectors in radioisotope scanning, *Br. J. Radiol.* **42**:705–709.

CHAPTER 3

Rectilinear Scanners

DENNIS D. PATTON

3.1. INTRODUCTION

The rectilinear scanner is a device for imaging the distribution of radioactive material within the body. It is a systematic point sampling device that forms its image by moving over (scanning) the field of interest. Basically, the rectilinear scanner is a rigid bar with a radiation detector at one end and a light and a stylus at the other end (Fig. 3-1). When the detector detects radiation, the light flashes, exposing some film, and the stylus taps, marking some paper. The rigid bar provides position data linking the radiation detector and the flashing light. The motion is boustrophedonic,* alternately left to right and right to left. Of course, this simple model of the rectilinear scanner becomes more and more complex as one introduces the ancillary

* I am indebted to James L. Quinn III for this word, from the Greek *bous* ("ox") and *strephein* ("to turn"), an ancient form of writing in which the lines run, as in plowing, alternately left to right and right to left.

DENNIS D. PATTON • Division of Nuclear Medicine, Health Sciences Center, University of Arizona, Tucson, Arizona 85724.

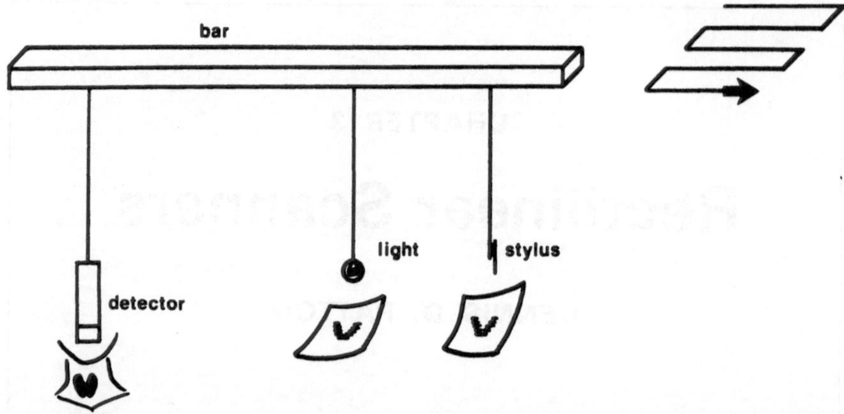

Fig. 3-1. Rectilinear scanner. The simplest model of a rectilinear scanner is a rigid bar with a radiation detector at one end, a light in the middle, and a stylus at the other end. When the detector detects radiation the light flashes and the stylus taps. The entire apparatus moves back and forth as shown in the figure. Modern rectilinear scanners have replaced the rigid bar with electronic circuitry, but the principle remains the same.

devices necessary to make the scanner operate properly. These will be covered in the following sections.

Anyone looking at radiographs and comparing them with radionuclide scans will notice immediately that the scan provides only the grossest depiction of anatomic structures, and is no way comparable to the X-ray in resolution. There are several reasons for this difference. First of all, the X-ray is an image made with radiation from a source that can be turned on and off rapidly, allowing a burst of several billion photons in a fraction of a second. The X-ray is made up of billions of image elements, and consequently has a high spatial resolution. The radionuclide scan, on the other hand, derives its image from radiation sources that are deposited within the body by metabolic processes, and cannot be turned on and off. In order to limit the radiation dose to the patient, it is necessary to limit the amount of radioactive material he receives. Consequently, within a reasonable imaging time only a million or less photons can be collected to make an image. Many scans are made of only a few tens of thousands of photons, and the spatial resolution is consequently low. A second reason is that while X-rays are emitted from a small source, internally deposited radionuclides form an extended (volume) source of radiation that is more difficult to image. In the radiograph each point on the film represents a well defined line passing through the body from the X-ray source to the film. In the radionuclide scan each point on the film represents a poorly defined irregular volume of uncertain depth within the body. The third reason is that X-ray energies can be selected electronically for optimum imaging of given structures, whereas gamma ray energies from radioactive sources are inherent to each radioactive isotope and cannot be adjusted. A fourth reason is that X-rays can be made to "illuminate" an area uniformly, whereas radiopharmaceuticals, being taken up by metabolic processes, are taken up unevenly to the extent that the processes themselves are uneven. It would be impossible to image a section of, say, bone that was completely dead or otherwise metabolically inactive. On the other hand, this feature of radionuclide imaging illustrates one basic difference between nuclear medicine images and X-rays: the radionuclide images are functional images in that they depict the level of metabolic activity, while radiographs depict levels of radiographic density. Functional images yield a different kind of information than morphologic images. As a matter of fact it would be impossible in most cases to tell from the radiograph of a femur whether the patient was alive or dead at the time the X-ray was taken, whereas a bone scan showing a femur establishes that the patient was alive at the time, and that the femur had metabolic activity. In this sense, the bone scan shows the "livingness" of bone in functional terms.

Most radionuclide scans show a single organ, whereas radiographs show every structure that is in the field of view. The challenge of designing radiopharmaceuticals that find their own way to a body organ by metabolic processes is one of the most important aspects of nuclear medicine. In order to image a body organ it is necessary to know some function it performs through which it could be induced into taking up a radioactive material. For example, one of the many functions of the liver is to filter out radioactive particles from the blood. Injecting a radioactive colloid into the blood stream would result in clearance of the colloid by the liver. When the radioactive colloid has accumulated in the liver to a sufficient extent, external detectors can be used to image the distribution of radioactivity. Focal defects in the distribution may suggest tumors, cysts, abscesses, or other abnormalities. Functional images based on active uptake of a radiopharmaceutical can be obtained in studies of bone, thyroid, lung, heart, liver, spleen, kidneys, and many other organs. In other cases it is possible to introduce the radioactive material directly, without waiting for metabolic processes; this forms the basis of studies of the cerebrospinal fluid and some other body spaces.

Invention of the rectilinear scanner is generally credited to Benedict Cassen (Cassen and Curtis, 1951; Cassen *et al.*, 1951), who developed the concept at the University of California at Los Angeles. A fairly similar rectilinear scanner was invented independently and almost simultaneously by the redoubtable Bernard Ziedses des Plantes (1950), then head of the Neurological Clinic, Municipal Hospital, Rotterdam. Prior to the advent of the scanner, the distribution of radioactive material within an organ was determined by placing the counter over a given point, observing the

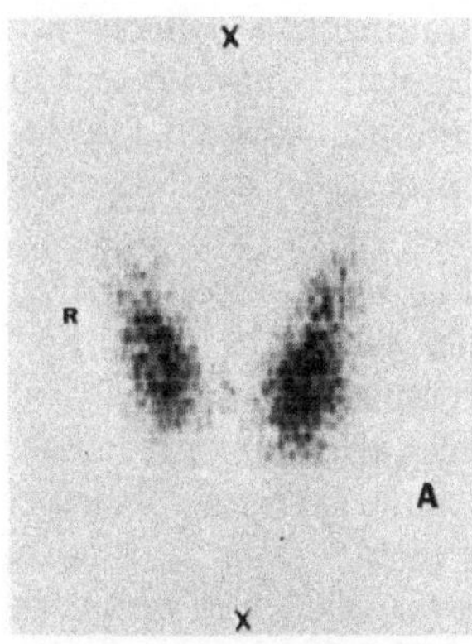

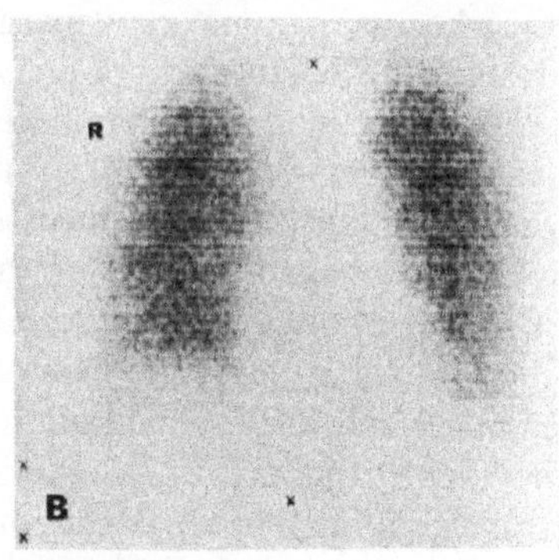

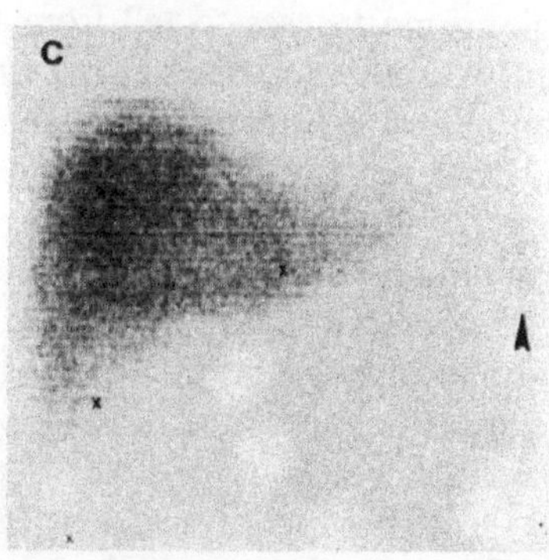

Fig. 3-2. Some typical rectilinear scans. Convention usually has the scan oriented as if the patient were actually there. Thus on anterior views the patient's right side would be to the viewer's left, and vice versa. On posterior views the patient's left side would be to the viewer's left, and the patient's right side would be to the viewer's right. This is in distinction to radiographic orientation which usually places the patient's left side at the viewer's right regardless of whether the view is AP or PA. Note that in nuclear medicine the images are emission images, with anterior, posterior, lateral, and other views. In nuclear medicine we do not speak of AP or PA views as in medical radiography, as this terminology refers to a beam of X-rays entering the body through one side and exiting through the other. Emission images, since they represent radiation originating deep within the body and exiting through one surface, have a simpler terminology. (A) Thyroid scan, anterior view. Note that the image is composed of horizontal lines, and that the density at any point along a line represents the count rate detected over the thyroid at that point. The photographic process has accentuated the contrast somewhat, and on the original image some background counts can be seen scattered throughout the image. The upper mark (×) identifies the patient's chin and the lower mark the manubrial notch, both being anatomic landmarks commonly used to refer the scan image of the thyroid to the patient's body. Note that in this type of image, as opposed to an X-ray, the only organ being imaged is the thyroid. Radioactive iodine (I-131) had been given to this patient 24 hr before the scan. Approximately 25% of the administered dose was taken up by the thyroid gland, and the gamma radiation from the I-131 was used to obtain the scan. (B) Lung scan, anterior view. Radioactive particles slightly larger than capillaries were injected into the patient's arm vein a few minutes before the scan was taken. The particles passed through the heart and into the lungs, where they were trapped in the capillaries of the lung. In this procedure only a tiny fraction of lung capillaries are blocked, and there is no hazard. The particles pass through the lung capillaries in a few hours. Note reasonably uniform activity in both lung fields, except for statistical fluctuations in count rate. Lung perfusion is normal in this case. The space between the two lungs is the mediastinum, containing the heart, which widens the mediastinum in its lower half, and many other structures. The upper anatomic mark is the manubrial notch, the lower mark the

count rate, recording this figure manually, and proceeding to the next point. The invention of the rectilinear scanner provided an instrument that would systematically sample all of the desired points, and record the count rate at each point in the form of an image. The earliest scanners formed their image by causing a stylus to make marks upon a piece of paper. The advent of photographic film provided a far superior image. It is interesting that Cassen and Ziedses des Plantes applied the rectilinear scanner first to images of the thyroid, since radioactive iodine was at that time the only widely available radiopharmaceutical. This early work with the thyroid influenced the development of the rectilinear scanner for years to come. Some typical scans are shown in Figs. 3-2 and 3-3.

3.2. THE DETECTOR

For the most part, currently available rectilinear scanners use a radiation detector that is composed of a sodium iodide crystal, a photomultiplier tube, and associated hardware and electronics. This type of radiation detector is essentially a two-stage transducer, converting high-energy photons (gamma rays, X-rays) into flashes of light, then converting flashes of light into pulses of electrons. It is beyond the scope of this chapter to discuss the crystal at great length, but basically the crystal consists of sodium iodide to which has been added a small amount of thallium as an activator (see Chapter 1). The presence of thallium in the sodium iodide crystal provides energy levels from which the transition to the ground state is forbidden, with the result that the return-to-ground transitions that do occur within the crystal after a high-energy photon has been absorbed tend to favor an allowed transition at 420 nm, a color that closely matches the spectral sensitivity of the photocathodes commonly used in photomultiplier tubes. Most scanner crystals have a thickness of approximately 2 in., and are available in diameters of 3, 5, 8 in., and other sizes for special applications.

The side of the crystal facing the photomultiplier tube is joined to it by a transparent optical coupling, but all other faces are rendered internally reflective so that light cannot exit the crystal except in the direction of the photomultiplier tube. Light is produced within the crystal by an indirect

---

umbilicus. This type of scan is used to investigate pulmonary blood flow in patients thought to have possible pulmonary emboli (blood clots in the lungs). (C) Liver scan, anterior view. A radioactive colloid had been injected into the blood stream of this patient about 20 min before the scan was taken. One of the functions of the liver is to filter out particles from the blood, and the radioactive particles have accumulated in the liver. Uptake is fairly uniform, again allowing for statistical fluctuations in the count rate. The spleen (arrowhead) is faintly visualized. The anatomic marks are at the lower rib margin and the lower mark is at the body wall.

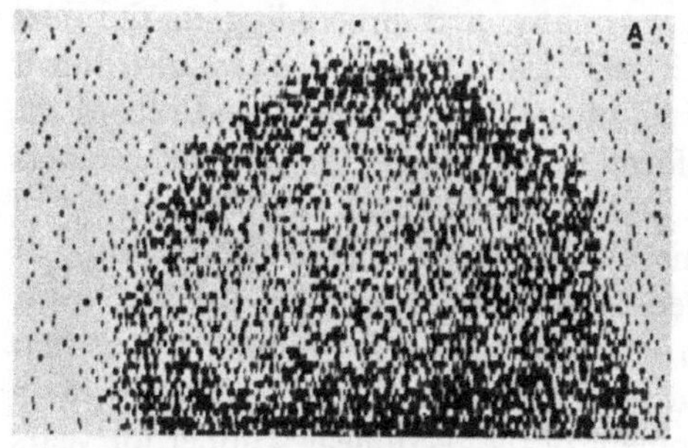

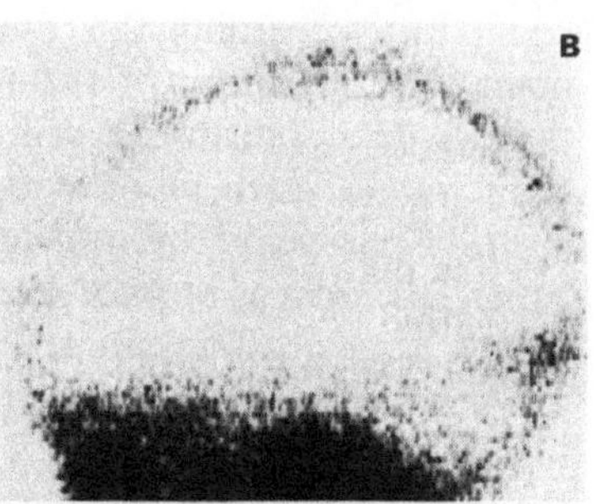

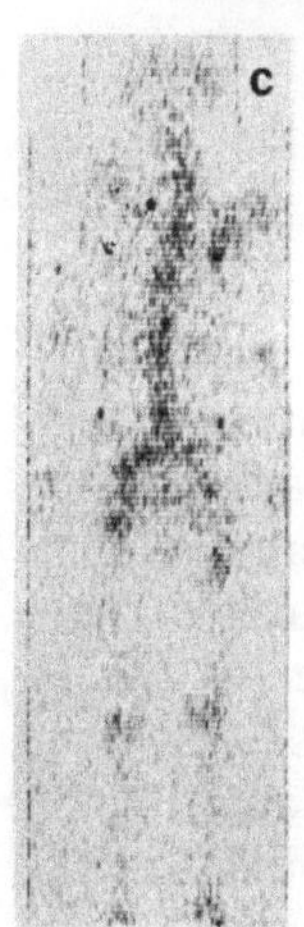

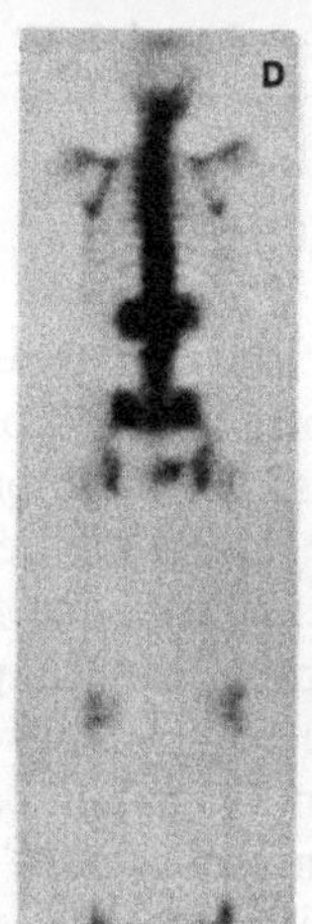

Fig. 3-3. Improvements in scanning technique. (A) Brain scan using ^{203}Hg chlormerodrin 100μCi. Scan took almost 1 hr per view and usually only two views were obtained. Radiation dose to the kidneys was about 100 rads. Note poor resolution and statistical fluctuation due to low count rate. (B) Brain scan using ^{99m}Tc DTPA 20 mCi. Each view takes 5–10 min and 4 or 5 views are obtained routinely. Radiation dose is low and image quality is high. (C) Bone scan using ^{85}Sr 100 μCi. (D) Bone scan using ^{99m}Tc diphosphonate 20 mCi. Note improvement in resolution. The lower radiation dose of ^{99m}Tc (despite the higher administered dose) allows its use in children, who could not be examined at all using ^{85}Sr.

process. A gamma ray is absorbed in the crystal primarily through ionizing interactions with the orbital electrons it encounters. These electrons, liberated from their atoms by photoelectric and Compton processes, cause secondary ionization and excitation. It is the recombinations that follow ionization and excitation that give rise to the light itself. Each keV of gamma ray energy is transformed into 20–30 such interactions, with the result that at the recombination step, hundreds or thousands of individual flashes of light may reach the photocathode all essentially at the same time.

3.3. COLLIMATOR

If the detector were exposed to radiation without some sort of shielding, there would be no way of knowing from which direction the radiation came. It is necessary to "direct the attention" of the detector to radiation originating from a known direction, so that a meaningful image can be obtained. This is done by surrounding the detector with shielding (usually lead), in which a hole, or holes, allow radiation to enter the detector from only one direction. The device is called a collimator. Its function is to block radiation, except that emanating from a preferred location.

For maximum sensitivity (maximum count rate for a given activity) one could make the hole quite large. However, a large hole makes it difficult to determine exactly from what direction the radiation entered the detector. To improve the resolution, i.e., to make the detector sensitive to radiation coming only from a specified direction, one would make a very small hole in the lead collimator. In actual practice the trade-off between sensitivity and resolution is one of the basic problems of collimator design and even at this time is still alive with controversy.

A single hole in the collimator could represent a reasonable trade-off between sensitivity and resolution, but would cause the detector to be most sensitive for radiation sources located very close to it. In medical practice the organs to be imaged are usually located not on the surface of the body but somewhat deeper within it, so that it would be disadvantageous to design a detector that was most sensitive to radiation originating at the skin (and less so for radiation originating deeper within the body). For this reason, collimators are designed with not one but a number of holes drilled in such a way that their axes converge at a point several inches away from the collimator face. The point at which these axes converge is called the *focal point*, and the distance from the face of the collimator to the focal point is called the *focal length* of the collimator. This type of collimator is called a "focused" collimator, which is somewhat of a misnomer as gamma rays cannot be focused in the usual sense. It rather refers to a type of collimator that has maximum sensitivity for a point a fixed distance away from it, and less sensitivity for points closer to it or farther from it. The reason for this is that radiation originating at the focal point can enter any of the holes, and will be detected with maximum sensitivity, while radiation originating at any other point can enter only a few holes. Even though the inverse square law favors the closer source, the overall sensitivity of the collimator is greatest at the focal point. This type of collimator is ideal for medical applications. Focused collimators are available with a variety of different focal lengths for various medical imaging applications.

The same trade-off between sensitivity and resolution applies to focused collimators. If the holes are very large, and the walls between them (septa) correspondingly thin, the collimator will have high sensitivity but poor resolution. Conversely, if the collimator has very small holes and thick septa, sensitivity will be reduced but resolution will improve. To some extent gamma rays will penetrate the septa (depending on their energy) and so the resolution of the collimator for gamma ray imaging is never as good as its optical resolution.

Figures 3-4 and 3-5 illustrate the focal point, focal length, sensitivity,

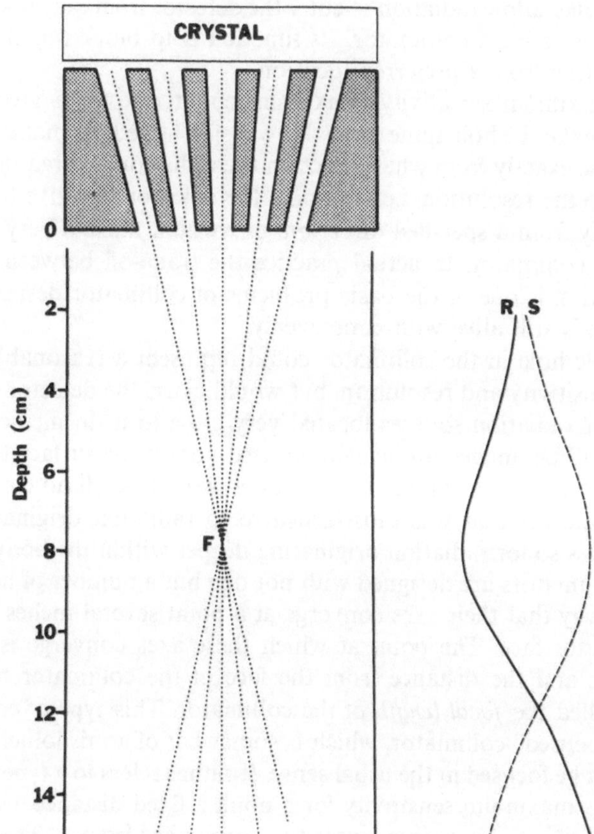

Fig. 3-4. Schematic drawing indicating some features of the focusing collimator (shaded area, top). The collimator is made of lead in which several holes have been drilled at such an angle that the axes converge at a point in space (F), called the focal point. In this hypothetical case the focal point is 8 cm from the face of the collimator. Radiation originating at the focal point can enter the detector through any of the collimator holes, and is therefore detected with maximum sensitivity. Radiation originating closer to the collimator than F, or farther away from it, can only enter the detector through some of the holes and is detected with less sensitivity.

The variation of sensitivity with distance from the collimator is shown by the dashed curve S. The sensitivity is maximum at the focal point. The resolution of the collimator for objects at different distances is shown by the solid curve R. In this example the best resolution, 2.5 mm, is obtained at the focal point. Resolution is poorer at closer and farther distances.

For most collimators the focal point represents the point both of maximum sensitivity and of optimum resolution.

and resolution of a focused collimator. Figure 3-5 was obtained by scanning back and forth across a point source of radiation while the collimator was moved farther and farther away from it, through a distance of 0–35 cm. The density of the image at any given point reflects the sensitivity of the

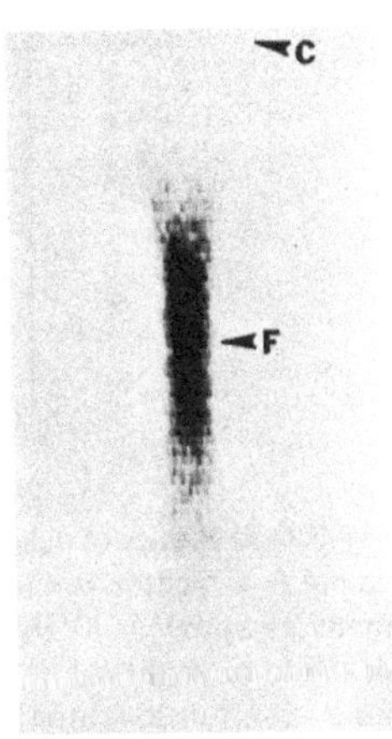

Fig. 3-5. Scan of point source, indicating response of collimator as a function of distance. The detector was made to pass back and forth in front of a point source as the distance between the detector and the source was increased. At distances close to the collimator (C) the sensitivity and resolution are both low, and the image is very faint. With increasing distance the count rate increases and the resolution improves, both becoming optimum in the region of the focal point (F). Note that this collimator has a fairly broad depth of focus. If it were used to scan an internal organ, its best response would be a slab of tissue several centimeters thick, at a distance of several centimeters from the collimator. At distances beyond the focal point both the sensitivity and the resolution are degraded.

detector, and it can be seen that the detector is most sensitive to radiation originating at the focal point. Sensitivity drops off at closer and farther distances. The width of the pattern is a measure of the resolution of the detector system. The resolution is best at the focal point. Sources closer to the detector, and sources farther away, are "blurred" and contribute less to the image, even though the counts are there.

With the use of the focused collimator, a given plane can be selected in which objects will be "in focus." By rescanning the same organ several times, setting the focal point at different planes, it is possible to prepare a series of tomograms in which successive planes are in focus. Visual inspection of this set of images allows one to reconstruct a three-dimensional concept of the original organ.

The sensitivity of the collimator is fairly easy to specify, being the number of counts per minute recorded from a point source of given activity located at the focal point. If there is very little septal penetration, high count rates will generally be associated with good images, though if the energy of the gamma ray is too high for the septal thickness, septal penetration will degrade the image. The "sensitivity" will be falsely elevated (see Fig. 3-6).

The resolution of the collimator is somewhat more difficult to specify. A point source of radiation will be imaged as a somewhat extended source, and the *point spread function* can be used to specify the degree to which this takes place. The *line spread function* is a similar way of describing resolution and is based on the response of the detector system to a line source perpendicular to it; the response will be the line spread function. The shape of the line spread function is the same as that of the point spread function.

It can be seen from Fig. 3-6 that the point spread function (or line spread function) is a somewhat bell-shaped curve generally suggesting a Gaussian

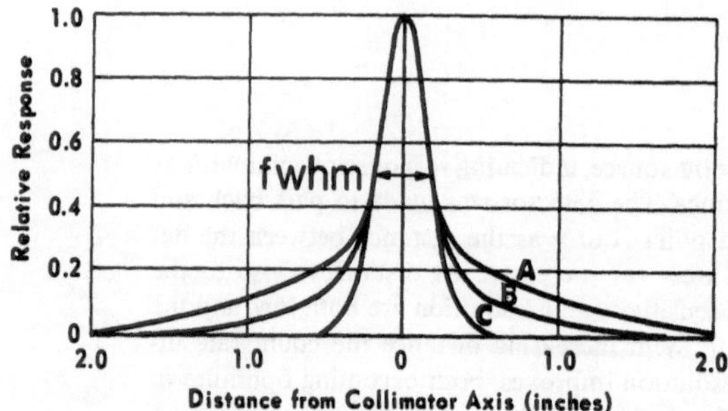

Fig. 3-6. Response of detector–collimator system to a point source for three scatter conditions. Curve A, air; curve B, 4 in. of backscatter; curve C, 4 in. of backscatter and 3 in. of frontscatter material. Source is ^{197}Hg, energy window is 65–100 keV, and scatter material is lucite. Septal penetration at these low energies is negligible, and the broadening of the base of the spread function is due to scattering only. Note that all three curves have the same FWHM; this number above would be insufficient in this case. Septal penetration by high-energy gamma rays causes a similar effect. [Reprinted from Rollo and Schulz (1970) with permission.]

distribution, symmetric about the detector axis. Since curves of this type have similar shapes, the entire curve can be specified by a single number: the width of the curve at a height equal to one-half of its maximum value (normalized to 100% for convenience). This number, the full width at half maximum (FWHM), is a frequently used indicator of resolution in detector systems and collimators; however, the shape of the point spread function is distorted by septal penetration and by scatter, so that the tails of the curve are longer than might be expected from the ordinary Gaussian distribution. Penetration varies with gamma energy.

The Fourier transform of the line spread function can be normalized, and is called the *system transfer function.* The absolute value of the system transfer function is called the *modulation transfer function* (MTF). For a fuller discussion of the theory of collimator resolution, the reader is referred to Gregg (1965), Harris *et al.* (1968), Knowles *et al.* (1972), Mozley (1968), Myhill and Hine (1967), Rollo and Schulz (1970), and Schulz *et al.* (1970).

In designing and selecting collimators, certain parameters are of foremost importance. The collimator must be selected with the gamma energy in mind. The septal thickness must be such as to exclude excessive penetration while allowing for reasonable sensitivity. The focal length of the collimator must be selected considering the target organ to be imaged. Finally, the trade-off between resolution and sensitivity may be different for different clinical applications. In lung scanning for pulmonary emboli, resolution is of lesser importance as the smallest significant areas to be imaged are 2–3 cm in diameter or larger, and the generally acute nature of the patients thought to have pulmonary embolism requires that the imaging time be brief, and therefore that the sensitivity of the detector be high. On the other hand, scans of the thyroid are sometimes done to look for nodules or space-occupying lesions that may measure 0.5–1 cm in diameter. The high resolution necessary for this type of study is obtained only at the expense of sensitivity, but the type of examination does not require high speed, and long imaging times are acceptable. Most nuclear medicine clinics using rectilinear scanners maintain a variety of collimators on hand for different clinical applications.

3.4. SCANNING MOTION

In order to maintain close correspondence between the position of the detector and the position of the light source, and in order to maintain a constant relationship between count rate and density, it is necessary that the drive mechanism be constructed with a high level of speed stability (Hine and Erickson, 1974). If a rigid bar connects the detector and the light source, the spatial relationship will always be maintained, but if the coupling is electronic, speed stability must be insured by the use of appropriate feedback systems. If the drive speed is uneven, the detector may spend more of its time imaging certain areas than others, and the count rate will appear to increase in the areas that are scanned more slowly. This discrepancy between count rate and film density will cause artifacts in which the count rate may appear to be higher or lower than is actually the case.

Usual scanning speeds in rectilinear scanners run from 20 to 500 cm/min, and higher speeds are available. Spacing between adjacent lines can be set so that the scanner increments exactly one line between passes, or exactly two lines, or one-half line (allowing for overlap of data). Line spacings usually run from 2 to 6. The limits of the field are set manually so as to include all areas of interest, with the constraint that the maximum field size (without minification) is 14 × 17 in., the size of the largest available X-ray film cassette. Some scanners provide a minified image, usually 1/2 to 1/5 of normal size, and a much larger portion of the body can be reduced to fit the film-cassette sizes available. With 5:1 minification, the entire body can be imaged on a single film, even if the patient is 7 ft tall.

3.5. INTERNAL ELECTRONICS

It was mentioned previously that the detector is a two-stage transducer, converting gamma rays into light (in the crystal) and light into electron pulses (in the photomultiplier tube). Once the electron pulses are formed, they are then amplified, measured, screened, and displayed (or discarded). The basic flow of data is shown in Fig. 3-7.

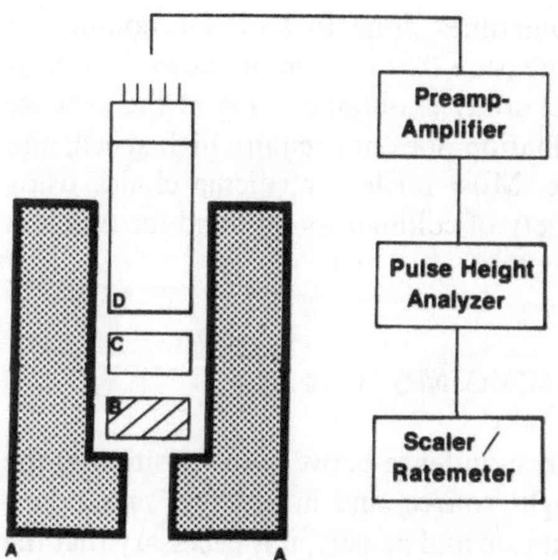

Fig. 3-7. Schematic drawing of electronics in a typical rectilinear scanner. The detector unit consists of a collimator (A), in this case shown as a single hole for simplicity, a crystal (B), a light pipe for optical coupling (C), and a photomultiplier tube (D). The detector is a two-stage transducer which converts gamma rays to light photons in the crystal, then converts light to electrons in the photomultiplier tube. The pulse of electrons is amplified and the height of the pulse is then analyzed. The height of the electron pulse depends on the number of electrons leaving the photomultiplier tube, which in turn depends (assuming constant multiplication factor) on the number of light photons impinging upon the photocathode. This number depends in turn on the number of light photons originating in the crystal, which depends in turn on the energy of the gamma rays absorbed in the crystal. Therefore the pulse height is a function of gamma ray energy, and the pulse height analyzer is a technique for registering only those events that correspond to the gamma ray energy of interest.

To operate the photomultiplier tube, a very stable source of high voltage is necessary. The stability is important because it is necessary to know the energy of an incident gamma ray in order to distinguish primary photons from scattered photons. If the high voltage in the photomultiplier tube is unstable, the multiplication factor will vary, and scattered photons may be imaged instead of being rejected.

The electronic circuitry that measures the energy of the incident gamma ray is called the *pulse height analyzer*. The pulse height analyzer selects pulses of a preset height, rejecting all others. The preset height is adjusted so that primary photons will be accepted and scattered photons, having a lower energy, will be rejected. The sequence of events is as follows: a high-energy photon is absorbed by the sodium iodide crystal, giving rise to a large number of flashes of light. The number of flashes depends on the energy of the gamma ray. These flashes are collected by the photocathode of the photomultiplier tube, and are converted into a corresponding number of electrons. The photomultiplier tube multiplies the number of electrons by a constant factor (the multiplication factor), and the output is a pulse of electrons, the number of electrons depending on the original photon energy. After amplification and pulse shaping, the pulse is presented to the pulse height analyzer to decide whether it should be accepted or rejected. In practice the pulse height analyzer is set to within a certain tolerance either way about a central value, and provides a "window" through which pulses of the correct height can pass. Without such a "window" a large number of scattered photons would be accepted for imaging. Since scattered photons generally do not come from directly in front of the collimator, but rather from some distance away from the axis, their inclusion in the image would degrade it. In practice it is not possible to reject all scattered photons. The window must be set to a certain finite width in order to accept a sufficient number of primary photons; imperfections in a crystal and electronic design, as well as the limited energy resolution of the sodium iodide itself, mean that the photopeak (energy spectrum of primary, unscattered photons) is a narrow, Gaussian-like curve rather than a sharp spike. A window of finite width, extending even slightly below the photopeak itself, must necessarily accept some scattered radiation. Within the body, gamma photons lose energy depending on the angle through which they are scattered. Small scattering angles are associated with relatively little energy loss. Thus photons with energies slightly below that of the photopeak have been scattered through small angles, while photons with energies much below the photopeak have been scattered through larger angles, or have undergone multiple scatter. Each increment in energy can be thought of as a cone extending out from the collimator. Within each cone the Compton scatter causes an energy loss no greater than $E^2(1\text{-}\cos\phi)/[511 + E(1\text{-}\cos\phi)]$, where E is the incident gamma photon energy in keV, and ϕ is the scattering angle. Widening the window will increase the count rate but will decrease the spatial resolution.

It is often useful to disregard those portions of the image in which the count rate is very low. The instrument can be instructed to disregard all count rates below a certain minimum value. This feature is called "background erase" or "background suppression." Figure 3-8 shows that without

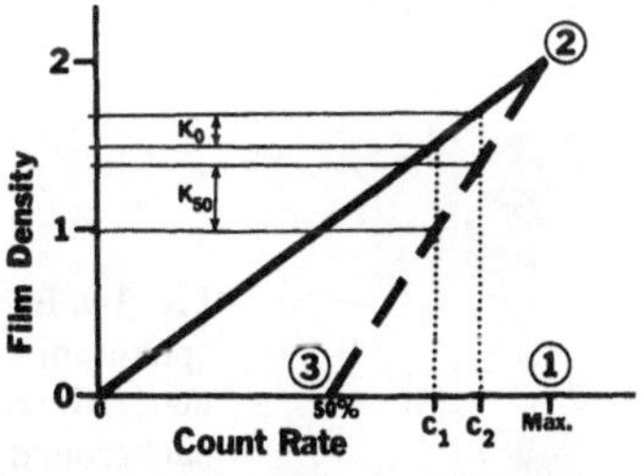

Fig. 3-8. Technique for setting up background suppression for the purpose of increasing contrast. Theoretically film density is a linear function of count rate (in actuality the relationship is much more complex but for the discussion we will assume the simple case). For two given count rates C_1 and C_2 the contrast in film density is the difference between the densities corresponding to the two count rates, here shown as K_0.

With background suppression the scanner is instructed to print nothing until the count rate is a preset percentage of the maximum count rate, in this illustration 50%. If 50% background suppresion is used, the difference in contrast between the count rates C_1 and C_2 is greater (K_{50}). Note that contrast will be greater throughout the range between the preset cutoff and the maximum count rate, but count rates below the cutoff will not be registered at all.

In practice the scanner can be set up by (1) observing the maximum count rate in the area of interest, (2) setting the film exposure factor such that the maximum film density corresponds to the maximum count rate, and (3) introducing background suppression if desired.

background suppression, the density of exposed film would (ideally) progress linearly from 0 density at 0 count rate, to maximum density at the maximum preset count rate. (In actual practice the relationship is not linear.) Introducing background suppression moves the foot of the curve to higher count rates. It also increases the contrast by providing a steeper relationship between film density and count rate. Thus background suppression is invariably associated with enhancement of contrast, a step that results in deceptively crisp-looking images which often contain less information than their less contrasty, unsuppressed counterparts. The effect of background suppression on the image is shown in Fig. 3-9.

It is often the case that certain ranges of count rate in an image contain most of the critical clinical information. Some manufacturers provide the option of altering contrast in different regions of count rate by altering the shape of the density/exposure curve. The steep portion of the nonlinear curve can be adjusted to high, medium, or low regions of count rate. Of course, it would be preferable to record the study linearly and introduce the nonlinear contrast enhancement subsequently, but this is not always practical.

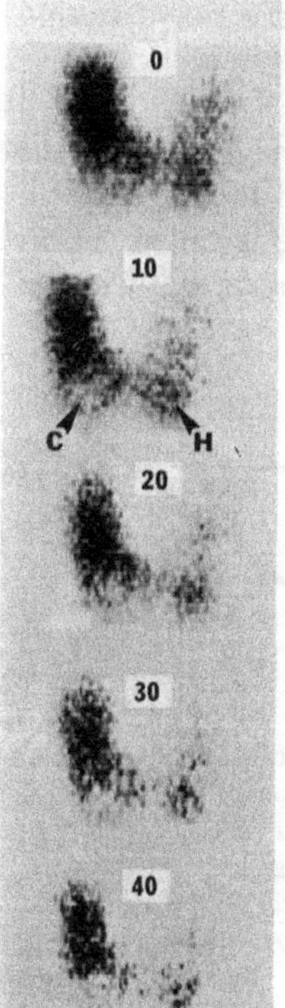

Fig. 3-9. Effect of background suppression on the image. A thyroid "phantom" (hollow plastic model) was filled with radioactive material and scanned. The figures above each image show the percent background suppression that was used. The "phantom" contained a filler to mimic a zone of decreased activity ("cold" nodule C) and a recess to mimic a region of increased activity ("hot" nodule H). Note that the contrast increases with increasing background suppression. The "nodules" are somewhat better seen in the enhanced scan than on the unenhanced, but the exaggerated fluctuations in count rate suggest irregularities and possible focal abnormalities when in fact there are none. In clinical practice little or no background suppression is used; suppression can later be added optically or electronically if desired.

3.6. DISPLAY

The display of the distribution of radioactive material within the body could take the form of a sketch or X-ray of the area of interest with the actual count rate superimposed over each point. If sufficient data are available, points having the same number of counts can be connected by contours (isocount contours), to give a semitopographic display.

With rectilinear scanners, the area of interest is automatically surveyed and count rates are displayed point by point either as a series of dots (or short bars) on a piece of paper, or as images of a light source on film. The earliest scanners used a display consisting of dots on a piece of paper. To even out the statistical fluctuation of the count rate, especially in areas of low count rate, a dot factor was introduced, by which each dot represents a predetermined number of counts. The degree of fluctuation of the count rate is represented by $\sigma = N^{1/2}$, where σ is the standard deviation and N is the number of counts. The fluctuation as actually observed by the eye is represented by the relative standard deviation, and is given by the expression $\sigma/N = N^{1/2}/N = 1/N^{1/2}$. It is evident from this last expression that increasing the number of counts by a factor of 2 will decrease the relative standard deviation by a factor of 1.4, i.e., by 40%. Increasing the number of counts by a factor of 4 will decrease the relative standard deviation by a factor of 2. The dot factor, by increasing the number of counts each dot represents, smooths out the fluctuation. On the other hand, the use of a large dot factor reduces resolution by making it necessary for the display device to accumulate more data before printing. Edges and fine detail are washed out by this technique.

Several methods have been advanced to improve the performance of the imaging device in areas of low count rate. One is to introduce a time constant by which a certain number of counts are stored, or integrated, before the display is activated. Use of the time constant results in somewhat smoother images but introduces other artifacts such as scalloping (Fig. 3-10). (The scalloping can be eliminated by having the scanner print only in one direction, returning between passes without printing.) Another technique is to convert the count rate into a frequency by means of a variable oscillator. The frequency output of the oscillator depends on the count rate. This method also tends to smooth out the image at the expense of introducing certain artifacts, and is not found in most modern rectilinear scanners.

The raster effect produced by dots results in a somewhat distracting image, and the image can be made more pleasing to the eye by replacing the dots with bars whose length is exactly equal to the width of the scan pass. In this way adjacent passes fill in the image so as to leave no intervening spaces. The resulting image is more pleasing to the eye, though the data remain the same.

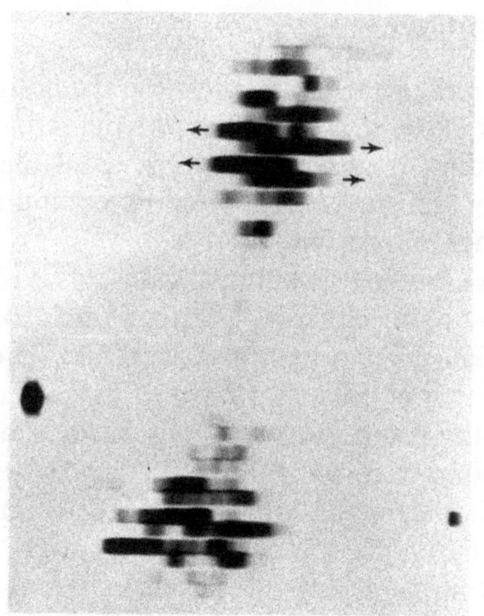

Fig. 3-10. Scalloping artifact. This is a small portion of a bone scan done on an infant. The time constant of the scanner was inadvertently set too high, and as a result the image corresponding to each scan line is displaced in the direction the detector was moving at the time (arrows). This exaggerated example was selected to illustrate the principle; an image like this would not be found in ordinary practice.

The physician's interpretation of the resulting scans depends upon his appreciation of differences in density. It became necessary, as techniques improved, to appreciate finer and finer differences in density (count rate). Because the eye is limited in being able to distinguish subtle differences in grey, shades of grey can be coded in different colors, different colors representing different count rates. This is done by using multicolor ribbon with the stylus advanced to the ribbon of the color corresponding to the count rate. By the use of color, it is possible to distinguish count rate differences more subtle than the eye can appreciate by grey alone. However, the amount of data in the scan remains the same. Color-coded count rate tends to exaggerate random fluctuations and is not in widespread use at this time.

An inherent limitation of scans made by marks on paper is that the dynamic range can vary only between dense black and the brightness of light reflected from the unmarked paper. A far greater dynamic range is possible with transilluminated photoscans. With transillumination the range of available densities runs from 0.3 (the density of unexposed film) to 2.0, or higher if desired. The introduction of a light source to make marks on film, rather than a tapper to make marks on paper, makes it possible to vary the display in ways that would not otherwise be possible. The intensity of the light source can be varied according to count rate or changes in count rate; the duration of the light source can be varied; and the waveform can be varied as well. In this way a scan can be produced in which areas of low count rate are relatively suppressed, and in which contrast can be enhanced from the very beginning.

It is obvious that neither the dots, the bars, nor the circular or square aperture used in photoscanning fairly represents the point spread function that the detector system actually "sees." Elimination of the image of the aperture (dot, bar, circle, or square) might enhance the interpretability of the image. A variety of techniques for "data blending" have been introduced. Physicians would remove their glasses to read scans, or alternatively, put on glasses if they did not normally wear them. Scans were read with diffusing screens in front of them (Christie *et al.*, 1965), or viewed at a distance through a lens (Leins *et al.*, 1969), or were produced by a light source that had been deliberately defocused (Christie *et al.*, 1965), or were reprocessed through photographic or video techniques that introduced a quasi-Gaussian defocusing (Oldendorf *et al.*, 1967).

The quality of the scan image depends in part on the number of data points it contains. Assuming that each count is recorded as one data point, one can define linear information density (LID) as the number of counts per centimeter along a given scan line. Area information density (AID) represents the number of counts in a given square centimeter of the scan image. The linear information density is expressed as follows:

$$\text{LID (counts/cm)} = \frac{\text{count rate (counts/min)}}{\text{scanning speed (cm/min)}}$$

The area information density is expressed as follows (assuming adjacent scan lines just touch):

$$\text{AID (counts/cm}^2\text{)} = \frac{\text{LID (counts/cm)}}{\text{line width (cm)}}$$

In setting up the scan it is advisable to select an appropriate LID or AID, and to set the scanning speed according to the count rate available. Figure 3-11 presents a chart that could be used to set up a rectilinear scan. First, the maximum count rate of interest is selected. Using the chart in Fig. 3-11, a "quality region" is selected that corresponds to a given LID. The scanning speed corresponding to this "quality region" is read off the ordinate, and the time that would be required to scan a 10 × 10 cm unit area is read off the right-hand side of the chart. Knowing the total area that is to be scanned, the time required can be estimated. If this time is excessive, one may expect that the image would be degraded by patient motion (if the study requires more than, say, 30 min for a single view). If the time is considered to be excessive, a shorter time can be selected, and the scanning speed and LID will be reestimated. The best compromise between image quality (LID) and total time required per view can be worked out from this chart. The effect of LID on image quality can be seen in Fig. 3-12.

After the scanning speed has been selected, the detector is placed over

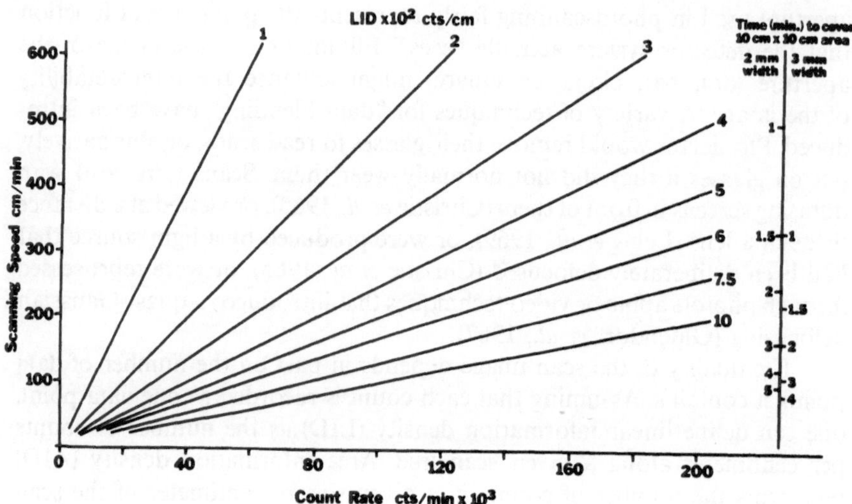

Fig. 3-11. Setting up a scanner. The chart shows the relationship between linear information density (LID), scanning speed, and count rate. With the patient in position under the scanner, the maximum count rate over the area of interest is noted. An LID figure is selected, the higher figures corresponding to higher image quality. The scanning speed corresponding to the intersection of the count rate and the LID is noted. The axis on the right shows the amount of time required to scan a unit 10 × 10 cm area, depending on whether the scan line width is 2 or 3 mm. If this time is acceptable, the scanning speed corresponding to this will be usable. If the time is excessive, a faster scanning speed will have to be used with a corresponding decrease in linear information density. The advantage of a chart like this is that it enables the operator to select the optimum scanning speed for the clinical situation, and to be able to expect in advance the image quality and time required to perform this study.

the region of maximum usable count rate, and the density of the film is set to the maximum usable density (usually 2.0). Using Fig. 3-8 background suppression can be set, if desired, as well as nonlinear contrast enhancement if this option is available.

A common line spacing for rectilinear scanners is three scan lines per centimeter. This introduces a raster effect which is sometimes distracting during interpretation. The smallest image that the detector system can realistically image is on the order of 1 cm. This means that the scan line itself, being much smaller than this, represents a totally useless artifact. Morgan (1966) has explored the response of the eye to different spatial frequencies, in the context of interpretation of radiographic images. Figure 3-13 shows the response of the retina to different spatial frequencies. It is seen that the maximum response occurs at a retinal spatial frequency of approximately ten cycles per millimeter. The size of the object that will yield the maximum response on the retina depends on the viewing distance. Figure 3-14 shows the object diameter as a function of viewing distance for

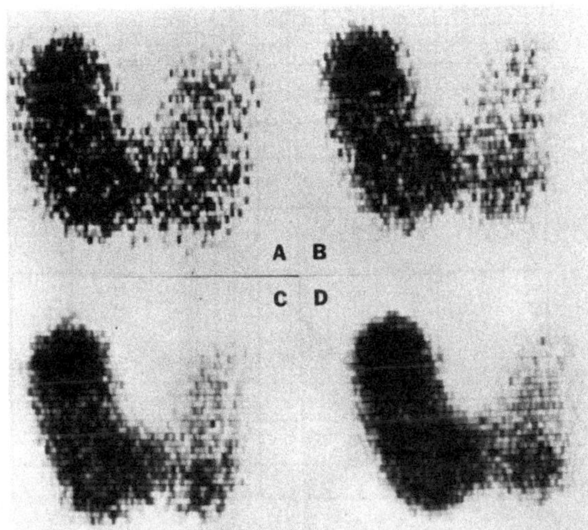

Fig. 3-12. Effect of linear information density on image quality. A thyroid phantom was scanned with four different linear information density levels. (A) LID = 100 counts/cm^2; (B) 300 counts/cm^2; (C) 600 counts/cm^2; (D) 1000 counts/cm^2.

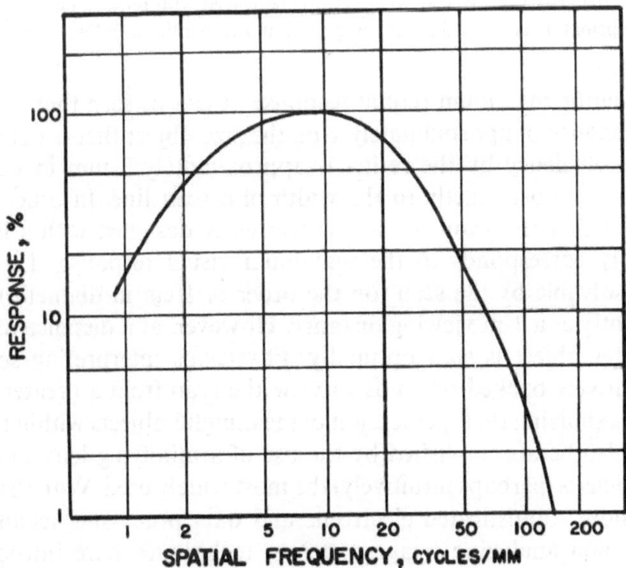

Fig. 3-13. Response of the retina to spatial frequencies. The retina has maximum visual response to spatial frequencies in the order of ten cycles per millimeter, falling off markedly on either side of this figure. Thus the eye is a band-pass filter for retinal spatial frequencies around 10/mm. [Reprinted from Morgan (1966) with permission.]

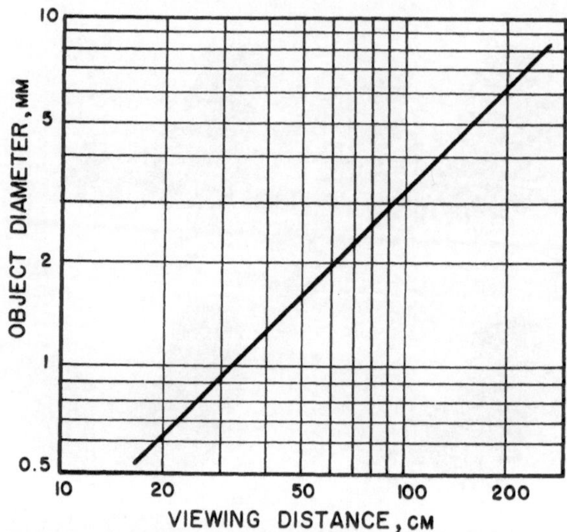

Fig. 3-14. Relationship of object diameter to viewing distance. In this case the object diameter is that which is perceived by the eye with maximum response. Normal viewing distances are between 50 and 100 cm. Note that the object diameter that is best perceived in this range is 1.7–3.2 mm. Very few scanning systems offer this kind of resolution. However, the width of the ordinary scan line is 2–3 mm, an object size that is visualized with greatest efficiency. In other words, the aspect of the scan image that is perceived with greatest efficiency by the eye is not the information contained in the image itself but rather the scan line raster.

objects eliciting maximum retinal response. It can be seen that at a normal viewing distance of approximately 1 m, the size object that is detected with maximum efficiency by the retina is approximately 3 mm in width. This corresponds almost exactly to the width of a scan line. In other words, it came about that the scanner was inadvertently designed with a line width that exactly corresponds to the maximum visual response. The smallest objects resolvable by the scan (on the order of 1 cm in diameter) are seen less efficiently at a 1-m viewing distance. However, at a distance of 3 m a 1-cm-diameter object is seen optimally. Physicians interpreting scans have often intuitively backed off so as to view the scan from a greater distance, thereby maximizing their perception of meaningful objects within the image. This can also be accomplished by the use of a minifying lens, and the 3:1 minifying lens is (perhaps intuitively) the most widely used. With the development of more sophisticated electronic and data processing techniques for modifying and analyzing images, various techniques were introduced for processing raw data. If a scan is obtained using no background suppression or contrast enhancement, and using a short time constant with essentially no preprocessing, the image can be "rescanned" using a scanning densitometer or closed circuit television, into which electronic modifications can be introduced. In this way the brightness, contrast, size, and other features can be manipulated. Raw data can also be recorded on magnetic tape or disks, if an encoder is available for recording the position of the scanner.

No matter what kind of processing is done on a scan image, it will always have inherent differences from X-ray radiographic images, and will probably always fall short of the expectations of those used to working with radiographs. Scans are basically different from radiographs in several respects. First of all, scans are functional images in that they depict the active metabolic function of the organ being imaged, whereas radiographs generally depict morphologic detail rather than function (though many exceptions exist). As was mentioned earlier, it would be impossible to tell from the radiograph of a femur whether the patient was alive or not at the time the study was done, but a bone scan of the same area would show life and metabolic activity. Secondly, the X-ray tube can be rapidly turned on and off, emitting a very large number of photons in a very brief period of time. Radionuclide images, on the other hand, are made from radionuclides deposited as internal emitters which cannot be turned on and off. In order to protect the patient from excessive radiation, it is necessary to limit the dose that is given, which in turn limits the number of photons available for imaging. A typical image consists of anywhere from 10^4 to 10^6 photons, whereas a typical radiographic image consists of several billion photons. Thirdly, the source of radiation in an X-ray is essentially a point source, whereas the source of radiation in a radionuclide study is an extended source giving rise to a great deal of scatter and background. Fourth, the distribution of activity in the radionuclide image reflects the normal irregularity present in biologic systems. And finally, the energy of an X-ray source can be varied by varying the voltage across the tube, and an optimum energy can be selected for any given imaging application. On the other hand, radionuclides are supplied by nature with gamma energies that are inherent and unvariable, and we must select those radionuclides that give the best compromise among a number of fixed parameters (gamma energy, particulate radiation, half-life, biologic activity, etc.).

3.7. MODIFIED SCANNERS

3.7.1. Multiple Detectors

Rectilinear scanners are available with more than one detector. A number of companies make scanners with two detectors, so that both anterior and posterior views may be obtained at the same time. If the two detectors are properly aligned, the geometric mean of the two count rates is fairly independent of depth. A four-detector scanner has been described (DiChiro *et al.*, 1968).

3.7.2. Sector Scanner

A sector scanner developed by Kuhl and Sanders (1971) consists of four detectors, each of which makes a single pass across the area to be imaged. The entire assembly is then rotated slightly and the pass is repeated at a slightly different angle. Data from a large number of passes is stored in a computer. The resulting reconstructed image displays a single slice through the body in a manner analogous to that of computed tomography (CT). Emission tomography has not found widespread application, but the images that have been published so far are images that could hardly have been produced any other way.

3.7.3. Positron Scanners

Positron-emitting radionuclides represent a special case of beta-emitting radionuclides, and make possible some unique applications in medical imaging. Positrons are positively charged electrons emitted from radioactive nuclei at the time of disintegration. After being slowed down by passage through matter, a positive electron interacts with an ordinary negative electron in a process of mutual annihilation, in which the mass of the two electrons is converted into electromagnetic energy. To conserve energy and momentum the two electron masses (each corresponding to an energy of 511 keV) are converted into two 511-keV gamma rays traveling in opposite directions. This "annihilation radiation" is what is actually imaged in the case of positron emitters, not the positrons themselves.

The fact that the two annihilation gamma rays travel in exactly opposite directions makes possible some interesting instrumentation for imaging. First of all, if two detectors are situated on opposite sides of a positron emitter, and if the two detectors are fed into a coincidence circuit such that only the pulses originating simultaneously in both detectors are counted, no shielding is necessary because the chance of spurious coincidences is extremely small. Since no shielding is required, the sensitivity of a positron imaging device is much higher than that of a conventional gamma ray imaging device, which requires collimators to absorb unwanted gamma rays (originating in the source and environment). For a single pair of detectors there is the usual trade-off between sensitivity and resolution: for small detectors the resolution will be high but with low sensitivity, while for large detectors the sensitivity will be high at the expense of resolution. It is possible to construct an array of multiple detectors (Brownell and Burnham, 1974) in which a number of detectors are situated on either side of the source. Coincidences occurring in any pair of detectors can be displayed as a line passing through the source, connecting one detector with the other. A large number of such lines passing through the object being imaged will identify the distribution of sources within it. This type of image contains some depth information from which a three-dimensional image could be reconstructed, although better techniques are available.

A different array of multiple coincidence detection devices was suggested by Rankowitz *et al.* (1961), using a ring of 32 detectors surrounding an object containing a positron emitter. This device records coincidences between any pair of detectors and prepares an image in which the two detectors are connected by a line. This device was developed into an advanced form by Ter-Pogossian (Phelps *et al.*, 1975; Phelps *et al.*, 1976; Ter-Pogossian *et al.*, 1975). The imaging device of Ter-Pogossian and co-workers uses a ring of 48 detectors with appropriate coincidence circuitry, and reconstructs an image representing a slice through the object. It is called the PETT (positron emission transaxial tomograph). In some ways this instrument bears a resemblance to the sector scanner of Kuhl (Kuhl *et al.*, 1973), but uses many stationary detectors (rather than a few moving detectors) to image annihilation radiation from positron emitters (as opposed to ordinary gamma emission). The PETT yields images that are somewhat analogous to those of the whole body CT scanner. However, the images are not morphologic images of radiographic density, as in the case of the CT scanner, but rather images of the distribution of radioactive materials that have been actively taken up by metabolic and physiologic processes within the body. Thus the PETT can be used to image physiologic processes and to detect physiologic abnormalities, features that are common to most nuclear medicine studies as opposed to radiographic studies.

Positron emitters give the potential of yet another innovation in imaging, called time-of-flight scintigraphy. When a positron in the object being imaged is annihilated, the two annihilation gamma rays travel in opposite directions. If they reach two detectors essentially at the same time, the coincidence circuit will register the count, and will, in its memory, construct a line connecting the two detectors and passing through the object. However, even though the two gamma rays reach the detectors at *essentially* the same time, they do not reach them at *exactly* the same time unless they originate at a point equidistant from the two detectors. Any other point of origin will result in one gamma ray reaching its detector slightly ahead of the other. Traveling the speed of light the gamma rays would travel 30 cm in 1 nsec. To resolve small distances within the object by this technique it would be necessary to have the capability of resolving two events in time to within a small fraction of a nanosecond. Work along this line is underway (Brownell and Burnham, 1974) and if successful, will open the way for three-dimensional imaging of positron-emitting objects.

3.7.4. Profile Scanning

Profile scanning is a technique yielding essentially a one-dimensional determination of the distribution of radioactivity within an object (Tothill,

1974). A detector large enough to view the full width of the body along a narrow slice samples the activity in the body from head to toe by moving parallel to the long axis of the body (or by having the body move past it along its long axis). It is faster and more sensitive than conventional scanning techniques, but gives no information about the distribution of radioactivity at right angles to the long axis of the body. Its use is restricted to those situations in which it is not necessary to image this distribution but rather to determine it in a quantitative way along the long axis. The technique has been used in skeletal surveys, mainly involving the spine (DeNardo *et al.*, 1967), which is essentially a one-dimensional object with finite thickness. Profile scans of the spine (in search for metastatic disease) are rapid and simple. Newer radiopharmaceuticals have made conventional scans of the entire skeleton fairly rapid, and profile scanning has not achieved widespread application.

3.7.5. Dual-Isotope Subtraction

It happens occasionally that a radiopharmaceutical is taken up not only by an organ of interest, but also by another organ adjacent to it in such a manner as to present an unacceptably high background. An example of this is scanning of the pancreas with selenium-75 selenomethionine, which is taken up both by the pancreas and by the liver. The liver is adjacent to the pancreas and in many cases overlaps it. Although the uptake of the radiopharmaceutical per gram of tissue is greater in the pancreas than in the liver, the larger bulk of the liver overshadows the pancreas and may obliterate its image. A method of getting around this problem was devised by Kaplan *et al.* (1966), who added a second radioisotope of different energy, which is taken up by the liver but not the pancreas. Counts from the liver-seeking radioisotope were subtracted from the total count (liver and pancreas combined) to enhance the image of the pancreas. To accomplish this a rectilinear scanner was equipped with two pulse height analyzers, one window of which was set to the energy of the selenium-75 and the other to that of gold-198, which (as gold colloid) was used to image the liver. Radiocolloids are taken up primarily by the liver and the spleen, and to a lesser extent by bone marrow and lung. Better radioactive colloids are now available for liver imaging but Se-75 selenomethionine is still used for the pancreas. By adjusting windows and scaling factors so that the net count rate over the liver (which contains both radioisotopes) is zero, the image of the pancreas (which contains no radiocolloid) is enhanced. Very satisfactory images of the pancreas can be obtained in this manner. Subtraction scanning has been used to image subphrenic abscesses, which are abscesses located between the liver and right hemidiaphragm (Damron *et al.*, 1976), by using a combination of gallium-67 citrate (which is taken up both by inflammatory tissue and by the normal liver) and technetium-99m sulfur colloid (which is taken up by the liver but not by inflammatory tissue). Subtracting the liver counts from the combined liver/abscess counts yields an enhanced image of the abscess. The subtraction scanning technique has been used to enhance the parathyroid gland, subtracting the thyroid, and to enhance bone scans after background vascular activity has been subtracted (Patton, 1970).

Subtraction scanning has been used with a dual-color display (Ben-Porath *et al.*, 1969), based on a video system. The use of two colors enables one to preserve the information in both images and to display them independently using a color addition technique.

3.8. CLINICAL CONSIDERATIONS: SCANNER OR CAMERA?

Each nuclear medicine clinic must decide what types of imaging devices would be most appropriate for its clinical needs. Both cameras and scanners have advantages and disadvantages that must be considered in making choices. Gamma cameras have the advantage of being faster, capable of dynamic images, capable of imaging a fairly large area all at once, and being easily set up. They can image patients in almost any plane. Disadvantages include a limited field per image (unless the moving whole body table is used), limited useful gamma energy range (resolution is very poor for gamma energies much below 90 keV or above 350 keV), greater sensitivity for activity in structures adjacent to the collimator than for activity deeper within the body (this is frequently a problem in brain scans), and somewhat higher cost. Rectilinear scanners have the advantage of tomographic capability by virtue of their focused collimator, by which they can image sources located deep within the body (Fig. 3-15); a thicker crystal, by which it can image a far wider range of gamma energies, ranging

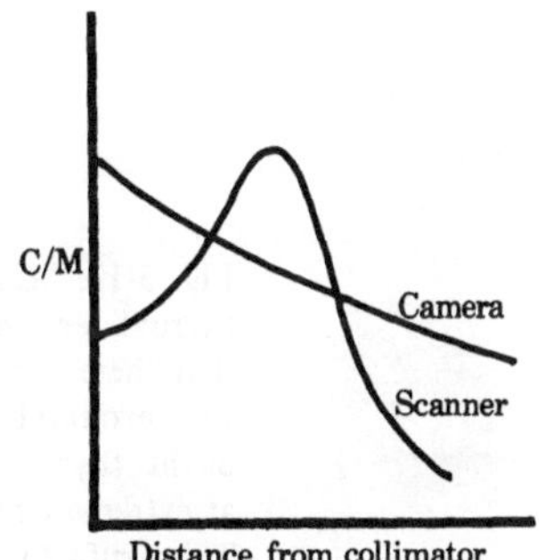

Fig. 3-15. The sensitivity of the rectilinear scanner and gamma camera as a function of distance from the collimator. Because of the focusing collimator the rectilinear scanner has maximum sensitivity for sources located at a certain depth. The gamma camera, on the other hand, has maximum sensitivity for sources located immediately adjacent to the collimator. In selecting which instrument to use for clinical imaging applications, one might select the rectilinear scanner to visualize an organ that lay at some depth beneath the surface, especially if there were some conflicting activity overlying it.

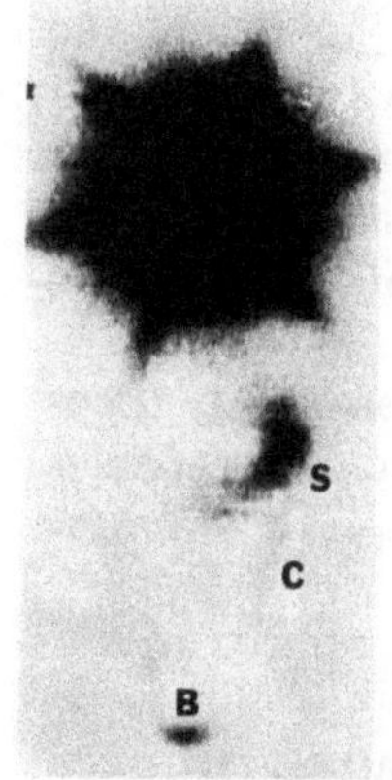

Fig. 3-16. Rectilinear "star" artifact. This is a whole body scan of a patient who received a large amount of I-131 to treat thyroid cancer. The scan was done to search for metastatic disease. The large focus of activity at the top of the picture represents activity in the remaining thyroid gland. The "star" artifact results from penetration of collimator septa by the high-energy radiation from I-131. The star assumes a six-pointed configuration because of the trilinear configuration of the collimator holes. Note the normal structures also visualized: the stomach (S), the colon (C), and the bladder (B). No metastatic disease was found.

from 30 keV to 1 MeV; and a large field of view albeit the field must be sampled point by point. Disadvantages of the rectilinear scanner include its limitations to static imaging only, its somewhat slower imaging speed, limitation to one plane, and somewhat more complex setup. Many nuclear medicine imaging facilities employ both cameras and scanners.

The rectilinear scanner can produce life-size images. This feature is useful as it enables the physician to superimpose the image on the patient, or on an X-ray of the patient. Rectilinear scans are sometimes used to guide biopsy or surgical procedures.

Rectilinear scans are subject to some characteristic artifacts, most of which can be eliminated by proper setup procedure. Scalloping has been discussed in a previous section. Septal penetration artifacts (Fig. 3-16) may occur when collimator septal thickness is not enough to absorb all of the off-axis radiation. The "overshoot" or "saturation" artifact (Fig. 3-17) is a result of detector dead time which limits the count rate the detector can handle. If the actual count rate exceeds the detector capability, the observed count rate will drop and the image will show an inappropriate decrease in density.

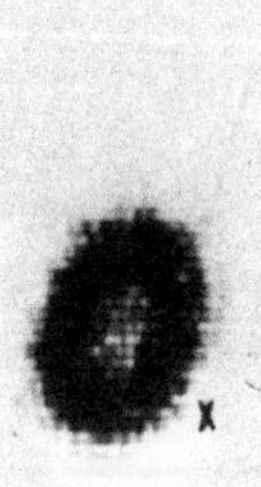

Fig. 3-17. "Overshoot" artifact. This patient had had one lobe of the thyroid removed. Scan was done to examine the remaining lobe. Note that there appears to be less activity in the central portion of the lobe than around the periphery. In actuality the activity is higher in the center of this thyroid gland. The artifact results from saturation of the detector at extremely high count rates, resulting in an apparent drop in activity. This artifact is eliminated by correct setting of the scanner controls.

3.9. RADIOPHARMACEUTICAL SELECTION

Radionuclides and their chemical forms (radiopharmaceuticals) must be selected so as to match the capabilities of the imaging instruments. In the case of rectilinear scanners, a wide range of gamma energies is usable (see preceding section). The half-life of the radionuclide within the body depends on its physical half-life, which is governed by the laws of radioactive decay, and its biological half-life, which is governed by metabolic processes. The physical half-life, of course, is independent of the fact that the material is inside the body, while the biological half-life is independent of the fact that the material is radioactive. The effective half-life must be chosen so as to match the time required for the study while giving an acceptable radiation dose to the patient. A radionuclide with a physical half-life of 1 sec would be unsuitable for studies of bone metabolism, while one with an effective half-life of 20 years would be unsuitable as it would linger in the body long after the study is completed, delivering radiation without benefit to the patient. An ideal effective half-life is one that is comparable to, and somewhat longer than, the time required to complete the study. Corrections for radioactive decay are complex but can be facilitated by the use of computers. Positron-emitting radionuclides comprise about half of all available radionuclides, and recent advances in positron imaging have spurred interest in them. Ideally, the radiopharmaceutical should emit neither alpha nor beta radiation: such radiation (particulate radiation) contributes to the radiation dose while contributing nothing to the image. Finally, the biological handling of the radiopharmaceutical must be such that the tracer accurately reflects the metabolic process being studied. For example, radioactive iodine in the form of iodide ion behaves exactly the same as stable iodine in the same chemical form; this is the tracer principle. On the other hand the metabolism of amino acids such as tyrosine cannot be evaluated by using radioiodinated forms, as radioiodinated tyrosine is not a tracer equivalent of tyrosine in terms of metabolic behavior.

The selection of radiopharmaceuticals available in nuclear medicine is changing rapidly. It is interesting to note that of 22 radiopharmaceuticals described as "frequently used" in a well known 1967 textbook on nuclear medicine (Brownell *et al.*, 1967), 16 (73%) are no longer in widespread use at the present writing.

3.10. PATIENT FACTORS

Imaging systems are generally developed and calibrated using radioactive phantoms. When the phantoms are imaged satisfactorily, the system is then used to image patients. There is a world of difference between imaging

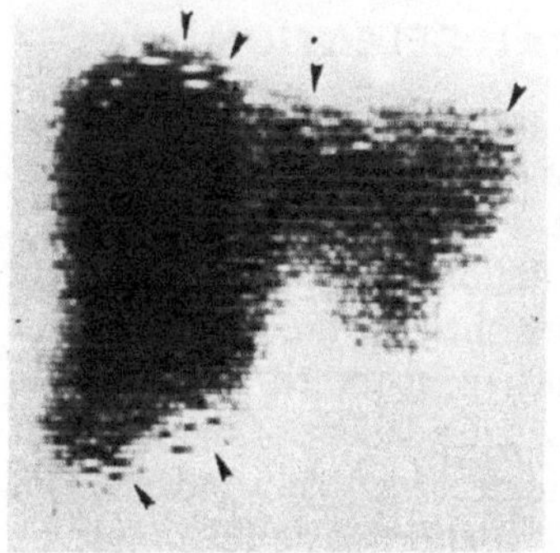

Fig. 3-18. Respiration artifact. Liver scan showing apparent irregularities along the superior and inferior surfaces (arrowheads). These irregularities result from movement of the liver in and out of the field as the patient breathes during the scan. Breathing, a vertical motion in this orientation, brings the liver in and out of the sensitive field of the detector which is moving in a horizontal direction. In actuality the entire liver suffers from the respiration artifact, but it is only at the superior and inferior surfaces where the liver actually moves in and out of the field of view that the artifact is most noticeable.

phantoms and imaging patients. People come in a variety of sizes and shapes. A liver scan of a patient who is very fat may look substantially different from one in a thin patient, and such differences must be taken into account. Large breasts may obscure underlying activity and resemble artifacts. Patient motion can obscure detail in radionuclide images, and in fact liver scans suffer from respiratory motion in a manner that is peculiar to rectilinear scanners (Fig. 3-18). The position the patient is in when scanned can affect the appearance of the organ being imaged. To obtain a lateral view with the rectilinear scanner (which can only image in the horizontal plane), it is necessary to place the patient on his side (decubitus position). Since the body is not a rigid box, structures inside the body such as the liver, lung, heart, kidneys, etc. tend to move in complex ways when the patient is on his side, and do not represent an orthogonal projection to that obtained in anterior or posterior views when the patient is supine or prone. Finally, the possibility of artifacts must be considered. Metal objects in the patient's clothing or worn about the body may introduce artifacts resembling focal defects. Prosthetic devices must be removed prior to scanning. Radioactivity excreted from the body in saliva or urine may contaminate the field and introduce confusing artifacts. Brain scans are subject to artifacts including lesions of the scalp or skull, metal plates in the skull, other metallic objects (bullets) in the head, hearing aids, and glass eyes. Liver scans may show apparent defects which in reality are artifacts caused by cigarette lighters, belts, coins, or other metal objects carried or worn about the body. The imaging technologist must be constantly aware of possible artifacts due to body build, motion, foreign objects, and all the other imaging pitfalls which, after all, are ordinary human attributes.

REFERENCES

Ben-Porath, M., Clayton, G.D., and Kaplan, E. (1969), Tape recording of dual-channel energy-modulated color scanning, *J. Nucl. Med.* **10**:155.

Brownell, G.L., Aronow, S., and Hine, G.J. (1967), Radioisotope scanning, in Hine, G.J. (ed.), *Instrumentation in Nuclear Medicine*, Vol. 1, Academic Press, New York.

Brownell, G.L., and Burnham, C.A. (1974), Recent developments in positron scintigraphy, in Hine, G.J., and Sorenson, J.A. (eds.), *Instrumentation in Nuclear Medicine*, Vol. 2, Academic Press, New York.

Cassen, B., and Curtis, L. (1951), The *in vivo* delineation of thyroid glands with an automatically scanning recorder, UCLA Report No. 130.

Cassen, B., Curtis, L., Reed, C., and Libby, R. (1951), Instrumentation for I-131 use in medical studies, *Nucleonics* **9:**46.

Christie, J.H., MacIntyre, W.J., Ferber, C.J., and King, R.L. (1965), Area recording and data blending in radioisotope scanning, *J. Nucl. Med.* **6:**333.

Damron, J.R., Beihn, R.M., and DeLand, F.H. (1976), Detection of upper abdominal abscesses by radionuclide imaging, *Radiology* **120:**131.

DeNardo, G.L., Horner, R.W., Leach, P.J., and Bowes, D.J. (1967), Radioisotope skeletal survey, *J. Am. Med. Assoc.* **200:**111.

DiChiro, G., Ommaya, A.K., Ashburn, W.L., and Briner, W.H. (1968), Isotope cisternography in the diagnosis and follow-up of cerebrospinal fluid rhinorrhea, *J. Neurosurg.* **28:**522.

Gregg, E.C. (1965), Information capacity of scintiscans, *J. Nucl. Med.* **6:**441.

Harris, C.C., Satterfield, M.M., Ross, D.A., and Bell, P.R. (1968), Moving-detector scanners *versus* stationary imaging devices, in Gottschalk, A., and Beck, R.N. (eds.), *Fundamental Problems in Scanning*, Charles C Thomas, Springfield, Illinois.

Hine, G.J., and Erickson, J.J. (1974), Advances in scintigraphic instruments, in Hine, G.J., and Sorenson, J.A. (eds.), *Instrumentation in Nuclear Medicine*, Vol. 2, Academic Press, New York.

Kaplan, E., Ben-Porath, M., Fink, S., Clayton, G.D., and Jacobson, B. (1966), Elimination of liver interference from the selenomethionine pancreas scan, *J. Nucl. Med.* **7:**807.

Knowles, L.G., Hart, E.F., and Schulz, A.G. (1972), Effect of line spacing and ratemeter averaging on lesion detection, *J. Nucl. Med.* **13:**191.

Kuhl, D.E., and Sanders, T.P. (1971), Characterizing brain lesions using transverse section scanning, *Radiology* **98:**317.

Kuhl, D.E., Edwards, R.Q., Ricci, A.R., and Reivich, M. (1973), Quantitative section scanning using orthogonal tangent correction, *J. Nucl. Med.* **14:**196.

Leins, P.A., Bodfish, R.E., and Patton, D.D. (1969), Simple pocket-sized data blender for scans, *J. Nucl. Med.* **10:**417.

Morgan, R.H. (1966), Visual perception in fluoroscopy and radiography, *Radiology* **86:**402.

Mozley, J.M. (1968), The modulation transfer function for scanners, in Gottschalk, A., and Beck, R.N. (eds.), *Fundamental Problems in Scanning*, Charles C Thomas, Springfield, Illinois.

Myhill, J., and Hine, G.J. (1967), Multihole collimators for scanning, in Hine, G.J. (ed.), *Instrumentation in Nuclear Medicine*, Vol. 1, Academic Press, New York.

Oldendorf, W.H., Palmer, J., and Patton, D.D. (1967), Quasi-gaussian defocussing of the radioisotope scan, in Fogel, L.J., and George, F.W. (eds.), *Progress in Biomedical Engineering*, Spartan, Washington, D.C.

Patton, D.D. (1970), Elimination of soft tissue from ^{87m}Sr bone scans by dual-isotope subtraction, *J. Nucl. Med.* **11:**348.

Phelps, M.E., Hoffman, E.J., Mullani, N.A., and Ter-Pogossian, M.M. (1975), Application of annihilation coincidence detection to transaxial reconstruction tomography, *J. Nucl. Med.* **16:**210.

Phelps, M.E., Hoffman, E.J., Coleman, R.E., Welch, M.J., Raichle, M.E., Weiss, E.S., Sobel, B.E., and Ter-Pogossian, M.M. (1976), Tomographic images of blood pool and perfusion in brain and heart, *J. Nucl. Med.* **17:**603.

Rankowitz, S., Robertson, J. S., Higinbotham, W. A., and Rosenblum, M. J. (1961), Positron scanner for locating brain tumors, *IRE Int. Conv. Rec.* **9**:49.

Rollo, F. D., and Schulz, A. G. (1970), A contrast efficiency function for quantitatively measuring the spatial-resolution characteristics of scanning systems, *J. Nucl. Med.* **11**:53.

Schulz, A. G., Knowles, L. G., Kohlenstein, L. C., Mucci, R. F., and Yates, W. A. (1970), Quantitative assessment of scanning-system parameters, *J. Nucl. Med.* **11**:61.

Ter-Pogossian, M. M., Phelps, M. E., Hoffman, E. J., and Mullani, N. A. (1975), Positron-emission transaxial tomograph for nuclear imaging (PETT), *Radiology* **114**:89.

Tothill, P. (1974), Profile scanning, in Hine, G. J., and Sorenson, J. A. (eds.), *Instrumentation in Nuclear Medicine*, Vol. 2, Academic Press, New York.

Ziedses des Plantes, B. G. (1973), Direct and indirect autoradiography, in (editors anonymous), *Selected Works of B. G. Ziedses des Plantes*, Excerpta Medica, Amsterdam. (Paper read at the Sixth International Congress of Radiology, London, 1950.)

CHAPTER 4

A Review of Gamma Camera Technology for Medical Imaging

RONALD E. McKEIGHEN

4.1. INTRODUCTION

The ability to visualize the uptake within the body of radio-labeled pharmaceuticals spawned the now clinically established field of nuclear medicine. Pioneering studies were done with single-crystal PMT detectors mechanically scanned over the patient in raster fashion. The practice of nuclear medicine achieved a milestone with the invention in 1956 by Hal Anger of the scintillation camera. With this, activity could be processed in real time making dynamic blood flow studies possible and greatly reducing imaging times for static studies. In a scintillation camera the x,y coordinate of each gamma ray interaction in the detector is determined and a spot of light is electronically generated in a corresponding position on the face of a display device (CRT). Each such spot contributes to the latent image on photographic film. The overlap of several of these spots results in a visible dot on the film whose brightness is proportional to the number

RONALD E. McKEIGHEN • Searle Diagnostics, Inc., 2000 Nuclear Drive, Des Plaines, Illinois 60018. *Present address*: K. B. Aerotech, P.O.Box 350, Lewistown, Pennsylvania 17044.

of overlapped events. The "image" of the object radioactive source distribution is consequently the result of hundreds of thousands of these dots recorded on the film. The perceived image brightness in any section is a combination of the number of dots per unit area and individual dot brightness which combination in turn is directly proportional to the number of detected gamma rays per unit area. Examples of gamma camera scintiphotos are illustrated in Figs. 4-9 through 4-12 taken from clinical studies. The Anger camera has been continually refined since its invention, but one normally expects that after 20 years a given technology or invention will be superceded by new advances in other approaches. Indeed there has been a veritable potpourri of schemes investigated or proposed for implementing a gamma camera. I will here review the more significant of the many schemes and discuss their features and drawbacks.

There are devices of limited versatility having unique characteristics for specific applications, for instance a device that has superb resolution but a small field of view or one that can handle tremendous count rates for dynamic studies but has poor resolution. Although one might build special purpose devices superior in a particular specification, a real replacement for the Anger camera must be a general purpose device superior in many respects to the overall performance of the Anger camera, and at a competitive cost. Technical performance features of a system to be considered are its (1) spatial resolution, which consists of the intrinsic camera resolution convolved with the collimator resolution; (2) count rate capability, or conversely, system dead time; (3) high detection efficiency for gamma rays of 100–500 keV energy; (4) field of view; (5) pulse height discrimination capability to eliminate image contrast degradation due to scattered gamma rays and background radiation; (6) uniformity of response over the field of view and freedom from distracting spatial distortions; (7) complexity; (8) cost. For clinical utility, the useful field of view should be 30–40 cm in diameter and imaging times for a given study should not be lengthened beyond currently accepted norms.

In this survey, in addition to the Anger camera, we will consider the following generic types of gamma camera systems: (1) image intensifier systems; (2) multiple-crystal cameras; (3) cameras using solid state (semiconductor) detectors; (4) multiwire proportional chambers (MWPC); (5) a camera using the light scintillations in liquid xenon; (6) hybrid scanner–cameras; and (7) techniques not requiring multichannel collimators.

4.2. IMAGE INTENSIFIER CAMERAS

Perhaps because of their excellent intrinsic electro-optical image resolution and their successful application in radiology, image intensifiers have attracted many workers seeking to build a successful gamma ray imaging device for nuclear medicine. Anger tried this approach initially in 1952–1954. However, the many designs have met with basic difficulties. Although some can give good images of phantoms or bar patterns, they are often plagued with a basic lack of contrast in a clinical situation. Good pulse height discrimination is also very difficult to attain. A good discussion of image intensifier cameras and their difficulties is given in a survey by Moody *et al.* (1970) and a good review by Anger (1966a).

The various approaches taken may be discussed under one of three basic groupings involving the use of (a) large-diameter image intensifier tube, (b) small-diameter intensifier viewing large-area scintillator minified through a lens, (c) image intensifiers with capability of estimating centroid of light distribution.

4.2.1. Large-Diameter Image Intensifier Systems

Gamma cameras built around image intensifiers of large diameter (~9 in.) have included that of the University of Toronto (Moody *et al.*, 1969, 1973), C. Kellershohn (Moody, 1970), the Magnacamera (Ter-Pogossian, 1969) marketed by Picker, and the Quantascope by Harshaw. Both the Quantascope and the University of Toronto (U.T.) cameras make use of a mosaic of thick scintillation crystal elements placed on the curved intensifier faceplate. The camera of Kellershohn uses a thin (3-mm) single-crystal disk of CsI(Tl) placed like a watchglass on the face of the first image intensifier, while the Magnacamera (Ter-Pogossian) has its 1.5-mm-thick CsI(Na) phosphor incorporated inside the first intensifier just behind the input window.

The University of Toronto approach features a CsI(Na) mosaic of some 1500 elements (0.16 in. square × 1 in. long) on a 9-in.-diameter image intensifier as illustrated in Fig. 4-1. After three years of research, they can now make 40-element (1.5 in. square × 1 in. deep) subunits in a single operation. The element spacing is 3/16 in. but the effective size is degraded by the glass faceplate (0.080 in.) and collimator to about 1/4 in. (6.4 mm). At 2 in. from the collimator a bar pattern of 1/4 in. separation was resolved. It should be noted, however, that at 4 in. the collimator resolution is about 9.6 mm FWHM. At the time of their Monaco report (1972) only 1/9 of the full mosaic area had been assembled for evaluation. In some situations the lines separating submosaics are visible and might prove a nuisance. Pulse height discrimination is achieved by switching on a later intensifier stage. After the first stage of intensification, light missing the lens coupling the later stage is collected by an elliptically shaped disk and measured by a PMT and single-channel analyzer. To compensate for a photocathode variation of 50% and the pulse height variation from crystal element to

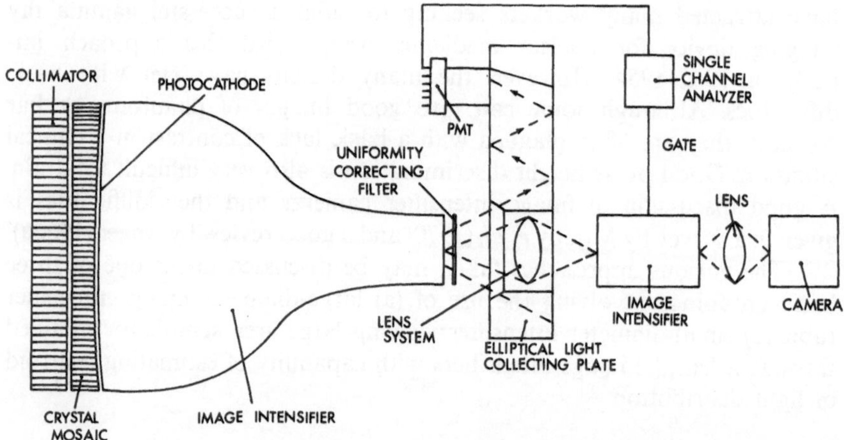

Fig. 4-1. University of Toronto image intensifier gamma camera illustrating crystal mosaic and pulse height determination scheme.

element, an equalizing filter transparency was introduced in front of the coupling lens to yield better uniformity. With the filter, an energy resolution of 18.5% FWHM was obtained for ^{203}Hg (279 keV), as compared to an energy resolution of about 11% for the Anger camera. The resolving time of the camera is limited by the decay time of the phosphors, i.e., of the scintillator convolved with each phosphor of the intensifier cascade (typically P15). Pulse height analysis is done on the first 30–40% of available light in a pulse ($\Delta\tau \simeq 0.5\ \mu$sec) and if accepted, the remaining stages are switched on to image the remaining available light. In the U.T. camera the tube is held on for 3 μsec for each accepted event. It should be noted though that the maximum count rate is not necessarily restricted by this parameter. In fast dynamic studies where scatter rejection may not be so important, the shutter tube could be left on so that the image intensifier becomes a parallel processor with essentially no limits on count rate.

The Quantascope developed by Harshaw used a 10-in.-diameter image intensifier with a diverging collimator giving it about a 16-in.-diameter field of view at 4 in. There were 2515 matched CsI(Tl) scintillation crystals aligned with the holes in the collimator. The 1/8-in.-diameter by 5/8-in.-long crystals were arranged in a hexagonal array on 3/16-in. centers. Application of the geometrical formulas for the resolution of a collimator indicates that for the collimator described, the resolution at 4 in. would be about 13 mm. Because of the discrete crystal mosaic, resolution is independent of gamma ray energy, in contrast to the Anger camera. Pulse height discrimination is achieved through the unique deflection-gating action of the specially designed tube (Fig. 4-2). Because of light losses in each crystal, pulse height resolution was worse than in the Anger camera. Dead time is again determined by the decay time of the scintillator in conjunction with the output phosphors and is a few microseconds, similar to the U.T. camera.

The instrument developed by Kellershohn (Moody, 1970) used a thin single-crystal disk (3 mm) of CsI(Tl) as opposed to thick individual crystals (Fig. 4-3) and is reported to yield 5-mm resolution at the gamma ray phosphor. Because of the thin crystal used, the photopeak detection efficiency for stopping 150-keV gamma rays will be about 65%, lower than the Anger camera's value of 80–90%. Pulse height discrimination is achieved by gating later intensifier stages in a manner similar to the U.T. camera, but with lower optical collection efficiency. To maintain good spatial resolution, an air gap had to be left between the scintillation crystal and the intensifier faceplate, reducing the yield of photocathode electrons. Consequently, pulse height resolution was poor, being on the order of 50%. Because of gating requirements and electronic difficulties, the count rate capability was also rather poor.

Ter-Pogossian's Magnacamera has its thin (1.5-mm) CsI(Na) phosphor incorporated inside the first-stage image intensifier in intimate contact with the photocathode. Because of the thin phosphor, the total gamma ray absorption efficiency is only 40% at 140 keV and falls to 10% at 270 keV. The intrinsic resolution of this camera is stated to be 2 mm, which, combined with the collimator, yielded an overall system resolution of 10 mm at 10-cm object distance. Here again the resolution is independent of gamma ray

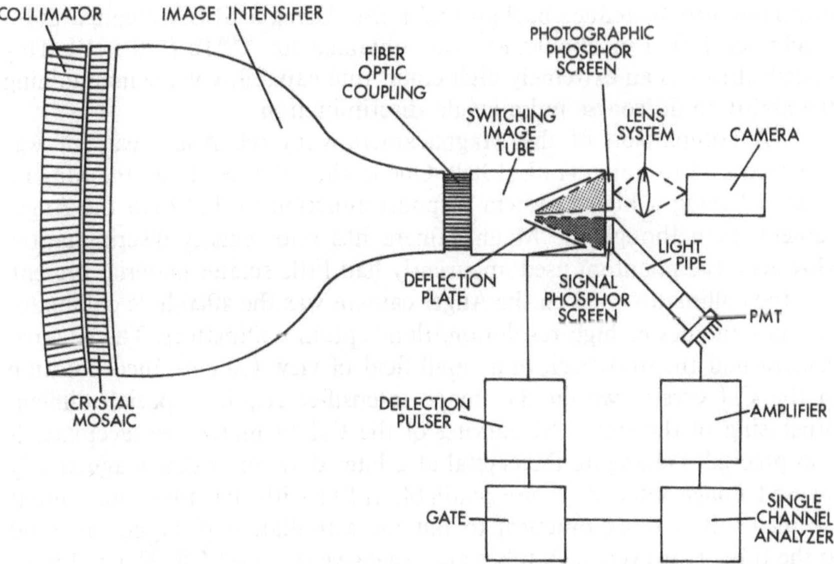

Fig. 4-2. The Quantascope by Harshaw. Special image intensifier tube with pulse height analysis and deflection circuitry is depicted.

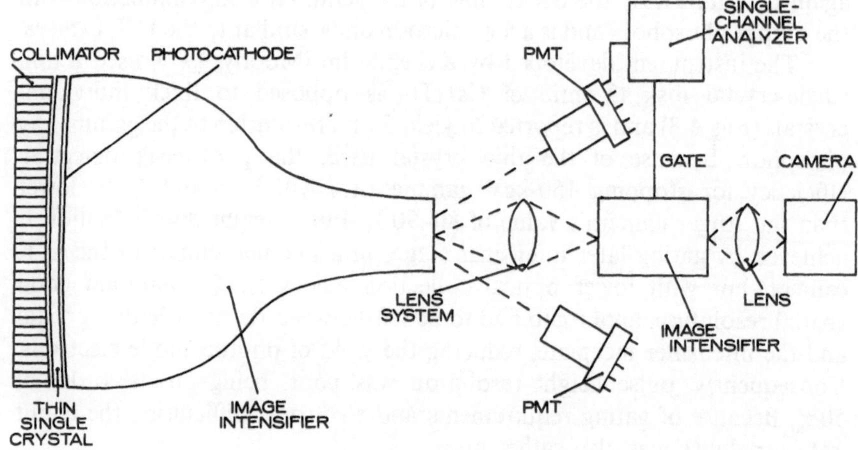

Fig. 4-3. Image intensifier camera of Kellershohn and Lansiart illustrating pulse height discrimination scheme. Magnacamera developed by Ter-Pogossian was similar except its scintillation crystal was incorporated within the vacuum envelope and did not have pulse height analysis.

energy. The output of the image intensifier was viewed through a lens by a TV camera. Although no satisfactory photopeak can be expected, the video signal from the vidicon can be subjected to upper- and lower-level discriminators to reduce background noise. Using a SEC vidicon, a pulse height resolution of about 58% was obtained for ^{99m}Tc (140 keV). This system thus has an extremely high count rate capability while maintaining the ability to do coarse pulse height discrimination.

A comparison of the Magnacamera with the Anger camera was reported by Freedman *et al.* (1969). One of their figures shows the Magnacamera having a higher system response function (MTF) than the Anger camera, even though the Magnacamera has poor energy discrimination. However, the phantom used apparently had little scatter material present, and the collimator used on the Anger camera was the 4000-hole collimator and not the newer high-resolution, thin-septum collimators. The Magnacamera had the drawback of a small field of view (20 cm). Incorporation of the CsI crystal within the image intensifier requires special, difficult processing of the tube and curving of the CsI to match the faceplate. It also precludes changing the crystal at a later date. Now that magnetically focused image intensifiers are available (ITT) with flat, fiber optic input faceplates, it is more practical to put the scintillation phosphor external to the tube. However, such tubes are expensive ($20,000–$40,000) and have rather limited diameters (~ 6 in.). The Magnacamera was plagued by uniformity problems which made the useful field of view even smaller, but apparently part of this problem was in the orthicon TV camera used. The Anger camera has better field sensitivity and uniformity and also includes two electronic features the Magnacamera does not: pulse height analysis and quantitative information storage and output. In addition, adaptation for digital computer processing is more difficult with the Magnacamera than with the Anger camera. On the other hand, video recording comes naturally and the image intensifier camera is well suited for handling high-count-rate fast dynamic studies with moderate resolution, especially when larger amounts of radioactive tracer can be safely administered to the patient to offset the decreased stopping power of the thin crystal used.

The image intensifier cameras described have pulse height discrimination capability inferior to that of the Anger camera. In the individual pulse-processing mode, the dead time will also be long because of the decay time of the phosphors in the various stages. However, if one is willing to forego pulse height discrimination, these systems are capable of handling very high count rates. The cameras using a mosaic of thick scintillation crystals have good gamma ray stopping power but the resultant resolution is no better than the Anger camera is capable of. The approaches using a thin scintillation crystal yielded good intrinsic resolution but the consequently lower gamma ray interaction probability means longer clinical imaging times and increased chance of resolution degradation due to patient motion. Also the range of useful isotope energies is restricted to 30–290 keV, whereas the useful range of the Anger camera is 70 keV to over 500 keV.

4.2.2. Small-Diameter Image Intensifier Viewing Large-Area Scintillator through Lens

Gamma cameras of this type are exemplified by the Aber-gammascope (Mallard and Wilkes, 1969; Mitchell *et al.*, 1973) and the one developed at the University of Michigan (Thomas *et al.*, 1969). The image intensifier used here is typically 1 or 2 in. in diameter. Light generated by a scintillation in a thick crystal is focused by a lens onto the input photocathode of the image intensifier (see Fig. 4-4). Good quantum detection efficiency is difficult to attain because of the constraints of light collection efficiency. A 140-keV photoelectric interaction in NaI(Tl) would typically yield 5600 optical photons. Considering the light collection efficiency of an *f*/0.87, 76-mm focal length lens with transmission losses, the average number of photons incident on the first photocathode of the image intensifier is only about 1.61 (Thomas *et al.*, 1969). If the front surface of the NaI crystal is mirrored this could be raised to about 2.42 photons reaching the photocathode. For a bialkali photocathode having 24% efficiency, on the average then, 0.58 photoelectrons are emitted for each 140 keV gamma absorbed. Assuming a

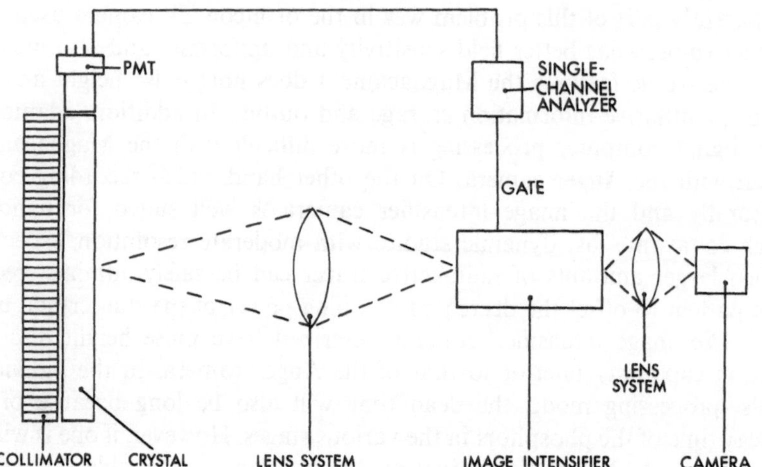

Fig. 4-4. Principle of gamma camera investigated at University of Michigan and University of Aberdeen (Aber-gammascope).

Poisson distribution, there is a probability of 0.44 for the emission of one or more photoelectrons. Actual experimental measurements at the University of Michigan for 140-keV gamma rays yielded values from 0.15 to 0.30 for the probability of one or more photoelectrons per event in the crystal. In effect this means that the quantum utilization of the activity emitted from the patient is low, increasing imaging time.

Mitchell *et al.* (1973), developing the Aber-gammascope, had worked with Varian Associates to increase the light collection efficiency and consequently the photoelectron per gamma ratio. Briefly, the greater the minification of the lens system, i.e., the bigger the field of view required, the smaller is the photoelectron per gamma efficiency. Conversely, if the diameter of the image intensifier is increased, the efficiency will also increase. Varian did computer calculations for a 10-cm(3.94-in.)-diameter intensifier in conjunction with an optical system giving a 14-in. field of view and employing two glass lenses, several acrylic lenses, and two mirrors, one between the crystal and collimator (Mitchell *et al.*, 1973). Assuming 12% light conversion efficiency in NaI, this gave 30 focused photons for a full energy 140 keV gamma event on axis. Further assuming 18% photocathode efficiency, the photoemission is 5.4 electrons on center, and 3.8 electrons for an event at field periphery. To obtain 15–20% energy resolution similar to the Anger camera would require the release of an average of about 240 photoelectrons per gamma ray event! Using a homemade plastic (Perspex) lens system of 9-in.-diameter at a minification of 7:1 and a 2-in.-diameter image intensifier, Mallard and Wilkes (1969) have estimated an average of 5.8 photoelectrons released per incident gamma ray, using a 1/2-in.-thick

NaI(Tl) crystal. This number is too small to get reasonable pulse height discrimination to reject scattered gamma rays. Therefore, to accomplish good pulse height discrimination, analysis is made on the light per scintillation that never reaches the image intensifier but is trapped in the scintillation crystal and piped to the edge of the crystal by total internal reflections. This amounts to 85% of the light produced per scintillation (Mitchell *et al.*, 1973). Light guides collect this light which is then measured by photomultipliers for pulse height analysis. The image intensifier is subsequently gated on when an acceptable event has occurred. After some work on the design of light guides, Mitchell *et al.* (1973) measured the FWHM for a point source of ^{99m}Tc (140 keV) to be 22%. Due to nonuniformities, the FWHM averaged over the full field of view would be expected to be higher than this value. (The University of Michigan obtained a FWHM of 30% within a 4-in. radius of center but was about 70% FWHM for the full field of view.) This was an improvement on the previous FWHM of 45% but the clinical results still proved to be disappointing because of the severe lack of contrast in clinical situations.

Subsequently, the three main components of the system, i.e., image intensifier, crystal, and lens, were studied to determine which one contributed most to the degradation. The results indicated that much of the problem was due to light trapped in the crystal escaping from scratches and imperfections and being imaged by the system as light spots well away from the original scintillation point. This contribution increases as the area of the scintillation crystal increases. For a 35-cm field flooded with gammas except for a small shielded area, the illumination of this cold area is 25% of the flooded field area. The contrast loss due to this phenomenon could be eliminated either by using a crystal with an optical quality polished finish or by employing a CCD imaging array to discriminate and read out the recorded image frame by frame. Fairchild recently announced a 488 × 380 CCD array sensitive down to an illumination of 1.5 × 10^{-5} ft cd sec. Even more recently RCA has come out with a 163,840 element array (512 × 320). The use of these arrays coupled to the output of the image intensifier would have several desirable properties: (1) High count rate capability. For example, at high frame readout rates such as 400 per second, data rates of several hundred thousand counts per second could be accommodated; (2) frame storage for high sensitivity—each diode integrates photocurrent for the entire frame time; (3) self-scanning in both X and Y for serial video output; (4) computer compatible outputs/inputs; (5) crude pulse height discrimination might be done on the contents of each photodiode cell as it is read out serially. This would minimize or eliminate the effect of the dark current of the image tube and other spurious signals since they would be accumulated only over one frame time after which they can be eliminated during frame readout by lower-level discrimination. The contrast loss due to spurious light scatter from the scintillation crystal could also be eliminated in the same manner. Mallard and co-workers (Mitchell *et al.*, 1973) concluded that:

> ...setting a discrimination to define at least 3 photoelectrons per event will reduce the total scatter (optical background) to 0.2%. For equivalent collimator sensitivity and crystal thickness, the large lens–image intensifier system operated in this mode will have sensitivity and contrast comparable to the Anger camera. The calculated intrinsic resolution for 140 keV gamma events at any position over the full 35 cm diameter field is 2 to 3 mm FWHM, depending on the image recording technique after the image intensifier.

The difficulty of this approach lies in achieving sufficiently good optical light collection efficiency in the process of minifying and projecting a satisfactorily large field of view onto the input of the image intensifier. Sufficient light photons must be collected to assure a high probability of more than one photoelectron being emitted per scintillation event, otherwise, quantum detection efficiency is lower than with the Anger camera and longer imaging time results. The problem of contrast degradation due to light scattered from the detecting phosphor must also be solved.

4.2.3. Image-Intensifier Systems with Capability of Generating Centroid of Light Distribution

The image intensifier cameras described in Section 4.2.1. obtain good detection efficiency by use of thick scintillation crystals and useful field of view by using large-diameter tubes which require thick glass faceplates (2–4 mm). However, light spreading in the thick crystal and glass faceplate degenerates the resolution obtainable. Good resolution could be maintained, however, if the system were capable of recording the event as happening at the centroid of the broadened light spot. One such scheme was investigated in our research department (Muehllehner, 1972). The system used a 8.6-in.-diameter first-stage minifying intensifier optically coupled to two small-diameter intensifiers. A flat, 0.5-in.-thick NaI(T1) crystal was coupled to the curved intensifier faceplate by a light guide. The output detector was a position-sensitive silicon photodiode coupled to the fiber optic output of the last intensifier stage. For each scintillation, four signals are generated whose values are related to the position at which the event occurred and whose sum is proportional to the energy deposited by the gamma ray interaction in the scintillator. With a 35% window, FWHM resolution of about 5 mm was obtained for the 122-keV ^{57}Co gamma. There were nonuniformities at the edge because of the light coupler and the useful field of view was 4–5 in. but could easily be made 7 in. out of the possible 8.6 with a good optical compensation mask. The count rate capability of the system is limited by the dead time determined by the decay time of the scintillator convolved with that of each phosphor in the intensification cascade, but could possibly be held to 2–3 μsec. The incorporation of a silicon position-sensitive detector within the vacuum envelope of the image intensifier has also been considered (Berninger, 1974) (Fig. 4-5). Today, with the availability of Polyscint™(NaI) from Harshaw, a thick scintillator could be molded to the face of the intensifier faceplate and eliminate the interposing light guide. Also, larger-image intensifiers are available. Thompson-CSF now has available image intensifiers with 34-cm (13.4-in.) input diameter and 20-mm output diameter with a 4-mm-thick faceplate. These tubes are billed as being designed for nuclear medicine applications with an S-20 photocathode and a P15 or E6 output phosphor. The noise background from photocathode thermal emission is given as 150–200 e^-/cm^2 sec. A closely related approach would be to read out the coordinate position of an event with four photomultipliers viewing the output phosphor of the image intensifier in place of the previously mentioned position-sensitive semiconductor device. This approach was described independently by both Lansiart *et al.* (1969) and Conrad (1969) and more recently by Driard *et al.* (1976). Siemens worked on such a device under the trade name "Scinticon." A zoom feature on the image intensifier allows one to blow the image up, increasing effective resolvable resolution. For a 32-cm field of view the resolution was said to be 5.4 mm (for ^{99m}Tc) and 3.6 mm for an 18-cm field of view. To summarize, the basic properties of these camera systems are (1) high detection efficiency (same as Anger camera) due to use of 0.5 inch NaI(Tl) crystal, (2) restricted but acceptable field of view, (3) energy discrimination capability, (4) count rate capability less than Anger camera, and (5) good spatial resolution when used in zoom mode to

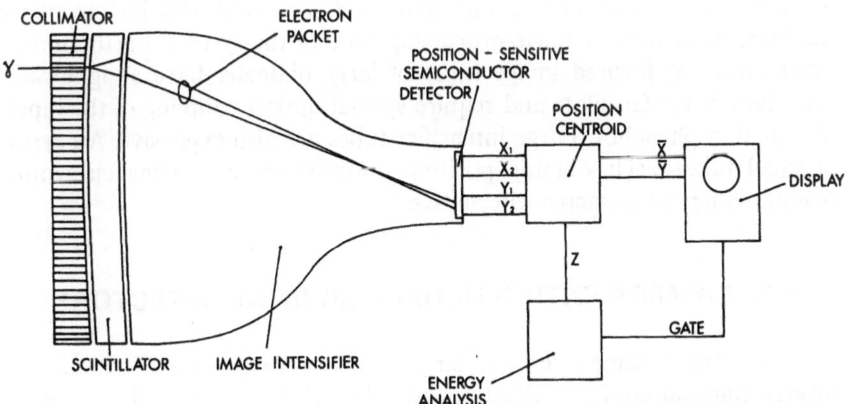

Fig. 4-5. Image intensifier camera with centroid determining capability provided by position-sensitive silicon detector incorporated within tube vacuum.

examine smaller areas. It should be noted that the Anger camera can also be used in a "zoom" mode by using a converging collimator to minimize the limiting effect of intrinsic resolution.

Astronomy researchers have had "one of a kind" image intensifiers made which incorporate one-dimensional self-scanned photodiode arrays inside the vacuum envelope as the readout device. The Electronic Vision Corporation of California made such a tube for the University of Texas, Austin, by incorporating a Reticon 256-element array inside a 1-in. image intensifier. A two-dimensional self-scanned array could be used to generate the centroid of the light distribution. There will be problems with the two-dimensional MOS arrays, however. Since the readout structures are intertwined with the detecting areas, their exposure to the electron beam may result in deterioration.

There is an alternative approach using image intensifiers whose output is capable of giving the centroid of a light distribution. Instead of using one large tube whose diameter is equal to the requisite field of view, one could conceive of using an array of small image tubes, each with a centroid-generating capability. In 1965, Anger (1966) proposed that a gamma camera of improved inherent resolution could be built by development of photomultipliers that give coordinate-indicating readouts. He suggested making the anode of a venetian blind PMT of four intertwined sections (fingers) that would interpolate signal location. Under AEC contract, Burns (1961) of the University of Chicago attempted to develop this tube in consultation with Anger. Unfortunately, the two prototypes built were plagued with breakage and field emission problems and the contract expired before any fruitful results were obtained.

To recapitulate, schemes using image tubes having centroid-calculating capability offer the possibility of improved resolution. However, an image intensifier whose output is a phosphor adds an additional increment to the basic dead time or pulse-processing time of the system. Furthermore, electrostatically focused image tubes of large diameter have a significant curvature of the faceplate and require special optical coupling of the input scintillation phosphor. Large intensifier tubes are also expensive. An array of small tubes, each yielding position information and giving electronic readout, offers an attractive alternative.

4.3. CAMERA WITH MULTIPLE-CRYSTAL DETECTORS

The Anger camera uses a large-diameter single crystal viewed by several photomultipliers. Bender and Blau (1963) developed a camera using 294 individual NaI(Tl) scintillation crystals coupled via a complex light pipe (DiRocco and Grenier, 1967) system to 35 photomultiplier tubes. The 1.1 × 1.1 × 3.8 cm crystals are arranged in 14 rows and 21 columns.

The camera is marketed by Baird Atomic under the trade name Autofluoroscope. Although one would expect that with the thicker discrete crystals, the detection efficiency for high-energy gammas would be higher than the Anger camera's 1.2-cm-thick crystal, Beck (1968) has pointed out that because of Compton scattering out of the individual crystal, the photofraction for events within a given crystal is less than for the Anger camera. Furthermore, since the total photopeak efficiency is a product of the interaction probability times the photofraction, it turns out that the photopeak efficiency of the Autofluoroscope and the Anger camera are equal. The basic image resolution of this system has been improved by placing the patient on a moving bed that increments through 16 steps to effectively generate unit cells smaller than the actual crystal dimensions. The count rate capability of the Autofluoroscope can be quite high if one accepts coarser resolution and uses a coarse collimator in a nonstepping mode. Data from the detector assembly is handled by a computer system and provides useable data at count rates up to 200,000 counts per second. Fast electronics have recently been implemented in the Anger camera and its count rate performance raised to the same limit. Pulse height resolution capability of the Autofluoroscope is only on the order of 50% and thus ability to reject scattered radiation is limited and will result in poor image contrast with the amount of scatter present in most organ studies. In short, this camera system is capable of high count rates but with only 1.5–2.0 cm resolution. At a sacrifice of count rate capability, in the scanning mode, resolution can be improved to about 1.0 cm. Grenier *et al.* (1974) have reviewed the design features and clinical utility of the Autofluoroscope (System 70). In many parameters it is competitive with the Anger camera but offers no advantages. Upgrading of its performance would require a significant increase in complexity and number of components.

4.4. CAMERAS USING SEMICONDUCTOR DETECTORS

Because of their superb energy resolution, semiconductors offer the potential of superior performance over scintillation detectors since less of the scatter fraction is included in the photopeak. The better energy resolution arises because the energy required to form an electron-hole pair is of the order of 3 eV instead of the 30 eV or more ionization potential of gas chambers and scintillation detectors. The state of the art in energy resolution is about 0.4% but crystals with 3–4% energy resolution are more easily attainable. The largest improvement in contrast with the use of semiconductor detectors is achieved in the visualization of cold lesions, because of the increased effectiveness of rejecting scattered radiation from the surrounding activity.

For the detection of gamma rays, there are a number of desirable properties a semiconductor detector should have: (1) high atomic number and density; (2) large detection volume (depletion layer); (3) long carrier life in the excited state (requires minimum trapping and indirect band gap); (4) carrier mobility (collection velocity); (5) low energy required to create an electron-hole pair; (6) large energy bandgap for room temperature operation. A summary of essential material characteristics is given in Table 5-1 of Palms (1971).

To date only silicon and germanium crystals have been developed to sufficient quality for versatile use as radiation detectors. The atomic number and density of silicon are too low for serious consideration as a gamma ray detector. However, lithium-drifted germanium detectors [Ge(Li)] of large volume (up to 100 cm^3) have been widely applied in gamma ray spectroscopy. The comparison between Ge and NaI in their relative efficiencies for gamma ray detection is complicated by the fact that while the effective atomic number of NaI (49.2) is higher than Ge (32), the density of Ge (5.33 g/cm^3) is higher than that of NaI (3.67 g/cm^3). This leads to the interesting fact that above 300 keV the linear attenuation coefficient of Ge is greater than NaI. Using position-sensitive Ge (Li) arrays in a gamma camera, technological problems suggest a limit of about 1.0 cm for the sensitive depth (Parker *et al.*, 1973). At 150 keV the total absorption efficiency of 1 cm of Ge would be about 55% as compared to about 90% for the 1.27-cm-thick NaI crystal used in the Anger camera. Germanium 5 mm thick would have an efficiency of about 33% for total absorption of 150-keV gammas.

The lower stopping power will result in longer imaging time in nuclear medicine applications. Furthermore, it has been shown with scanners that the results of a Ge(Li) detector can be simulated using NaI with the lower-level discriminator set high in the photopeak to eliminate the major portion of scatter (Hoffer and Beck, 1971, and Glass *et al.*, 1973). This results in image quality and detection efficiency comparable to Ge when the NaI energy window baseline is set at 145 keV for the 140-keV technetium photopeak. Glass *et al.* (1973) indicated that when used in scanners, the availability of large Ge crystals with two to three times the sensitivity of their prototype detectors would give the edge to Ge over NaI. In lithium-drifted detectors the high mobility of the lithium ion at room temperature requires the continual cryogenic cooling (liquid nitrogen) of the detectors once fabricated. Germanium of sufficiently high purity that lithium drifting (compensation) is not required is now becoming available, and would permit periodic warming to room temperature.

Although high-purity germanium allows one the liberty of periodic warming to room temperature, there is a fundamental problem of encapsulating the crystals. Crystals encapsulated in a simple vacuum have exhibited a disturbing and dramatic deterioration of detector properties with a time constant varying from a few hours to days. This is due to the formation of a P^+ inversion layer on the surface which shunts the junction. This degradation phenomenon has been traced by Armantrout *et al.* (1974) to the absorption of hydrogen on the surface. Ironically the source of this hydrogen is from within the crystal itself and arises from out diffusion or migration to the surface, in the vacuum environment. This problem could potentially be solved by growing the crystals in hard vacuum. However, all currently available detector-grade high-purity germanium has been grown in hydrogen at atmospheric pressure. Armantrout *et al.* mention two alternatives to vacuum growth which show promise for solving the dilemma of encapsulating high-purity germanium gamma ray detectors by including catalyst and getter materials or driving out the hydrogen with heat. The problem can also be minimized in actively pumped vacuum systems. The presence of an optimum concentration of water vapor in the detector environment prior to cool down has also been shown to improve stability.

Several groups have worked on the development of a gamma ray camera using germanium as the detector (Ter-Pogossian and Phelps, 1973). Three basic designs of semiconductor cameras have been tested to date: the orthogonal strip (Parker *et al.*, 1973; Detko, 1973; McCready *et al.*, 1971; Kaufman *et al.*, 1975; Schlosser *et al.*, 1974), polar coordinate design (Strauss and Sherman, 1972) and resistive divider (Owen and Awcock, 1968; Berninger, 1974). In the orthogonal strip design, the position of an event is determined by the X, Y coordinates of two orthogonal strips. The inherent resolution of these devices is limited by the distance between strips and is approximately twice this distance. Schlosser *et al.* (1974) estimate that for 122 keV, an energy resolution of less than 4 keV and a spatial resolution less than 4 mm are conceivable in these systems. Conceptually, a camera with a large field of view could be constructed using an array of subunits, say, $4 \times 4 \times 1.0$ cm thick. However, germanium detectors are extremely sensitive to surface and environmental effects. The reliable fabrication of detectors whose performance does not degrade in time is still a technical problem to solve and will be compounded in an array scheme (Gelezunas, 1974). Also, pure germanium requires cryogenic cooling in operation in order to reduce leakage currents.

A continuing search is under way for semiconductors with a higher stopping power for gamma rays than silicon or germanium, and that have good detector properties. A tabulation of the properties of various semiconductors is given in Tables I and II of Malm (1972) and Tables 5-1 and 5-2 of Palms (1971). Of these, CdTe and HgI_2 are the ones seen as most likely to have application in nuclear medicine. They both offer the advantage of operation at room temperature.

Cadmium telluride detectors are available in sizes of about 1 cm in diameter and 2 mm thick at a prototype cost of \$1000–\$1500. CdTe has a linear attenuation coefficient at 100 keV about 50% higher than NaI and is typically doped with either chlorine or indium. The chlorine-doped detectors have exhibited undesirable deterioration in time of their pulse height and pulse height resolution and gamma ray counting efficiency. This is due to polarization effects (Malm and Martini, 1974) caused by charge trapping on deep-lying trap states. These effects can be minimized by periodically switching the bias to zero. This may be inconvenient to the user, however. Although the polarization effect is a bulk phenomenon, the use of platinum contacts has also helped reduce the polarization problem (Entine, 1974, private communication). Recently, halogen-doped CdTe exhibiting no polarization effects has been made giving 7% energy resolution at 122 keV at room temperature (Serreze *et al.*, 1974). Undoped CdTe crystals have also been grown which do not exhibit polarization effects and have given energy resolution of 4.2 keV for a 122-keV gamma at room temperature (Siffert *et al.*, 1975). In applications where timing is important, such as the positron camera, the low charge-carrier velocity in CdTe compared to Ge leads to poorer timing performance. A FWHM of 15 nsec is quoted (Siffert *et al.*, 1975) which is ten times poorer than Ge(Li). The long collection time and limited mobility–lifetime product of CdTe also mean that leakage and energy resolution will be worse in larger-volume crystals. Useful detectors will probabily be limited to a few millimeters' thickness. In summary, CdTe undoubtedly will find use in small medical detector probes but its utility for a large detector array camera system seems limited.

Mercuric iodide has recently made its appearance on the scene and appears very attractive because of the very high Z (80 for Hg and 53 for I) and consequent stopping power, about three times as high as NaI. Detectors of a few mm^2 in area and thickness of about a millimeter have been made. The extremely poor hole mobility will limit its usefulness as a detector, however. The crystal studied by Malm (1972) had a hole mobility estimated at 4 cm^2/V sec, which appeared to be limited by trapping. Exciton formation also appears to play a key role in charge transport properties of HgI_2 (Llacer *et al.*, 1974). The consequences of its low mobility are that for detectors thicker than 1 mm, energy resolution will be poor and the count rate possible will be limited. But for detectors less than 500 μm thick, a resolution of 3.1 keV has been measured for the ^{57}Co 122-keV gamma. With a mobility of 4 cm^2/V sec in a field of 10^3 V/cm, a hole would require 0.025 msec to traverse a 1-mm depletion depth. Polarization effects similar to those noted in CdTe have also been observed in HgI_2. Improvements in these detectors will depend strictly on growing better crystals, and all past experience with compound semiconductors indicates that improvements in this field are quite tedious and difficult to achieve, as pointed out in the review paper of Bertolini *et al.* (1973).

Along with a gamma ray detection efficiency lower than desirable, currently useable semiconductor detectors have the drawback of being very expensive. Even with detector-grade germanium available at about \$10 per gram or about \$55 per cm^3, a composite array of 10-in.-diameter by 0.5 cm thick would contain \$13,900 worth of germanium. This is just the basic cost of the raw material alone. Fabrication and encapsulation of the array detector would cost much more. While this price discourages the development of a full scale general purpose germanium camera, a special purpose camera with small field of view might find application. The key characteristics a germanium detector has to offer are the fast timing for coincidence events as in a positron camera and its better ability to discriminate against scattered radiation. In studies of organs such as the liver, up to 40% of the events included in the image can come from scattered gamma rays. While the detection efficiency of a germanium camera for ^{99m}Tc 140-keV gammas may be only one-third to one-half that of the Anger camera, Parker *et al.* (1973) have pointed out that a system with better energy discrimination yields better contrast perceptibility in the image using fewer photons. However, statistical image quality requirements must still be met in order to convey the resolution a system is capable of and this means longer imaging times for a germanium camera because of the lower gamma detection efficiency (Llacer, 1973). This may be unacceptable to the clinician and also gives greater chance for image degradation due to patient movement. If the improved energy resolution is all that one desires, it should be kept in mind that the performance of a germanium detector in rejecting scatter can be mimicked by raising the lower threshold of the energy window on a NaI detector. While Ge is better at rejecting scattered gamma rays from the patient, the Compton scatter of the gamma rays within the detector itself may compromise this advantage. In attempting to fabricate a germanium camera detector with resolution of a few millimeters, one finds that a large fraction of incident gamma rays do not deposit their full energy within a radius of 2 mm of where they enter the crystal. This has interesting consequences. Strauss and Sherman (1975) define an imaging efficiency parameter which is related to image signal-to-noise ratio for a given imaging time, and conclude that even compared to a Ge detector 2 cm thick, the imaging efficiency of the NaI Anger camera is as good as their germanium camera of polar coordinate design. The germanium camera does offer better intrinsic spatial resolution but this is always compromised by collimator resolution, and the payoff of good scatter rejection is highest for deep-lying "cold" lesions such as are found in the liver, a situation where respiratory motion of the organ may override the better camera intrinsic resolution. The required vacuum-mounting chamber and cryogenic cooling of a germanium camera also complicate the operation and maintenance of a clinical gamma camera.

Long-term reliability and avoidance of degradation of detector characteristics also has to be achieved.

4.5. MULTIWIRE PROPORTIONAL CHAMBERS

4.5.1. Gas-Filled Chamber

Gas-filled multiwire proportional chambers (MWPC) have been widely used in high-energy physics as position-sensitive detectors with high spatial resolution (Charpak *et al.*, 1971). An excellent review is given by Charpak (1970). Spatial resolution is basically related to (not necessarily equal to) wire spacing. Position readout can be either analog or digital and some elegant readout schemes have been devised (Dhawan, 1973; Bonazzol *et al.*, 1972). Efforts have been made to coordinate the development of commercially available special integrated circuits for proportional wire chamber readout (Larsen, 1972, 1973). Lap Yen Lee (1973) has described binary coding schemes for position-sensitive radiation detectors that might have application in multiwire proportional chambers for reducing the number of amplifiers and pulse height analyzers required. In general, N amplifiers could code (2^N-1) wires. Consequently $2N$ amplifiers could handle a $(2^N-1) \times (2^N-1)$ array.

To avoid the complexity of reading out each wire individually, some systems capacitively couple each wire to an electromagnetic delay line (Kaplan *et al.*, 1973; Grove *et al.*, 1972; Rindi *et al.*, 1970; Swanson *et al.*, 1973). The position of an event is determined by the time it takes to travel down the delay line and is determined with differentiation and zero-crossing techniques using a time-to-amplitude converter. This can be done in each of two dimensions to give X_i, Y_i position information. Held and Weisskopf (1973) described interpolation circuitry to locate the centroid of a low-energy X-ray (few keV) event with an accuracy of approximately 1/8 the cathode-wire spacing. The dead time due to the delay line was about 1 μsec for the 30.5 × 30.5 cm chamber built by Kaufman *et al.* (1972).

Borkowski and Kopp (1970, 1972) developed a new method for determining the position of ionizing events by measuring the risetime of output pulses from detectors having high resistance collectors. These detectors were treated as infinite RC lines with distributed parameters, and the position-dependent rise time of the output pulses was measured by cross-over timing after double RC differentiation. This can be contrasted with other schemes (Owen, 1968) which use relatively low resistance collectors that are virtually shorted at both ends, and where the position of a detected event is determined from the ratio of the currents at the detector ends. Since the timing techniques effectively measure the position of the centroid of the charge distribution, displacements smaller than one wire spacing in the direction across the anode wires can be detected. However, when imaging gamma rays, resolution is degraded by phenomena to be discussed below. The spatial sensitivity expressed in the units of time it takes a pulse to move a unit length depends on the gain of the time analyzer, the resistance and capacitance per unit length of the cathode lines, and the center frequency of the filter network. The chamber assembled by Borkowski in 1972 had a pulse-processing time of less than 5 μsec for a 20 × 20 cm chamber. The processing time (maximum) will of course increase with the linear dimensions of the chamber, and limit the data rate handling capability of such chambers. The energy resolution obtained for 22-keV photons was 35% FWHM.

The key deficiency gas chambers have for medical radioisotope imaging is the very small stopping power (detection efficiency) for gamma rays above 50 kdV. For a 90% xenon–10% CO_2 gas mixture at 1 atm, the detection efficiency for the 140 keV technetium gamma is only 1.5% (Kaufman *et al.*, 1972). A chamber pressurized to 4 atm yielded a detection efficiency of about 5.5% at 150 keV (Kaufman *et al.*, 1973). St. Onge (1973) described a chamber filled to greater than 10 atm (absolute) pressure and claimed a corresponding counter efficiency ten times that at 1 atm. The detection efficiency of such a gas chamber is still an order of magnitude too low for nuclear medicine. Furthermore, when imaging higher-energy gamma rays, resolution is deteriorated due to the increased range of the photoelectrons. In addition, even though collimated, the gammas will enter the chamber at some angle. There is a probability a gamma ray will interact anywhere along a given length of traversal. The oblique projection on the collecting plane of this range of possible interaction points gives a measure of the resolution smearing from this additional phenomenon.

Muehllehner (1972, private communication) proposed placing a photocathode layer in close proximity to a large-area, thick scintillation crystal. The photocathode would be inside the environment of a multiwire gas proportional chamber and the electrons ejected from the photocathode would be accelerated and collected in the plane of the anode wires. The coordinates of the centroid of their distribution would be determined with good precision leading to a high intrinsic camera resolution. Little is known, however, about the problems that would arise from the presence of a photocathode in the environment of a proportional counter, such as optical feedback, ion bombardment, and quantum efficiency. Westinghouse Research Laboratories have recently reported on the development of silicon field emission arrays which are extended-area (2–3 cm^2) photosensitive cold cathode devices and are air stable. Multitudes of "stalagmite" field emission tips are etched on a silicon wafer by photolithographic techniques. Unfortunately, they presently require cooling to about 15°K to reduce the dark current.

4.5.2. Liquid Xenon Chamber

It was because of the deficiencies of a gas-filled chamber for gamma ray imaging that it was suggested that one could decrease the thickness of the chamber and increase the density of the detecting medium by replacing the gas in the chamber with a liquefied noble gas (Muller, 1971). Liquid xenon is the only known liquid in which ionization electrons both remain free and can be avalanched reliably to give a fast electronic pulse. The range of a 200-keV photoelectron in liquid xenon is only 0.057 mm so that resolution smearing from this is negligible. Zaklad *et al.* (1972) studied the avalanche process near fine wires (3.5–25 μm) at fields $\geq 10^6$ V/cm and at voltages > 2000 V. Pulse rise times of 150 nsec were observed for the proportional pulses and $\simeq 20$ nsec for the Geiger-type pulse. Liquid xenon has a density of 3.06 g/cm^3, an atomic number of 54, liquifies at -107.1°C, and solidifies at -111.9°C at 1 atm. Thus there is a narrow range over which the temperature of the chamber must be held to avoid crystallization or frosting of the xenon. The working range of temperature will be wider for higher pressures. The gross detection efficiency and photofraction of liquid xenon are presented in Zaklad *et al.*, (1972). The electron drift velocity in liquid xenon is 3×10^5 cm/sec at fields greater than 1000 V/cm. The positive xenon ion mobility is 3×10^{-4} cm^2/V sec. These parameters are important in determining pulse-processing time and consequently camera dead time. Charpak (1970) points out that a common misconception is that the pulse on the wires is due mainly to the collection of the electrons from the avalanches produced against the wire: "The important fact is that since the pulses on the wire are produced mainly by the drifting of the positive ions away from the wire, positive pulses are induced on the neighboring electrodes, i.e., on the wires and high-voltage planes."

For detector operation the impurity problems in liquid xenon are quite severe. The presence of only a few parts per million of electronegative impurities can seriously impair the performance of the chambers. A sufficient amount of electronegative impurity can suppress the avalanche by capturing the free electrons. Oxygen is a culprit but some materials have much larger electron attachment cross sections. For instance compounds like C_6F_{14} and SF_5 in concentrations of parts per billion are as effective as oxygen in concentrations of parts per million (Zaklad, 1971). After extensive work, the Berkeley group reports to have reduced the impurity problem to the point where the electron attachment is less than 1% per millimeter of drift. Purification is accomplished by a combination of continuous recirculation purification of the gas followed by purification of the liquid by electronegative ion pumping (ENIP) (Zaklad *et al.*, 1972). The xenon gas continuously circulates for several hours over a hot copper catalyst (200°C) and cold (-77°C) molecular sieve. The copper reacts with oxygen while the molecular sieve traps other unknown electronegative impurities. Every few weeks of operation, excess nitrogen is removed by passing the gas over hot calcium chips (600°C). There are safety considerations in operating such a system because of the potential generation of hydrogen, especially during initial operation. When a fresh change of calcium turnings is heated, absorbed water is broken up and hydrogen is released. The copper catalyst can remove this hydrogen by catalyzing its conversion to water. The copper catalyst is available by its commercial name, BTS. This catalyst is supplied in the oxidized state only and it must be reduced by flowing hydrogen and helium over it at 150°C. Since a great deal of heat is released, the amount of hydrogen must carefully be increased from 4% to 100% over a few hours.

With continuous recycling purification, Zaklad (1971) found that for oxygen in argon, impurity levels of about 10 ppb were attainable. The oxygen and nitrogen level attained in xenon was put at below 10 ppb. In xenon, it appeared that some unknown impurity was the worst impurity present. The source of these impurities in xenon was attributed to a catalytic reaction over hot calcium.

The Berkeley group has built a prototype liquid xenon camera with a sensitive volume 7 × 7 × 1.5 cm (Zaklad *et al.*, 1973a). The chamber contained 24 anode wires 5 μm in diameter spaced 2.8 mm apart and had 24 orthogonal cathode strips. The chamber was maintained in a liquid state as long as 24 hr. By the method of electronegative ion pumping over a 12-hr period a clean liquid was obtained. During a run this process had to be repeated every hour, but it is hoped this requirement will be relaxed in future designs. The energy resolution for 279 keV (^{203}Hg) was 19% FWHM.

Whereas the multiplication in a gas proportional chamber is of the order 10^4–10^5, in the liquid-filled chamber the gain falls in the range 10–70. To get the high fields required, very thin wires (diameter 3–5 μm) must be used in the liquid medium. For 5-μm-diameter wires at voltages above 6.5 kV, oscillating instabilities and breakage occur because of the high electrostatic forces. The breakage problem can be minimized by supporting them with quartz fibers. Irregularities on the surface of the anode wires will result in locally higher electric fields and consequent variations in pulse height. For a single-wire proportional counter, these hot spots averaged one per centimeter and the gain corresponded to that of a field 30% greater (Muller, 1971). In general, the construction of a multiwire proportional chamber requires close tolerances. For wires of 20-μm diameter and 2-mm spacing, a displacement in the plane of the wires of 0.01 mm leads to a difference in amplification of 30% between the two wires adjacent to the displaced wire. For certain gas-filled chambers, a 10% change in the diameter of a single wire will change the amplification by 20% (Charpak, 1970).

With wires spaced 2.8 mm, the spatial resolution (intrinsic) of the chamber was stated to be better than 4 mm FWHM. There can be "ghosting" problems. Because of the electrostatic focusing properties of the anode wires, when a point source is not aligned exactly over one wire it will be imaged as two points. Zaklad *et al.* (1973a) suggested that this pattern produced by the anode wires could be eliminated by moving the detector during exposure and making the corresponding correction to the image in the manner of a Potter–Bucky filter.

To keep the cost and complexity of the electronics down, a readout scheme based on charge division was initially used (Owen, 1968). However, this was found to suffer from the effects of chamber capacitance and it was found necessary to go to a system using a preamplifier per wire (Zaklad *et al.*, 1973b). One advantage of using an amplifier and single-channel analyzer (SCA) per wire is that the count rate capability could effectively be $N \times 10^5$ per second, where N is the number of wires in the chamber. Also, the variation of pulse height from wire to wire would not be crucial. A chamber 15 × 15 in. with wire spacing of 2 mm would have 190 wires and preamplifiers in each of two directions.

Another important consideration in the commercial development of a liquid xenon gamma camera is the cost and availability of xenon. Presently, xenon comes from conventional liquid air processing sources. Current prices are \$15/liter of gas. In large quantities this price might drop to \$7–\$10/liter of gas. A price of \$10/liter of gas equates to a cost of \$5.23/cm^3 of liquid. A chamber 15 in. × 15 in. × 1 cm thick would have a volume of 1451 cm^3 and require \$7600 worth of liquid xenon (at the price of \$10/liter of gas). The production of 50 such chambers a year would require some 38,000 liters of xenon gas a year. The data indicate that an air separation plant capable of yielding 1000 tons of oxygen per day should be able to recover about 90,000 liters of xenon gas per year (Rohrmann, 1971). One supplier (Sarocka, 1973, private communication) has stated that to process 50,000 liters of xenon gas even after collection would take about two years, with their present facilities! It has been suggested that the problem of cost and availability of large quantities of xenon will be solved by the collection of fission product xenon from nuclear fuel reprocessing plants, of which an increasing number will come on line during the next 10 years (Rohrmann, 1971). Estimates as optimistic as \$1.00/liter of xenon gas from this source have been made, but as Rohrmann points out the low projected prices must assume that facilities are required for krypton trapping and retention as a pollution control effort. The main domestic uses of xenon are as an inert atmosphere in long-lived tungsten filament incandescent lamps and as an anesthetic. However, for use in incandescent lamps xenon does have to compete with krypton. Furthermore, for applications as a radiation detector, there might be problems with ^{85}Kr contaminant in fission product recovered xenon gas. Present rare gas processing techniques can insure separations down to the few parts per million level, normally 20 ppm, with 5 ppm achievable. Based on the assumption that fission product krypton contains 6% ^{85}Kr and a xenon product contains 5 ppm of total krypton contamination, the background activity from ^{85}Kr would be 8.7×10^6 cts/sec/cm^3 of liquid! Recent work at Oak Ridge yielded material containing only 2 μCi of ^{85}Kr per liter of xenon. This would still equate to an activity of 3.88×10^4 cts/sec/cm^3 of liquid! ^{85}Kr has a half-life of 10.76 years and emits a gamma of 514 keV with 0.41% abundance. The decay is to the ground state of ^{85}Rb 99.6% of the time with beta emission of 670 keV end point energy. This level of background activity due to the intrinsic detector medium itself would be unacceptable in a gamma camera. More recently, Zaklad *et al.* (1973a,b) state that they have gotten the krypton impurity down to the level of about 60 pCi/liter with a repetitive dilution technique. This would reduce the background count rate to about one count per second, and be acceptable.

Despite the difficulties, the Berkeley group did obtain useful data on a liquid xenon camera. But to date only a small-scale chamber has been evaluated. The numerous problems and complexity associated with this technology make the development of a commercial camera both quite risky and expensive. The need for frequent purifying by electronegative ion pumping during the course of a day would be a hindrance in a clinical environment and the frequency this is required must be greatly reduced. The main improvements to be offered by a liquid xenon camera are increased count rate capability (assuming an amplifier and SCA per wire) and improved intrinsic resolution (2–4 mm depending on the number and spacing of wires). These gains must be weighed against the complexity and technical problems of such a system and other considerations such as the cost and availability of high-quality xenon gas.

4.6. XENON SCINTILLATION DETECTOR

The characteristics of the light luminescence or "scintillation" following an interaction in liquid xenon may also have potential application as the detecting medium of a gamma ray camera. The decay constant of the luminescence from liquid xenon is about 10 nsec (Lavoie, 1973), 23 times as fast as that of NaI(Tl). Some researchers indicate that the light output is comparable to that of NaI(Tl) (Northrup and Nobles, 1956; Northrup *et al.*, 1958). Indications are that the light output can be increased by application of an electric field to produce electron multiplication (Dolgosheim *et al.*, 1967). Application of an electric field to a gas mixture such as Ar–5% Xe can increase the light output to about 250 times that of CsI(Tl) and NaI(Tl) scintillators, but the rise time of the pulse is slow ($\sim$10 μsec)

(Policarpo *et al.*, 1968; Conde *et al.*, 1968). The primary scintillation spectrum of liquid xenon is about 220 Å wide and is centered about 1780 Å and thus would require UV-transmitting windows for measurement (Lavoie, 1973). The use of a liquid xenon scintillation detector held between optically polished UV-transmitting plates would perhaps eliminate the scatter background buildup that has plagued image intensifier cameras such as the Aber gammascope. It should be noted that xenon gives rise to a visible emission continuum as well as the ultraviolet (Morucci and Lansiart, 1970). The short decay constant of the intrinsic scintillation from liquid xenon would make possible higher count rates when used in an Anger camera.

An interesting combination that might have application in a gamma camera is a "two-phase" detector consisting of a xenon gas proportional (amplification) region over a liquid xenon interaction or stopping layer. This would combine the good stopping power of the dense liquid xenon medium with the multiplication gain of a proportional chamber with applied electric field. It has been proven that electrons can escape the liquid phase and drift to the gaseous phase (Allemand *et al.*, 1971). Such a chamber would always have to be used in a horizontal plane, however. This combination could be useful as the input phosphor of a coded aperture camera because of its high stopping power and high light output. In systems where events are not processed pulse by pulse, the increased dead time would not be detrimental and the increased light output that comes with application of an electric field would be useful in darkening the film faster and reducing imaging time. Alternatively, event location could be read out electronically from the wires used to generate the multiplying fields and energy discrimination done on a pulse by pulse basis.

Perhaps the application most likely to make use of the characteristics of a liquid-xenon-filled chamber would be a positron camera. Liquid xenon scanners used in pairs as positron imaging detectors can accept five times the activity of similar NaI(Tl) devices for the same accidental coincidence rate (Lavoie, 1973). The number of coincidences is proportional to the square of the photofraction (Zaklad *et al.*, 1972). In thin liquid xenon chambers the photofraction at 500 keV is about five times larger than in germanium.

4.7. HYBRID SCANNER–CAMERA

The hybrid scanner is intermediate in speed and complexity between a mechanical rectilinear scanner and a stationary camera device. A long rod-shaped detector or "bar" is scanned longitudinally across the patient. In the schemes tried so far (Davis and Martone, 1966; Miraldi and DiChiro,

1970; Crawley and Veall, 1973) resolution in the direction along the detector is determined by the ratio of the signals received by photomultipliers placed at the ends of the scintillation crystal. The light intensity in a long rod of scintillator falls off exponentially with distance from its point of origin (Miraldi and DiChiro, 1970). Therefore the event is located by the log of the ratio of the two photomultiplier signals. The resolution in this direction should be proportional to the length of the crystal. David and Martone (1966) found their resolution to be about 10% of the crystal length (8 in.) but felt this could be significantly improved by proper design of the scintillation crystal package. The resolution in the direction of scan will be determined solely by the collimator characteristics and will not necessarily be the same as in the transverse direction. A "low-energy" version with a lightweight collimator making it possible to take the scanner to the patient's bed has been constructed (Planiol *et al.*, 1973). Such a device might be very useful for screening for pulmonary emboli or deep-vein thrombosis. The position of the event along a bar scanner can also be determined by placing several photomultipliers side by side on top of the bar crystal, analogous to a one-dimensional Anger camera (Bok and Fonroget, 1975).

While the hybrid scanner–camera could be used for many procedures, it is not suitable for fast dynamic studies. A well-designed system based on this principle could possibly compete with the Anger camera in static imaging but could hardly be considered to be the device which will replace it. Perhaps the bar detector will find its role in a system circling the patient for radionuclide emission computerized section imaging.

4.8. APPROACHES ELIMINATING THE NEED OF A COLLIMATOR

Somewhat analogous to the image-forming lens of an optical camera, the "lens" of a gamma ray camera is the collimator in front of the detector. The collimator "forms" the image but unfortunately also greatly reduces the flux of photons contributing to the image. Since conventional parallel hole collimators typically only let one in 10^4 of the gammas emitted by the source reach the detector, it has motivated the investigation of schemes that would eliminate the collimator. A great deal of anticipation was stimulated by the work of Barrett and Rogers which suggested that a high collection efficiency two or three orders of magnitude over a parallel hole collimator could be achieved by replacing the collimator with a coded aperture such as a Fresnel zone plate (Barrett, 1972; Rogers *et al.*, 1972). Although the collection efficiency is higher in these shadow-casting schemes, conversely many photons are required to well define the shadow cast by a point source. Further analysis of the signal-to-noise ratio of the resultant images has brought the realization that the same imaging time will be required to obtain the same signal to noise ratio as the Anger camera (Jaszczak, 1974, private communication; Barrett and DeMeester, 1974).

A second gamma ray imaging scheme which requires no collimation has been proposed (Todd *et al.*, 1974) and also independently by the present author (1973). In essence two detector planes are used, one right behind the other (see Fig. 4-6). The first detector is such that the most probable interaction is a Compton scatter event and the scattered photon is stopped in the second detector. From the positions of the events in the two detectors and the deposited energies one can calculate the scattering angle and backproject onto the object the vector along which the gamma traveled. It turns out that the gamma for a given event could have originated from inside the object anywhere along a locus of points defining an ellipse. To image the object, for each event a corresponding ellipse is generated on a CRT. The image of a point source results from the intersection of many of these ellipses. Because of the way the image is formed, there will be a significant background and image contrast for small or "cold" lesions will be marginal. The image is a tomographic one with out-of-focus information

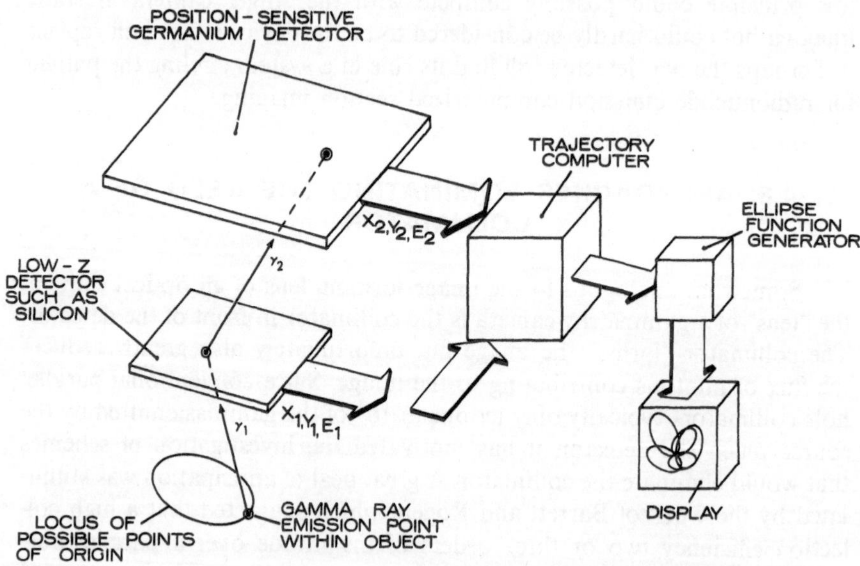

Fig. 4-6. Illustration of gamma camera principle requiring no collimation. Since in the first detector Compton scattering events are used, a low Z detector such as silicon is desirable. It is also desirable that both detector planes have good energy resolution as well as good spatial resolution. An image of an object distribution is generated by backprojection of ellipses onto the image plane, giving tomographic images of a plane at a particular depth.

from other planes overlying the plane chosen to be in focus. However, for studies of hot objects against an activity-free background, such as skeletal imaging or blood pool studies, this scheme might have utility. An interesting feature of one embodiment permits a large object to be imaged with a small-area semiconductor detector (Todd, 1975). Since the device uses Compton scattering, a silicon position-sensitive detector could possibly be used without working at cryogenic temperatures.

The most viable camera system which eliminates the need of multihole collimation is the positron camera. When an electron–positron annihilate, two 511-keV gammas are emitted in opposite directions. These may be detected in diametrically opposed detectors so that the event's origin within the source may be estimated, yielding tomographic images with a finite depth of focus. Two opposed Anger camera detector heads may be used to implement such a positron camera, giving huge geometric collection efficiency since the scintillation crystal no longer requires an interposing collimator (Anger, 1967; Kenney, 1971). However, earlier versions of such a positron camera could not handle electronically the data rates generated by such good detector geometry and clinically useful count rates were limited to about 200 per second. Vastly improved performance characteristics making useful clinical data rates of 8000 cts/sec possible, depending on the amount of scatter have recently been described (Muehllehner, 1975; Muehllehner *et al.*, 1976). This has been achieved through a combination of new fast dc-coupled electronics, suppression of scatter from the patient via energy selective absorbers, and including in the coincidence counting, gamma rays which do not manage to deposit their full energy in the detector. The performance of these systems is primarily limited by the amount of background generated by random coincidences and is given by $N_c = 2\tau N_1 N_2$. Although the positron camera allows a much higher fraction of the gammas emitted by the source to reach the detector, still with a "scattering" patient as the source, only about 2% of the gammas hitting a given detector will actually be in coincidence with an event at the other detector and contribute to the image. Furthermore, the ratio of random coincidences to true coincidences can be on the order of 20% for a τ of 10 nsec. Even so, the photon utilization of a positron camera is now such that a sensitivity of 200 cts/sec/μCi can be achieved.

It is perhaps in a positron camera that the properties of a germanium gamma camera might have their highest payoff. A germanium camera has two things to offer: coincidence resolving time τ ten times smaller than NaI, thus reducing random coincidence background, and better intrinsic resolution capability, which becomes more significant when it is not degraded by a parallel hole collimator. With a better understanding of charge collection properties in germanium, new techniques have been developed which indicate that time resolutions of a fraction of a nanosecond should be possible. This means that with 10^6 counts per second incident on the detector, true to random coincidence ratios of 1000:1 can be achieved. The excellent time-resolving capability of germanium could make feasible the time-of-flight estimation of depth of the source, yielding true three-dimensional imaging with image planes of about 2.25-cm thickness (Llacer and Cho, 1973). Furthermore, by including Compton scattered events occurring in the detector when looking for coincidences, the detection efficiency of a germanium detector for 511-keV gammas can be quite comparable to that of a NaI detector (Llacer and Cho, 1973). As pointed out earlier, above 300 keV the interaction probability in Ge is higher than that in NaI. Improvements in intrinsic camera resolution translate directly to improved clinical resolution in a positron camera, whereas in a standard gamma camera, improvements are masked by the resolution of the parallel hole collimator. Although germanium cameras can ostensibly be made with improved resolution one must also remember that the resolution of the Anger camera at 511 keV is much better than it is at the 140-keV gamma of technetium. To summarize, the positron camera has now become a viable clinical imaging tool and one can look for continued technical innovation in improving its performance.

4.9. THE ANGER CAMERA

A discussion of the principle of the Anger scintillation camera is appropriate since it is the bench mark against which other systems are compared in this review. More detailed descriptions are given in Anger (1958, 1966b, 1967). H.O. Anger developed some of his ideas while working on position-sensitive radiation detection devices for monitoring the beam position in accelerators. In high-energy physics, such detectors are usually referred to as hodoscopes. The Anger camera consists of a large-diameter assembly with a single crystal of NaI(T1) typically a half an inch thick. Upon the flat surface of the assembly are placed several photomultiplier tubes (PMT) side by side in a close-packed array. The original camera used a 4-in.-diameter crystal and seven photomultipliers (Anger, 1958). Commercial versions have employed crystals from 12.25 inches to 17.5 inches in diameter and with either 19, 37, or 61 phototubes. In Fig. 4-7 is shown a modern Anger camera system with control console, multiformat image-recording accessory, and scanning bed. The sodium iodide crystal has a thin aluminum cover on the side the gamma rays enter and a thick glass cover plate on the opposite side to let the light from the scintillation reach the phototubes and also give structural rigidity to keep the crystal from cracking. Also, to place the phototubes at the right distance from the scintillation to get the appropriate response, a disk of Plexiglas is optically coupled to the glass cover of the crystal and it is on the surface

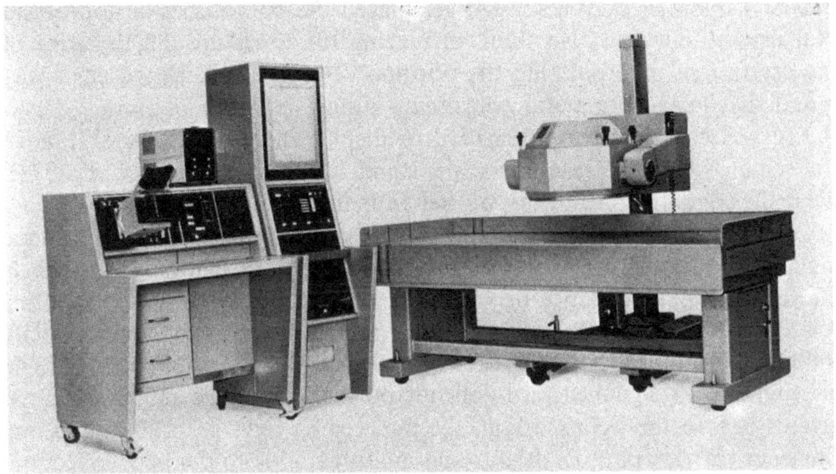

Fig. 4-7. Anger gamma camera. Imaging unit and stand are at right, with scanning table; console and imaging accessories are at left. This is a large field of view camera with a 15-in.-diameter field. (Courtesy of Searle Radiographics.)

of the Plexiglas that the photomultiplier tubes are actually coupled. Since round tubes do not fully cover the crystal area with active photocathode it is in some cases beneficial to cut conical pads into the surface of the Plexiglas, upon which the phototubes are placed. The intervening layers from scintillation to PMT of crystal, Pyrex, and Plexiglas constitute a "light guide."

A scintillation of light occurs in the crystal when a gamma ray interacts transferring energy to a photoelectron or Compton scattered electron. These electrons excite the lattice structure of the crystal and these levels deexcite by the isotropic emission of optical photons. The position of each such event is determined by the interpolation of the signals generated by the phototubes. This is the essence of the Anger principle. Each phototube contributes to the calculation with a weight proportional to its position. Thus the event is displayed as occurring at the centroid of the light distribution created by each scintillation. Subsequently, thousands of discrete event positions can be localized using a small number of photomultipliers. The early cameras used a matrix of capacitors to give each tube its appropriate weight in the calculation (Anger, 1967); most commercial cameras have used a matrix of resistors to generate the appropriate weighted signals. An algorithm for optimizing both linearity and resolution has been used and it was found that the algorithm could be approximated by feeding the PMT signals into a tapped delay line followed by double delay line clipping (Tanaka *et al.*, 1970). It can be shown that in the vicinity of the scintillation, the functional dependence of the Anger algorithm approaches that of Tanaka *et al.* Whereas Anger placed the phototubes on top of the NaI crystal, one can also think of placing the tubes around the edge of the crystal and interpolating the position of each event. However, it was found that for such a polar coordinate system using 16 photomultiplers, the response was rather insensitive to displacements of the source near the center, where the resolution was some 20 mm (Ben Zeev *et al.*, 1973). Near the edges the resolution was better, being about 7 mm.

Factors which affect the intrinsic resolution of the Anger camera include the statistical variation of photoelectrons emitted from each photocathode, the distance between tube centers, variation in depth of the scintillation in the crystal, energy of the gamma ray, and to a small extent multiple Compton scattering events in the crystal. The statistics of each photomultiplier signal in turn depends on the solid angle subtended by a given PMT to the light's origin, the intervening light path, the quantum efficiency of the photocathode, and photocathode-to-dynode collection efficiency. To make the camera resolution independent of where the scintillation occurs in the crystal and independent of pulse-to-pulse variations, it was noted that the calculated position should be divided by the sum of all PMT signals in a "ratio circuit" (Mallard and Myers, 1963). This of course is the way a normalized centroid should be calculated.

Other characteristics of the Anger camera have been a noticeable "barrel distortion" for line sources lying near the edge of the field of view and a phenomenon called "edge packing." Edge packing is the bright ring observed around the periphery when the crystal face is flooded with a uniform distribution of gamma rays. It occurs because for gamma ray interactions near the edge of the crystal, there are no longer any PMTs farther out to help locate the event and the inboard PMTs pull the events location inward, piling them up along the periphery. Scattering the light off the edge of the crystal back toward the center also plays a role. The only problem caused by edge packing is a reduction in the effective field of view. Also observed in a flood image is an area of increased activity higher than average, in the center of the crystal. However, this nonuniformity is much less pronounced in recent cameras using more phototubes of smaller diameter. One feature that has given the Anger camera such utility is the ease with which its effective diameter and field of view can be increased.

Another key event in molding gamma camera technology was the introduction in 1964 of the radioisotope technetium 99m. The isomeric transition with a half-life of 6 hr results in the emission of a 140-keV gamma. This energy is enough to allow it to escape from the body yet low enough to make detection relatively easy. Early cameras were designed to cope with a range of energies from 70 to 511 keV. The predominant use of ^{99m}Tc makes possible the use of less shielding in the tub holding the detector head, thus making lightweight, mobile camera heads feasible. Furthermore, a camera specifically designed for the energy of ^{99m}Tc can use a thinner light guide and hence achieve better resolution. This is because higher-energy gammas typically penetrate deeper into the crystal on the average and a camera designed for all energies has to have the PMTs farther back to make the solid angle subtended less dependent upon depth of interaction. The use of low energies such as the 140-keV gamma of ^{99m}Tc also made possible major improvements in collimator design (Muehlleher and Luig, 1973). The use of thin-wall septa made possible the fabrication by corrugation techniques of collimators optimized for both efficiency and resolution and greatly improved image quality attainable with the Anger camera.

Although there have been attempts at theoretical analysis for the purpose of optimization of Anger camera design, such has actually been achieved in practice primarily by empirical optimization. This is in part due to the fact that, although seemingly straightforward, the electro-optical analysis is complicated by the various boundaries of differing indices of refraction, by scattering and refraction, and by edge effects. Even so, it has been found that the signal at each photomultipler is directly proportional to the solid angle which that PMT subtends at any scintillation position (Scrimger and Baker, 1967). It has been concluded that light guide thickness should be scaled with photomultiplier diameter such that light guide thickness is equal to the radius of the PMT (Baker and Scrimger, 1967). However, when smaller tubes and thinner light pipes are used, hot spots over each tube appear in a flood image and nonlinearities worsen. Light pipe design can help minimize this and it has been found that placing dots or patterns under each PMT at the interface between Pyrex cover and Plexiglas can help significantly in improving flood uniformity and linearity (Martone *et al.*, 1974). A similar effect can be simulated electronically by use of a nonlinear preamplifier which rolls off the gain for the stronger signals.* Factors affecting resolution and linearity of the Anger camera have been thoroughly investigated (Anger, 1966b; Svedberg, 1973). It has been found that distortion can be minimized by use of adjusted weighting factors, rather than the nominal linear weighting matrix (Svedberg, 1969). Both analytical and computer modeling of the Anger camera's characteristics have been accomplished (Svedberg, 1972, 1975). Commercial versions use a sodium iodide crystal with a surface ground for diffuse scattering with a layer of MgO for good reflection. However, a substantial improvement in resolution was obtained when a light pipe material of refractive index closer to that of the NaI crystal was used, and also a polished specular reflecting surface on the entrance side of the crystal further improved performance (Svedberg, 1972). For good uniformity and linearity,

*Ohio Nuclear Corporation, Solon, Ohio.

the photomultipliers must be adjusted to gain to "tune" the camera. Early versions were adjusted to obtain constant count rate as a source is held at different positions across the face of the crystal. Best results are obtained if the camera is tuned for constant energy pulse from the sum of all PMT's and at least one commercial camera has included a multichannel analyzer to facilitate this tuning process.

What is most notable about the Anger camera is that while alternative camera systems were being developed promising improved resolution, the resolution of the Anger camera itself continued to improve. This history is traced in Fig. 4-8. In 1966 the introduction of higher quantum efficiency bialkali photocathodes in place of S-11 photocathodes improved camera resolution from 13.5 mm to 10.2 mm. Rather than include all photomultiplier

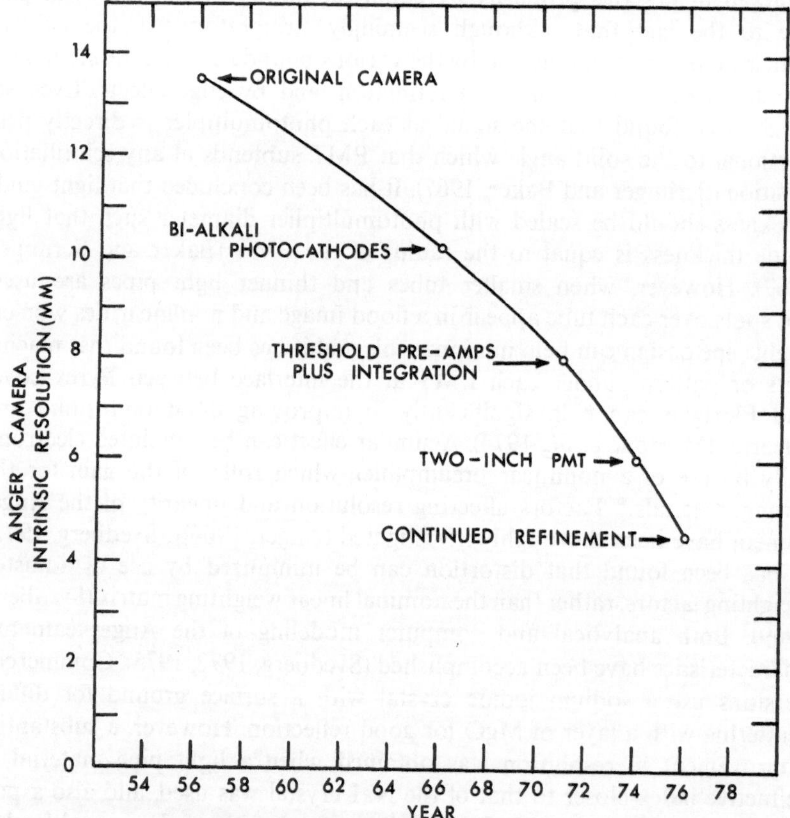

Fig. 4-8. History of evolutionary improvement in intrinsic resolution of Anger scintillation camera through the years. Resolution values are full width at half maximum for a gamma ray energy of 140 keV and values plotted represent approximate values only, so variations from camera to camera can be expected.

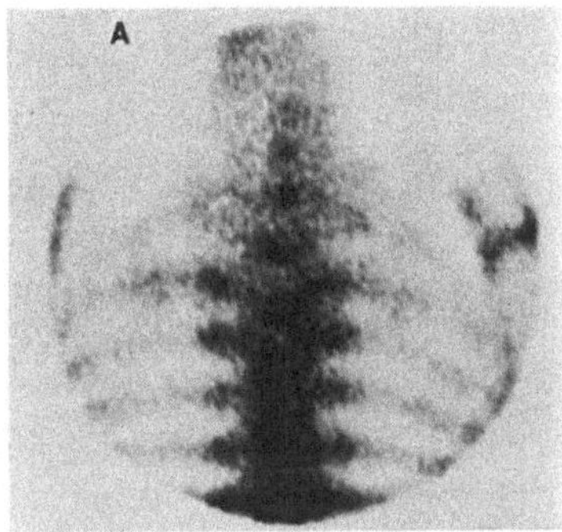

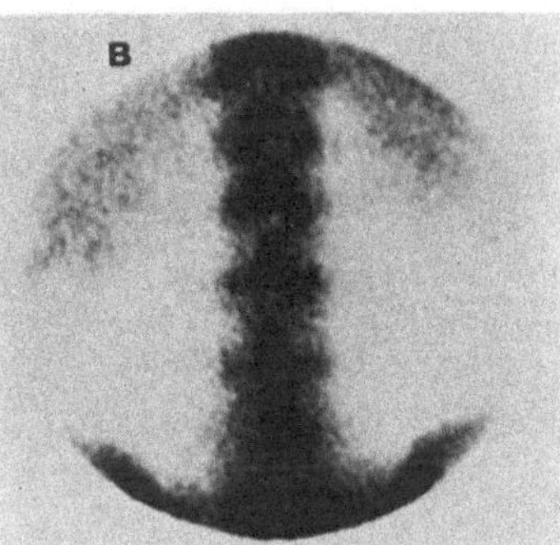

Fig. 4-9. Bone scan. Patient was given 20 mCi Tc-99m diphosphonate 4 hr prior to the scan. A, posterior view of upper thoracic spine. B, posterior view of lumbar spine. Note vertebral bodies, ribs, and other bone detail. Kidneys are faintly seen in upper field of B.

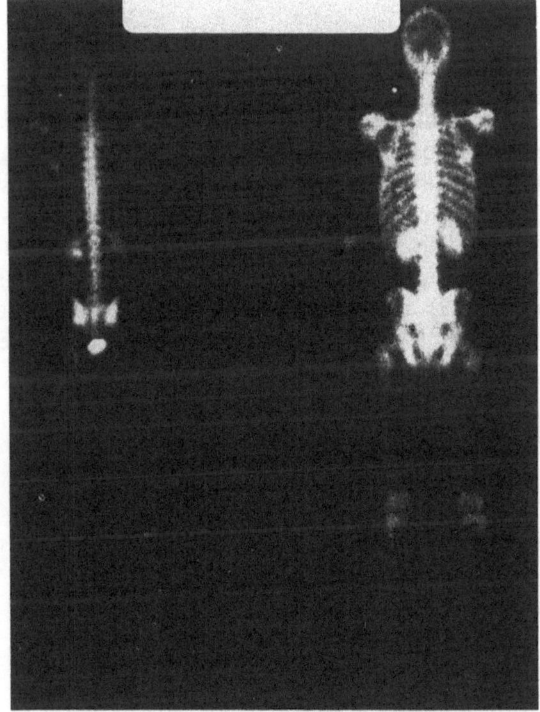

Fig. 4-10. Bone scan (posterior view) using whole body scanning table. Table moves linearly while camera electronics moves image in synchrony, giving a single image of the whole body. The two images are identical except that different light-spot intensity was used; some detail not evident in one image is clear in the other.

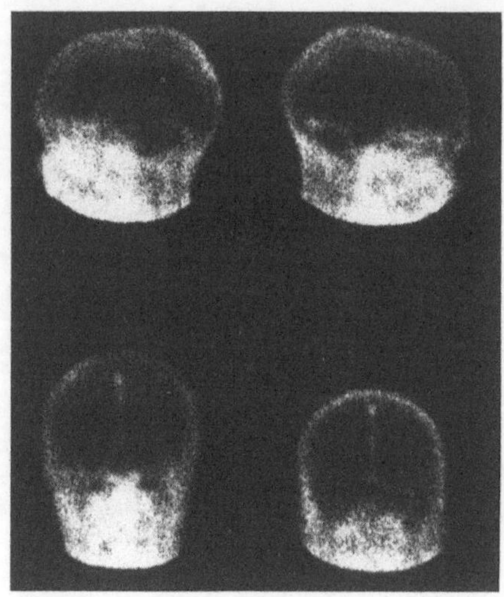

Fig. 4-11. Brain scan. Top row: left lateral, right lateral. Bottom row: anterior, posterior.

signals in the calculation, it was recognized that the PMTs far from the scintillation have weak, noisy signals and resolution is actually improved by excluding them from the centroid estimate (Kulberg *et al.*, 1972). Thus, in 1971, the introduction of thresholded preamplifiers in conjunction with increasing pulse integration time from 0.4 to 0.8 μsec improved resolution another 25% down to about 8 mm. Introduction of cameras with 37 2-in. photomultipliers in 1974 further improved resolution down to about 6.0 mm. Limiting resolution for the Anger camera of about 4 mm seems feasible with improvements in components and design. Use of large-diameter crystals and converging collimation can further reduce the influence of

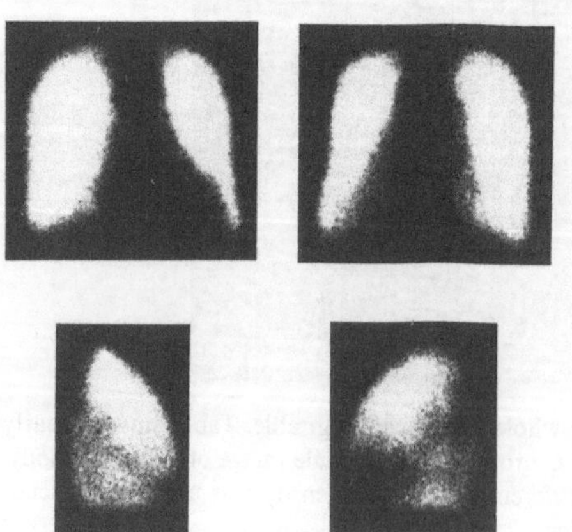

Fig. 4-12. Lung scan. Top row: anterior, posterior. Bottom row: right lateral, left lateral.

the camera's intrinsic resolution (Murphy *et al.*, 1975). Performance capability of the Anger camera at high data rates has also been vastly improved by new dc-coupled fast electronics so that count rates up to 200,000 cts/sec are possible. Comparisons between various commercially available Anger cameras have been made (Luc Moretti *et al.*, 1976; Hine and Paras, 1975), but the vitality of Anger camera system development is such that comparisons are probably only valid at the time they are made. Considering the Anger camera "system" one should include display technology as well as basic detector technology (Whitehead, 1978).

Examples of clinical studies done with the Anger camera are shown in Figs. 4-9 through 4-12.

4.10. DISCUSSION

The salient features of the various camera systems considered here are presented in Table 4-1. Semiconductor detectors have been plagued with reliability and stability problems. One must also note that in the orthogonal strip readout schemes, spatial resolution is limited to about twice the strip spacing. Some of the image intensifier schemes are potentially capable of about 3-mm resolution when a small field of view is blown up with the zoom feature of the intensifier tube. A similar resolution-enhancing "zoom" effect can also be implemented on the Anger camera, however, by use of a converging collimator to magnify the image. Quite often an experimental camera scheme will give beautiful images of test phantoms in the laboratory only to give marginal images in a real life clinical patient. This is because of the additional factors affecting the clinical image, such as scattering of gamma rays within the patient and movement of the patient or organ. One can conceptualize the clinical or resultant system resolution R_S as being influenced by several factors:

$$R_S \cong (R_I^2 + R_C^2 + R_M^2 + R_{ST}^2 + R_{SC}^2 + R_{CX}^2)^{1/2}$$

where the various blurring factors are related to R_I, intrinsic camera resolution; R_C, collimator resolution; R_M, blurring factor due to motion; R_{ST}, blurring factor related to statistical image quality (Vetter and Pizer, 1971); R_{SC}, a blurring factor related to scatter fraction; and R_{CX}, a blur factor related to multiple Compton scattering in the detector. Even if intrinsic camera and collimator resolutions are the only contributing factors it becomes evident that there is a point of diminishing returns in efforts to reduce intrinsic camera resolution. Consider Fig. 4-13 which graphs system resolution as a function of intrinsic camera resolution for a typical parallel hole collimator with 8 mm resolution at 10 cm. Reducing the intrinsic resolution from 8 mm down to 1 mm will only reduce resultant

Table 4-1. Comparison of Alternative Gamma Camera Systems

Camera system	Spatial resolution (intrinsic) (mm)	Dead time or count rate	Energy resolution (FWHM)	Detection efficiency (140 keV)	Field of view	Uniformity	Comments
Anger	5–7	2 μsec	14%	90% (NaI)	10–16-in. diameter	Good	1. Versatile 2. Resolution has continually improved
Semiconductor: germanium	3–5	~ 0.5 μsec	1–5%	55% (1 cm thick)	Matrix of subunits	?	1. Good scatter rejection but can be simulated by NaI 2. Cryogenic cooling required 3. Reliability a problem 4. Potential for fast timing in positron camera
Semiconductor: cadmium telluride	3–5	~ 1 μsec	5–10%	50% (2 mm thick)	Matrix of subunits	?	1. Degradation of response due to polarization effects but has recently been improved 2. Noise and leakage will probably limit useful device to 2–4-mm thickness 3. Room temperature operation
Image intensifier: large diameter	3–9	Several μsec or parallel processing	20–50%	40–90%	10–14-in. diameter	± 25%	1. Pulse height discrimination difficult 2. High count rate possible with no energy discrimination
Image intensifier: large diameter with centroid readout	3–6	Several μsec	10–15%	90%	14 in.	± 15% 5% (corrected)	1. Zoom mode can yield better resolution for smaller field of view

Image intensifier: small diameter viewing scintillator through lens	3–6	Several μsec	30–70 %	Low	Large	?	1. Low quantum detection efficiency because of lens coupling 2. Poor clinical image contrast because of light diffusion and scatter in crystal
Multicrystal dectector	10–20	2 μsec	40–50 %	90 %		± 15 %	1. Two operating modes: High count rate—low resolution Low count rate—high resolution 2. Resolution improved by stepping mode
Gas MWPC	1–4	1 μsec	17–35 %	1.5 % @ 1 atm	Large	?	1. Low detection efficiency: ~ 15 % at 10 atm
Liquid xenon MWPC	2–4	1–10 μsec or $10^5/10^6$ cts/sec per wire	11–22 %	90 %	Large	?	1. Gas purification problems 2. Refrigeration required 3. Safety concerns 4. Cost and availability of xenon uncertain
Liquid xenon scintillation	4–6	Luminescent decay time 1/23 that of NaI	?	90 %	Large	?	1. Refrigeration required 2. Light emitted in UV 3. Gas purity no so stringent as MWPC
NaI bar detector	6–8	2 μsec	20 %	90 %	Large	Good	1. Useful for whole body scanning 2. Several could be placed around patient for computerized section imaging

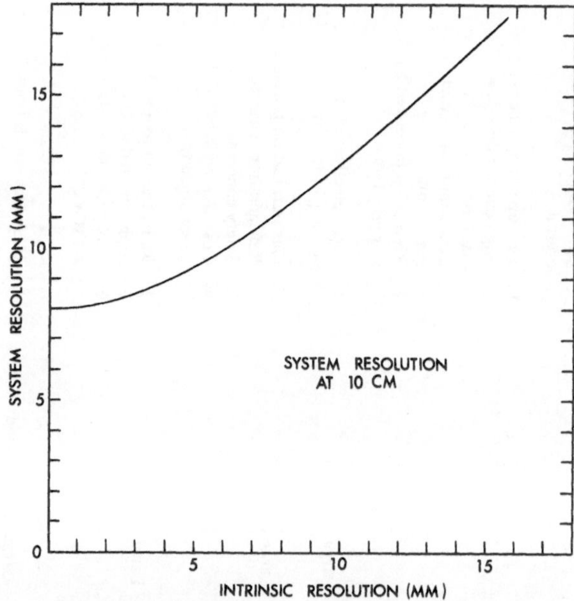

Fig. 4-13. System resolution (FWHM) at 10 cm as function of intrinsic camera resolution, $R_S = (R_I^2 + R_C^2)^{1/2}$, using parallel hole collimator with $R_C = 8$ mm.

system resolution from 11.3 mm down to 8.06 mm, a reduction of only 29%. Furthermore, there are statistical image quality factors to be taken into account. To maintain image statistical quality and take full advantage of an improved resolution capability one must accumulate the same number of counts per resolution element (Llacer, 1973), which will mean longer imaging times for a given source strength and collimator efficiency. Consider a case where the camera has perfect intrinsic resolution and system resolution is limited solely by the collimator. If the collimator resolution is improved by a factor of 2, the geometric collection efficiency will be cut by a factor of 4. Also, there will be four times as many resolution elements in the image. Therefore, in this hypothetical example one would have to image a factor of 16 times longer in order to maintain statistical image quality and actually convey the improved resolution. Lengthened imaging times make it more likely that the patient cannot tolerate lying still that long and that movement will reduce image quality. If clinicians will not accept any increase in imaging times, then 5–8 mm (due to collimator) seems to be an asymptotic limit of resolution for nuclear medicine imaging devices using parallel hole collimators and currently popular radioisotopes. In general, nuclear medicine cannot image with the same morphological detail possible with X-ray radiology or ultrasound. It would thus seem that positron imaging will become increasingly important because it eliminates the resolution-limiting effect of the collimator and also because the metabolically important elements have positron-emitting isotopes, making imaging related to physiology a closer reality, something nuclear medicine has always promised.

Although there have been some systems developed which compete favorably with the Anger camera, none offer any superiority for a general purpose imaging system. One normally expects the lifetime of a given invention or technical system to be no more than 20 years before it is superceded by advancing technology. Such does not seem to be the case with the Anger camera. The Anger camera has proven to be an inherently viable configuration with potential for improvement. This is because of its intrinsic characteristics as a detector. Its detection quantum efficiency is excellent over the range of gamma energies (100–600 keV) relevant to nuclear medicine. Energy resolution is good enough to allow discrimination against the contrast degradation of scattered gammas. Camera intrinsic resolution has continuously improved over the years from 10 mm to under 6 mm. Major improvements in phototube photocathodes translated directly to better resolution in the Anger camera. The camera's dead time is fundamentally limited only by the decay time of NaI (230 nsec) and recent implementation of fast electronics has made image count rates up to 200,000 cts/sec possible, depending on the scatter present. The field of view of the Anger camera is quite adequate. Recent introduction of 17-in.-diameter NaI crystals has made it possible to image both lungs or liver/spleen with parallel hole collimation. The use of converging collimation on the larger cameras can yield noteworthy improvements in collection efficiency and resolution. The field uniformity and linearity of the Anger camera are quite acceptable and have continually improved. Perhaps the cardinal characteristic of the Anger camera is its ubiquitous versatility. As opposed to a scanner, it can generate hemodynamic flow studies (Fig. 4-14) as well as high-quality static images. Two Anger detectors can be used facing each other to form a positron camera. Mounted above and below the patient, two Anger heads can be moved across the patient after the fashion of a scanner and the data arranged to produce longitudinal tomographic images of several planes simultaneously. Alternatively, in a simpler mode of operation, moving the detector head over the patient has found great utility in whole body scanning for bone lesions and metastases. Furthermore, high-contrast section images can be computer derived from data collected by rotating the camera head around the patient. Use of the Anger camera in this mode can generate several sections simultaneously (Oppenheim *et al.*, 1976; Jaszczak *et al.*, 1976). The field of nuclear medicine has built upon the strength of the Anger gamma camera.

The photomultipliers of the Anger camera are spaced from the scintillation crystal by a lucite light guide. The resolution of the camera may be improved by using a thinner light guide and moving the phototubes closer

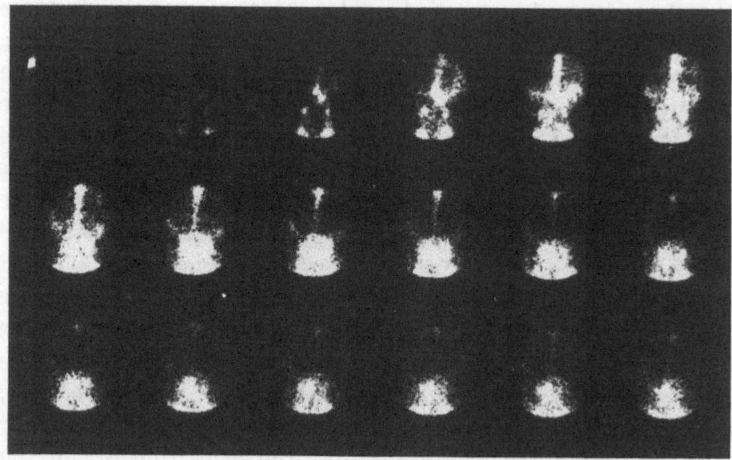

Fig. 4-14. Dynamic flow study of cerebral circulation. Radioisotope is injected rapidly into an arm vein, and pictures of the head are taken when the radioisotope is first seen there, usually about 10–15 sec after injection. Sequential images at 1-sec intervals show decreased perfusion of the right hemisphere (left side of image) in a patient with a stroke.

to the crystal. However, this is always at the expense of generating hot spots in the flood field and distortions in image linearity. Consequently, a compromise is always made and the phototubes placed to yield the best combination of resolution, uniformity, and linearity. Now with the advent of microprocessors, fast ADCs, and ROMs it becomes feasible to move the phototubes closer to the crystal and correct for the distortions digitally. Advances in large-scale integrated microelectronics have continually increased device speed and density and brought down prices. It is becoming feasible now to think of digitizing each PMT signal early and processing data digitally. An event-by-event pattern recognition scheme for locating an event's origin has been discussed (Blum, 1974) but would require massive computer memory. Nonetheless, a digital system would open up the possibility of implementing new positioning algorithms other than the simple centroid estimation arithmetics that Anger originally used. Hand in hand with advances in electronics we can thus expect improvements in gamma camera technology.

Acknowledgments

The author acknowledges the helpful suggestions and stimulation given by Dr. Gerd Muehllehner during the course of this review. Special thanks go to Linda Walker for typing the manuscript.

REFERENCES

Allemand, R., Laval, M., Prunier, J. F. (1971), The use of liquefied noble gases: a new prospect for x-ray and λ-ray localization detectors, *Int. J. Appl. Radiat. Isot.* **22:** 633–634.

Anger, H. O. (1958), Scintillation camera, *Rev. Sci. Instrum.* **29** (1): 27–33.

Anger, H. O. (1966a), Survey of radioisotope cameras, *ISA Trans.* **5** (4): 311–334.

Anger. H. O. (1966b), Sensitivity, resolution, and linearity of the scintillation camera, *IEEE Trans. Nucl. Sci.* **NS-13** (3): 380–391.

Anger, H. O. (1967), Radioisotope cameras, in Hine, G. J. (ed.), *Instrumentation in Nuclear Medicine*, Vol. 1, Academic Press, New York, pp. 485–550.

Armantrout, G. A., Wichner, R., and Swierkowski, S. P. (1974), Encapsulation of high-purity germanium detectors, *IEEE Trans. Nucl. Sci.* **NS-21** (1): 344–346.

Baker, R. G., and Scrimger, J. W. (1967), An investigation of the parameters in scintillation camera design, *Phys. Med. Biol.* **12** (1): 51–63.

Barrett, H. H. (1972), Fresnel zone plate imaging in nuclear medicine, *J. Nucl. Med.* **13:** 382–385.

Barrett, H. H., and De Meester, G. D. (1974), Quantum noise in fresnel zone plate imaging, *Appl. Opt.* **13** (5): 1100–1109.

Beck, R. N. (1968), A note on crystal efficiency, in *Fundamental Problems in Scanning*, Charles C. Thomas, Springfield, Illinois, pp. 229–230.

Ben Zeev, D., Kelin, Y., Sabbah, B., *et al.* (1973), New concepts for imaging instruments, *J. Nucl. Med.* **14:** 379, 380.

Bender, M. A., and Blau, M. (1963), The autofluoroscope, *Nucleonics* **21** (10): 52–56.

Berninger, W. H. (1974), Monolithic gamma detector arrays and position sensitive detectors in high purity germanium, *IEEE Trans. Nucl. Sci.* **NS-21:** 374–378.

Berninger, W. H. (1974), Pulsed optical and electron beam excitation of silicon position sensitive detectors, *IEEE Trans. Nucl. Sci.* **NS-21** (1): 386–389.

Bertolini, G., Cappellani, F., and Restelli, G. (1973), Current state of the art in semiconductor detectors, *Nucl. Instrum. Methods* **112:** 219–228.

Blum, A. S. (1974), A scintillation camera, *IEEE Trans. Nucl. Sci.* **NS-21** (1): 695–696.

Bok, B. D., and Fonroget, F. (1975), A new whole-body unidirectional moving scanner: comparative study of performance, *J. Nucl. Med.* **16:** 516.

Bonazzola, G. C., Bressani, T., Chiavassa, E., *et al.* (1972), A simple coding system for multiwire proportional counters, *Nucl. Instrum. Methods* **98:** 273–277.

Borkowski, C. J., and Kopp, M. K. (1970), Some applications and properties of one and two dimensional position sensitive proportional counters, *IEEE Trans. Nucl. Sci.* **NS-17** (3): 340–349.

Borkowski, C. J., and Kopp, M. K. (1972), Proportional counter photon camera. *IEEE Trans. Nucl. Sci.* **NS-19** (3): 161–168.

Burns, J. (1961), Imaging multiplier phototube for a gamma-ray pinhole camera, TID-14559.

Charpak, G. (1970), Evolution of the automatic spark chambers, in *Ann. Rev. Nucl. Sci.* **20:** 195–254.

Charpak, G., Fischer, G., *et al.* (1971), Some features of large multiwire proportional chambers, *Nucl. Instrum. Methods* **97:** 377–388.

Conde, C. A. N., Policarp, A. J. P. L., and Alves, M. A. F. (1968), Gas proportional scintillation counter with xenon and xenon mixtures, *IEEE Trans. Nucl. Sci.* **NS-15** (3): 84–91.

Conrad, B. (1969), A detector for determining the distribution of radioactive materials, Great Britain patent No. 1,174,558 awarded to Siemens Aktiengesellschaft, December 1969.

Crawley, J. C. W., and Veall, N. (1973), The design and some clinical applications of a hybrid scanner, in *Medical Radioisotope Scintigraphy*, Vol. 1, IAEA, Vienna, pp. 105–112.

Davis, T.P., and Martone, R.J. (1966), The hybrid radioisotope scanner, *J. Nucl. Med.* **7**: 114–127.

Detko, J.F. (1973), A prototype, ultra pure germanium orthogonal strip gamma-camera, in *Medical Radioisotope Scintigraphy*, Vol. 1, IAEA, Vienna, pp. 241–254.

Dhawan, S. (1973), A survey of proportional wire chamber electronics and readout systems, *IEEE Trans. Nucl. Sci.* **NS-20** (1): 166–171.

DiRocco, J.V., and Grenier, R.P. (1967), Addressing of the 294 crystal mosaic of the digital autofluoroscope, *IEEE Trans. Nucl. Sci.* **NS-14** (1): 204–210.

Dolgosheim, B.A., Lebedenko, V.N., and Rodionov, B.V. (1967), Luminescence induced by alpha particles in liquid xenon in an electric field, *JETP Lett.* [English Transl.] **6**: 224.

Driard, B., Rozieres, G., and Verat, M. (1976), A large field image intensifier tube for scintillation cameras, *IEEE Trans. Nucl. Sci.* **NS-23** (1): 502–506.

Entine, G. (1974), Radiation Monitoring Devices, Inc., private communication.

Freedman, G.S., Goodwin, P.N., Johnson, P.M., *et al.* (1969), The image intensifier camera and single-crystal camera: a comparative evaluation, in *Medical Radioisotope Scintigraphy*, Vol. 1, IAEA, Vienna, pp. 31–42.

Gelezunas, V.L. (1974), The effect of exposure to various gaseous environments on the subsequent performance of high purity germanium gamma ray detectors, *IEEE Trans. Nucl. Sci.* **NS-21**: 360–369.

Glass, H.I., Hudson, F.R., French, M.T., *et al.* (1973), A 70 mm diameter germanium detector medical radioisotope scanner, in *Medical Radioisotope Scintigraphy*, Vol. 1, IAEA, Vienna, pp. 79–103.

Grenier, R.P., Bender, M.A., and Jones, R.H. (1974), A computerized multi-crystal scintillation gamma camera, in Hine, G., and Sorenson, J.A. (eds.), *Instrumentation in Nuclear Medicine*, Vol. 2, Academic Press, New York, pp. 101–134.

Grove, R., Ko, I., *et al.* (1972), Phase compensated electromagnetic delay lines for wire chamber readout, *Nucl. Instrum. Methods* **99**: 381–385.

Held, D., and Weisskopf, M.C. (1973), A position sensitive x-ray detector for the HEAO-A satellite, *IEEE Trans. Nucl. Sci.* **NS-20** (1): 140–144.

Hine, G.J., and Paras, P. (1975), Performance of scintillation cameras, *J. Nucl. Med.* **16**: 1206–1207.

Hoffer, P.B., and Beck, R.N. (1971), Effects of minimizing scatter using Ge(Li) detectors on phantom models and patients, in Hoffer, P.B., Beck, R.N., and Gottschalk, A. (eds.), *Semiconductor Detectors in the Future of Nuclear Medicine*, Society of Nuclear Medicine, New York, pp. 131–143.

Jaszczak, R.J. (1974), Searle Analytic, Inc., private communication.

Jaszczak, R.J., Huard, D., Murphy, P.H., *et al.* (1976), Radionuclide emission computed tomography with a scintillation camera, *J. Nucl. Med.* **17**: 551.

Kaplan, S.N., Kaufman, L., Perez-Mendez, W., *et al.* (1973), Multiwire proportional chambers for biomedical application, *Nucl. Instrum. Methods* **106**: 397–406.

Kaufman, L., Perez-Mendez, W., *et al.* (1972), A multiwire proportional chamber for nuclear medicine applications, *IEEE Trans. Nucl. Sci.* **NS-19** (3): 169–172.

Kaufman, L., Perez-Mendez, W., Stoker, G. (1973), Performance of a pressurized xenon filled multiwire proportional chamber, *IEEE Trans. Nucl. Sci.* **NS-20** (1): 426–428.

Kaufman, L., Hattner, R., Price, D., *et al.* (1975), Imaging with a small ultra pure germanium gamma-camera, *IEEE Trans. Nucl. Sci.* **NS-22** (1): 395–403.

Kenny, P.J. (1971), Spatial resolution and countrate capacity of a positron camera: some experimental and theoretical considerations, *Int. J. Appl. Radiat. Isot.* **22**: 21–28.

Kulberg, G.H., van Dijk, H., Muehllehner, G. (1972), Improved resolution of the Anger scintillation camera through the use of threshold preamplifiers, *J. Nucl. Med.* **13**: 169–171.

Lansiart, A., Lequais, J., Roux, G., Morucci, J.P., and Gaucher, J.C. (1969), Detecteur stationnaire a gaz et nouveau type de gammascope, in *Medical Radioisotope Scintigraphy*, Vol. 1, IAEA, Vienna, pp. 87–98.

Larsen, R.S. (1972), Interlaboratory development of an integrated circuit for multiwire proportional chambers, *IEEE Trans. Nucl. Sci.* **NS-19** (1):483–494.

Larsen, R.S. (1973), A hybrid integrated circuit for multiwire proportional chambers, *IEEE Trans. Nucl. Sci.* **NS-20** (1):172–181.

Lavoie, L. (1973), Use of inert element scintillators in nuclear medicine. Published in *Proceedings of the symposium on Advanced Technology Arising from Particle Physics Research*, held at Argonne National Laboratory, May 17, 1973 (Conf-730541-2).

Lee, Lap Yen (1973), Optical-binary coded position sensitive radiation detector, U. S. Patent No. 3,758,780, September 11, 1973.

Llacer, J. (1973), Ultimate capabilities of detectors with high energy resolution in radioisotope scanning, *IEEE Trans. Nucl. Sci.* **NS-20** (1):273–281.

Llacer, J., and Cho, Z.H. (1973), Preliminary study of a germanium three dimensional camera for positron emitting radioisotopes, *IEEE Trans. Nucl. Sci.* **NS-20** (1):282–293.

Llacer, J., Watt, M., Schieber, M., *et al.* (1974), Preliminary studies of charge carrier transport in mercuric iodide radiation detectors, *IEEE Trans. Nucl. Sci.* **NS-21** (1):305–314.

Luc Moretti, J., Mensch, B., Guey, A., *et al.* (1976), Comparative assessment of scintillation camera performance, *Radiology* **119:**157–165.

Mallard, J.R., and Myers, M.J. (1963), The performance of a gamma camera for the visualization of radioactive isotopes *in vivo*, *Phys. Med. Biol.* **8** (2):165–182.

Mallard, J.R., and Wilkes, P.J. (1969), The Aber-gammascope, an image intensifier gamma camera, in *Medical Radioisotope Scintigraphy*, Vol. 1, IAEA, Vienna, pp. 3–16.

Malm, H.L. (1972), A mercuric iodide gamma-ray spectrometer, *IEEE Trans. Nucl. Sci.* **NS-19** (3):263–265.

Malm, H.L., and Martini, M. (1974), Polarization phenomena in CdTe nuclear radiation detectors, *IEEE Trans. Nucl. Sci.* **NS-21** (1):322–330.

Martone, R.J., Goldman, S.C., and Wolczek, W. (1974), Scintillation camera with improved light diffusion, U. S. Patent No. 3,814,938, June 1974.

McCready, V.R., Parker, R.P., Gunnersen. E.M., *et al.* (1971), Clinical test on a prototype semiconductor gamma-camera, *Br. J. Radiol.* **44:**58.

Miraldi, F., Di Chiro, G. (1970), Tomographic techniques in radioisotope imaging with a proposal of a new device: the Tomoscanner, *Radiology* **94:**513–520.

Mitchell, J.G., Mallard, J.R., *et al.* (1973), Towards a fine resolution image intensifier gamma camera: the Aber-gammascope, in *Medical Radioisotope Scintigraphy*, Vol. 1, IAEA, Vienna, pp. 157–167.

Moody, N.F., Paul, W., and Joy, M. (1969), A versatile gamma-ray camera for dynamic or static studies in medicine, *IEEE Trans. Nucl. Sci.* **NS-16** (2):3–18.

Moody, N.F., Paul, W., and Joy, M. (1970), A survey of medical gamma-ray cameras, *IEEE Proc.* **58** (2):217–242.

Moody, N.F., Joy, M., and Paul, W. (1973), An image intensifier gamma-ray camera, and its variants, in *Medical Radioisotope Scintigraphy*, Vol. 1, IAEA, Vienna, pp. 255–267.

Morucci, J.P., and Lansiart, A. (1970), Investigation of light emission by electron avalanches in binary mixtures where xenon is the parent constituent. Attempted interpretation of the visible continuum emitted by xenon, *IEEE Trans. Nucl. Sci.* **NS-17** (3):95–106.

Muehllehner, G. (1972), Searle Analytic, Inc., private communication.

Muehllehner, G. (1972), Radiation imaging apparatus, U. S. Patent No. 3, 683, 185. August 1972.

Muehllehner, G. (1975), Positron camera with extended counting rate capability, *J. Nucl. Med.* **16:**653–657.

Muehllehner, G., and Luig, H. (1973), Septal penetration in scintillation camera collimators, *Phys. Med. Biol.* **18** (6):855–862.

Muehllehner, G., Buchin, M.P., and Dudek, J.H. (1976), Performance parameters of a positron imaging camera, *IEEE Trans. Nucl. Sci.* **NS-23** (1):528–537.

Muller, R.A., Derenzo, S.E., Alvarez, L.W., *et al.* (1971), Liquid filled proportional counter, *Phys. Rev. Lett.* **27**:532–535.

Murphy, P.H., Burdine, J.A., and Moyer, R.A. (1975), Converging collimation and a large-field-of-view scintillation camera, *J. Nucl. Med.* **16**:1152–1157.

Northrup, J.A., Nobles, R.A. (1956), Some aspects of gas scintillation counters, *IRE Trans. Nucl. Sci.* **NS-3**:59–61.

Northrup, J.A., Gursky, J.M., and Johnsrud, A.E. (1958), Further work with noble element scintillators, *IRE Trans. Nucl. Sci.* **NS-5** (3):81–87.

Oppenheim, B.E., Hoffer, P.B., and Gottschalk, A. (1976), Nuclear imaging: a new dimension, *Radiology* **118**:491–494.

Owen, R.B., and Awcock, M.L. (1968), One and two dimensional position sensing semiconductor detectors, *IEEE Trans. Nucl. Sci.* **NS-15** (3):290–303.

Palms, J.M. (1971), Newer developments in detector design and materials, in Hoffer, P.B., Beck, R.N., and Gottschalk, A. (eds.), *Semiconductor Detectors in the Future of Nuclear Medicine*, Society of Nuclear Medicine, New York, pp. 59–77.

Parker, R.P., Gunnersen, E.M., Ellis, R., and Bell, J. (1973), A semiconductor gamma-camera: assessment of results, in *Medical Radioisotope Scintigraphy*, Vol. 1, IAEA, Vienna, pp. 193–216.

Planiol, T.H., Floyrac, R., Itti, R., *et al.* (1973), La scintigraphie au lit du malade. Résultats obtenus à l'aide d'un scintigraphe hybride portatif, in *Medical Radioisotope Scintigraphy*, Vol. 1, IAEA, Vienna, pp. 113–119.

Policarpo, A.J.P.L., Conde, C.A.N., and Alves, M.A.F. (1968), Large light output gas proportional scintillation counters, *Nucl. Instrum. Methods* **58**:151–156.

Rindi, A., Perez-Mendez, V., and Wallace, R.I. (1970), Delay line readout for proportional chambers, *Nucl. Instrum. Methods* **77**:325–327.

Rogers, W.L., Han, K.S., Jones, L.W., *et al.* (1972), Application of a Fresnel zone plate to gamma-ray imaging, *J. Nucl. Med.* **13**:612–615.

Rohrmann, C.A. (1971), Fission product xenon and krypton, an opportunity for large scale utilization, *Isot. Radiat. Technol.* **8** (3):253–260.

Sarocka, L. (1973), Air Products and Chemicals Inc., Specialty Cases Department, private communication.

Schlosser, P.A., Miller, D.W., Gerber, M.S., *et al.* (1974), A practical gamma-ray camera system using high-purity germanium, *IEEE Trans. Nucl. Sci.* **NS-21** (1):658–664.

Scrimger, J.W., and Baker, R.G. (1967), Investigation of light distribution from scintillations in a gamma camera crystal, *Phys. Med. Biol.* **12** (1):101–103.

Serreze, H.B., Entine, G., and Wald, F.V. (1974), Advances in CdTe gamma-ray detectors, *IEEE Trans. Nucl. Sci.* **NS-21** (1).

Siffert, P., Cornet, A., Stuck, R., *et al.* (1975), Cadmium telluride nuclear radiation detectors, *IEEE Trans. Nucl. Sci.* **NS-22** (1):211–225.

St. Onge, R. (1973), A high resolution, high efficiency proportional counter X-ray camera, *IEEE Trans. Nucl. Sci.* **NS-20** (1):333.

Strauss, M.G., and Sherman, I.S. (1972), Gamma-ray camera using a coaxial germanium detector, *J. Nucl. Med.* **13**:767.

Strauss, M.G., and Sherman, I.S. (1975), Imaging efficiency of Ge and NaI(Tl) gamma-ray detectors, *IEEE Trans. Nucl. Sci.* **NS-22** (1):331–343.

Svedberg, J.B. (1969), Improved pulse arithmetics for a gamma camera system, in *Medical Radioisotope Scintigraphy*, Vol. 1, IAEA, Vienna, pp. 125–134.

Svedberg, J.B. (1972), On the intrinsic resolution of a gamma camera system, *Phys. Med. Biol.* **17** (4):514–524.

Svedberg, J.B. (1973), Computed intrinsic efficiencies and modulation transfer functions for gamma cameras, *Phys. Med. Biol.* **18** (5).

Svedberg, J.B. (1975), Computer simulation of the Anger gamma camera, *Comput. Programs Biomed.* **4**:189–201:189–201.

Swanson, F., Kuehne, F., and Favale, A. (1973), High spatial resolution MWPC systems using electromagnetic delay line readouts, *IEEE Trans. Nucl. Sci.* **NS-20** (1):160–165.

Tanaka, E., Hiramoto, T., and Nohara, N. (1970), Scintillation cameras based on new position arithmetics, *J. Nucl. Med.* **11**:542–547.

Ter-Pogossian, M. (1969), The magnacamera, an image-intensifier radioisotope camera, in *Medical Radioisotope Scintigraphy*, Vol. 1, IAEA, Vienna, pp. 151–159.

Ter-Pogossian, M.M., and Phelps, M.E. (1973), Semiconductor detector systems, *Semin. Nucl. Med.* **3** (4):343–365.

Thomas, F.D., Beierwaltes, W.H., *et al.* (1969), A new scintillation camera, in *Medical Radioisotope Scintigraphy*, Vol. 1, IAEA, Vienna, pp. 43–55.

Todd, R.W. (1975), Methods and apparatus for determining the spatial distribution of a radioactive material, U. S. Patent No. 3, 876, 882, April 1975.

Todd, R.W., Nightingale, J.M., and Everett, D.B. (1974), A proposed γ-camera, *Nature* **251**:132–134.

Vetter, H.G., and Pizer, S.M. (1971), A measure for radioisotope scan image quality, *J. Nucl. Med.* **12**:526–529.

Whitehead, F.R. (1978), Minimum detectable gray scale differences in nuclear medicine images, *J. Nucl. Med.* **19**:87–93.

Zaklad, H. (1971), A purification system for the removal of electronegative impurities from noble gases for noble-liquid nuclear particle detectors, thesis, Lawrence Radiation Laboratory Report UCRL-20690, April 1971.

Zaklad, H., Derenzo, S.E., Muller, R.A., *et al.* (1972), A liquid xenon radioisotope camera, *IEEE Trans. Nucl. Sci.* **NS-19** (3):206–213.

Zaklad, H., Derenzo, S.E., Muller, R.A., *et al.* (1973a), Initial images from a 24 wire liquid xenon gamma camera, *IEEE Trans. Nucl. Sci.* **NS-20** (1):429–431.

Zaklad, H., Derenzo, S.E., and Smits, R.G. (1973b), Liquid-xenon gamma camera—Progress report, *J. Nucl. Med.* **14**:645.

CHAPTER 5

Tomography

J.A. PATTON

5.1. INTRODUCTION

Typical radioisotope imaging devices have, as an inherent drawback, limited information as to lesion depth. Knowledge of the exact depth, location, and size of tumors are prime variables determining surgical approaches prior to operative removal, implantation of radioactive sources, or direction of external beams used in radiation therapy. Information involving source (i.e., lesion) depth is very difficult to obtain, especially when sources lie deep to superficial areas of activity as is the general case in the human body.

As has been described in previous chapters, the typical nuclear medicine image obtained with a rectilinear scanner is a crude tomogram of a preselected depth, while that obtained with a gamma camera is an image of primarily superficial structures. Figure 3-15 shows the relationship between

J. A. PATTON • Department of Radiology, Vanderbilt University, Nashville, Tennessee 37232.

the two types of imaging modalities with regard to the dependence of sensitivity with depth. If better tomographic information could be obtained, there would be several clinical advantages.

First of all, improved tomographic imaging would be expected to result in better detection of abnormalities. The usual liver scan, for example, presents approximately half of the liver to the viewer on a single image. A small defect located in the liver may be missed because overlying or underlying normal liver activity "fills in" the abnormality and hides it from view. The same would be true in scans of the thyroid, kidney, lung, and other solid organs. Scans of the body using gallium-67 (a radioisotope that is taken up by some tumors and by inflammatory tissues) would benefit from tomographic presentation, as one could then see more clearly whether there are differences between normal structures and areas of unusual accumulation of radioisotope.

Second, tomographic imaging, by giving information on the anatomic location of a lesion, would aid in a more specific diagnosis. For example, a filling defect in the anterior region of the liver may actually be a lesion located outside the liver, giving the effect of a liver defect by an extrinsic mass effect. Such a lesion may be an enlarged gall bladder, or a tumor in the colon located anterior to the liver. Tomographic imaging, by showing more exactly the anatomic location of the abnormality, could aid in making a diagnosis. Similarly, other organs located near the liver (kidney, adrenal, pancreas, small intestine) could, if enlarged or abnormal, cause extrinsic mass effects which on ordinary images may be indistinguishable from filling defects within the liver itself. Tomographic images could separate lesions in the brain from lesions in the skull, and lesions in the heart muscle itself (myocardium) from lesions in the sac surrounding the heart (pericardium). In gallium-67 scans done for the detection of tumor or inflammatory disease, tomographic images could help decide whether abnormal activity, if present, is located in lymph nodes vs. in the peritoneal cavity, or in the lung vs. the mediastinum.

Finally, detection and localization are not sufficient; the disease must be staged, that is, the physician must reach an understanding of the degree and severity. For metastatic disease it is essential to know the extent of disease for planning therapy. In diseases involving lymph nodes it is essential to know the distribution of the involved nodes. The clinical questions one asks in staging disease are fairly straightforward, and a good system of tomographic imaging would contribute greatly to the staging procedure.

In the past few years, several different attempts have been made to develop a system to obtain images of planes of activity within the body. These instruments have been given the name of tomographic imaging devices because their goal is the same as their counterparts with the same

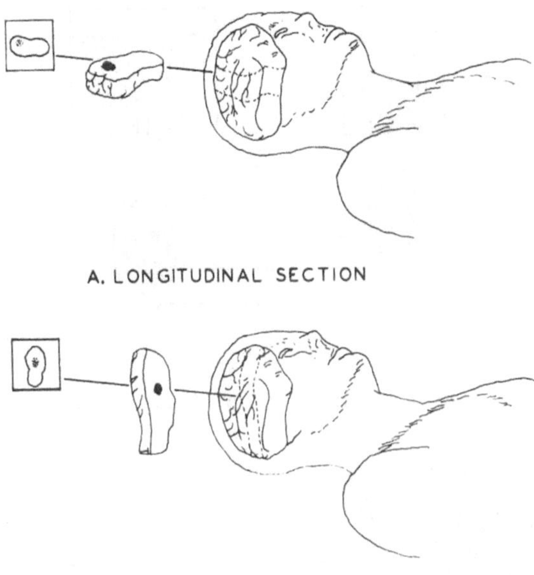

Fig. 5-1. Illustration of the concepts of longitudinal and transverse section tomography. (Courtesy of Searle Diagnostics, Inc.)

name in diagnostic radiology. However, the problem of radionuclide tomography is more difficult to solve than that of X-ray tomography because the photon distribution originates within the body (i.e., from many discrete points) instead of a single point outside of the body, as with an X-ray tube. The concept of a tomographic scanner was first proposed in 1963 (Kuhl, 1963) and two techniques of radionuclide tomography were defined. The procedures of longitudinal and transverse section tomography are illustrated in Fig. 5-1 with images of the brain used as an example.

5.2. LONGITUDINAL SECTION IMAGING

In longitudinal section imaging, the goal is to divide the human body into planes parallel to its length and image the radioactivity in each of these planes separately. Rectilinear scanners with focused collimators were actually the first longitudinal section imaging devices (see Chapter 3). This capability is due to the fact that focused collimators have a point in the field of view with maximum sensitivity and optimum resolution (the focal point) which maps out a plane of interest (the focal plane) when the collimated detector is moved in a rectilinear raster (see also Chapter

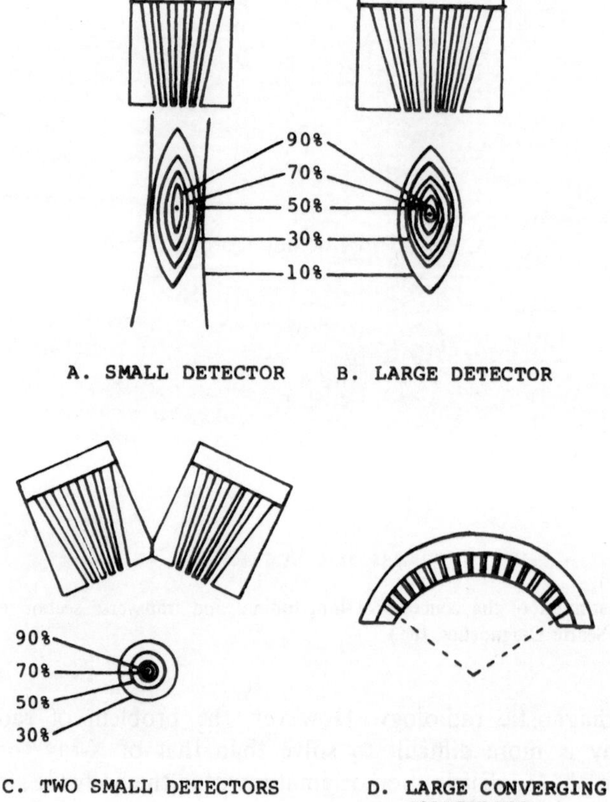

Fig. 5-2. (A) The point of maximum sensitivity and optimum resolution in the field of view of a detector with a focused collimator is the focal point. The depth of response (i.e., thickness of the focal plane) can be reduced by using large detectors (B), multiple detectors with intersecting focal points (C), or converging collimators (D).

2—Scintillation Camera Collimators). The depth or thickness of the plane may be several centimeters for small detectors (Fig. 5-2A) due to the long depth of response. But as detectors increased in size in order to increase sensitivity (8-in.-diameter detectors soon became available), the thickness of the plane became smaller (Fig. 5-2B). In fact this phenomenon actually was a disadvantage of the large scanning detectors because these instruments were being used for routine frontal plane scanning and lesions outside of this thin focal plane were being missed. Images of different depths required repeat scans after changing the patient-to-detector distance so that the time required for multiple sections became prohibitive. In addition, activity in the planes not being imaged interfered with data collection from the plane of interest resulting in images of relatively poor contrast (i.e., these images were not true section images).

One way of enhancing the focal plane response was to use multiple detectors with intersecting focal points and simply sum the outputs of the different detectors together as shown in Fig. 5-2C. Raytheon actually marketed a rectilinear scanner with this capability; however, this technique was not widely utilized. It is obvious how the focal plane response is improved by this arrangement. The addition of more detectors would further increase this enhancement. Longitudinal section scanning was performed in 1965 with a variation of this multiple detector concept to enhance the focal point response (Cassen, 1965). A wide-angle converging collimator was mounted on a rectilinear scanner as shown in Fig. 5-2D. The detector consisted of irregular pieces of activated sodium iodide immersed in chlorinated diphenyl liquid. Views of different planes within the body were obtained by varying the detector-to-patient distance and repeating the scan. Even though an event recorded by the detector most probably originated at the focal point, sources of radiation outside of the focal plane led to degradations in the quality of the tomographic sections obtained. Multiple scans were still required in order to image multiple planes.

With the development of the scintillation camera, much of the work in radionuclide tomography focused on attempts to modify this instrument for section imaging due to its wide acceptance as a routine imaging device.

The longitudinal section imaging capability of the scintillation camera was developed by Muehllehner in 1971. The technique utilizes a rotating collimator having parallel holes which are slanted 20° from the vertical. The concept is shown schematically in Fig. 5-3 where Fig. 5-3B shows the collimator rotated 180° about its center relative to the position shown in Fig. 5-3A. In practice, the collimator is in constant motion. Thus photons emitted from a location within the region of interest will pass through different holes, in accordance with the rotational position of the collimator. This results in photons interacting at different positions in the crystal despite the fact they originate from the same point. Therefore, as shown in Fig. 5-3, different image patterns are produced. In this example, image A is a routine frontal plane image of the activity distribution with the collimator in position B. In both cases, the images are comparable to those obtained with a conventional parallel hole collimator rotated to the appropriate oblique angles. It was found by Muehllehner that he could optimize information from a given plane by performing a translation of coordinates of recorded events in each of the two images followed by a superposition of the transformed images. Thus, to reconstruct plane 1, image A is translated a distance $d1$ to the right and image B is translated a distance $d1$ to the left. The images are then added together. The distance of translation $d1$ is a function of the angle of inclination of the holes ϕ as well

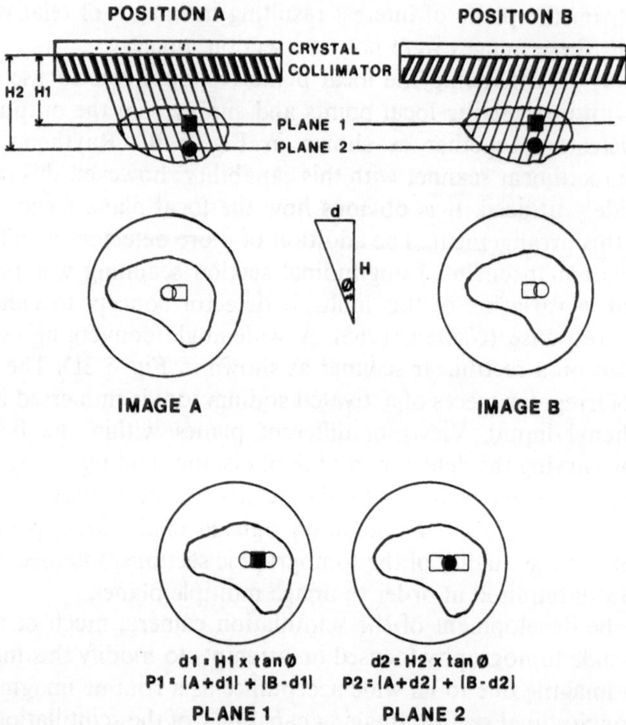

Fig. 5-3. Longitudinal section tomography with a rotating collimator and a scintillation camera. Positions A and B of the slant hole collimator differ by 180°. Reinforcement of the information from a particular plane is obtained by translating each separate image a distance d determined by the distance between the plane and the crystal face and the angle of inclination ϕ of the collimator holes from the vertical. Note that in actuality d is a vector quantity. The signs of $d1$ and $d2$ in the equations $P1$ and $P2$ are provided for clarity.

as the distance from the plane of interest to the crystal as shown in the figure. Two reconstructed images are shown. On the left, plane 1 is reinforced. Thus the cube is well seen and the sphere of plane 2 is blurred out. In the reconstruction shown on the right, plane 2 is reinforced. Therefore the sphere is well defined, while the cube is defocused. In practice, multiple images are obtained for all other possible angular positions of the collimator. It should be noted that for the more involved case, the simple translation described above has to be extended to a two-dimensional translation to accomodate the additional angular positions of the collimator. In Muehllehner's system the translations are performed by means of analog circuits such that the positions of scintillations displayed on the CRT display are electronically altered in relation to the position of the collimator. Data are collected continuously as the collimator rotates about its center.

Four simultaneous images are obtained for each of four preselected planes within the object being studied. A scanning bed is moved in synchrony with the collimator rotation in order to increase the useful field of view. The system was commercially available as an attachment to the Searle scintillation camera.

Freedman, working independently of Muehllehner, developed a very similar system for longitudinal section tomography (Freedman, 1970). The primary differences were that in his system 12 arrays of data were collected in a digital computer corresponding to rotational increments of 30° of the collimator. Images were reconstructed by the computer after completion of the study by performing two-dimensional translations on the data. Thus an image of any plane of interest could be obtained by simply entering the corresponding depth dimension into the computer.

Miraldi and Di Chiro (1970) constructed a system based on the rotating collimator or circular tomography concept. The system consisted of a $1 \times 1 \times 11$-in. bar of NaI(Tl) collimated with tapered channels. Varying degrees of angulation could be obtained by pivoting the detector about its long axis.

Anger (1971) has developed a longitudinal section scanning instrument consisting basically of two small scintillation camera devices fitted with focused collimators which scan in a rectilinear raster. In the latest version of this system the position of each scintillation corresponding to each detected photon in the 9.3-in.-diameter by $\frac{1}{2}$-in.-thick crystal is determined by an array of 19 photomultiplier tubes (see Fig. 5-4). The system contains a multi-image format display device (Microdot) and the appropriate electronics for displaying information from 12 planes simultaneously on separate sections of the display. For each image plane, information from other planes are blurred and diminished in intensity. The display system works on the principle that point sources in different planes in the field of view of the detector appear to move across the crystal face at different velocities as the detector moves across the patient. The velocities are proportional to the distances of the sources from the focal plane of the collimator. The electronics of the display system are fabricated such that if a source lies in a particular plane, it will appear to move in the images of all planes except the image corresponding to that plane. Thus the source will appear in focus in that image and be blurred out in the other images. This is actually a backprojection technique accomplished by the instrument keeping track of the coordinates of the center of the detector in its rectilinear raster, the coordinates of each interaction within the crystal, the distance from the crystal to the focal plane, and the distance from the focal plane to the plane being reconstructed. The end result is a film containing 12 images (6 from each detector) corresponding to 12 planes at preselectable distances and separations. A typical example of the images obtained with such a system

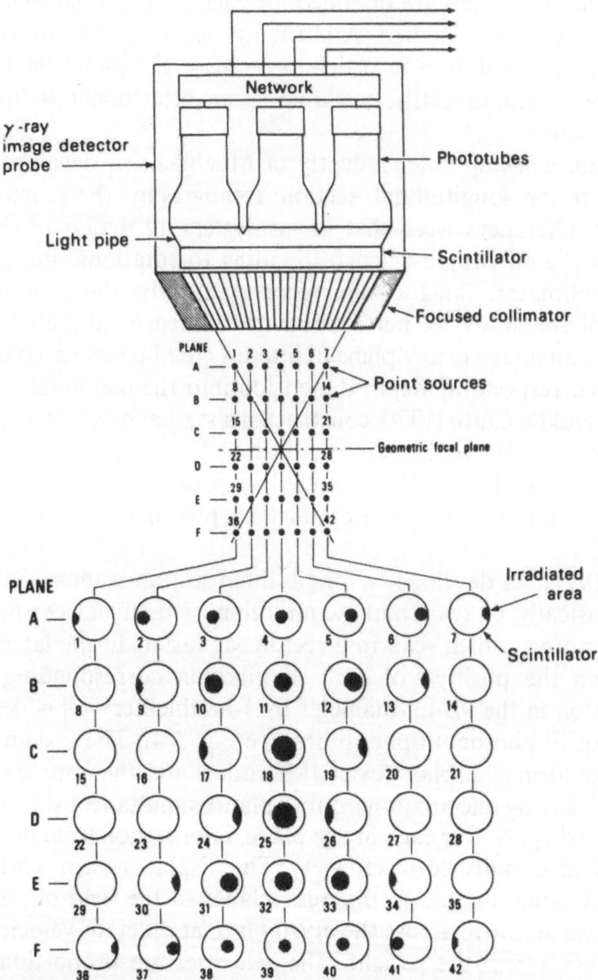

Fig. 5-4. Schematic diagram showing the stationary response of Anger's multiplane tomographic scanner to point sources placed at 42 different locations in six planes within the field of view. Note the apparent difference in sizes of the sources in the different planes. As the system scans, the sources appear to move across the crystal face at different velocities in the imaging of different planes. An image of each plane is reconstructed on a film moving in synchrony with the probe by an optical system that reduces the source to the proper size for that plane. (Anger, H.O., 1974, with permission.)

is shown in Fig. 5-5. This system is now being marketed by Searle Radiographics, Inc., under the trade name Pho/Con.

All longitudinal section imaging techniques are inherently low in contrast due to the fact that activity in planes outside of the plane of interest interfere with data collection from the plane of interest. Although the

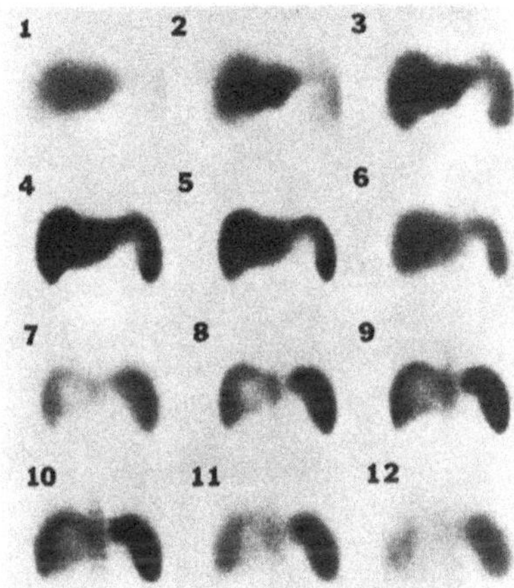

Fig. 5-5. Longitudinal section images of the liver and spleen obtained with Anger's multiplane tomographic scanner. Images 1–6 were obtained with the anterior probe and images 7–12 with the posterior probe. (Courtesy of Searle Diagnostics, Inc.)

systems described here tend to blur out or distort these contributions, they are still significant and lead to an overall degradation in image quality.

5.3. TRANSVERSE SECTION IMAGING

Transverse section imaging produces maps of radioactivity in a cross-sectional slice through the body. The advantage of this procedure is that areas adjacent to regions of high radioisotope content can be mapped with little or no interference. Transverse section imaging is accomplished by recording data from the patient from as many different angles as possible either with moving detectors or stationary systems such as the scintillation camera. Image reconstruction is then accomplished by projecting the data back along lines through the image array corresponding to the direction from which the data were collected. This process can be demonstrated by illustrating a research prototype transverse section imaging system built at Vanderbilt University (Patton *et al.*, 1973) and shown schematically in Fig. 5-6A. The system consists of eight detectors arranged in a circle and permitted to pivot about axes perpendicular to the support rings. Data are collected at preset angular increments from each detector as its field of view is swept through the scanning area at a constant angular velocity by a precision stepping motor and timing belt assembly. Data are stored in a computer until completion of the study and then the image is reconstructed. Data collected from a single point source at the center of the scan field are shown to illustrate how the data are manipulated. The data from each detector are an activity profile or projection of the two-dimensional image into a one-dimensional representation (Fig. 5-6B). To build the image, the simplest technique is to project the data from

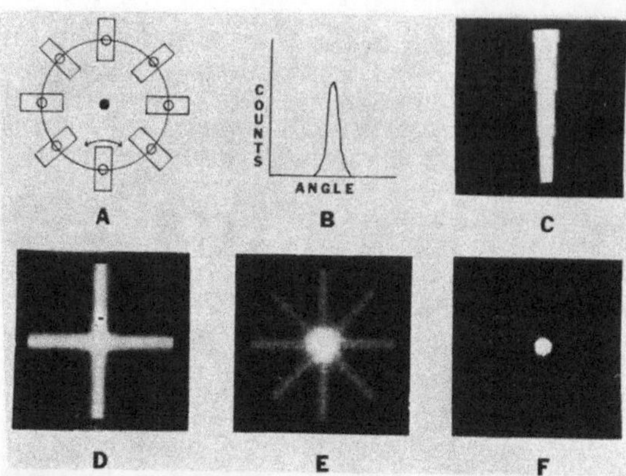

Fig. 5-6. Image construction of a point source by linear superposition of back projections from data obtained with the Vanderbilt University tomographic scanner. Data are collected as a one-dimensional profile from each detector (B) and projected back into the image array (C) assuming equal probabilities of occurrence along each ray. The superposition of images from four orthogonal detectors is shown in D and all eight detectors in E. A background cutoff can then be used to enhance the image (F).

each detector back onto the array and distribute the data assuming equal probabilities of occurrence along each ray (Fig. 5-6C). This is done for each detector in succession until the final image is obtained which shows the "star" effect due to this type of construction (Fig. 5-6E). A baseline cutoff can then be used to enhance the image (Fig. 5-6F). This method is called linear superposition of backprojections and was first applied to transverse section imaging by Kuhl and Edwards (1963), who were the pioneers in this area. The resulting images are relatively low in contrast and may contain artifacts. Several mathematical techniques can be applied to improve the image quality and have been developed by several investigators and applied to systems currently in use. Iterative techniques can be used in which an initial image is generated (such as a simple backprojection image) and corrections are applied successively in order to force the image into better agreement with the data from each of the detectors. This process can be continued until the image converges to a final status in which further corrections cause no change in the image. These corrections can be made simultaneously, ray by ray, or point by point. Analytical reconstruction can also be used in which exact equations can be solved in order to obtain the final images. Two-dimensional Fourier reconstruction is one such analytical technique. This technique is implemented by taking the one-dimensional transform of the projections and plotting them at the corresponding angles in the Fourier plane, then interpolating to provide a two-dimensional array of Fourier coefficients (necessary because the Fourier coefficients obtained from the projections do not fall on a rectangular

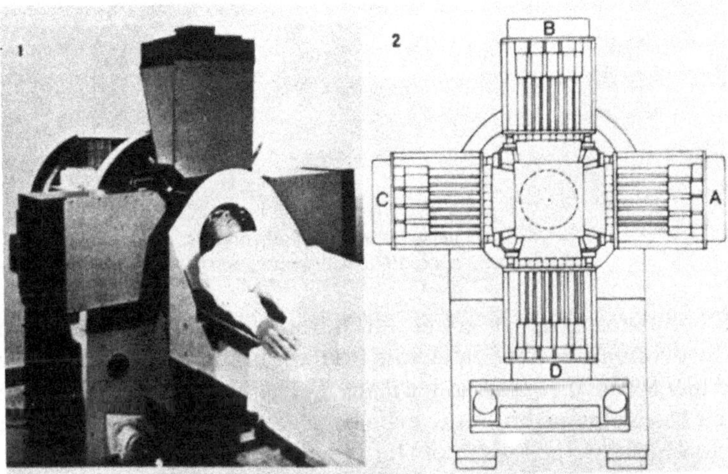

Fig. 5-7. The Mark IV system constructed for transverse section radionuclide emission imaging of the brain. (From Kuhl, D. E., *et al.*, 1976, with permission.)

matrix), and finally taking the inverse two-dimensional transform to obtain the final image. Another analytical technique is filtered backprojection, in which the individual projections are altered or filtered before being projected back into the image array where they are again summed together. Review articles by Brooks and Di Chiro (1976) describe all of those mathematical reconstructions in detail and provide an excellent working bibliography.

The most effective work to date in the field of transverse section radionuclide tomography has been accomplished by Kuhl and Edwards. Their first studies were obtained in 1963 with a two-detector system (Kuhl and Edwards, 1963). The latest version of their system to be developed is the Mark IV (Kuhl *et al.*, 1976) and is shown in Fig. 5-7. It consists of four linear arrays, each containing eight detectors, and is optimized for brain scanning. The detectors are fixed in place and different projections are obtained by rotating the entire frame such that the fields of view of the detectors are interlaced to provide a linear sampling interval of 0.8 cm. The data are buffered into 7.5° increments in a computer and an image is reconstructed after a complete rotation. The rotation continues with the image being updated at the end of each revolution on the basis of the additional data collected. Each revolution requires 50 sec, and five revolutions (4.2 min) are required for most clinical studies. Images are reconstructed by an iterative technique called cumulative additive tangent correction (CATC), an additive correction process in which corrections are based on pairs of orthogonal projections.

Since the system consists of 32 detectors, it is necessary to correct for

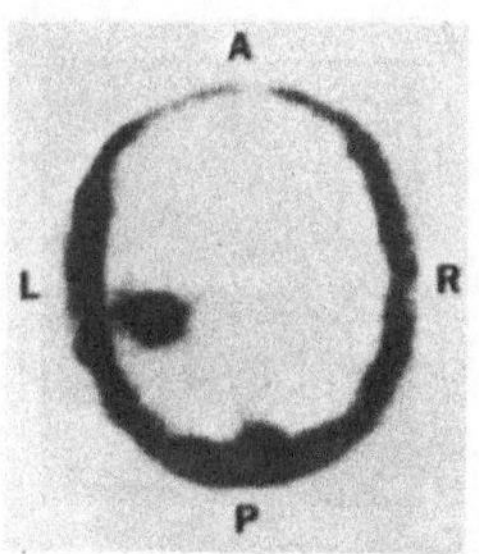

Fig. 5-8. Transverse section image of the brain in a patient with brain metastases from bronchogenic carcinoma. (From Kuhl, D.E., *et al.*, 1976, with permission.)

slight nonuniformities in count rates from different detectors. This is done by obtaining correction factors from calibrations performed each day with a plane source of radioactive material placed in front of each detector. Also an 18-cm.-diameter plastic cylinder of activity is scanned each day in order to obtain correction factors for attenuation within patients. A typical transverse section image of the brain obtained with this system is shown in Fig. 5-8.

Transverse section imaging has also been accomplished by several investigators using the scintillation camera with the parallel hole collimator coupled to a computer (Muehllehner, 1971; Freedman, 1970; Keyes and Simmon, 1973; Budinger *et al.*, 1975; Jaszczak *et al.*, 1976). Static images are collected at multiple angles about the patient and then these data are used to reconstruct multiple sections through the patient employing the various reconstruction techniques described earlier. Data for these studies have been obtained both by moving the camera about the patient and rotating the patient in front of a stationary camera. Problems associated with this technique include difficulties in registration of the multiple images and loss of spatial resolution with depth. Keyes has overcome the former problem by mounting a scintillation camera on a rotating frame, and transverse section images of the brain have been obtained showing excellent registration (Keyes *et al.*, 1976). Advantages of using the scintillation camera are high sensitivity and the ability to record images simultaneously from multiple planes.

The use of positron emitters lends itself very well to transverse section imaging. This is due to the fact that a positron (positively charged electron) is a very unstable particle with an extremely short lifetime. Thus when a positron is emitted from a nucleus, it travels only a very short distance before uniting with a negatively charged electron. The electrons are mutually annihilated and their masses are converted to energy in the form of two 511-keV gamma rays (see Fig. 5-9). These two photons leave the site of their production in opposite directions. Thus if they are detected simultaneously in two opposed detectors, it is known that their origin lies somewhere along a straight line drawn between the two detectors. This phenom-

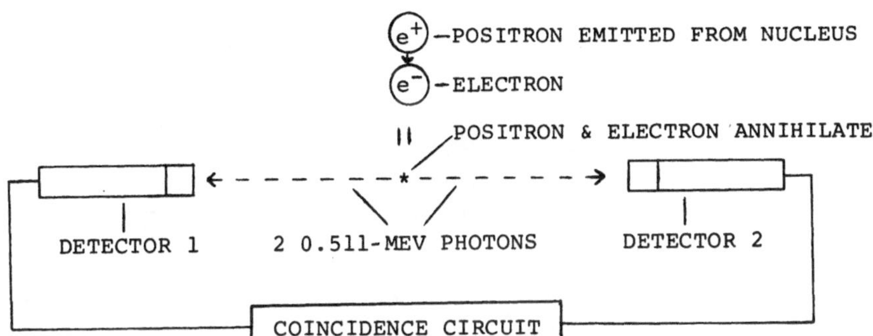

Fig. 5-9. Illustration of the production of two 0.511-MeV photons from the annihilation of a positron with an electron.

enon can be used in transverse section imaging because each recorded pair of 511-keV gamma rays is immediately reduced to a one-dimensional problem in determining their origin. Also since the origin of the detected emissions is determined by the physical characteristics of the annihilation process, the need for conventional radionuclide collimators is eliminated.

A positron coincidence imaging system has been constructed consisting of 32 detectors arranged in a circle with corresponding coincidence circuitry (Robertson *et al.*, 1973).

A 64-detector system using the same circular geometry is currently under development (Cho *et al.*, 1976). One system (ECAT) is commercially available from Ortec, Inc. This is an updated version of the PETT III system built by Phelps and Ter-Pogossian and is shown in Fig. 5 10 (Phelps *et al.*, 1977; Hoffman *et al.*, 1976). The new system consists of 66 detectors arranged in a hexagonal array with 11 detectors in each of six banks. The 11 detectors in a bank are wired in coincidence with the 11 detectors in the opposite bank. Thus there are a total of 363 lines of response for the system. Data are collected by moving the detector banks in synchrony to perform linear scans over a distance of 3.5 cm. The system is rotated 5° and the linear scan is repeated. This process is continued until the entire system has been rotated 60° and an image is then reconstructed using the Fourier techniques of linearly superimposing filtered back projections. Since no collimator is necessary, a high detection efficiency is obtainable. It has been demonstrated that this type of system has distinct advantages over the single-photon detection systems described earlier (Hoffman *et al.*, 1976). One such advantage is that the resolution is spatially invariant. It is determined by the size of the crystals used, whereas with single-photon detection systems the resolution is a function of the detector collimator and varies with distance from the collimator face. The ECAT system has an inherent resolution of 1.5 cm (FWHM). This is improved to 1 cm by adding shadow shields which limit the thickness of the cross section being imaged. In

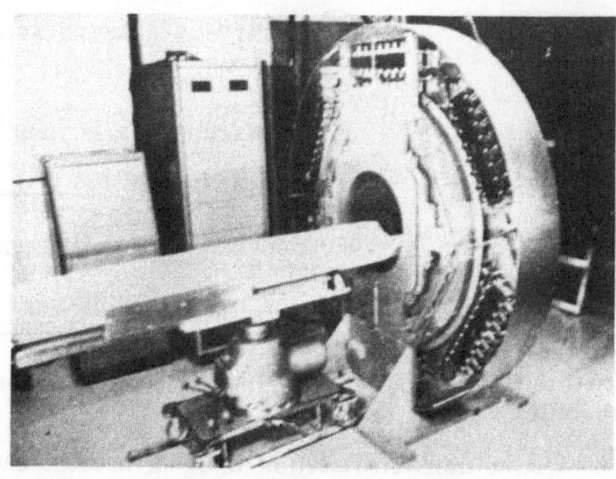

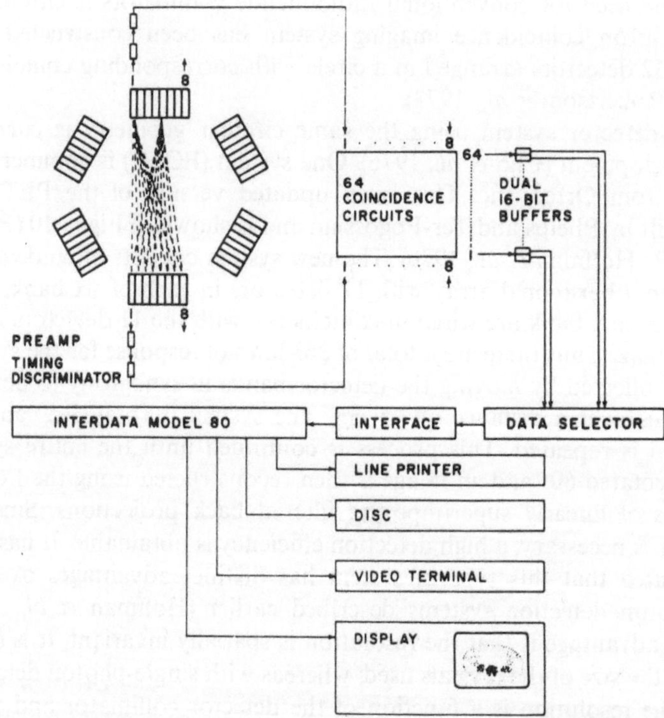

Fig. 5-10. The PETT III system for transverse section imaging of distribution of positron emitters within the body. This system is the forerunner of the commercially available ECAT system. (From Hoffman, E.J., *et al.*, 1976, with permission.)

addition, since a pair of 511-keV photons always travel the same total path length between detectors, the sensitivity of this system is depth independent (i.e., the attenuation and solid-angle efficiency are constant). Thus the positron systems can be used for obtaining transverse section images of any plane in the body and are not limited to the head as are most single-photon detection systems.

As is the case with single-photon emission tomography, camera-type devices have also been used for transverse section tomography with positrons. One such imaging device is the Massachusetts General Hospital (MGH) positron camera (Burnham and Brownell, 1972). This system consists of two opposed detector arrays, each containing 127 small NaI(T1) crystals and 72 phototubes. Each crystal is wired in coincidence with 25 crystals in the opposite array. Thus as a stationary imaging system the detector arrays can produce images of longitudinal sections. If multiple images are obtained as the system is rotated about the patient, the data can then be used to reconstruct transverse section images using the same concepts described earlier for the ECAT system (Chesler, 1971).

A dual-opposed scintillation camera system (Muehllehner *et al.*, 1976) has also been used for both longitudinal and transverse section imaging with positrons. Two large-field-of-view (15.25-in.-diameter) scintillation cameras were mounted on a gantry and wired in coincidence. The advantage of camera-type systems such as these are that data for reconstructing multiple sections can be obtained with one pass of the detectors.

5.4. OTHER APPROACHES

The positron techniques can be taken one step further by introducing time measurements into the coincidence detection circuitry. With this positron time-of-flight measurement, not only are the two 511-keV photons detected in two opposed detectors, but the actual time difference between the recording of the two events is also measured. Thus the origin of the photons is reduced to a one-dimensional problem by isolating the point of production to a line between two detectors. The one-dimensional problem can then be solved uniquely by knowing the difference in arrival times of the photons at the two detectors. This technique has been limited in the past due to the time resolution available with current systems. Recent studies (Dunn, 1975) have shown that by using plastic scintillators and ultrafast photomultipliers, amplifiers, and discriminators, time resolutions are now available on the order of 180 psec, which would correspond to FWHM spatial resolutions of 2.5 cm. The advantage of this system would be that the determination of the origin of each emission would be uniquely defined electronically and thus true transverse section images could be obtained directly with no need for complex reconstruction algorithms. This may be a promising approach for the future.

Another interesting approach to tomography is the use of Fresnel zone plates as coded apertures for the collection of coded data which can then be decoded to produce section images. This technique is discussed in detail in Chapter 8 of this book.

One area that has received relatively little attention is the area of three-dimensional displays. In general, the section images are displayed as two-dimensional representations. Three-dimensional effects have been obtained in displays by obtaining multiple (36) routine frontal plane images as the patient is rotated in front of the scintillation detector (Handmaker *et al.*, 1973). The information is then sequentially photographed on 16-mm film and projected as a continuous loop. By observing the rotating radioactive distribution a degree of depth perception is obtained. This same type of information could also be obtained by recording the images sequentially on a video disk with a television camera, eliminating the need for film processing.

5.5. SUMMARY

Much research has been done in the area of radionuclide tomography since its conception around 1963. The interest in this area has been stimulated by the recent developments in X-ray-computed axial tomography and work is continuing actively in many laboratories. The use of radionuclide-emission-computed tomography to provide functional information to complement the high-resolution anatomical information obtainable with X-ray transmission systems should prove to be extremely useful in the future. The development of new display systems based on holographic techniques should also significantly enhance these capabilities.

REFERENCES

Anger, H.O. (1971), Tomographic gamma-ray scanner with simultaneous readout of several planes, in Gottschalk, A., and Beck, R.N. (eds.), *Fundamental Problems in Scanning*, Charles C Thomas, Springfield, Illinois, pp. 195–211.

Anger, H.O. (1974), Tomography and other depth-discrimination techniques, in Hine, G.J., and Sorenson, J.A. (eds), *Instrumentation in Nuclear Medicine*, Academic Press, New York.

Brooks, R.A., and Di Chiro, G. (1976), Principles of computer-assisted tomography (CAT) in radiographic and radioisotopic imaging, *Phys. Med. Biol.* **21**:689–732.

Budinger, T.F., DeLand, F.H., Daggan, H.E., *et al.* (1975), Dynamic time-dependent analysis and static 3-dimensional imaging procedures for computer-assisted CNS studies, in *Non-Invasive Brain Imaging, Computed Tomography and Radionuclides*, Society of Nuclear Medicine, New York, pp. 45–66.

Burnham, C.A., and Brownell, G.L. (1972), A multi-crystal positron camera, *IEEE Trans. Nucl. Sci.* **NS-19:**201–205.

Cassen, B. (1965), Section scanning with a large solid angle collimator, *J. Nucl. Med.* **6:**767.

Chesler, D.A. (1971), Three-dimensional activity distribution from multiple positron scintigraphs, *J. Nucl. Med.* **12:**347–348.

Cho, T.H., Chan, J., and Ericksson, L. (1976), Circular ring transaxial positron camera for 3-D reconstruction of radionuclide distributors, *IEEE Trans. Nucl. Sci.* **NS-23:**613–622.

Dunn, W.L. (1975), Time of flight localization of positron-emitting isotopes, M.S. thesis, Vanderbilt University, 1975.

Freedman, G.S. (1970), Tomography with a gamma camera theory, *J. Nucl. Med.* **11:**602–604.

Handmaker, H., Anger, H.O., and McRae, J. (1973), Rotational cinescintiphotography as a means of obtaining three-dimensional organ images, in Freedman, G.S. (ed.), *Tomographic Imaging in Nuclear Medicine*, Society of Nuclear Medicine, New York, pp. 196–199.

Hoffman, E.J., Phelps, M.E., Mullani, N.A., *et al.* (1976), Design and performance characteristics of a whole-body positron transaxial tomograph, *J. Nucl. Med.* **17:**493–502.

Jaszczak, R., Huard, D., Murphy, P., *et al.* (1976), Radionuclide emission computer tomography with a scintillation camera, *J. Nucl. Med.* **17:**551.

Keyes, J.W., and Simmon, W. (1973), Computer techniques for radionuclide transverse section tomography in quantitative spatial (3-dimensional) imaging, in *Sharing Computer Programs and Technology in Nuclear Medicine*, USAEC Report Conf-730627, pp. 190–201.

Keyes, J.W., Orlandea, N., Heetderks, W.J., *et al.* (1976), The humongotron–gamma camera transaxial tomography, *J. Nucl. Med.* **17:**552.

Kuhl, D.E., and Edwards, R.Q. (1963), Image separation radioisotope scanning, *Radiology* **80:**653–661.

Kuhl, D.E., Edwards, R.Q., Ricci, A.B., *et al.* (1976), The Mark IV system for radionuclide computed tomography of the brain, *Radiology* **121:**405–413.

Miraldi, F., and Di Chiro, G. (1970), Tomographic techniques in radioisotope imaging with a proposal of a new device: the tomoscanner, *Radiology* **94:**513–520.

Muehllehner, G. (1971), A tomographic scintillation camera, *Phys. Med. Biol.* **16:**87–96.

Muehllehner, G., Buchin, M.P., and Dudek, J.H. (1976), Performance parameters of a positron imaging camera, *IEEE Trans. Nucl. Sci.* **NS-23:**528.

Patton, J.A., Brill, A.B., and King, P.H. (1973), Transverse section brain scanning with a multicrystal cylindrical imaging device, in Freedman, G.S. (ed.), *Tomographic Imaging in Nuclear Medicine*, Society of Nuclear Medicine, New York, pp. 28–43.

Phelps, M.E., Hoffman, E.J., Coble, C.S., *et al.* (1977), Some performance and design characteristics of the PETT III, in *Reconstruction Tomography in Diagnostic Radiology and Nuclear Medicine*, University Park Press, Baltimore, Maryland.

Robertson, J.S., Marr, R.B., Rosenblum, M., *et al.* (1973), 32 Crystal positron transverse section detector, in Freedman, G.S. (ed.), *Tomographic Imaging in Nuclear Medicine*, Society of Nuclear Medicine, New York, pp. 142–153.

CHAPTER 6

Quantitative Analysis of Minimum Detectable Uptake Ratios for Nuclear Medicine Imaging Systems

F. R. WHITEHEAD

6.1. INTRODUCTION

A diagnostic medical image is nothing more, nor less, than a display of measured data, and specifically for nuclear medicine it is a display of radiopharmaceutical uptake as a function of position within some object. As with any measuring device, the important characteristics of an imaging system are its precision, accuracy, and range of measurement scale. When the output of an imaging system is viewed by a human observer, the measured quantity of interest is contrast, or incremental change of input signal level divided by the average signal level. Thus the precision of the imaging systems' measurement capability is determined by the minimum detectable contrast which can be observed, the imaging system's accuracy, which is determined by the fidelity with which a specific object contrast is repre-

F. R. WHITEHEAD • Searle Diagnostics, Inc., 2000 Nuclear Drive, Des Plaines, Illinois 60018. *Present address*: General Electric Medical Systems Division, 11505 Douglas Road, Rancho Cordova, California 95670.

sented in the image, and the range of measurement scale, which is simply the dynamic range, as determined by the largest value of object contrast which can be accurately reproduced in the image.

With medical imaging systems, an important difference from most other types of imaging systems is that accurate representation of the object contrast is not needed. In fact, it is usually undesirable. One is not familiar with viewing the objects of medical imaging systems by using the unaided eye, so there is no "natural" reference for the image contrasts. Instead, the physician establishes his reference by viewing images of normal (i.e., healthy) individuals, and then wishes to determine if the image of an individual with some symptomatic complaint deviates from the normal. Thus it is usually desired that extremely low contrast should be perceptible to the observer, and this dictates the use of high-contrast, and therefore "inaccurate," gray scale transfer functions for the imaging system.

Previous chapters have discussed the important parameters used to describe the performance of an imaging system, such as resolution, detective quantum efficiency, and photographic gamma. The characteristics of minimum detectable contrast, signal-to-noise ratio, and dynamic range, which describe output image quality, have also been discussed. In this chapter, the mathematical relationships between system performance parameters and image quality parameters will be developed for nuclear medicine imaging systems. Once these relationships are known, it becomes a relatively simple matter to work backwards from the human visual system threshold contrast and signal-to-noise requirements for detection of a spherical lesion in an image, to determine the minimum detectable uptake ratios, or amount of activity per unit volume, which can be measured in various objects using a given nuclear medicine imaging system.

6.2. LINEAR SYSTEM ANALYSIS OF NUCLEAR MEDICINE IMAGING SYSTEMS

Various types of nuclear medicine imaging systems have been described in Chapters 2, 4, and 5. The two systems in widespread clinical use are the Anger camera and the rectilinear scanner. Both of these systems are described by the linear system model shown in Fig. 6-1. The complete imaging system may be divided into two important subsystems; a basic imaging system which determines the overall spatial resolution characteristics of the complete system, and a display system which determines the overall gray scale characteristics of the complete system.

The scintillation detector and associated electronics make up the basic imaging system. For low-energy radionuclides, such as ^{99m}Tc, over 90% of the gamma photons striking the scintillation crystal produce a detectable

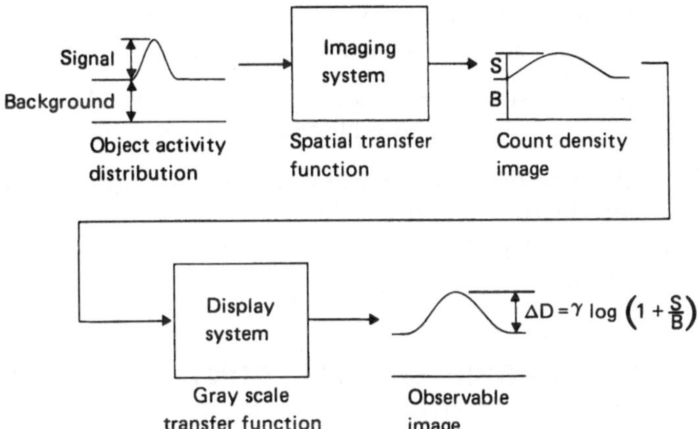

Fig. 6-1. The linear system model for a nuclear medicine imaging system. The signal-to-background ratio in the object is related to the observable image density difference by means of the appropriate transfer functions for the imaging system.

pulse from the photomultiplier tubes. These pulses are processed one by one in the electronics and a spot is generated on the face of a CRT at appropriate x, y coordinates, corresponding to the location where the gamma photon struck the scintillation crystal. Thus the basic imaging system is a quantum counter, and its DQE is over 90%, due to the fact that all internal sources of noise are completely negligible. The pattern of dots generated on the CRT represents a count density image—i.e., so many counts per unit area—and the relationship between contrast in this image and the corresponding contrast in the object is determined by the MTF of the imaging system. The statistics of this image are simply the Poisson statistics of the input gamma photon flux from the object.

To produce an observable image, the count density image is passed through a display system which integrates and stores the time-sequential pattern of dots generated on the CRT. Although a persistence CRT may be used to generate a quick-look image for patient orientation, the image used for diagnostic reading is usually made by allowing the dots on the CRT to expose a piece of photographic film. Since all integration and storage functions are performed by the film, the image gray scale characteristics, such as gamma and dynamic range, are determined mainly by the film characteristics. This is true, however, only when the CRT spot size and shape, as well as the development procedure for the film, are properly adjusted and carefully controlled. The MTF of the display system is always much better than that of the basic imaging system, so the display system MTF may be ignored in all calculations of image contrast.

Thus a nuclear medicine imaging system may be modeled by a simple cascading of a basic imaging system, consisting of the scintillation detector and electronics, plus an image display system which is usually photographic film. The final image contrast is related to the input object contrast by

$$\text{image contrast} = \text{object contrast} \times \text{MTF contrast factor} \times \text{gray scale contrast factor} \tag{6-1}$$

The MTF contrast factor is determined by the basic imaging system, and the gray scale contrast factor is determined by the gamma of the image display system. The relationships for both of these contrast factors will now be developed in detail.

6.3. RELATIONSHIP BETWEEN CONTRAST IN THE OBJECT AND THE COUNT DENSITY IMAGE

Recall that linear system analysis of an imaging process assumes that the input object function is convolved with the impulse response of the imaging system to generate the output image. The mathematical operation of convolution describes the physical process of blurring the image in relation to the object, due to the fact that the imaging system does not have infinite resolution, i.e., perfect physical separation of adjacent points in the object. Although the convolution integral represents the direct mathematical model of the imaging process, in practice it is usually awkward for numerical calculations. Such calculations are often more easily accomplished by the method of Fourier analysis.

With Fourier analysis, the input object function is analyzed as a sum of sine and cosine functions where the relative magnitudes and phases of these spectral components provide the unique description of any specific input function. For the input function of a single lesion on a uniform background level, as shown in Fig. 6-1, the ratio of the maximum signal from the lesion to the average background level is called the *contrast* of this lesion signal. Thus

$$C = \frac{S}{B} \tag{6-2}$$

In a similar manner, the ratio of the magnitude of an individual sine or cosine component, in the Fourier spectrum of this lesion signal, to the background level is called the *contrast modulation* of that component. Figure 6-2 shows an example of a sinusoidal pattern and the calculation of its contrast modulation as defined by

$$C_M = \frac{I_{max} - I_{min}}{I_{max} + I_{min}} \tag{6-3}$$

When the appropriate expressions for I_{max} and I_{min} are substituted in Eq.

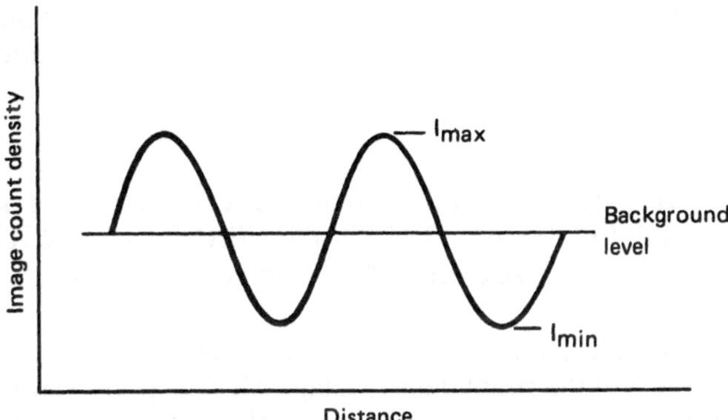

Fig. 6-2. Definition of contrast modulation, and signal-to-background ratio for a cosine pattern. The contrast of a lesion distribution is calculated by adding up all the contrast modulation values of the sine and cosine components in its Fourier transform. I_{max} = background + peak signal; I_{min} = background − peak signal; contrast = $(I_{max} - I_{min})/(I_{max} + I_{min})$ = (peak signal)/(background).

(6-3), the contrast modulation expression reduces to a simple signal-to-background ratio. Recall that the integral of the Fourier spectrum of a function is its peak value, so it follows that the peak signal-to-background ratio, or contrast, of a single source in a uniform background is just the sum of the *contrast modulation* values for all its sine and cosine components.

Note that contrast modulation values for an actual image of a sine or cosine pattern can never be greater than 1, because negative intensity levels are physically unrealizable. This restriction does not necessarily apply to contrast modulation values for individual Fourier components of a complex image, however, because these components are not imaged independently of each other. A well-known example of this is the square wave bar pattern often used to measure the resolution of imaging systems. The contrast modulation value of the pattern itself is 1, while the contrast modulation value of its fundamental Fourier component is approximately 1.3. Not infrequently, an error in the measurement of the MTF for an imaging system occurs due to neglect of this fact.

Once the contrast modulation values for the object signal distribution are known (by computing its Fourier transform and dividing by the background level) the contrast modulation values for the image signal distribution are calculated by multiplying the object values by the MTF of the imaging system. Integration of the resulting values then yields the count density image signal-to-background contrast. The MTF of most nuclear medicine imaging systems is closely approximated by a Gaussian function, so that for spherical lesions, the image contrast can be computed from knowledge of the object contrast and a transfer factor determined by the ratio of lesion diameter to full width at half maximum of the imaging system line spread function. The detailed procedure for this calculation, plus the procedure needed to account for the effects of gamma-ray scattering and attenuation, is given in Appendix 6.A.

6.4. THE GREY SCALE TRANSFER FUNCTION AND PERCEIVED GRAY SCALE DIFFERENCES IN THE OBSERVABLE IMAGE

The MTF calculation described in the previous section determines only the contrast of the count density image which is never viewed directly. Instead, this count density image is used as the input to a display system, such as photographic film, or a persistence CRT, which provides the final observable image. The relationship between the contrast in the count density image and the contrast in the observable image is determined by the gray scale transfer function of the display system. For photographic film, the familiar D vs. $\log E$ curve represents its gray scale transfer function. It will now be shown that knowledge of the count density image signal-to-background ratio, and the D vs. $\log E$ curve for the film, allows direct calculation of the visually perceived gray scale difference between lesion and background regions of the final image.

Return to Fig. 6-1, and consider the count density image. The lesion appears as an increased signal of magnitude S on a lower background activity of level B. When a photographic image is recorded from the CRT of an Anger camera, the relative exposure between the tumor and background regions is directly proportional to the relative count densities in these two regions. Analytically, the reflectance of a positive print in the respective regions will be given by

$$R_{\text{signal}} = R_0 \left(\frac{S + B}{I_0} \right)^{\gamma}$$
$$R_{\text{background}} = R_0 \left(\frac{B}{I_0} \right)^{\gamma} \tag{6-4}$$

where R_0 is a reference reflectance value at the count density of I_0, S and B are the respective count density contributions from the lesion and background, and γ is the slope of the D vs. $\log E$ curve for the film. The ratio of reflectance values between these two regions is

$$\frac{R_s}{R_b} = \left(1 + \frac{S}{B} \right)^{\gamma} \tag{6-5}$$

The visual system responds to the logarithm of the incident light level, so that to obtain the *perceived gray scale difference* between the lesion and background it is necessary to take the *logarithm* of this ratio. The logarithm of the reflectance ratio, however, is simply the density difference, on the film, between the signal and background regions. Therefore,

$$\Delta D = \gamma \log\left(1 + \frac{S}{B}\right) \tag{6-6}$$

Thus the density difference, ΔD, between the lesion and background regions of the image is given by the product of the film gamma and the logarithm of the quantity 1 plus the signal-to-background ratio. It is merely necessary to look at a calibrated photographic step wedge to see that equal density differences on film are perceived as equal steps of gray scale in the image.

Visual perception of the lesion in the image depends upon two factors. First, the density difference between lesion and background must be sufficient to exceed the threshold of detection for the human visual system. Second, quantum fluctuations in the image must be low enough that no random deviations in background density level are greater than approximately 25% of the density difference between lesion and background. The numerical value for this second requirement is relatively easy to determine from a calculation of the allowable false positive rate in the image, as will be shown later. The numerical value for the detection threshold of the human visual system is much more difficult to determine, however, because it depends upon several parameters, such as image size, resolution, lesion shape, and the illumination level used for viewing.

Schade (1956) has developed an extensive analysis of the human visual system, and measured both its gray scale and modulation transfer functions for various levels of illumination. At normal illumination levels, the eye has a rather unique MTF which approaches zero in the low-frequency region. Because of this, the eye operates primarily as an edge detector, and threshold contrast for sharp edges is considerably less than the value required for edges of gradual slope. Schade has measured the threshold contrast value for sharp edges in a noisy background at approximately 12% (Schade, 1964). In another experiment, Revesz and Haas (1972) found that reliable detection of a disk lesion in a chest radiograph also required approximately 12% contrast between lesion and background.

Since the edge sharpness of spherical lesions in nuclear medicine images, displayed in the conventional format on Polaroid film, is considerably less than that of the images used by Schade and by Revesz and Haas, the required threshold contrast value should be greater. Although extensive measurements have not been made, the author's experiments with images of phantoms containing spherical lesions show that threshold contrast for the eye is approximately 17–20% with these images. More appropriately, since the eye's response is logarithmic, threshold contrast is a density difference of approximately ± 0.07 units. Using Polaroid film, which has a gamma of 1.3 (Polaroid, 1976), inversion of Eq. (6-6) shows that these values of visual contrast correspond to contrasts of approximately 13–15% in the count density image.

Thus the analysis of contrast transfer through a nuclear medicine imaging system requires a two-step calculation. The first step is to compute the effect of the imaging system MTF upon lesion contrast. The result of this step yields the contrast between lesion and background in the count density image, which is the image produced by the detector and processing electronics of a nuclear medicine camera or scanner. The second step of the analysis is to compute the effect of the display system gray scale transfer function upon lesion-to-background contrast. This calculation accounts for the effect of using different films or CRT display systems with a given camera or scanner. The result yields the density difference between lesion and background which is presented to the observer's visual system. If this final image density difference is above the threshold of the human visual system, then the lesion will be seen in the image, provided an adequate signal-to-*noise* ratio* is maintained by collecting a sufficient number of counts in the image. This additional requirement of adequate signal-to-noise ratio is the next topic of discussion.

6.5. EFFECT OF QUANTUM NOISE ON IMAGE QUALITY

If the input gamma flux to a nuclear medicine imaging system were deterministic in nature, then the conceptual analysis discussed in the previous sections would be all that was necessary to evaluate the comparative performance of different imaging systems. Unfortunately, it is not sufficient to determine whether or not a given value of object contrast will be visible in the image, but it is also necessary to determine whether or not the corresponding value of image contrast is statistically significant. This is done by calculating the probability of having a particular contrast value occur accidently in the image due to statistical variations in the number of photons collected. If this probability is higher than desired, then visible image structure at this contrast value must be rejected with regard to being a true representation of object structure. Thus the ability of a medical imaging procedure to detect the differences between normal and abnormal patients is a direct function of the statistical noise present in the image.

An analysis of the effects of statistical noise with any type of imaging

* From this point on, the reader must carefully note the distinction between signal-to-*noise* ratio and signal-to-*background* ratio.

system has been given by Rose (1974). In this section, his analysis will be applied to nuclear medicine imaging systems, and it will be shown that this analysis leads directly to a specification of the maximum useful count density in a nuclear medicine image, in terms of the number of counts per resolution element. This maximum useful count density value varies with the gamma of the gray scale transfer function for the image display system, as one would expect from intuitive considerations, and is an important consideration in the selection of the type of film to be used for a particular imaging procedure.

Suppose one is imaging an object which consists of a large uniform background distribution plus a small lesion located somewhere within the imaging system's field of view. Let the difference in *average count rate* between lesion plus background and background alone be 15%. If the observation time is such that an average of 500 counts per resolution element are collected in the image, then the difference between the resolution element containing the lesion, and one containing only background is 75 counts. For Poisson-distributed noise, the probability of a statistical accident causing a 75-count deviation in a resolution element containing only background is approximately 0.0008. Standard nuclear medicine cameras with a 10-in. field of view have about 500 resolution elements, so that the average number of errors in a single image is 0.4. (Probability of an error times the number of chances for it to happen.) Using a table of the summed Poisson probability function, the probability of the image having one or more deviations in the background level with the same contrast value as the lesion is found to be 33%. A similar calculation for a camera with a 15-in. field of view results in a 60% chance of having one or more errors in a single image, simply because there are more resolution elements. Obviously, reliable detection of the lesion is impossible under these conditions.

For an average count density of 500 counts per resolution element, the rms variation in count density is 22 counts per resolution element. The lesion variation of 75 counts per resolution element is approximately three times this rms value, so that, in effect, one has a signal-to-noise ratio of 3 to 1 in the example considered. Calculation of the probability of an error has shown that this is inadequate for reliable detection of the lesion, and this calculation did not include the statistical deviations on the signal itself. When statistical deviations on both the signal and background are considered, it can be shown (Appendix 6.B) that a signal-to-noise ratio between 4 and 4.5 to 1 does provide reliable detection of the lesion. A signal-to-noise ratio of 4 to 1 yields a probability of error of approximately 5% for detection of a 15% contrast lesion within a 10-in. field of view, while a signal-to-noise ratio of 4.25 to 1 reduces the error to approximately 1%. Finally, one can determine that specification of an error rate of 1% in the image from a 15-in.-field-of-view camera requires a signal-to-noise ratio of approximately 4.5 to 1. *Thus the minimum detectable lesion contrast value in a nuclear medicine image is between 4 and 4.5 times the rms noise level divided by the average background level.*

Now consider the density difference which a lesion at this minimum detectable contrast value produces on film. The signal level, for a background level of N counts per resolution element, and a signal-to-noise ratio of k is

$$S = kN^{1/2} \tag{6-7}$$

so that the lesion contrast, or signal-to-background ratio, is

$$\frac{S}{B} = \frac{k}{N^{1/2}} \tag{6-8}$$

Substitution of this expression into Eq. (6-6) yields a density difference of

$$\Delta D = \gamma \log\left(1 + \frac{k}{N^{1/2}}\right) \tag{6-9}$$

Thus the density difference produced by the minimum detectable contrast value is reduced in magnitude as more counts are collected in the image, and smaller differences in radionuclide uptake are observed at higher image count densities. Obviously, the appropriate number of counts in the image will yield a minimum detectable contrast value which produces the visual threshold density difference of 0.07 units on the film. At this point, accumulation of more counts in the image is simply a waste of time, because no perceptible increase in image quality will occur. Even though lower-contrast lesions will become statistically significant with more counts, they will not be perceptible to the observer, because their final image density differences will be below visual threshold.

To calculate this maximum useful image count density for any given film, observer, and signal-to-noise ratio, one simply inverts Eq. (6-9) to obtain

$$N = \frac{k^2}{(10^{\Delta D/\gamma} - 1)^2} \tag{6-10}$$

where k is the required signal-to-noise ratio, ΔD is the threshold of visibility for the observer, γ is the slope of the D vs. $\log E$ curve for the film, and N is in counts per resolution element. Note that the denominator of Eq. (6-10) is actually the square of the minimum detectable contrast value for the count density image.

Now consider the display of nuclear medicine images on Polaroid type 107 film. This film has a gamma of 1.35 (Polaroid, 1976) so that with a visual threshold of ± 0.07 density units, and a signal-to-noise ratio of 4.25 to 1, the maximum useful count densities obtained from Eq. (6-10) are approximately 1100 counts per resolution element for hot lesions, or 1400 counts per resolution element for cold lesions. The corresponding minimum detectable contrast values in the count density image are about 13% for hot lesions and 11% for cold lesions.

When a higher-contrast film is used with the same imaging system, the maximum useful count density is increased, and lower-contrast lesions can be detected. For example, high-contrast transparency film, such as Kodak type SO-179, has a gamma of approximately 2, and with a signal-to-noise ratio of 4.25 to 1, the maximum useful count densities are approximately 2600 counts per resolution element for hot lesions and 3000 counts per resolution element for cold lesions. The corresponding minimum detectable contrast value in the count density image is now approximately 8% for both hot and cold lesions.

It must be emphasized that these numerical values are extremely sensitive to slight changes in the assumed values of observer visual threshold, signal-to-noise ratio, and film gamma. Both observer threshold and signal-to-noise ratio are determined from statistical averages, and they cannot be specified with high precision. Correlation of the calculated count densities and minimum detectable contrast ratios with empirically determined values from established nuclear medicine imaging procedures is quite good, however, so that Eq. (6-8), (6-9), and (6-10) provide a useful basis for calculation of "trial" values to use when establishing procedures for new films and imaging systems.

6.6. MINIMUM DETECTABLE LESION-TO-BACKGROUND UPTAKE RATIOS FOR SPHERICAL LESIONS

In the previous sections, the important relationships between the characteristics of an imaging system and final image contrast and signal-to-noise ratio were discussed. In this section, these relationships will be used to determine the approximate theoretical limits of detectability for spherical lesions of various sizes, using a high-quality nuclear medicine imaging system. This will be done by calculating the minimum ratio of activity per unit volume between lesion and background needed to make a given size lesion visible in the final image from a particular system. Such calculations provide a convenient method for evaluation of nuclear medicine imaging systems, as well as a guide in the development of new clinical procedures.

As shown in Appendix 6.A, the minimum detectable uptake ratio for spherical lesions may be determined from

$$\mu = 1 + \frac{(1 + S_F)(10^{\Delta D/\gamma} - 1)\, L \sinh(\alpha_b L/2) \exp(-\alpha_b L/2)}{D\,\mathrm{CF} \exp(-\alpha_p z_0)(\alpha_b L/2)} \qquad (6\text{-}11)$$

where μ is the target-to-nontarget uptake ratio, S_F is the Compton scatter fraction, ΔD is the visual threshold density difference, γ is the slope of the D vs. $\log E$ curve for the film used, L is the thickness of the background activity, α_b is the "effective" background attenuation coefficient for the selected detector energy window width (see Appendix 6.A), D is the diameter of the lesion, CF is the MTF contrast factor (from Table 6.A-1), α_p is the attenuation coefficient for the primary energy gamma rays, and z_0 is the depth of the lesion in the attenuating medium.

Now consider a hypothetical brain-scanning problem where it is required to estimate the minimum lesion-to-background uptake ratio which will allow detection of a 3-cm lesion, 5 cm deep, in a background distribution 15 cm thick. The imaging system is an Anger camera, with a parallel hole collimator, and the image will be displayed on Polaroid film with a gamma of 1.35. The total system resolution *at the depth of the lesion* is 10 mm FWHM.

For a 30% energy window, the background attenuation coefficient is 0.1, and the scatter fraction for a 5-cm-deep lesion is 0.5 (Dresser, 1972). The attenuation factor $\exp(-\alpha_p z_0)$ for the lesion is 0.47. For a 3-cm lesion, imaged by a system with 1.0 cm FWHM, the calculated MTF contrast factor (using Eq. (6.A-18) and Table 6.A-1) is 0.91. Finally, it is convenient to choose a value of 0.08 units as the required density difference between lesion and background in the final image. Use of this value, which is slightly higher than the visual threshold value of 0.07 units or less, allows some margin of error for experimental problems, such as nonuniformity in the imaging system, or measurement error in filling of a phantom.

Calculation of the required target-to-nontarget uptake ratio is now a matter of appropriate substitution of these numerical values into Eq. (6-11). Thus

$$\mu = 1 + \frac{1.5(10^{0.08/1.35} - 1)\, 15 \sinh[(15/2)(0.1)] \exp[-(0.1)(15/2)]}{3(0.91)(0.47)[(15/2)(0.1)]} = 2.33 \qquad (6\text{-}12)$$

Therefore if the lesion has 2.33 times the activity per unit volume of the background, it will be just visible in the final image, provided a sufficient number of counts are collected to prevent statistical fluctuations from masking its presence. An estimate of the required image count density can be obtained from Eq. (6-10), and for this case

$$N = \frac{(4.25)^2}{(10^{0.08/1.3} - 1)^2} = 780 \text{ counts per resolution element} \qquad (6\text{-}13)$$

If a different film is used with the same camera, the minimum detectable uptake ratio, and required count density values will change. For example, Kodak type SO-179 film has a gamma of about 2, and use of this value in Eq. (6-11) yields a required lesion uptake ratio of

$$\mu = 1.87 \qquad (6\text{-}14)$$

The corresponding image count density requirement from Eq. (6-10) is now

$$N = 1940 \text{ counts per resolution element} \qquad (6\text{-}15)$$

Thus the use of higher contrast film and increased image count density allows the detection of smaller differences between lesion and background activity levels. Further comparison of theoretically estimated, minimum detectable target-to-nontarget ratios versus lesion diameter are given in Figs. 6-3 and 6-4, for Kodak type SO-179 and Polaroid type 107 films, used with a high-quality Anger camera.

Although potential lesion detectability is always better with high-contrast film than with low-contrast film, it does not follow that high-contrast film is always the correct film to use with every nuclear medicine procedure. Effective use of a high-contrast film requires that the image count density used be sufficient to suppress the visibility of statistical noise

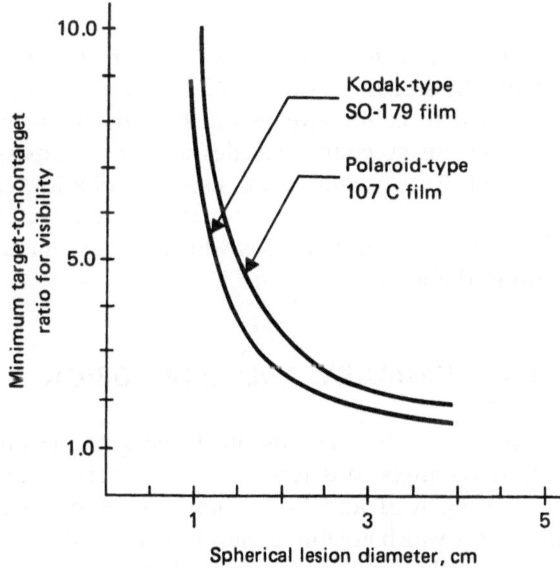

Fig. 6-3. Minimum detectable uptake ratios for various-size hot, spherical lesions. The lesions are 5 cm deep, in a 15-cm-thick background. The imaging system uses a parallel hole collimator, has a 10 mm FWHM line spread function, and a 30% energy window. Required count densities are 1300 cts/cm^2 for Polaroid film, and 3000 cts/cm^2 for SO-179 film. Note that lesion size–activity ratio combinations *above* the curve for each film will be visible in the final image.

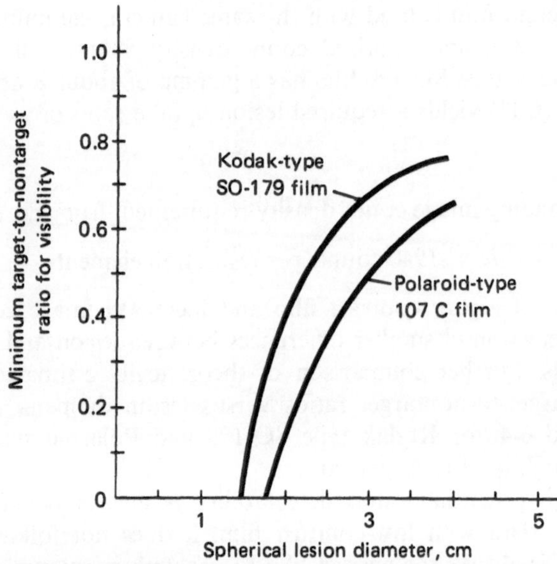

Fig. 6-4. Minimum detectable uptake ratios for various-size cold, spherical lesions. The lesions are 2.5 cm deep, in an 8-cm-thick background. All other parameters are the same as in Fig. 6-3. Note that lesion size–activity ratio combinations *below* the curve for each film will be visible in the final image.

in the image. If this is not done, then it is necessary for the observer to mentally determine the statistical validity of observed detail in the image, and this would appear to be inconvenient at best, or impossible at worst. Therefore, when high image count densities are either impossible or unnecessary, because of the procedure being used, use of a low-contrast film can suppress the visibility of distracting statistical fluctuations without reducing the detectability of those lesions which do have an adequate signal-to-noise ratio in the image.

6.7. SUMMARY AND DISCUSSION

When a physician reads a nuclear medicine scan, he must perform two tasks. First, he attempts to determine the presence of differences between the image being read and his memorized set of normal images. Second, any differences which are found must be explained, either as normal variants, or as a clinically significant finding related to the patient's symptoms and medical history. The key to this process is the ability to detect differences between images, and this in turn, relies upon the ability to differentiate structures within a single image. Thus the diagnostic information content of a nuclear medicine image is, among other things, directly proportional to its minimum perceptible contrast ratio and the statistical reliability of that contrast ratio.

The preceding analysis of the measurement characteristics of a nuclear medicine imaging system has shown that these characteristics determine the minimum detectable lesion-to-background uptake ratio displayed in the final image. For simple phantom objects, such as one or two lesions in a uniform background distribution of activity, one can obtain reasonably accurate, quantitative estimates of the minimum detectable uptake ratio versus lesion size from knowledge of the imaging system line spread function width and the gamma of the gray scale transfer function. Comparison of the minimum detectable lesion-to-background uptake ratio for various imaging systems then provides a useful estimate of the relative diagnostic image quality which can be expected from each system.

Although the usefulness of any diagnostic imaging procedure obviously depends upon more than the minimum detectable contrast ratio, optimum design and use of medical imaging systems can occur only when such simple, objective characteristics of image quality are understood by both equipment manufacturers and practicing physicians. Only then is it possible to access the relative advantages of sacrificing performance in one area in order to gain increased performance in another. In addition, direct measurement of objective image characteristics provides the best way to assure reliable, consistent performance of any imaging system.

Acknowledgments

Although the existence of direct literature references is of obvious importance in any area of research, such references can never provide an author with the stimulation and critical review that is possible in a discussion with others. Several of the author's colleagues in the research department of Searle Diagnostics were of assistance in this respect during the research for this work. In particular, Drs. Ronald Jaszczak, Gerd Muehllehner, and Ronald McKeighen provided information which helped to confirm the validity of our analytical model. Diane Huard quickly provided the computer programs for solving the two numerical integrations necessary to obtain quantitative predictions from the theory. Mark Groch aided with technical criticism, experimental verification, and review of the manuscript. Jay Wolff provided several stimulating discussions on the effects of photographic film. Robert Beck, of the University of Chicago, has given much encouragement during this research, and of course, provided many fundamental contributions to knowledge in this area with his own publications. Finally, Dr. H. H. Barrett of the University of Arizona receives the credit for showing us the correct procedure of calculating total image error probability from the error rate for a single resolution element.

Special thanks are due Dr. William White and Mr. Philip Shevick, management of Group Research, Searle Diagnostics, who not only initiated our research, but continuously encouraged that more time be devoted toward a better understanding of basic fundamentals.

Preparation of the manuscript was done with the assistance of Linda Walker, who patiently typed several drafts, and Anton Smudde, who gave considerable assistance with the illustrations.

APPENDIX 6.A. CALCULATION OF MINIMUM DETECTABLE LESION-TO-BACKGROUND UPTAKE RATIOS FOR SPHERICAL LESIONS

6.A.1. Calculation of the Input Lesion Contrast

Consider the three-dimensional object distribution

$$O(x, y, z) = B(x, y, z) + (\mu - 1)\, S(x, y, z) \qquad (6.\text{A-1})$$

which consists of a background volume, $B(x, y, z)$, with unit activity per unit volume, and a lesion distribution, $S(x, y, z)$, with activity per unit volume of $(\mu - 1)$. Note that μ represents the target to nontarget ratio of the radiopharmaceutical, and that when $\mu = 1$, there is no differential between lesion and background uptake. When $\mu > 1$, the lesion is hot, and when $\mu < 1$, the lesion is cold.

The projection of this three-dimensional object into an "effective" two-dimensional object distribution for any particular imaging system is given by

$$O(x, y) = \int_{-z}^{0} G(z)\, O(x, y, z)\, e^{\alpha z}\, dz \qquad (6.\text{A-2})$$

where $G(z)$ is the collimator sensitivity for a point source (which may vary with depth) and α is the attenuation coefficient of the object medium (including both scattering and absorption). The limits of integration correspond to assuming that the object is to the left of the plane $z = 0$.

This integral is, in general, rather difficult to evaluate; however, there are some useful, simple cases. For parallel hole collimators, the sensitivity is independent of the distance from the collimator, and therefore we may ignore collimator sensitivity for this case. (Resolution, however, is not independent of distance, and this will be considered later.) The problem then reduces to finding useful object distributions, which not only can be integrated into Eq. (6.A-2), but are also amenable to easy derivation of a

Fourier transform for the resulting two-dimensional object. This latter requirement is necessary in order to calculate the effect of the imaging system spatial transfer function on the signal-to-background ratio. There are at least three object distributions which can be easily used in this manner: a uniform background distribution containing either a point source, a Gaussian-shaped lesion, or a spherical lesion. Of these three, the uniform background containing a spherical lesion seems to be most representative of a "true" clinical object. Therefore, consider the following distribution:

$$O(x, y, z) = \mathrm{rect}\left(\frac{x}{L}, \frac{y}{L}, \frac{z}{L}\right) + (\mu - 1)\, S\left(\frac{x}{a}, \frac{y}{a}, \frac{z}{a}\right) \tag{6.A-3}$$

where $\mathrm{rect}(x/L, y/L, z/L)$ represents a cube of length L on all sides, and with unit activity per unit volume. $S(x/a, y/a, z/a)$ represents a sphere of radius a, with activity per unit volume of $\mu - 1$, where μ is the target-to-nontarget ratio for the radionuclide. Note that when $\mu = 1$, the object degenerates to a uniform cube at the background activity level.

To determine the "effective" two-dimensional signal and background, the respective terms from (6.A-3) must be substituted into (6.A-2) and the integration carried out. For the background term, this procedure yields an effective sheet source of dimensions $L \times L$, and activity per unit area of

$$B = L\,\frac{\sinh(\alpha_b L/2)}{\alpha_b L/2}\exp(-\alpha_b L/2) \tag{6.A-4}$$

Note that a subscripted attenuation coefficient, α_b, has been used in Eq. (6.A-4). The reason for this will be given shortly, when the effect of gamma-ray scattering on image contrast is considered.

For the signal term, consider a small cylindrical distribution cut along the z-axis diameter of the sphere, like the core of an apple. If the center of the sphere is located at $z = -z_0$ from the surface of the collimator, the two-dimensional projection of this cylinder becomes a disk source of activity per unit area given by

$$S(0) = (\mu - 1)\, D\,\frac{\sinh(\alpha_p D/2)}{\alpha_p D/2}\exp(-\alpha_p z_0) \tag{6.A-5}$$

where $S(0)$ refers to the peak height of the resulting two-dimensional distribution, D represents the diameter of the sphere, and α_p represents the attenuation coefficient for primary gamma rays.

Note that without attenuation, the complete two-dimensional projection of the sphere would be a hemisphere described by

$$S(r) = 2(a^2 - r^2)^{1/2}, \qquad r \le a \tag{6.A-6}$$

where $r^2 = x^2 + y^2$, and again, a is the radius of the sphere. The $(\sinh x)/x$

factor in (6.A-5) is approximately unity for any sphere less than 4 cm in diameter, so that for spherical lesions of interest, distortion of the shape function caused by attenuation may be ignored, and the two-dimensional projection of the spherical lesion may be approximated by

$$S(r) = 2(\mu - 1)(a^2 - r^2)^{1/2} \exp(-\alpha_p z_0) \tag{6.A-7}$$

including the effects of attenuation. From (6.A-7) and (6.A-4), the effective two-dimensional object distribution which represents the input to the nuclear medicine imaging system has a signal-to-background ratio given by

$$\frac{S}{B} = \frac{D(\mu - 1)\exp(-\alpha_p z_0)}{L\dfrac{\sinh(\alpha_b L/2)}{\alpha_b L/2}\exp(-\alpha_b L/2)} \tag{6.A-8}$$

where μ is the target-to-nontarget ratio, L is the thickness of the background distribution, α_p is the attenuation coefficient for primary gamma rays, α_b is the "effective" attenuation coefficient for the background activity (this depends upon detector energy window width), D is the diameter of the lesion, and z_0 is the depth of the lesion.

Equation (6.A-8) represents an analytical expression for the input contrast to a nuclear medicine imaging system from a spherical lesion at a depth of z_0 in a background volume of thickness L. Note, all that has been done is to calculate the projection onto a plane of the original three-dimensional object distribution. Attenuation has been included by weighting the contribution from each incremental volume element with an appropriate factor. At this point, there have been essentially no approximations other than dropping the hyperbolic sine factor from the lesion projection. The error from this procedure is about 6% on a 4-cm lesion, so that this approximation does not appear unreasonable compared to other possible sources of error such as visual system threshold and gamma ray scatter fraction—important parameters which will enter into the calculation shortly.

6.A.2. Calculation of Contrast in the Count Density Image

Once the input signal-to-background contrast ratio is known, the next step is to calculate the contrast in the count density image. As discussed in the main text, this is done using the MTF of the imaging system. Since the two-dimensional projection of a spherical lesion is rotationally symmetric, the calculation is most conveniently done using polar coordinates. Thus

$$C_{\text{image}} = 2\pi \int_0^\infty \tilde{C}(\rho)\,\tilde{H}(\rho)\,\rho\,d\rho \tag{6.A-9}$$

where ρ represents a radius in spatial frequency coordinates, $\tilde{C}(\rho)$ is the input lesion contrast as a function of spatial frequency, and $\tilde{H}(\rho)$ is the MTF of the imaging system. Equation (6.A-9) is equivalent to the contrast efficiency function of Rollo and Schulz (1970) and interested readers are referred to this reference for a complete discussion of its meaning.

For radionuclide imaging systems, the MTF may usually be approximated by a Gaussian, or at least a sum of Gaussians, so that the transfer functions have the form

$$\tilde{H}(\rho) = \exp(-2\pi^2\sigma^2\rho^2) \tag{6.A-10}$$

where σ is related to the FWHM of the imaging system line spread function by

$$\sigma = \frac{\text{FWHM}}{2.355} \tag{6.A-11}$$

The input lesion contrast function, $\tilde{C}(\rho)$, is determined by computing the Fourier transform of the effective two-dimensional lesion distribution from Eq. (6.A-7), and then dividing by the effective background level given by Eq. (6.A-4). Although somewhat involved, this step is relatively straightforward, because rotational symmetry of the projected lesion distribution makes it possible to derive its two-dimensional Fourier transform with a simple one-dimensional integral. From Eq. (6.A-6), one may write the two-dimensional projection of a sphere as

$$S(x, y) = 2(a^2 - x^2 - y^2)^{1/2}, \qquad x^2 + y^2 \leq a^2 \tag{6.A-12}$$

Integrating out the y dependence yields

$$S(x) = \pi(a^2 - x^2), \qquad |x| \leq a \tag{6.A-13}$$

which represents a one-dimensional projection of the sphere. Computing the Fourier transform of $S(x)$ results in a *profile* through the two-dimensional transform of the expression for $S(x, y)$ given in Eq. (6.A-12). Because of circular symmetry, this profile is identical to the expression in polar coordinates for the two-dimensional transform of $S(x, y)$. The Fourier transform of $S(x)$ may be easily computed, and the result is

$$\tilde{S}(\rho) = 4\pi a^3 \left[\frac{\sin(2\pi a\rho)}{(2\pi a\rho)^3} - \frac{\cos(2\pi a\rho)}{(2\pi a\rho)^2} \right] \tag{6.A-14}$$

where ρ is the radial spatial frequency coordinate, and has dimensions of line pairs per unit distance. By using the series representations for the sine and cosine functions, it is easy to determine that

$$\tilde{S}(0) = \frac{4\pi a^3}{3} \tag{6.A-15}$$

which is the volume of the sphere.

Table 6.A-1. Contrast Factors for Spherical Lesions

β	Contrast factor	β	Contrast factor	β	Contrast factor
0.00	1.00	0.22	0.89	0.44	0.54
0.02	1.00	0.24	0.86	0.46	0.51
0.04	0.99	0.26	0.83	0.48	0.49
0.06	0.99	0.28	0.80	0.50	0.46
0.08	0.98	0.30	0.77	0.52	0.44
0.10	0.98	0.32	0.74	0.54	0.41
0.12	0.97	0.34	0.70	0.56	0.39
0.14	0.96	0.36	0.67	0.58	0.37
0.16	0.94	0.38	0.63	0.60	0.35
0.18	0.93	0.40	0.60		
0.20	0.91	0.42	0.57		

The output lesion contrast may now be calculated using Eq. (6.A-9). Thus

$$C_{\text{image}} = \frac{2\pi}{B}\int_0^\infty \tilde{S}(\rho)\,\tilde{H}(\rho)\,\rho\,d\rho \tag{6.A-16}$$

where B is the background level given by Eq. (6.A-4), $\tilde{S}$ is the lesion transform given by Eq. (6.A-14), $\tilde{H}$ is the MTF of the imaging system as given by Eq. (6.A-10). Substituting the appropriate expressions into (6.A-16) and performing some algebraic simplification results in

$$C_{\text{image}} = \frac{1}{B}\int_0^\infty \exp(-\beta^2 x^2)\,\frac{\sin x - x\cos x}{x^2}\,dx \tag{6.A-17}$$

where $\beta = 2^{1/2}\sigma/D$, $x = 2\pi a\rho$, σ is the standard deviation of the line spread function, D is the diameter of the spherical lesion, and B is the effective background level. A closed form solution for this integral could not be found (at least by the author) so it was computed by numerical integration. The result is a contrast percentage factor, CF, in terms of the parameter β. Numerical values of CF, for values of β up to 0.6, are given in Table 6.A-1. Use of the table allows rapid calculation of the output lesion contrast for any given combination of lesion size and imaging system FWHM. For example, suppose a 2-cm lesion is imaged with a system which has a line spread function of 1.0 cm FWHM. (Note that lesion diameter and system FWHM must both be expressed in the same dimensional units, i.e., centimeters or millimeters.) The value of β is given by

$$\beta = \frac{2^{1/2}\text{FWHM}}{2.355D} = 0.3 \tag{6.A-18}$$

which yields a corresponding contrast factor of

$$\mathrm{CF} = 0.77 \tag{6.A-19}$$

Thus the output image contrast is 77% of the input object contrast.

6.A.3. The Effect of Compton Scatter

The last step in the calculation of lesion contrast is to determine the effects of gamma-ray scattering. Scattering degrades lesion contrast by two mechanisms. The most important mechanism is the production of broad tails on the imaging system line spread function, which tend to blur the entire image by convolution of the object distribution function with this broad line spread function. Beck *et al.* (1969) have shown that a useful quantitative approximation for the loss of lesion contrast by this mechanism is given by

$$\text{contrast with scatter} = \frac{\text{contrast without scatter}}{1 + S_{\mathrm{F}}} \tag{6.A-20}$$

where S_{F} is the scatter fraction, or ratio of scattered to unscattered gamma rays, in the energy window of the scintillation detector. Note that this is a "worst case" approximation, so that for large lesions, or for hot lesions in a relatively cold background, the procedure will overestimate the loss of lesion contrast. The approximation is most valid for small cold lesions in a large volume of background activity, and since this is an extremely important problem in liver scanning, the approximation in Eq. (6.A-20) is useful in practical cases of interest.

Scatter also degrades image contrast because it produces an "apparent" difference in the attenuation coefficient for background and lesion activity (Jones, 1975). Any gamma ray from the background volume which is an accepted event in the energy window produces a "good" background count in the image. Scattered gamma rays from a hot lesion, however, do not aid in the formation of a lesion image, so that, in effect, the lesion activity produces a lower ratio of "good" events to "bad" events in the detector energy window than does the background activity. Thus the appropriate attenuation coefficient for the lesion activity is the listed value for unscattered gamma rays (e.g., 0.15 for 140-keV gamma rays in water), while the value needed for calculation of the background projection [Eq. (6.A-4)] depends upon the energy window width, and is always less than the value for the lesion. An easy way to determine the numerical value of the background attenuation coefficient is to measure the number of counts collected in equal times from a source at various depths in water, using a parallel hole collimator. With this data, one can compute the attenuation coefficient from

$$\alpha = \frac{1}{z} \ln \frac{N(z)}{N(0)} \tag{6.A-21}$$

where z is the depth of the source, $N(z)$ is the number of counts collected for some convenient time T, when the source is located at the depth of z, and $N(0)$ is the number of counts collected in time T for the source at the depth $z = 0$. Care must be used not to move the source so far away that a significant fraction of gamma rays are scattered out of the field of view of the camera. Also, it is necessary to correct for source decay in any experiment over 15 min with ^{99m}Tc. As an example, a 30% window for a 140-keV source in water yields an "effective background" attenuation coefficient of approximately 0.1.

6.A.4. Minimum Detectable Target-to-Nontarget Ratios for Spherical Lesions

From the expressions in Eqs. (6-6), (6.A-8), (6.A-17), and (6.A-20), it is possible to determine the minimum detectable target-to-nontarget ratio for a spherical lesion in a uniform background activity distribution. This is done by combining these equations and solving for μ. The result is

$$\mu = 1 + \frac{(1 + S_F)(10^{\Delta D/\gamma} - 1)\, L \sinh(\alpha_b L/2) \exp(-\alpha_b L/2)}{D\, \mathrm{CF} \exp(-\alpha_p z_0)(\alpha_b L/2)} \tag{6.A-22}$$

where μ is target-to-nontarget uptake ratio, S_F is the Compton scatter fraction, ΔD is the visual threshold density difference, γ is the slope of the D–$\log E$ curve for the film used, L is the thickness of the background activity, α_b is the "effective" background attenuation coefficient for the detector energy window width, D is the diameter of the lesion, CF is the MTF contrast factor (from Table 6.A-1), and α_p is the attenuation coefficient for the primary energy gamma rays.

APPENDIX 6.B. CALCULATION OF THE PROBABILITY OF A FALSE POSITIVE LESION IN A NUCLEAR IMAGE

Given an image with a uniform background distribution of average value $\bar{B}$ and a signal with the expected value of $\bar{S}$, where both B and S are Poisson-distributed random variables, the false-positive error rate is the probability that the random variable B is greater than the sum of its average value $\bar{B}$ and the random variable S.

Let the probability density functions for B and S be $f(B)$ and $f(S)$, respectively. Then for any given value of $S = S_0$,

$$\text{prob}\{B > \bar{B} + S_0\} = \int_{\bar{B}+S_0}^{\infty} f(B)\,dB \tag{6.B-1}$$

But the probability that S is within the interval dS around S_0 is given by

$$\text{prob}\left\{|S - S_0| \le \frac{dS}{2}\right\} = f(S_0)\,dS \tag{6.B-2}$$

So the percentage of times that $S = S_0$ and B exceeds $\bar{B} + S_0$ is given by

$$\text{fractional error} = f(S_0)\,dS \int_{\bar{B}+S_0}^{\infty} f(B)\,dB \tag{6.B-3}$$

The total error for all possible values of S is then given by

$$\text{total error} = \int_{-\infty}^{\infty} f(S)\,dS \int_{\bar{B}+S}^{\infty} f(B)\,dB \tag{6.B-4}$$

To determine explicit expressions for $f(S)$ and $f(B)$ in terms of the image contrast and signal-to-noise ratio, recall that image contrast is simply

$$C = \frac{\bar{S}}{\bar{B}} \tag{6.B-5}$$

and the *average* signal-to-noise ratio is just

$$k = \frac{\bar{S}}{\bar{B}^{1/2}} \tag{6.B-6}$$

Using (6.B-5) and (6.B-6) along with the fact that S and B are Poisson distributed,

$$\text{prob}\{\text{error}\} = \frac{C^{3/2}}{2\pi k^2} \int_{-\infty}^{\infty} \int_{S}^{\infty} \exp\left[\frac{-(S - k^2/C)^2}{2k^2/c}\right] \exp\left[\frac{-B^2}{2k^2/C^2}\right] dB\,dS \tag{6.B-7}$$

where the average value of $\bar{B} = k^2/C^2$ has been removed by a shift of the origin because it is irrelevant in the integration.

With numerical integration, this expression yields a family of curves for probability of error vs. image contrast at various values of signal-to-noise ratio, as shown in Fig. 6-5. Note that this graph represents the probability of an error for a *single resolution element.* The probability of having one or more errors in an image of n resolution elements is given by

$$\text{prob}\{\text{image error}\} = 1 - (1 - p)^n \tag{6.B-8}$$

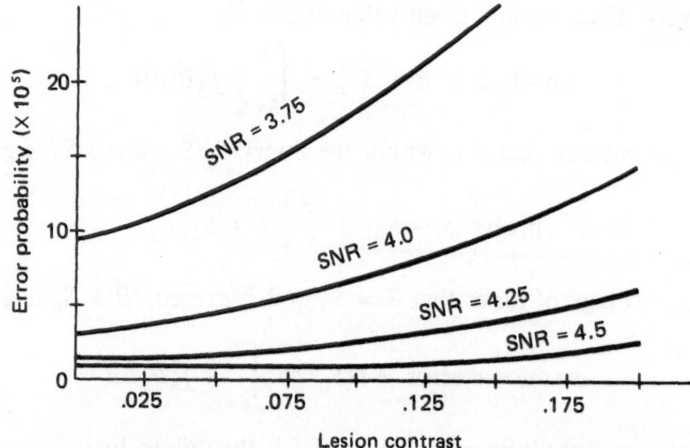

Fig. 6-5. Probability of the background level exceeding the signal in one resolution element. Values from this graph are used in Eq. (6.B-8) to compute the probability of error in an image containing n resolution elements.

where p is the single resolution element probability of an error obtained from Fig. 6-5.

For the example, in the main text, of detecting the presence of a 15% contrast lesion in the count density image, choice of a signal-to-noise ratio of 4 to 1 yields a single resolution element error of

$$p \approx 1 \times 10^{-4} \tag{6.B-9}$$

so that with a standard 10-in.-field-of-view nuclear medicine camera, containing approximately 500 resolution elements, the probability of one or more errors occurring somewhere in the image is found to be

$$P = 1 - (1 - 1 \times 10^{-4})^{500} \approx 0.05 \tag{6.B-10}$$

In other words, there is only a 5% chance that an image with a signal-to-noise ratio of 4 to 1 will contain a resolution element with a statistical deviation in the background that is greater than the signal from a 15% contrast lesion.

REFERENCES

Beck, R.N., Schuh, M.W., Cohen, J.D., and Lembares, N. (1969), Effects of scattered radiation on scintillation detector response, *Medical Radioisotope Scintigraphy*, Vol. 1, p.595. IAEA, Vienna.

Dresser, M.M. (1972), Scattering effects in radioisotope imaging, Ph.D. dissertation, University of Michigan (available from University Microfilms, Ann Arbor, Michigan).

Jones, J.P., Brill, A.B., and Johnston, R.E. (1975), The validity of an equivalent point source (EPS) assumption used in quantitative scanning, *Phys. Med. Biol.* **20**:3,455.

Polaroid Corporation, Technical Publication T570-1, June 1976.

Revesz, G., and Haas, C. (1972), Television display of radiographic images with superimposed simulated lesions, *Radiology* **102**:1,197.

Rollo, F. D., and Schulz, A. G. (1970), A contrast efficiency function for quantitatively measuring the spatial resolution characteristics of scanning systems, *J. Nucl. Med.* **11**:2,53.

Rose, A. (1974), *Vision, Human and Electronic*, Plenum Press, New York.

Schade, O. H., Sr. (1956), Optical and photoelectric analogue of the eye, *J. Opt. Soc. Am.* **46**:9, 721.

Schade, O. H., Sr. (1964), An evaluation of photographic image quality and resolving power, *J. Soc. Motion Pict. Telev. Eng.* **73**:2,81.

CHAPTER 7

X-Ray Fluorescence Imaging

J.A. PATTON

7.1. INTRODUCTION

X-ray fluorescence imaging is a relatively new technique for imaging distributions of nonradioactive elements within the body. The emission of characteristic X-rays (fluorescence) is induced by irradiation with an external source of photons as shown in Fig. 7-1. If the photons from the exciting source have an energy close to but greater than the *K*-shell binding energy of the atom being irradiated, there is a high probability that the photon will undergo photoelectric absorption by one of the *K*-shell electrons. The electron would then be ejected with a kinetic energy equal to the energy of the incoming photon minus the *K*-shell binding energy. The atom is left in an excited state with a vacancy in the *K* shell. This vacancy is promptly filled by an electron (most probably from the *L* shell) with the excess energy carried off by an Auger electron (which is absorbed within a short distance), or by a characteristic X-ray whose energy is equal to the difference between

J.A. PATTON • Department of Radiology, Vanderbilt University, Nashville, Tennessee 37232.

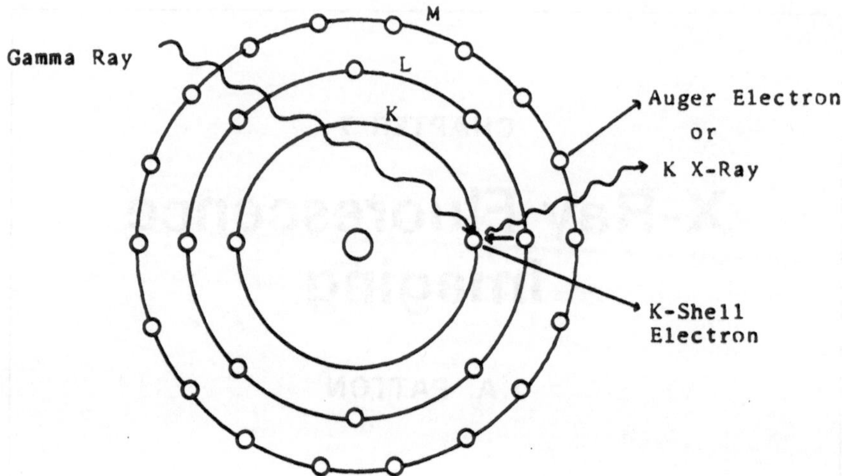

Fig. 7-1. Diagram of an atom showing a photon undergoing photoelectric absorption by a *K*-shell electron.

the binding energies of the *K* and *L* shells (28.5 keV for iodine). For elements with relatively high atomic numbers this X-ray is of sufficient energy to escape the patient and be counted by an external detector (Tinney, 1971).

7.2. USE OF X-RAY FLUORESCENCE IMAGING IN EVALUATING THYROID DISORDERS

This technique was first applied to imaging the stable iodine distribution within the thyroid by Hoffer and his associates at the Argonne Cancer Research Hospital (Hoffer, 1968). The ionization energy of the *K* electron of iodine is 33.2 keV. Sources emitting gamma radiation only slightly higher than this value would be very efficient in giving rise to fluorescent iodine X-rays, but the radiation would be severely attenuated in the neck tissue. A somewhat higher energy would be less efficient but would give greater penetration, so that the thyroid gland would be uniformly irradiated. Two kinds of radiation sources have been used: radioactive americium-241 ($^{241}_{95}$Am, half-life 450 years, gamma energy 60 keV, available in 1-Ci metal slugs), and an X-ray tube with special filters (effective energy 40–60 keV) (Johnson, 1979). Two systems are now commercially available for performing X-ray fluorescence imaging of the thyroid and are shown schematically in Fig. 7-2. The system developed by Hoffer *et al.* (1971) consists of an outrigger-type source holder and an uncollimated detector as shown in Fig. 7-2A. This system is commercially available from Kevex, Inc. The

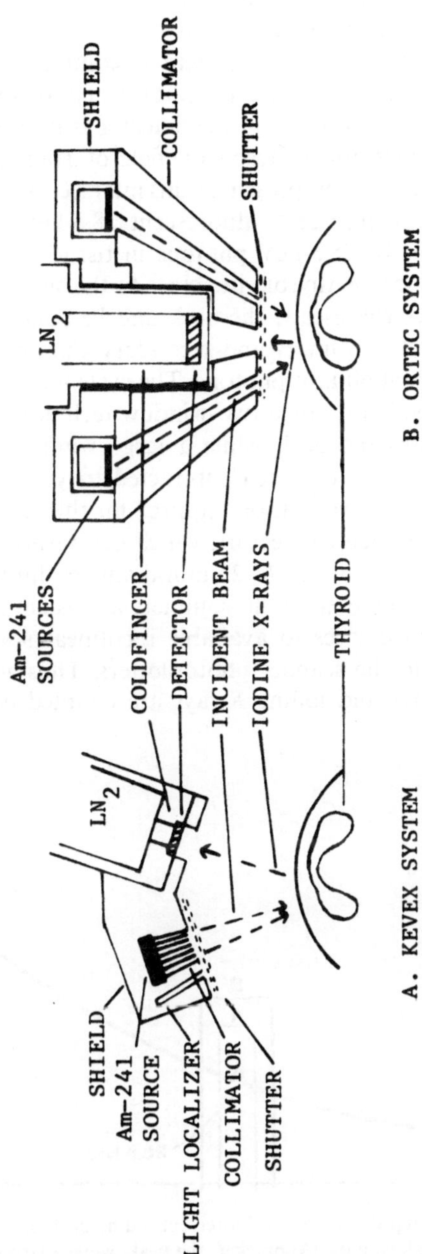

Fig. 7-2. Diagrammatic comparison of the Kevex (A) and Ortec (B) fluorescent systems that are commercially available as add-on devices to rectilinear scanners.

system developed by Patton *et al.* (1973) consists of multiple disk sources arranged in a circle concentric with a coarsely collimated detector as shown in Fig. 7-2B, and is a modified version of the system originally used by Hoffer (Hoffer *et al.*, 1968). This system is commercially available from Ortec, Inc. Both systems collimate the photons emitted from the source or sources (10–20 Ci of Am-241), and the detector is positioned such that the field of view of the detector intersects the field of irradiation of the sources. Thus if there are iodine atoms present at this intersection the 60-keV photons may be absorbed, giving rise to fluorescent 28.5-keV iodine X-rays. The half-value thickness for 28.5-keV photons in tissue is 2 cm (i.e., 50% absorbed in 2 cm). Since the thyroid lies close to the surface of the skin many of the iodine X-rays will escape the neck and be counted by the detector. There is a great deal of primary and secondary Compton scattering in the neck from the incident 60-keV photons. The system detects the subtle peak of fluorescent iodine X-rays by a two-window technique (Fig. 7-3): a small window encompasses the peak while a large window averages adjacent background scatter, which is then subtracted to yield an enhanced fluorescent peak. The energy resolution required for this technique can only be achieved by semiconductor detectors, which can resolve the iodine X-rays from the scatter background. A 25-mm-diameter lithium-drifted silicon [Si(Li)] detector is used in both commercial systems. The systems are marketed as add-on devices to available rectilinear scanners and can be interfaced directly to the scanner photoplotters. Thus as the system scans in a rectilinear raster and iodine X-rays are counted by the detector, an

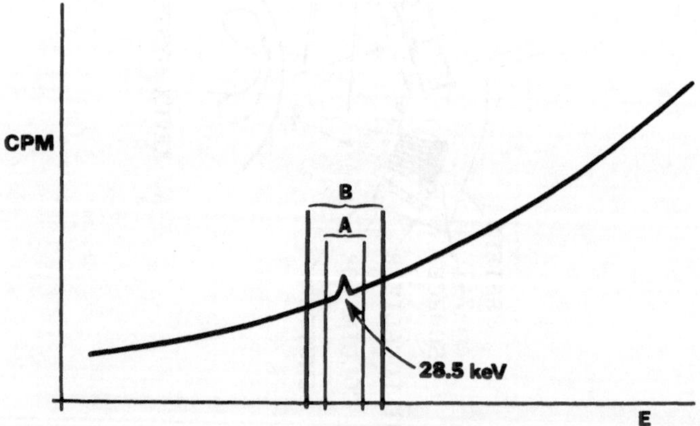

Fig. 7-3. Diagrammatic representation of fluorescent iodine peak on scatter curve. Only the K_α peak is shown. A small window (A) brackets the peak, while a larger window (B) averages adjacent scatter, which is then subtracted so as to enhance the peak.

intensity-modulated image appears on film depicting the stable iodine distribution within the thyroid gland.

There are many advantages of this technique over conventional radioisotope imaging procedures. The information obtained from the study provides new information on iodine storage properties of the gland as opposed to iodine uptake and turnover properties which are measured by radioisotope studies. No stable or radioactive materials are introduced into the body. The radiation dose is very low, i.e., 15–60 mrads as compared to 200–250 mrads with Tc-99m and 2–20 rads with I-131, and is limited entirely to the neck region. Patients with flooded iodine pools from radioopaque dye studies and patients on short-term thyroid suppression cannot be studied using conventional radionuclide procedures, but can be evaluated using the fluorescent technique since these factors do not affect the iodine content immediately as they do the iodine uptake of the thyroid.

The fluorescent technique is also a quantitative procedure in that the number of iodine X-rays detected is proportional to the amount of iodine present in the thyroid. A fluorescent system has been interfaced to a computer (Patton *et al.*, 1976) and the procedure calibrated by scanning thyroid phantoms containing known quantities of iodine in a simulated neck geometry. Thus direct measurements of the iodine content in milligrams can be made in patients. Mean values of thyroid iodine content of 33.3 mg have been reported for a hyperthyroid group, 1.5 mg for a hypothyroid group, and 10.7 mg for a group of normals (Patton *et al.*, 1976). This quantitative information is useful in following the course of various diseases such as thyroiditis and the effects of therapy on disease states such as I-131 therapy in hyperthyroidism. It may also be possible to use the iodine content in some way to predict the outcome of I-131 therapy and this is under study.

One of the most important applications of fluorescent thyroid scanning is the evaluation of the solitary "cold" thyroid nodule. A "cold" nodule in a conventional thyroid scan is a palpable mass that does not take up radioiodine like normal thyroid tissue. "Cold" nodules have a high probability of being malignant, but could also represent adenomas (benign tumors), colloid cysts (nonfunctioning accumulation of stored iodine-containing thyroid hormone), or other rarer entities. The ratio of the iodine content in solitary thyroid nodules to that in normal thyroid tissue has been suggested as a possible indicator of malignancy (Patton *et al.*, 1976). Colloid cysts were found to have a high iodine content ratio, benign adenomas normal or slightly decreased, and malignant tumors markedly decreased. The fluorescent scan distinguished benign from malignant nodules in 80% of the cases. Thus the fluorescent scan furnishes valuable new information in evaluating thyroid disorders.

7.3. OTHER APPLICATIONS OF FLUORESCENT SCANNING

One of the newest developments in fluorescent scanning is the capability of performing fluorescent scans simultaneously with radioisotope emission scans using Tc-99m. To accomplish this, the Si(Li) detector has been replaced by a high-purity germanium detector (HpGe) of the same size. The efficiency of the Si(Li) detector is 100% up to about 20 keV and then falls off very rapidly with increasing energy. The HpGe detector is 100% efficient up to about 90 keV and is about 60% efficient at 140 keV (the energy of Tc-99m) due to the higher atomic number of germanium (32 vs. 14 for silicon) and greater density (5.4 vs. 2.4 for silicon). A seven-hole focused collimator was added to the detector shown in Fig. 7-2B to focus the 140-keV photons of Tc-99m and to reduce the amount of scattered radiation entering the detector. The output of the single-channel analyzer, set on the 28.5-keV X-ray peak of iodine, was coupled to one photoplotter and the output of a second-single channel analyzer, set on the 140-keV peak of Tc-99m, was coupled to a second photoplotter of a dual system. Two images obtained simultaneously from a patient are shown in Fig. 7-4. The advantage of this new technique is that the fluorescent and emission images are obtained simultaneously with the same collimation (i.e., identical resolution) on the same imaging devices with the same display factors, and with the patient in the same position. Thus the two images can be overlaid for direct comparisons of regional uptake vs. iodine content. Also, by collecting the data in a computer, quantitative or numerical comparisons can be made on a regional basis and functional maps can be generated.

The possible application of X-ray fluorescence for imaging stable bismuth that would be introduced into the body and taken up by brain tumors has been studied (Patton, 1971). However, the systems currently available for this application are not sufficiently sensitive to image quantities that can be safely administered.

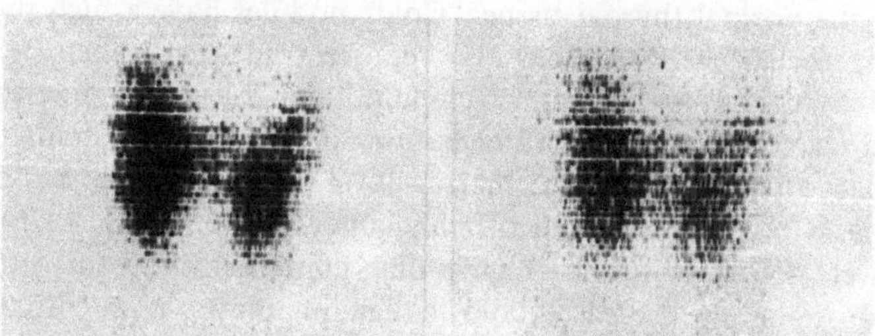

Fig. 7-4. X-ray fluorescent image (left) of the stable iodine in the diffusely enlarged thyroid of a patient collected simultaneously with the radioisotope emission scan (right) obtained by injecting a routine dose of Tc-99m pertechnetate. The detector used was a high-purity germanium detector (HpGe).

Dynamic studies have been performed by X-ray fluorescence techniques in which a sensitive volume is defined by the intersection of the field of irradiation of a collimated source or X-ray tube and the field of view of a collimated detector placed perpendicular to the source. This sensitive column can be positioned within a region of interest in the body, and X-ray fluorescence radiation induced from stable tracers (such as iodine) passing through the volume can be measured as a function of time. This technique has been applied to cerebral blood flow and blood volume measurements (Ter-Pogossian *et al.*, 1971), to cardiac output measurements (Kaufman *et al.*, 1973), and to measurement of iodine concentration in the liver (Koehler *et al.*, 1976).

REFERENCES

Hoffer, P.B., Jones, W.B., Crawford, R.B., *et al.* (1968), Fluorescent thyroid scanning: A new method of imaging the thyroid, *Radiology* **90**:342–344.

Hoffer, P.B., Bernstein, J., and Gottschalk, A. (1971), Clinical results in fluorescent thyroid scanning, in *Semiconductor Detectors in the Future of Nuclear Medicine*, Society of Nuclear Medicine, New York, pp. 239–250.

Johnson, P.M., Esser, P.D., and Lister, D.B. (1979), Fluorescent thyroid imaging: Clinical evaluation of an alternative instrument, *Radiology* **130**:219–222.

Kaufman, L., Shames, D.M., Greenspan, R.H., *et al.* (1973), A new method of measuring cardiac output using fluorescent excitation, in *Semiconductor Detectors in Medicine*, Oak Ridge, Tennessee, USAEC Conf-730321, pp. 353–408.

Koehler, R.E., Kaufman, L., Brito, A., *et al.* (1976), *In vivo* measurement of hepatic iodine concentration using fluorescent excitation analysis, *Invest. Radiol.* **11**:134–137.

Patton, J.A., Brill, A.B., and Johnston, R.E. (1971), Potential use of fluorescent scanning for brain tumor identification, in *Semiconductor Detectors in the Future of Nuclear Medicine*, Society of Nuclear Medicine, New York, pp. 258–270.

Patton, J.A., Brill, A.B., Blanco, J., *et al.* (1973), Experiences with semiconductors in imaging and function studies at Vanderbilt, in *Semiconductor Detectors in Medicine*, Oak Ridge, Tennessee, USAEC Conf-730321, pp. 254–294.

Patton, J.A., Hollifield, J.W., Brill, A.B., *et al.* (1976), Differentiation between malignant and benign solitary thyroid nodules by fluorescent scanning, *J. Nucl. Med.* **17**:17–21.

Patton, J.A. (1971), unpublished data.

Ter-Pogossian, M.D., Phelps, M.E., Lassen, M., *et al.* (1971), *In vivo* measurements of regional cerebral blood flow and blood volume by means of stimulated X-ray fluorescence, in *Semiconductor Detectors in the Future of Nuclear Medicine*, Society of Nuclear Medicine, New York, pp. 240–251.

Tinney, J.F. (1971), *In vivo* X-ray fluorescence analysis—concepts and equipment, in *Semiconductor Detectors in the Future of Nuclear Medicine*, Society of Nuclear Medicine, New York, pp. 214–229.

CHAPTER 8

Coded-Aperture Imaging

R.G. SIMPSON and H.H. BARRETT

8.1. INTRODUCTION

In a photographic camera, the camera lens forms an image of the object and the image is detected by the photographic film. In the Anger camera described in Chapter 4, the pinhole aperture or the multihole collimator performs the imaging operation while a detector system consisting of a scintillation crystal and an arrangement of photomultiplier tubes detects the image. The detector system in the Anger camera is very efficient and records almost every X-ray or γ-ray photon that arrives with an energy within the preselected energy window. Unfortunately, the imaging system severely limits the number of photons that arrive. A collimator typically passes only 0.01 % of the radiation emitted by the object. Since the statistical quality of the images formed in this way is dependent on the number of photons collected from a single element of the object, one needs to collect as many photons as possible. Patient-dose restrictions limit the number of

R.G. SIMPSON and H.H. BARRETT • Optical Sciences Center, University of Arizona, Tucson, Arizona 85721.

photons available, while exposure time is limited by temporal–resolution requirements in a dynamic study, by image degradation due to patient motion, by patient fatigue, or by the expense involved in tying up a clinical instrument for extended periods.

With a pinhole aperture or multihole collimator, the only way to collect more photons if the object radiance and the exposure time are fixed is to make the openings larger. That in turn degrades the resolution in the image. This inevitable trade-off between collection efficiency and resolution also occurs in other fields such as radar technology (Klauder *et al.*, 1960), X-ray astronomy (Mertz and Young, 1961; Young, 1963; Mertz, 1965; Abels, 1968; Dicke, 1968), and infrared spectroscopy (Golay, 1949, 1951; Girard, 1963; Harwitt, 1971). In these areas, techniques are used in which the resolution in the detected signal is sacrificed in order to increase the total amount of signal detected. Increasing the amount of detected signal improves the statistical quality of the signal. If the way in which the resolution is degraded is chosen carefully, it is possible to postprocess the signal to recover the resolution and still enjoy improved statistical quality in the processed signal. When these concepts are applied to nuclear medicine, they result in what are known as coded-aperture imaging techniques.

It must be understood from the start that coded-aperture imaging is distinct from conventional imaging techniques in that the detected image is not a recognizable representation of the object. Information about the object has been encoded in the detected image and must be decoded before a recognizable image can be obtained. The processing or decoding step is an essential part of the imaging system; it is not an optional enhancement process. Coded-aperture imaging systems differ from conventional imaging systems in a second important way. Collimators and pinholes form two-dimensional images of three-dimensional object distributions. In virtually all coded-aperture systems, the nature of the coding process allows the reconstruction of an object plane at a particular depth in the object while blurring other planes in the object. This tomographic capability is a very useful property and will be discussed in more detail later in this chapter.

All coded apertures share the same basic encoding operation that is described in the next section of this chapter. A particular coded aperture is chosen for use in a coded-aperture system because some property of the aperture allows effective decoding of the coded image. Interest in the Fresnel zone plate results from its ability to focus light. Nonredundant pinhole arrays are used because of the favorable shape of their autocorrelation function. The behavior of several coded-aperture systems will be discussed in later sections of this chapter in order to illustrate both the good and bad features of a coded-aperture system that employs a particular coded aperture. The chapter concludes with a discussion of the effects of noise in a coded-aperture system and a review of the factors and trade-offs that are important in the selection of a particular coded-aperture imaging system.

8.2. ENCODING PROCESS

The term "coded-aperture imaging" implies a two-step operation. In the first step, referred to as the encoding step, the coded aperture is placed between the object and the detector and the output of the detector is recorded. For coded apertures which have no time-varying properties,† it is essential that the detector be able to record the spatial distribution of the quanta incident upon it. A commonly used detector for coded-aperture systems is the scintillation-crystal detector system in the Anger camera; film has also been employed as the detector in some coded-aperture systems. In either case, the recorded coded image becomes the input in the second, or decoding, step. The exact nature of the decoding step is dependent on the aperture used and is discussed in later sections. The two-step nature of coded-aperture imaging has an important effect on the noise in the final image. For the present, statistical fluctuations in the coded image will be ignored; presence of random errors in the coded image will be taken into account in a later section on noise. The encoding step is common to all systems and is discussed here.

The encoding step is simply a shadow-casting operation. The basic arrangement is shown in Fig. 8-1. The aperture is placed between the object and the detector such that the aperture plane is parallel to the detector plane. The coded aperture consists of a layer of material that is effectively opaque to the radiation of interest. Certain regions of the opaque layer are removed to form the aperture.‡ While it is possible to modulate the thickness of the opaque layer to achieve a desired transmission function for the aperture, investigations to date have concentrated on aperture transmission functions that are binary; the aperture is either transparent or opaque at a given location.

Each point in the object casts a shadow onto the detector. The shadow will have the same shape as the aperture pattern. The size of the pattern on the detector will depend on the distance from the object point to the aperture plane, denoted s_1, as well as the distance from the aperture plane to the detector, denoted s_2. The shadow on the detector will be larger than the aperture pattern by a factor of $(s_1 + s_2)/s_1$. Since the size of the shadow is dependent on s_1, the coded image then contains information about the distance from the object to the aperture plane. The ability to successfully

† The time-varying coded-aperture system described in Section 8.6 encodes spatial information as a temporal signal. Spatial resolution in the detector is required only if tomographic information is desired.

‡ The term "aperture" is used quite often in this chapter as a shortened version of the term "coded aperture." Consequently, "aperture" usually refers to the entire coded aperture consisting of opaque and transparent regions, rather than to a single transparent region of the coded aperture. The usage should be quite clear from context and should cause no confusion.

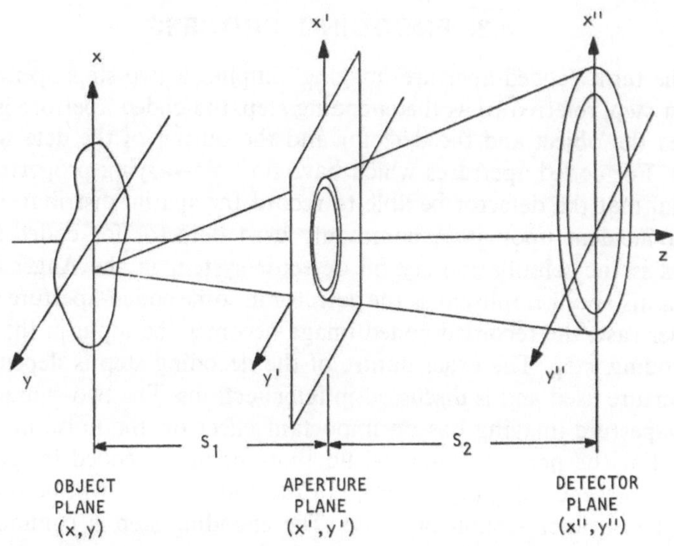

Fig. 8-1. Basic encoding geometry employed in a coded-aperture system.

decode this information results in the tomographic capability of coded-aperture systems.

All object points located a distance s_1 from the aperture plane will produce shadows of the coded aperture with the same scale factor, $(s_1 + s_2)/s_1$. Restricting our attention to an object plane (x, y) that is a distance s_1 from the aperture plane, let the shadow of the aperture due to an object point at $(x = 0, y = 0)$ be described by $h(x'', y''; s_1)$. The scale factor and all solid-angle factors that affect the actual collection efficiency of the aperture are contained implicitly in $h(x'', y''; s_1)$ through the parameter s_1; s_2 is assumed to be a known constant. The solid-angle factors are important when apertures are compared but can be neglected during discussions of the encoding and decoding processes for a single aperture. The shadow due to an object point at (x_0, y_0) is a shifted version of $h(x'', y''; s_1)$ centered at the point (x_0'', y_0'') in the detector plane. This is strictly true only if all obliquity factors and the thickness of the aperture material are neglected; such factors will be assumed negligible here and omitted. From the simple geometry involved, the two pairs of coordinates are related by

$$x_0'' = \frac{-s_2}{s_1} x_0 \tag{8-1a}$$

$$y_0'' = \frac{-s_2}{s_1} y_0 \tag{8-1b}$$

The aperture shadow due to an object point at (x_0, y_0) is then described by $h[x'' + (s_2/s_1)x_0, y'' + (s_2/s_1)y_0; s_1]$.

Suppose now that the object is planar and made up of n points located at (x_i, y_i), $i = 1, \ldots, n$, and the strength of the ith point is a_i. The pattern on the detector, $g(x'', y'')$, will be the sum of the individual shadows, given by

$$g(x'', y''; s_1) = \sum_{i=1}^{n} a_i h\left(x'' + \frac{s_2}{s_1} x_i, y'' + \frac{s_2}{s_1} y_i; s_1\right) \tag{8-2}$$

If the detector is linear, free of spatial distortion and capable of perfect resolution, $g(x'', y''; s_1)$ will describe the functional form of the output of the detector. In the limit of a continuous planar object, Eq. (8-2) becomes an integral expression written as

$$g(x'', y''; s_1) = \iint_{-\infty}^{\infty} o(x, y)\, h\left(x'' + \frac{s_2}{s_1} x, y'' + \frac{s_2}{s_1} y; s_1\right) dx\, dy \tag{8-3}$$

where $o(x, y)\, dx\, dy$ is the strength of the object in an infinitesimal area element. If a change of variables is made such that $\alpha = (-s_2/s_1)x$ and $\beta = (-s_2/s_1)y$, Eq. (8-3) becomes

$$g(x'', y''; s_1) = \left(\frac{s_1}{s_2}\right)^2 \iint_{-\infty}^{\infty} o\left(\frac{-s_1}{s_2}\alpha, \frac{-s_1}{s_2}\beta\right) h(x'' - \alpha, y'' - \beta; s_1)\, d\alpha\, d\beta \tag{8-4}$$

This is a special kind of integral known as a convolution integral.

Convolution integrals occur so frequently in engineering and the physical sciences that a special shorthand notation has evolved to handle them (Bracewell, 1965; Gaskill, 1978). If

$$f_1(x) = \int_{-\infty}^{\infty} f_2(\alpha)\, f_3(x - \alpha)\, d\alpha \tag{8-5}$$

then in shorthand notation,

$$f_1(x) = f_2(x) * f_3(x) \tag{8-6}$$

where the asterisk indicates the convolution integral that appears explicitly in Eq. (8-5). The function f_2 is said to be convolved with f_3 in order to obtain f_1.

Convolutions arise in linear circuit theory in electrical engineering. The output of a circuit $g(t)$ is related to the input $f(t)$ by a convolution with the impulse response of the circuit $h(t)$,

$$g(t) = f(t) * h(t) \tag{8-7}$$

In the analysis of optical imaging, the image $i(x, y)$ is found to be related to the object $o(x, y)$ by a two-dimensional convolution with the point spread function (PSF) $p(x, y)$:

$$i(x, y) = \iint_{-\infty}^{\infty} o(\alpha, \beta)\, p(x - \alpha, y - \beta)\, d\alpha\, d\beta \tag{8-8}$$

which in the shorthand notation becomes

$$i(x, y) = o(x, y) ** p(x, y) \tag{8-9}$$

where the double asterisk indicates the two-dimensional convolution.

Before Eq. (8-4) can be written in this shorthand notation, we must decide how to handle scaled functions such as $o[-(s_1/s_2)\,x, -(s_1/s_2)\,y]$. The function $f(x/a)$ is said to be scaled by the factor a; features in the function $f(x)$ that are separated by a distance d will be separated by a distance ad in the function $f(x/a)$. When scaled functions are used in the shorthand notation, the following interpretation will be assumed:

$$f_2(x/a) * f_3(x/b) = \int_{-\infty}^{\infty} f_2(\alpha/a)\, f_3\left(\frac{x - \alpha}{b}\right) d\alpha$$

It is important to realize that even though Eq. (8-6) might be true for the unscaled functions, it does not follow that $f_2(x/a) * f_3(x/b) = f_1(x/c)$. In the shorthand notation then, Eq. (8-4) becomes

$$g(x'', y''; s_1) = \left(\frac{s_1}{s_2}\right)^2 \left[o\left(-\frac{s_1}{s_2}x'', -\frac{s_1}{s_2}y''\right) ** h(x'', y''; s_1) \right] \tag{8-10}$$

The function $h(x'', y''; s_1)$ is called the point response function to distinguish it from the system PSF that results after the decoding operation. The arguments of the object function are scaled to take into account the magnification of the image relative to the original object. The minus sign accounts for the fact that the image will be upside-down relative to the object orientation. The leading factor of $(s_1/s_2)^2$ conserves object strength. If s_1 is larger than s_2, the scale of $o[-(s_1/s_2)\,x, -(s_1/s_2)\,y]$ is smaller than $o(-x, -y)$ and therefore the strength of the scaled object must be increased so that the total strength of the scaled object remains unchanged as the scale changes.

When a physical process is describable by a convolution operation, it is possible to take advantage of some powerful theorems from Fourier transform theory. The Fourier transform of the function $f(x)$ is defined as

$$F(\xi) = \int_{-\infty}^{\infty} f(x)\, e^{-i2\pi\xi x}\, dx \tag{8-11}$$

$$= \mathscr{F}\{f(x)\}$$

where $\mathscr{F}\{\cdot\}$ indicates the Fourier transform operation, not to be confused with the function $F(\xi)$. The variable ξ has units that are the reciprocal of the units of x. If x were a time variable with units of sec, ξ would be a temporal–frequency variable and have units of cycles/sec or Hz. If x were a spatial variable with units of cm, ξ would be a spatial–frequency variable and have units of cycles/cm or line-pairs/cm. When x is a time variable, the function $f(x)$ is said to exist in the time domain, while the function $F(\xi)$ is said to exist in the temporal–frequency domain. When x is a space variable, $f(x)$ is said to exist in the space domain, while the function $F(\xi)$ is said to exist in the spatial–frequency domain. Since $F(\xi)$ describes the frequency content of $f(x)$, it is often referred to as the Fourier spectrum of $f(x)$.

The relationship in Eq. (8-11) is invertible so that

$$f(x) = \int_{-\infty}^{\infty} F(\xi)\, e^{i2\pi\xi x}\, d\xi \tag{8-12}$$

The two functions $f(x)$ and $F(\xi)$ form a Fourier transform pair and knowledge of either one is sufficient to describe everything there is to know about both functions.

There is an important theorem in Fourier transform theory that involves convolutions. If

$$g(x) = f(x) * h(x) \tag{8-13}$$

and

$$\mathscr{F}\{g(x)\} = G(\xi) \tag{8-14a}$$

$$\mathscr{F}\{f(x)\} = F(\xi) \tag{8-14b}$$

$$\mathscr{F}\{h(x)\} = H(\xi) \tag{8-14c}$$

then

$$G(\xi) = F(\xi)\, H(\xi) \tag{8-15}$$

The convolution operation in Eq. (8-13) becomes a multiplication in the frequency domain. If $f(x)$ is the input into a circuit and $h(x)$ is the impulse response, the spectrum of the output $G(\xi)$ is equal to the spectrum of the input times the spectrum of the impulse response. If $H(\xi) = 1$, $F(\xi) = G(\xi)$ and the output signal will be identical to the input. If $H(\xi)$ is some non-constant function of ξ, the spectrum of the output will differ from the spectrum of the input. The function $H(\xi)$ describes what happens to a given frequency component of the input signal. $H(\xi)$ is therefore referred to as the transfer function; it transfers a given frequency component from the input to the output with the amplitude or phase change indicated by $H(\xi)$.

If $H(\xi) = 0$, an input signal with frequency ξ will not produce any output signal.

This formalism can be easily extended to two dimensions so that

$$F(\xi, \eta) = \iint_{-\infty}^{\infty} f(x, y)\, e^{-i2\pi(\xi x + \eta y)}\, dx\, dy \tag{8-16}$$

The convolution in Eq. (8-10) will become (letting $s_1 = s_2$ for simplicity)

$$G(\xi, \eta; s_1) = O(-\xi, -\eta)\, H(\xi, \eta; s_1) \tag{8-17}$$

The spectrum of the object is modified by the spectrum of the aperture shadow thanks to the encoding process. The form of $H(\xi, \eta; s_1)$ will indicate how much information about the object is contained in the coded image. Unfortunately, $H(\xi, \eta; s_1) = 1$ corresponds to the case of a very small pinhole, which is exactly the situation from which we are trying to escape.

In summary then, for planar objects, the encoding process is described by a convolution of the point response function for that plane with the magnified and inverted object. Objects that are not contained entirely in a single plane can be considered as several planar objects at different distances from the aperture. Assuming that the radiation emitted from a given plane is unaffected by passage through other object planes (i.e., scattering and attenuation can be ignored), the coded image is the summation of the coded images that would result from each plane of the object acting alone. For a three-dimensional object distribution $o(x, y, s_1)$, the coded image would be

$$g(x'', y'') = \int_{-\infty}^{\infty} \left(\frac{s_1}{s_2}\right)^2 \left[o\left(-\frac{s_1}{s_2}x'', -\frac{s_1}{s_2}y'', s_1\right) ** h(x'', y''; s_1) \right] ds_1 \tag{8-18}$$

As a result of this integration over s_1, a single object plane cannot be reconstructed totally free of contributions from other object planes. This complication will be ignored for most of the discussion in the rest of this chapter. Attention will be directed at the decoding of coded images of planar objects. For this reason, the parametric dependence of $h(x'', y''; s_1)$ on s_1 will usually be ignored. Once planar objects can be decoded, the effect of additional object planes can be easily calculated. The general result is that the additional planes produce a blurred background which is added to the decoded image of the in-focus plane.

8.3. DECODING—GENERAL REMARKS

It might seem that decoding of the coded image would consist of merely dividing the spectrum of the coded image by the spectrum of the coded aperture. Such an approach is known as inverse filtering and turns out to be very sensitive to noise in the recorded coded image. For all coded apertures with increased collection efficiency over a pinhole, the function $H(\xi, \eta)$ will be much less than 1 for many values of (ξ, η). Dividing by $H(\xi, \eta)$ at these points will highly amplify the noise and seriously degrade the resulting image. Fortunately, other options are available.

The basic requirement of any decoding method for coded-aperture images is the accurate estimation of the strength of an object point and its position based on the coded image. For an object consisting of a single point, this amounts to summing all the counts collected and estimating the center of the detected shadow. This is quite easy to do for a point object. Knowing the shape of the shadow in the limit of a large number of detected quanta, a template can then be made so that when the template is laid over the coded image and correctly centered, all of the counts can be seen and regions in the coded image that received no counts will not be visible. The decoding task then amounts to laying the template over the coded image and positioning it so that the largest number of counts is visible. The location of the center of the template is then the location of the object point, and the strength of the object point is proportional to the number of detected quanta visible through the template.

This template decoding method can be automated in the following way. The template is placed over the coded image and the number of counts visible through the template is measured as a function of the position of the template. Figure 8-2 shows the output that would result if an annular shadow is processed via template matching. Since the annulus is circularly symmetric, a plot of the output vs. the distance between the centers of the shadow and the template is sufficient to describe the output.

The process of template matching can be described mathematically by the correlation integral. The correlation $f_1(x)$ of the functions $f_2(x)$ and $f_3(x)$ is defined as

$$f_1(x) = \int_{-\infty}^{\infty} f_2(\alpha)\, f_3(\alpha - x)\, d\alpha \tag{8-19}$$

Just as for convolution integrals, there is a shorthand expression for the correlation integral

$$f_1(x) = f_2(x) \star f_3(x) \tag{8-20}$$

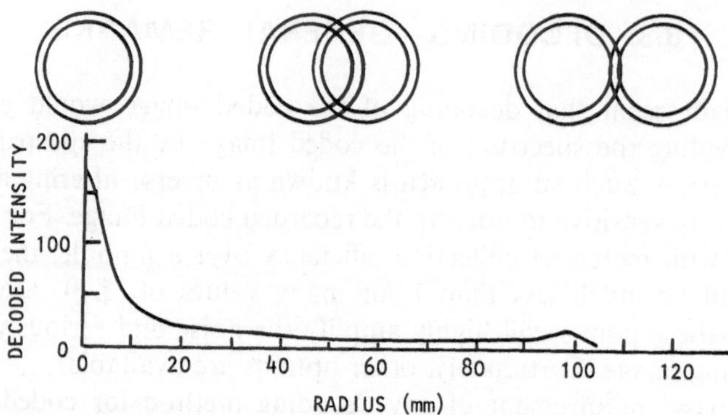

Fig. 8-2. Radial slice through the decoded image of a point source that was imaged with an annular-coded aperture and decoded by template matching.

where the star indicates the correlation integral. If either or both of the functions $f_1(x)$ and $f_2(x)$ are symmetric about the origin, correlation and convolution are identical. The definition generalizes to two dimensions just as for convolution:

$$f_1(x, y) = \iint_{-\infty}^{\infty} f_2(\alpha, \beta)\, f_3(\alpha - x, \beta - y)\, d\alpha\, d\beta \tag{8-21}$$

with the obvious shorthand notation

$$f_1(x, y) = f_2(x, y) \star\star f_3(x, y) \tag{8-22}$$

When $f_2(x, y)$ and $f_3(x, y)$ are the same function, the correlation operation is often referred to as an autocorrelation operation. If $f_2(x, y)$ describes the coded image of a point and $f_3(x, y)$ describes the template with values of 0 or 1, the evaluation of the correlation integral involves shifting the template by an amount (x, y) relative to the coded image and summing the coded image in those locations where the template has values of unity. The integral is repeated for all locations (x, y). This is exactly what is done in the automated template-matching operation described above. The resulting output is the decoded representation of the object. For a point object, the decoded image is the effective point spread function of the imaging system.

Template matching, or correlation of the detected signal with a desired signal waveform, is also performed in radar systems, where it is referred to as matched filtering. In the radar application (Klauder *et al.*, 1960), a known time-varying signal is transmitted and one is interested in detecting the return signal in the presence of all sorts of other signals. Suppose the detected signal is processed with a matched filter designed for the desired return-signal waveform. Provided that the return signal and any other detected signal have the same energy E defined as

$$E = \int_{-\infty}^{\infty} |\text{signal}|^2 \, dt \tag{8-23}$$

it can be shown that the matched filter guarantees that none of the other signals will produce a correlation peak larger than the peak resulting from the return signal (Papoulis, 1962). While this allows for possible false alarms to occur, it guarantees that the return signal will not be lost. Equally important is the fact that the value of the autocorrelation can never exceed the value obtained when there is no relative shift between the functions in the correlation integral.

If coded-aperture patterns are selected so that the only major peak in the autocorrelation of the aperture is located at $x = 0$, the detection of a single point is then quite easy with matched-filtering techniques. Unfortunately, point objects are rather scarce in nuclear medicine. In order to see what happens when the object is not a single point, consider Eq. (8-10) for the coded image of a planar object. For simplicity, let $s_1 = s_2$. If the coded image $g(x, y)$ is correlated with the template $h_2(x, y)$, the output $i(x, y)$ is then

$$\begin{aligned} i(x, y) &= g(x, y) \star\star h_2(x, y) \\ &= o(-x, -y) ** h_1(x, y; s_1) \star\star h_2(x, y) \end{aligned} \tag{8-24}$$

where the primes on the coordinates have been omitted. The function $h_1(x, y; s_1)$ is the shadow function formerly designated by $h(x'', y''; s_1)$ and $h_2(x, y)$ has the same functional form and scale as $h_1(x, y; s_1)$, differing only by a proportionality constant. The convolution and correlation operations are associative since the integrals they imply can be performed in either order. If the correlation is done first, such that

$$p(x, y; s_1) = h_1(x, y; s_1) \star\star h_2(x, y) \tag{8-25}$$

then

$$i(x, y) = o(-x, -y) ** p(x, y; s_1) \tag{8-26}$$

and $p(x, y; s_1)$ is seen to be the net point spread function for the entire coded-aperture imaging system. Imaging-system point spread functions should be as close as possible to a Dirac delta function. The Dirac delta function has the following two important properties:

$$\delta(x) = 0, \qquad x \neq 0 \tag{8-27}$$

$$\int_{-\infty}^{\infty} f(\alpha)\, \delta(x - \alpha)\, d\alpha = f(x) \tag{8-28}$$

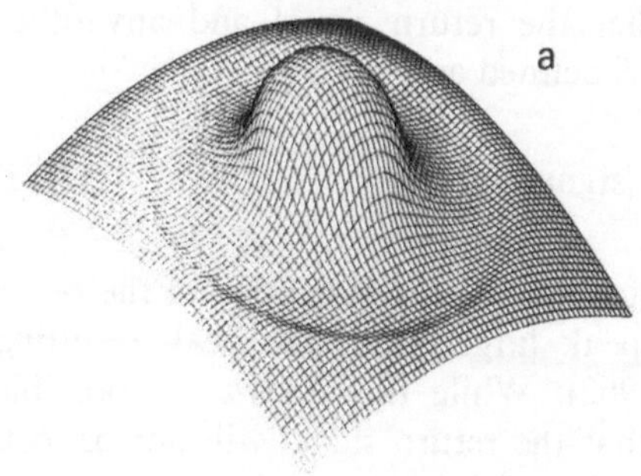

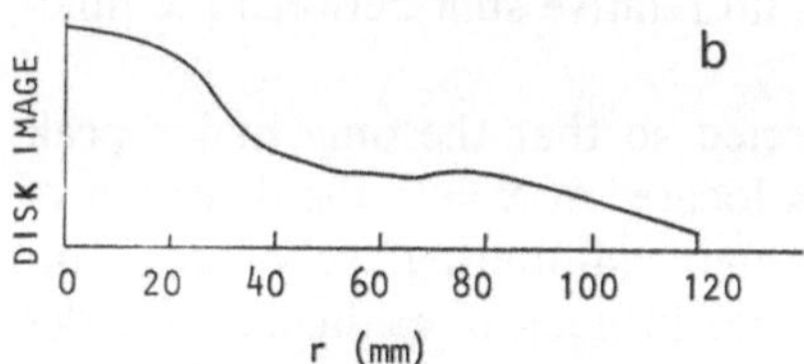

Fig. 8-3. (a) Isometric plot of a disk object imaged with an annular-coded aperture and decoded by template matching. (b) Radial slice through (a). The effect of the sidelobes in the PSF shown in Fig. 8-2 are quite evident.

The matched-filter operation guarantees a sharp central spike, but it does not guarantee that the net PSF returns to a zero away from the spike at $x = 0$. Recall the autocorrelation of an annulus shown in Fig. 8-2. When a disk object is imaged with this net PSF, one obtains the image in Fig. 8-3. Clearly the sharp peak in the PSF resulting from template matching is not sufficient to guarantee a good image. This is a very important concept. Matched filtering is great for single sources but may perform very poorly for extended objects.

Despite the caveat in the preceding paragraph, most coded-aperture decoding methods developed for the decoding of a single coded image are closely related to matched filtering. Departures from strict matched filtering occur in attempts to create a PSF that has improved imaging properties (i.e., made more like a delta function), or to take advantage of some analog means of performing the decoding operation. The reasons for a particular departure from matched filtering as well as the type of modification are as varied as the apertures that are used. Therefore, the precise decoding methods used will be discussed individually in the following sections for each of several apertures.

8.4. DECODING ALGORITHMS FOR SINGLE CODED IMAGES

In the discussions that follow, decoding algorithms for use with Fresnel-zone-plate apertures, annular apertures, and multiple-pinhole arrays will be discussed. While these apertures do not exhaust all the possible apertures or even all the apertures reported in the literature, they are representative of the majority of apertures and will serve to illustrate the types of problems that arise in developing a decoding process. For the present, attention will be restricted to coded-aperture systems that record a single coded image. Systems which use a sequence of apertures to record a sequence of coded images have proven quite valuable (Macdonald *et al.*, 1974; Barrett and DeMeester, 1974; Barrett *et al.*, 1974; Tanaka, 1975; Simpson, 1976; Simpson *et al.*, 1976). Discussion of these multicoding systems can be found in later sections.

8.4.1. The Fresnel Zone Plate

The pattern of black and white concentric annular regions shown in Fig. 8-4 is a Fresnel-zone-plate pattern. In order for a set of concentric annuli to qualify as a Fresnel zone plate, each annular region, or zone, whether it be black or white, must have the same area as the central disk. Numbering the zones outward from the central disk, the area constraint requires that the radius of the nth zone r_n be given by

$$r_n = n^{1/2} r_1 \tag{8-29}$$

where r_1 is the radius of the central disk. The Fresnel-zone-plate pattern can be constructed around either a white or a black central disk. In either case, all of the even-numbered zones must be the same color and all of the odd-numbered zones must be the other color.

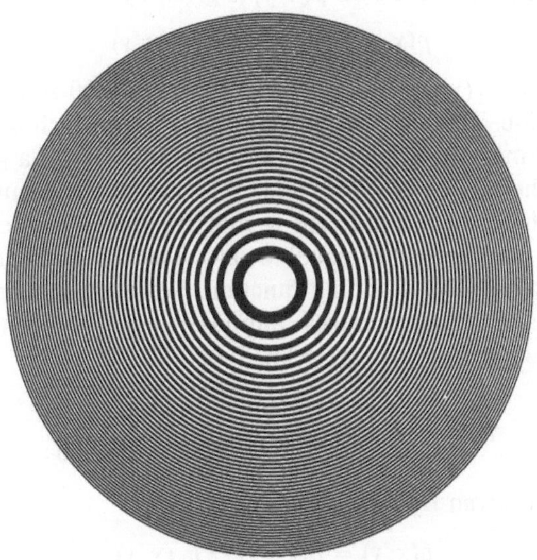

Fig. 8-4. On-axis Fresnel-zone-plate pattern.

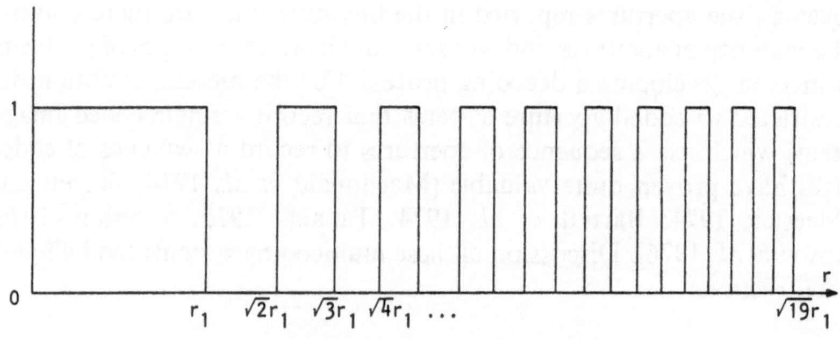

Fig. 8-5. Radial plot of γ-ray transmission of an ideal on-axis Fresnel zone plate with 20 zones.

A Fresnel-zone-plate coded aperture can be constructed so that it is opaque to the high-energy radiation where the zone plate is black and transparent to the high-energy radiation where the zone plate is white. In the limit of a large number of collected photons, the image of a point source formed with a Fresnel-zone-plate coded aperture is a scaled version of the pattern in Fig. 8-4. The correlation-decoding techniques discussed in the preceding section can be applied here. Let $h_1(x, y)$ describe the zone-plate shadow with values of 1 and 0 instead of white or black (parametric dependence of h_1 on s_1 will be ignored). A radial slice through $h_1(x, y)$ is shown in Fig. 8-5. If we ignore normalization constants for the time being, the matched-filter-decoded PSF $p(x, y)$ is given by

$$p(x, y) = h_1(x, y) \star\star\, h_2(x, y) \tag{8-30}$$

where $h_2(x, y) = h_1(x, y)$. The decoded PSF for a 20-zone zone plate is shown in Fig. 8-6. There is a very nice central peak which is unfortunately surrounded by many nonzero values that extend outward a great distance. The problem here is even worse than the case of the annulus shown in Fig. 8-2. The heart of the problem is that the functions being correlated have values all greater than or equal to zero. The coded image is inherently a positive function; the decoding function, however, can be modified to have positive and negative values. Suppose that $h_2(x, y)$ in Eq. (8-30) is replaced by the function $\bar{h}_2(x, y)$ defined as

$$\bar{h}_2(x, y) = \begin{cases} +1 & \text{when } h_1(x, y) = 1 \\ -1 & \text{when } h_1(x, y) = 0 \end{cases} \tag{8-31}$$

The PSF is now given by

$$p(x, y) = h_1(x, y) \star\star\, \bar{h}_2(x, y) \tag{8-32}$$

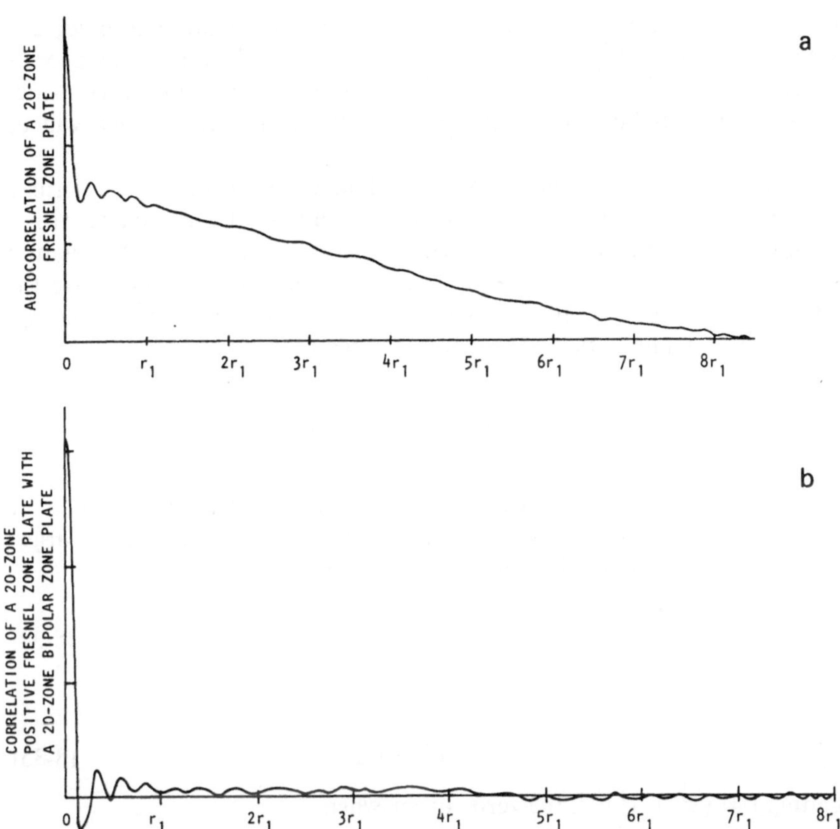

Fig. 8-6. (a) Radial slice through the two-dimensional autocorrelation of a 20-zone Fresnel zone plate containing values of 1 and 0. The radius of the central zone is r_1. (b) Radial slice through a two-dimensional correlation of a 20-zone positive Fresnel zone plate containing values of 1 and 0 with a 20-zone bipolar Fresnel zone plate containing values of $+1$ and -1. Peak value in both curves is $10\pi r_1^2$.

The PSF for a 20-zone zone plate processed in this manner is shown in Fig. 8-6b. This latter PSF is a significant improvement over its predecessor.

In order to perform the decoding by correlation with $\bar{h}_2(x, y)$ from Eq. (8-31), there must be a way to implement a template that has positive and negative values. This is no problem if the processing is performed on a digital computer (Budinger and Macdonald, 1975; Wilson *et al.*, 1975; Dance *et al.*, 1975). If template masks are used, two masks can be used, one which is transparent only where $\bar{h}_2(x, y)$ is positive and a second which is transparent only where $\bar{h}_2(x, y)$ is negative. Correlating the coded image with each of these masks and subtracting the two decoded images will give the desired result. It turns out that a reasonable approximation to correlation with $\bar{h}_2(x, y)$ is possible in an analog manner. The physical process involved is the diffraction of light, which should come as no surprise since the zone plate is known to have certain optical properties which will be discussed shortly.

The propagation of light from one plane to another can be described in terms of a convolution of the light amplitude in the first plane with a complex exponential $e^{i(\pi/\lambda d)(x^2+y^2)}$, where λ is the wavelength of the light, d is the distance between the two planes along the z axis and (x, y) are the coordinates in the two planes, both referred to the same z axis (Gaskill, 1978). The complex exponential can be written as

$$e^{i(\pi/\lambda d)(x^2+y^2)} = \cos\left[\frac{\pi}{\lambda d}(x^2 + y^2)\right] + i\sin\left[\frac{\pi}{\lambda d}(x^2 + y^2)\right] \quad (8\text{-}33)$$

The imaginary part of this expression is of particular interest. A plot of $\sin[(\pi/\lambda d)(x^2 + y^2)]$ is shown in Fig. 8-7; it has zeros whenever the argument of the sine function is an integral multiple of π:

$$\frac{\pi}{\lambda d}(x^2 + y^2) = n\pi \quad (8\text{-}34)$$

or

$$x^2 + y^2 = n\lambda d \quad (8\text{-}35)$$

Letting $r = (x^2 + y^2)^{1/2}$, the zeros occur when

$$r = (n\lambda d)^{1/2} \quad (8\text{-}36)$$

Referring back to Eq. (8-29), the zeros of the imaginary part of the complex exponential in Eq. (8-33) will coincide with the zone-plate radii if $r_1 = (\lambda d)^{1/2}$. Since the sine function in Eq. (8-33) has both positive and negative

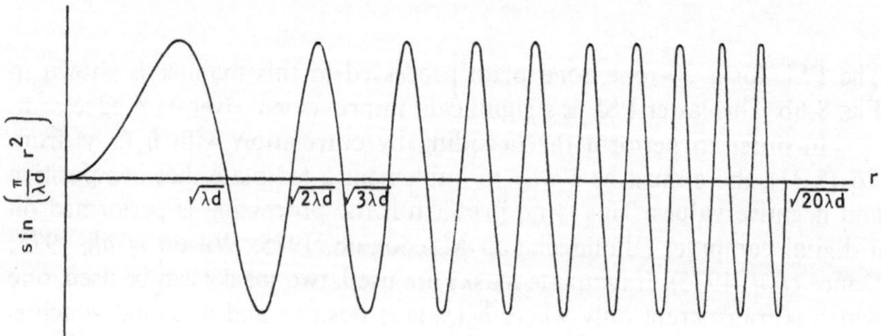

Fig. 8-7. Radial plot of $\sin[(\pi/\lambda d)(x^2 + y^2)]$ with $r^2 = x^2 + y^2$.

values and matches the zeros in $\bar{h}_2(x, y)$, it is a reasonable approximation to $\bar{h}_2(x, y)$. Therefore, if a transparency whose transmission is given by $h_1(x, y)$ is illuminated with a collimated beam of light, the light amplitude in a plane a distance $d = r_1^2/\lambda$ from the zone plate will be proportional to the convolution of $h_1(x, y)$ with

$$\cos\left[\pi\left(\frac{x^2 + y^2}{r_1^2}\right)\right] + i\sin\left[\pi\left(\frac{x^2 + y^2}{r_1^2}\right)\right]$$

Unfortunately, the amplitude of the light cannot be easily measured; only the intensity which is the squared magnitude of the light amplitude is directly detectable. It is therefore essentially impossible to observe only the convolution of $h_1(x, y)$ with $\sin\{\pi[(x^2 + y^2)/r_1^2]\}$. While the problems resulting from the cosine function in the real part of Eq. (8-33) and the fact that $\sin\{\pi[(x^2 + y^2)/r_1^2]\}$ is not an exact matched filter can be treated mathematically, the analysis would lead us far afield. All of the resulting behavior of optically decoded zone-plate images can be understood conceptually through physical arguments based on the well-known optical properties of zone plates. This approach allows for conceptual understanding with a minimum of cumbersome mathematics.

In order to understand the optical-decoding method, it is necessary to understand what happens when a parallel beam of light is incident on a transparency whose transmission is given by the function $h_1(x, y)$ shown in Fig. 8-5. Thanks to the physical phenomenon known as diffraction, part of the light that gets through the transparency is brought to a focus. In fact, there is a whole series of foci whose distance from the zone plate f_m is given by

$$f_m = r_1^2/m\lambda \tag{8-37}$$

where r_1 is the radius of the central zone of the zone plate, λ is the wavelength of the light being used, and m is an odd integer that has both positive and negative values. There is also a portion of the light that is undiffracted. The undiffracted light (or dc light in optical jargon) and the foci associated with $m = -3, -1, 1, 3$ are shown schematically in Fig. 8-8. Note in particular that the foci lie along a line passing through the center of the zone plate and that the focal lengths depend on the physical size of the central zone. If one looks at a plane containing the $+1$ focus and parallel to the zone plate, there will be a bright spot due to the focused light and a surrounding halo or blur due to the dc light, the -1 beam (also referred to as the twin image) and the plus and minus beams with larger m values. In this way, a Fresnel zone plate can be changed into a pattern with a sharp central peak via optical means. This is the basis for optical decoding of zone-plate coded images.

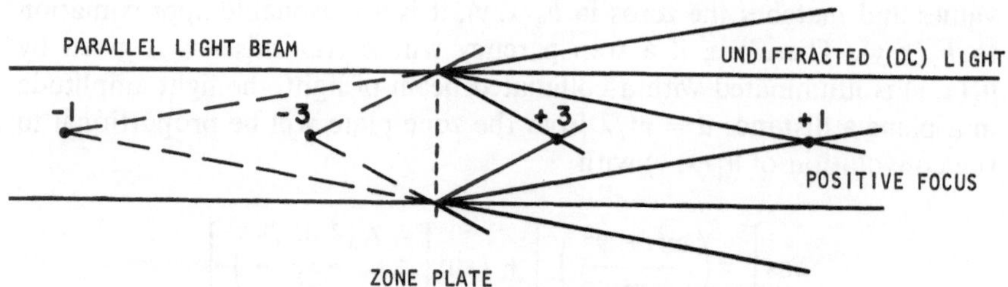

Fig. 8-8. Illustration of the focusing properties of an on-axis Fresnel zone plate. Both real and virtual foci are produced, in addition to an undiffracted beam.

The preceding discussion of diffraction and zone plates should be understood to apply only to the reconstruction process. The encoding process involves no diffraction; the structure in the zone-plate aperture is so coarse compared to the wavelength of the γ- and X-rays involved that diffraction is totally negligible. After the coded image is recorded it is reduced photographically so that the structure in the zone plate becomes finer and is capable of diffracting the light beam used in the decoding process.

In both Fresnel-zone-plate coded-aperture imaging and Gabor holography, a point source in the object is recorded as a correctly scaled and shifted zone-plate pattern. As far as the decoding process is concerned, there is no difference between the photographically reduced coded image and an on-axis Gabor hologram. The coded-image reconstruction possesses all the features of a Gabor hologram reconstruction, including the presence of three-dimensional information. Lateral position information is recorded by the lateral position of the zone-plate shadow and its associated focus while depth information is recorded in the scale of the zone-plate shadow. Since the focal length of a zone plate depends on the size of the central zone, object points at two different axial distances from the coded aperture will produce zone plates with different focal lengths. Only one object plane can be sharply in focus in the reconstructed image plane. Optical decoding therefore affords a method for recovering tomographic information from the coded images.

The lateral resolution and the tomographic resolution in the decoded image depend on how sharply the light is focused. Since each zone plate in the coded image behaves like a lens, the lateral and tomographic resolution can be determined from well-known formulas for lenses. The lateral resolution δ, based on the Rayleigh criterion, is

$$\delta = \beta\lambda(f/D) \tag{8-38}$$

where $\beta = 1.22$ for lenses with circular apertures,† λ is the wavelength of the light, f is the focal length of the lens, and D is the diameter of the lens. The depth of focus δz, which determines tomographic resolution, is given by

$$\delta z = \beta' \lambda (f/D)^2 \tag{8-39}$$

where $\beta' \simeq 2$ if the depth of focus is defined, following Born and Wolf (Born and Wolf, 1975), as the displacement from the focal plane that gives a 20% reduction in intensity at the center of the focal spot. A somewhat more practical value for this application would be $\beta' \simeq 3$, which corresponds to an ~50% reduction in the intensity at the center of the focal spot.

The ratio f/D for the zone plate in the photographically reduced copy of the coded image can be calculated in terms of the actual aperture dimensions, the scale factor $(s_1 + s_2)/s_1$ and the magnification m_p ($m_p < 1$) associated with the photographic-reduction step. For an N-zone zone plate with an outer radius of r_N, the diameter of the zone plate in the reduced coded image is

$$D = m_p \left(\frac{s_1 + s_2}{s_1} \right) 2r_N \tag{8-40}$$

Combining Eqs. (8-29), (8-37), and (8-40), we obtain

$$f_1 = \frac{m_p^2 r_N^2}{\lambda N} \left(\frac{s_1 + s_2}{s_1} \right)^2 \tag{8-41}$$

Therefore,

$$f_1/D = \frac{s_1 + s_2}{s_1} \frac{m_p r_N}{2\lambda N} \tag{8-42}$$

Using the relation

$$\begin{aligned} \Delta r_N &\equiv r_N - r_{N-1} \\ &\approx \frac{dr_N}{dN} \Delta N \\ &= r_1/2N^{1/2} \\ &= r_N/2N \end{aligned} \tag{8-43}$$

† The lateral resolution and depth-of-focus expressions used here are for incoherent light. When coherent light is used, β should be increased to about 1.6 and β' should be increased to about 2.9.

($\Delta N = 1$), we can write f_1/D as

$$\frac{f_1}{D} = \frac{s_1 + s_2}{s_1} \frac{m_p \Delta r_N}{\lambda} \tag{8-44}$$

Substituting Eq. (8-44) into Eqs. (8-38) and (8-39), we have

$$\delta = \beta \left(\frac{s_1 + s_2}{s_1} \right) \Delta r_N m_p \tag{8-45}$$

and

$$\delta z = \beta' \left(\frac{s_1 + s_2}{s_1} \right)^2 \frac{\Delta r_N^2}{\lambda} m_p^2 \tag{8-46}$$

These values for δ and δz are the resolution parameters in the decoded image. In order to determine the associated values in the original object, the relations between δx in the object and δ in the decoded image, and δs_1 in the object and δz in the decoded image must be established. The lateral-resolution quantities δ and δx are related quite simply by

$$\begin{aligned} \delta x &= -\left(\frac{s_1}{s_2} \right) \frac{\delta}{m_p} \\ &= -\beta \left(\frac{s_1 + s_2}{s_2} \right) \Delta r_N \end{aligned} \tag{8-47}$$

which is just β times the width of the smallest zone projected back onto the object from the detector plane. The lateral resolution of the zone-plate system is then equivalent to a pinhole system with a pinhole diameter of $\beta \Delta r_n$.

The relationship between z and s_1 is given by Eq. (8-37) with f_1 replaced by z:

$$z = \frac{m_p^2 r_N^2}{\lambda N} \left(\frac{s_1 + s_2}{s_1} \right)^2 \tag{8-48}$$

Since

$$\delta s_1 = \frac{ds_1}{dz} \delta z \tag{8-49}$$

Eq. (8-48) can be solved for s_1 and the resulting expression differentiated with respect to z. Substituting Eq. (8-48) for z, we obtain

$$\frac{ds_1}{dz} = \frac{-s_2}{2} \left(\frac{\lambda N}{r_N^2 m_p^2} \right) \left(\frac{s_1}{s_1 + s_2} \right) \left(\frac{s_1}{s_2} \right)^2 \tag{8-50}$$

resulting in

$$\delta s_1 = -\frac{s_1(s_1 + s_2)}{s_2}\frac{\beta'}{8N} \tag{8-51}$$

which implies that the tomographic resolution is determined by the number of zones and is independent of the size of the zone plate, scale factors, photographic-reduction factors, and the wavelength of the light used in decoding the coded image.

Those who are familiar with Gabor holography will recognize immediately that there are some problems with the optical decoding method. Referring back to Fig. 8-8, it is easy to understand why the reconstruction of a point is not perfect; all of the light is not in focus. While it will not be proven here, the total energy in the in-focus spot is considerably less than the total energy in the halo or background. For a point source this is no problem. However, for large objects, the background light adds up and reduces the contrast in the decoded image. This problem is compounded further since coherent light is being used in the reconstruction. When coherent light is present in an experiment, the light field must be described by the complex light amplitude. If the recording process is linear, the complex-amplitude patterns due to each zone plate in the coded image are added together in the decoded image. Due to the background, contrast in the complex-amplitude pattern is diminished.† However, intensity, not complex amplitude, is the measurable quantity, and in order to get intensity the squared modulus of the complex amplitude must be taken. This squaring operation further decreases the final contrast in the decoded image. For large extended objects, the image contrast becomes so small that the image can no longer be seen.

The fact that coherent light is involved in the decoding step has been used by Tipton (Tipton *et al.*, 1973) to produce decoded images that are dark on a light background. His method takes advantage of the fact that an opaque-central-zone zone plate produces focused light that is out of phase with the undiffracted beam. These two components interfere destructively to produce a dark rather than a bright reconstruction. In order to work properly for small objects, the contrast in the photographically reduced copy of the coded image has to be altered so as to allow additional undiffracted light. While this method allows the loss in contrast due to undiffracted light to be avoided, light from the twin image, which is also out of phase with the undiffracted light, will reduce the contrast, placing

† The term contrast is used very loosely here to indicate the ratio of the signal-to-background level. The usual definition of contrast is not applicable here since the light field is described in terms of a complex-valued field rather than real-valued intensity.

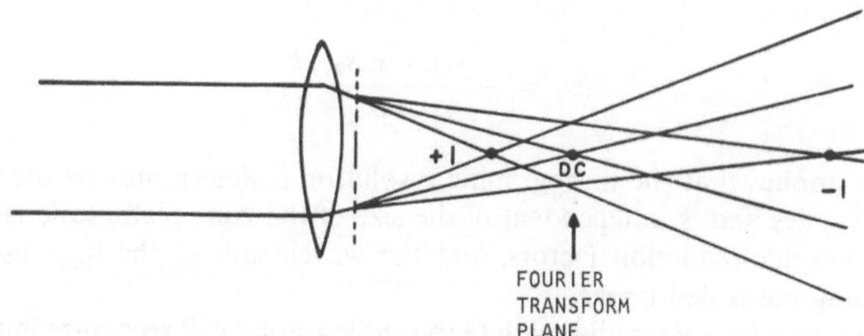

Fig. 8-9. Focusing properties of an on-axis Fresnel zone plate in combination with a lens. The undiffracted beam and the −1 virtual image are refocused by the lens, producing real images.

an upper limit on the size of the object that can be successfully reconstructed with adequate contrast.

The background problem could also be reduced without the use of any coherence tricks if some of the out-of-focus light could be eliminated. It is possible to eliminate the undiffracted light by altering the decoding system slightly. If a lens is placed in contact with the zone plate, the lens reimages the zone-plate foci and also brings the undiffracted light to a focus (see Fig. 8-9). If a small stop is used to block the dc light, and we look now at the −1 focus, the undiffracted light no longer contributes to the background. Unfortunately, the plane containing the focused dc spot is a very special sort of plane. The distribution of light in that plane is the Fourier transform of the coded image. Since the coded image is the convo-

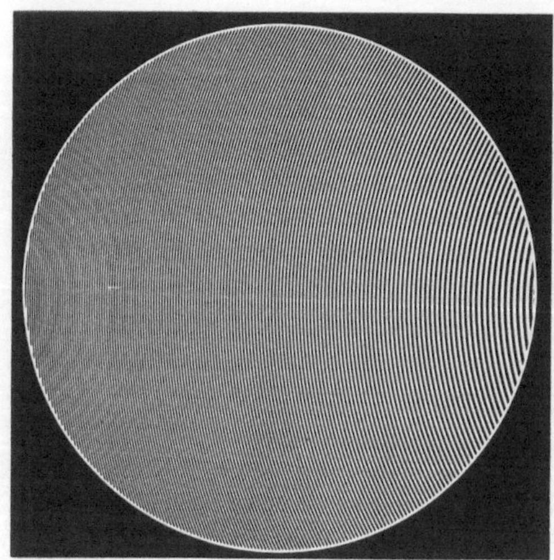

Fig. 8-10. Off-axis Fresnel-zone-plate pattern formed by taking an off-axis section of a large zone plate whose center is to the right of the figure.

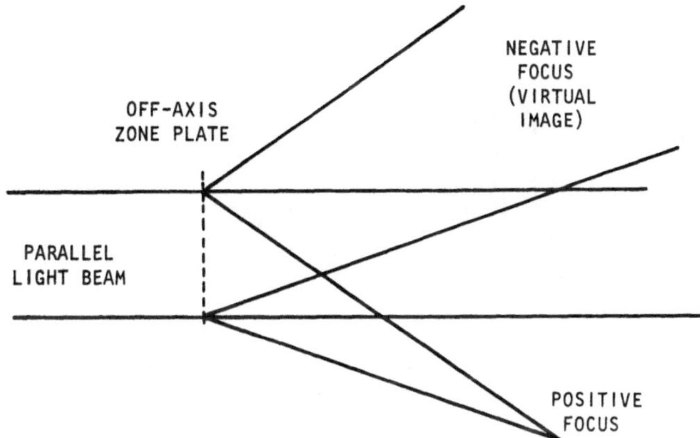

Fig. 8-11. Focusing properties of an off-axis Fresnel zone plate. The center of the parent zone plate is assumed to be located in the plane of the paper and beneath the off-axis segment.

lution of the coded aperture with the object, the Fourier transform of the coded image is the product of the Fourier transforms of the object and the coded aperture. The zero-spatial-frequency components of this product coincide with the focused dc spot. Therefore, the stop that blocks out the dc light will also eliminate the low-spatial-frequency components of the object. Since large objects have a lot of information in their low-frequency components, the dc stop causes a problem for just the sort of objects that it is intended to help.

There is a better way to eliminate the dc spot. If an off-axis section of a Fresnel zone plate is used for the coded aperture (see Fig. 8-10), it is possible to separate the beams. The focal points for the off-axis zone plate are the same as for the entire zone plate from which the off-axis section is taken. Since the foci are located on the axis of the zone plate, the light distribution to the right of the zone plate will be as shown in Fig. 8-11. The

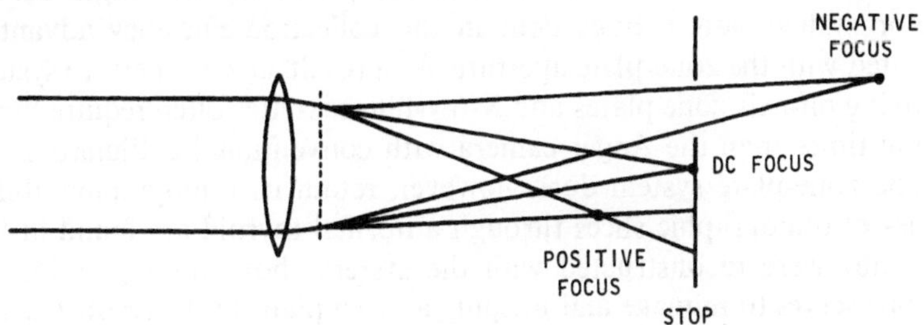

Fig. 8-12. Focusing properties of an off-axis Fresnel zone plate in combination with a lens. As in Fig. 8-11, the center of the parent zone plate is located beneath the aperture and in the plane of the paper.

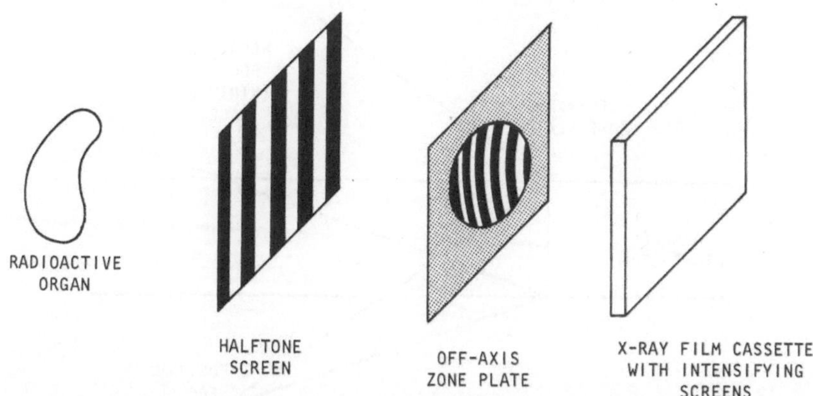

Fig. 8-13. Encoding geometry for the off-axis zone-plate system. The halftone screen is necessary in order to introduce a spatial carrier frequency into the object distribution.

undiffracted light goes straight through and the light from the +1 and −1 foci is diffracted in different directions. If a lens is placed in contact with the zone plate, the arrangement shown in Fig. 8-12 can be used to select out a single focus. Unfortunately, the transform of the object is still centered on the dc spot. In order to shift the object transform up into the open iris, it is necessary to place a halftone screen in front of the object. In electrical engineering terms, this halftone screen acts as a spatial carrier frequency which heterodynes the object transform into the "passband" of the system (Barrett *et al.*, 1972). The final encoding arrangement is shown in Fig. 8-13.

The coded image will now have much finer structure than in the on-axis zone-plate configuration. Unfortunately, the resolution required to ensure successful decoding exceeds the capability of the Anger camera detector system.† Off-axis zone-plate cameras require X-ray-film cassettes in order to obtain the necessary detector resolution. The diminished detection efficiency of the film cassettes compared to the Anger camera detector system puts a huge dent in the collection-efficiency advantage associated with the zone-plate aperture. As a result, coded-aperture systems employing off-axis zone plates and X-ray-film cassettes often require longer imaging times than the Anger camera with conventional collimators.

The zone-plate system does, however, retain its tomographic ability. A series of tomographic slices through a normal thyroid are found in Fig. 8-14. They were reconstructed with the system shown in Fig. 8-15. The telescope serves to reimage and magnify a given plane in the reconstruction onto a ground glass for viewing.

† The Anger camera detector system consists of the scintillation crystal, photomultiplier tube arrangement, and associated electronics; it is an Anger camera with the collimator removed.

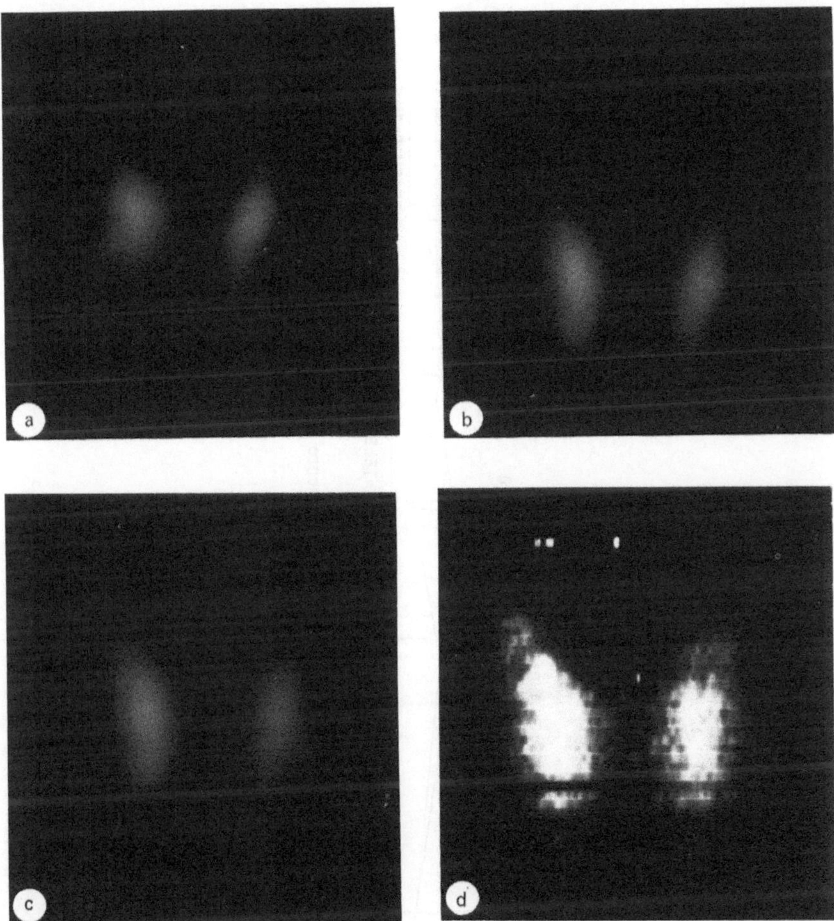

Fig. 8-14. Normal thyroid images. (a), (b), and (c) are three different tomographic cuts, separated by 0.6 cm, obtained from a single coded image. (d) Conventional rectilinear scan. Imaging agent was ^{123}I. The coded images involved a dose-exposure time product of 20 mCi min. The rectilinear scan has a peak count density of 1000 counts/cm^2 (Farmelant, 1975).

As mentioned earlier in this section, the use of coherent light in the decoding operation can result in interference between the diffracted beams. It is especially important to keep this in mind when viewing the tomographic reconstruction of a multiplanar object. Light from an out-of-focus plane can interfere with other light from the same plane, with light from other out-of-focus planes or with light from the in-focus plane. Constructive interference can produce spurious bright spots, while destructive interference can produce spurious dark spots. Referred to as coherent artifacts, their possible presence must be kept in mind when interpreting an optically

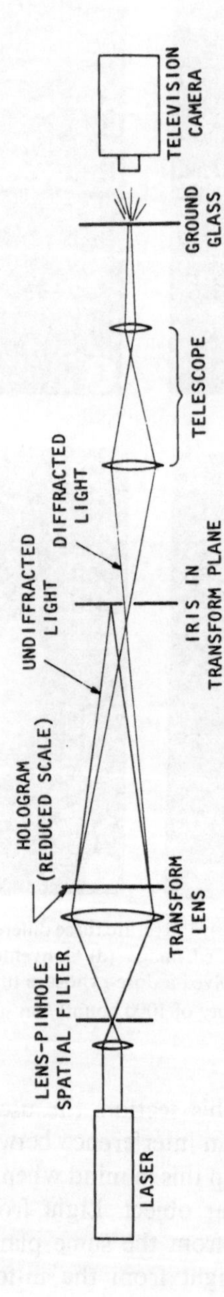

Fig. 8-15. Optical reconstruction system for use with an off-axis zone-plate camera. The absence of a collimated beam of light incident on the transform lens has no effect on the physical behavior of the decoding technique.

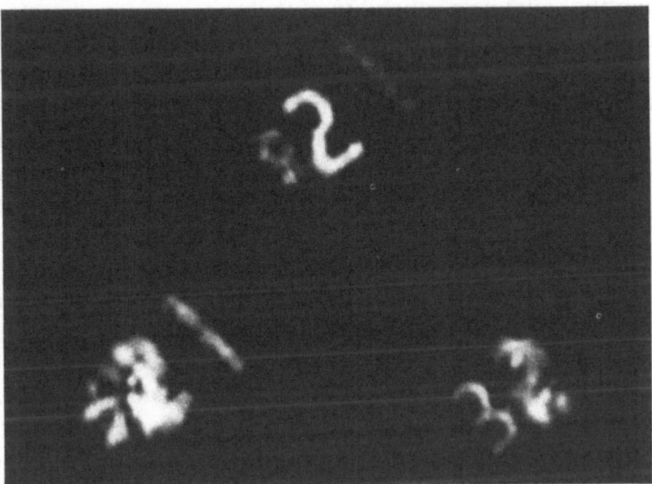

Fig. 8-16. Tomographic reconstructions of object containing radioactive numerals in three different planes separated by 1 inch. Note the presence of out-of-focus artifacts (Barrett *et al.*, 1973a,b).

decoded zone-plate coded image. Figure 8-16 shows a tomographic reconstruction in which some coherent artifacts can be seen. They seem to be more of a problem with high-contrast objects like the numeral phantom in Fig. 8-16 than with the clinical image in Fig. 8-14.

There is still another way to eliminate the problem of dc light while still using the on-axis zone plate. It involves taking a sequence of coded images using a slightly different aperture for each image. This concept will be discussed in the section on multicoding.

8.4.2. The Annulus

The annulus has been described as a one-zone zone plate. This is adequate to describe the form of the aperture, but the analogy comes to an end right about there. The annulus does not possess any enticing optical properties similar to those of the zone plate. The annulus also has a lower collection efficiency than the zone plate. At first glance, there are no apparent features of the annulus that would entice one to consider it a reasonable coded aperture. The annulus does, however, have some redeeming features which warrant its consideration as a possible coded aperture.

One problem with using the Anger camera detector system to record coded images formed with on-axis zone plates is the high count rate that results because of the large collection efficiency. Moderately sized objects can swamp the count-rate capability of the Anger camera detector system. The number of zones in the zone plate can be decreased, but that diminishes both the transverse and longitudinal resolution [see Eqs. (8-43), (8-45), and (8-46)]. To maintain the resolution, Δr_N needs to be kept the same. That suggests then that if the collecting area of the aperture is to be decreased in order to make the count rate more compatible with the Anger camera detector system, the central zones should be sacrificed first. The annulus represents the extreme case where all of the central zones have been eliminated.

There are also important features associated with the annulus when the effect of noise in the coded image is considered. When the object consists of more than one point such that shadows in the coded image overlap, the noise in the decoded image increases with the amount of area in the overlap region. More will be said about this in the section on noise, but clearly the annulus seems to have an advantage over the zone plate in this regard since the overlap area will be much less.

Suppose matched-filter decoding is considered as a starting point for developing a decoding procedure for annular-coded-aperture images. The resulting decoded PSF has the shape illustrated previously in Fig. 8-2. In fact, the first reported work using annular apertures in nuclear medicine employed just this sort of decoding process. The decoding operation was implemented using electronics and an image storage tube (Walton, 1973). As one might expect, it worked well for point objects. For extended objects like a disk, the nonzero values outside of the central peak of the autocorrelation behave like background terms that add up and diminish the contrast in the decoded image. The magnitude of this problem is illustrated in the disk reconstruction in Fig. 8-3.

Based on experience with the zone plate, it might appear that, in order to improve the decoded PSF, the decoding function should be changed to have both positive and negative values. This is in fact correct, only it is not as clear in the case of the annulus where the negative values should go. While there is no optical analogy to point the way as with the zone plate, there is an imaging system that provides a clue to what needs to be done. That system is the computerized axial-tomography (CAT) system that is revolutionizing radiology.

In computerized axial tomography, a sequence of one-dimensional projections through a two-dimensional object are recorded (see Fig. 8-17a). Each projection is performed at a certain angle relative to the coordinates of the planar object. In a process known as backprojection, each one-dimensional projection is projected back along the path along which the original projection was performed. For a discrete number of projections, the reconstructed image of a single point would have the spoke pattern shown in Fig. 8-17b. In the limit of projections along every angle through

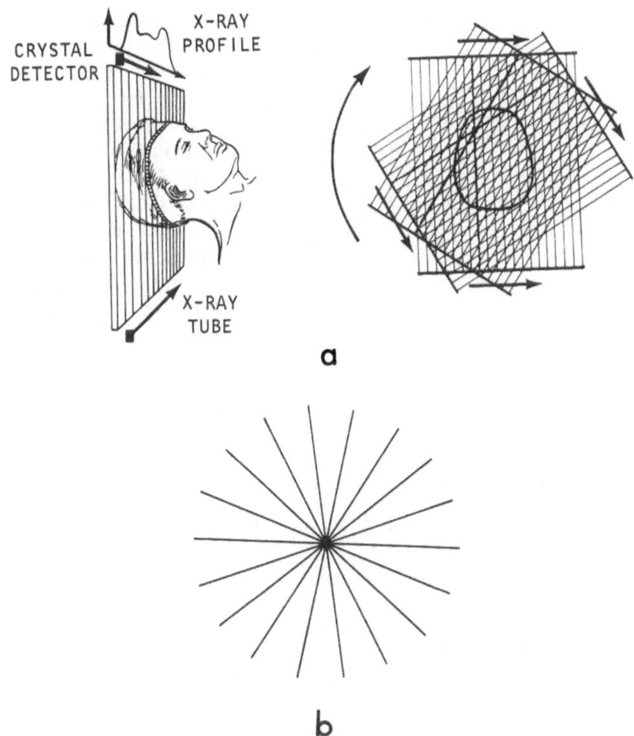

Fig. 8-17. (a) Data collection geometry for CAT scanning. (This figure is reproduced with permission from ACTA-Scanner: *The Whole Body Automatic Computerized Transverse Axial Tomographic Scanner*, R. S. Ledley, National Biomedical Research Foundation, 1974.) (b) PSF obtained by simple backprojection of a small finite number of projection data sets.

the point, the PSF would be

$$p(x, y) = A/r \tag{8-52}$$

where $r = (x^2 + y^2)^{1/2}$ and A is a normalization constant (Barrett and Swindell, 1977). A function with a $1/r$ fall-off makes a very poor two-dimensional PSF. The success of CAT scanners results from the existence of a method for changing the $1/r$ function into a function approximating a Dirac delta function. This operation is known in the literature as a ρ filter. The image formed by backprojection is convolved with a filter function $h(x, y)$ whose two-dimensional Fourier transform is

$$\begin{aligned} H(\xi, \eta) &= \mathscr{F}\{h(x, y)\} \\ &= (\xi^2 + \eta^2)^{1/2} \equiv \rho \end{aligned} \tag{8-53}$$

where ρ is the magnitude of the spatial-frequency vector.

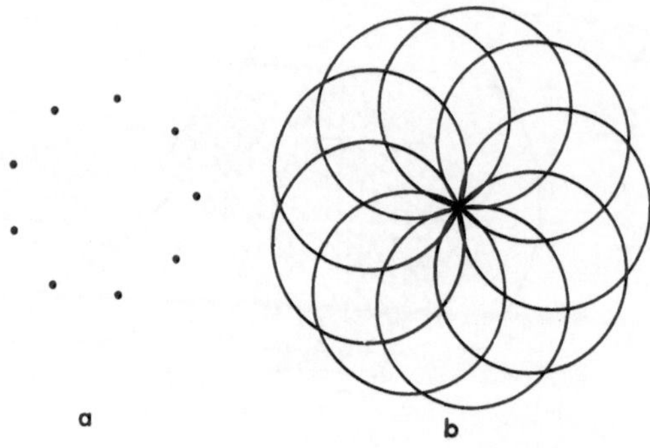

Fig. 8-18. (a) A discrete approximation to a thin annulus. As the number of pinholes around the circle increases, the approximation approaches the true annulus. (b) PSF obtained by correlating the discrete annulus in (a) with a continuous, thin annulus. As the number of pinholes in (a) approaches infinity, the PSF obtained by summing the annular patterns in (b) will approach the PSF in Fig. 8-2.

CAT scanning may not seem to have much to do with annular-coded apertures, but consider the matched-filter decoding operation for the annulus. The final PSF after decoding is

$$p(x, y) = h_1(x, y) \star\star\, h_2(x, y) \tag{8-54}$$

where $h_1(x, y)$ and $h_2(x, y)$ are given by

$$h_1(x, y) = h_2(x, y) = \begin{cases} 0 & (x^2 + y^2)^{1/2} > r_2 \quad \text{or} \quad (x^2 + y^2)^{1/2} < r_1 \\ 1 & r_1 \leq (x^2 + y^2)^{1/2} \leq r_2 \end{cases} \tag{8-55}$$

Writing out the integral for $p(x, y)$ we have

$$p(x, y) = \iint_{-\infty}^{\infty} h_1(\alpha, \beta)\, h_2(\alpha - x, \beta - y)\, d\alpha\, d\beta \tag{8-56}$$

The integral can be conceptualized as an addition of the functions $h_2(\alpha - x, \beta - y)$ weighted by $h_1(\alpha, \beta)$. This addition of shifted and weighted annuli is indicated in Fig. 8-18 for nine discrete values of (α, β). For a region near the center, this pattern looks very much like the spoke pattern in Fig. 8-17b. If the matched-filter-decoded annular-aperture PSF is ρ filtered, one obtains the PSF shown in Fig. 8-19. The damped oscillations near the central

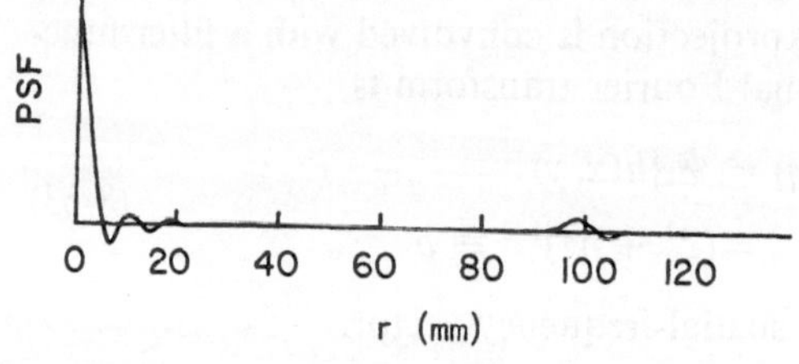

Fig. 8-19. PSF obtained by correlating an annular-coded aperture with an annular template and ρ-filtering the result.

core can be eliminated by introducing an apodizing function which returns the ρ filter smoothly to zero above a maximum spatial frequency. The PSF then returns to near-zero values outside the core except for the bipolar wiggle at $2\bar{r}$, where $\bar{r} = (r_1 + r_2)/2$. Provided that the object is not too large, this artifact will be outside the object reconstruction and can easily be ignored. The disk reconstruction shown in Fig. 8-3 is shown again in Fig. 8-20 after processing with an apodized ρ filter.

The net PSF is then given by

$$p(x, y) = h_1(x, y) \star\star h_2(x, y) ** h(x, y) \tag{8-57}$$

where h_1 and h_2 are defined in Eq. (8-55) and $h(x, y)$ is defined in Eq. (8-53). This expression can be regrouped as

$$\begin{aligned} p(x, y) &= h_1(x, y) \star\star [h_2(x, y) ** h(x, y)] \\ &= h_1(x, y) \star\star h_3(x, y) \end{aligned} \tag{8-58}$$

where

$$h_3(x, y) = h_2(x, y) ** h(x, y) \tag{8-59}$$

Instead of a two-step process, the decoding of the function $h_1(x, y)$ can be considered as a correlation operation with the function $h_3(x, y)$. The effective decoding function $h_3(x, y)$ is shown in Fig. 8-21. The essential features of this function are the positive lobe at the mean radius $\bar{r}$ and the negative

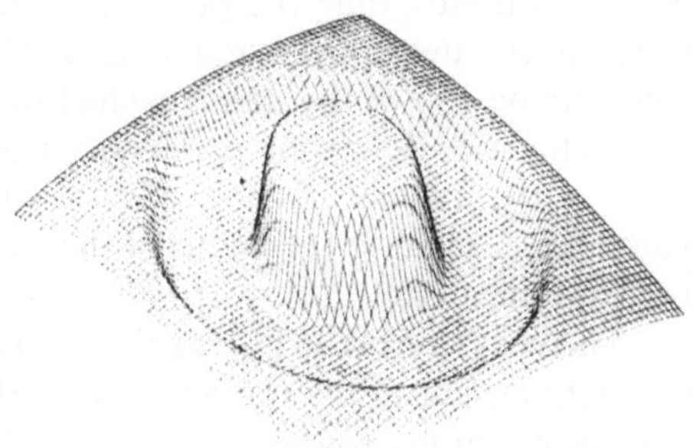

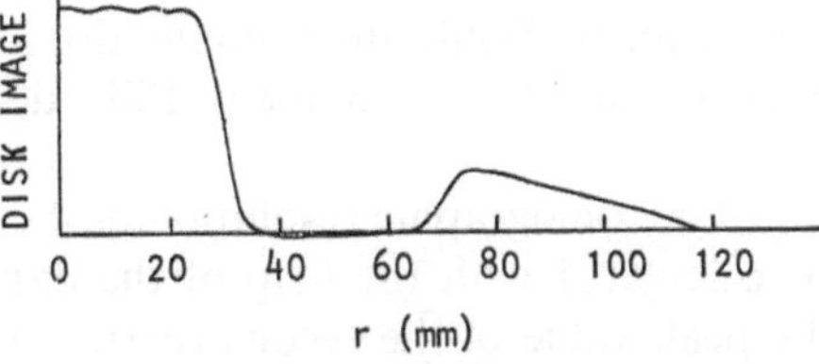

Fig. 8-20. Reconstruction of the same disk object as in Fig. 8-3 but with an apodized ρ filter included.

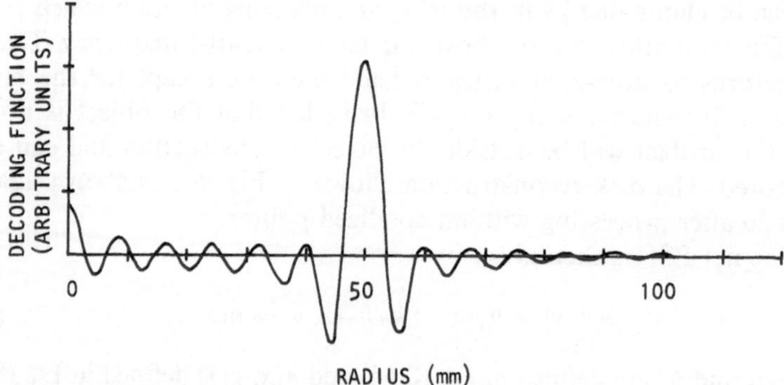

Fig. 8-21. The effective decoding filter which corresponds to decoding by correlating with an annulus and ρ filtering. If this function is correlated with an annulus, the decoded PSF shown in Fig. 8-19 is obtained.

sidelobes on each side of the positive lobe. The other oscillations result from limitations in realizing the ρ filter.

The analogy with CAT scanners was presented to motivate the use of the ρ filter. The need for the ρ filter can also be established by spatial-frequency-domain arguments (Simpson *et al.*, 1975). In either case, the ρ filter indicates where the negative values need to be added to the decoding template.

When the decoding function $h_3(x, y)$ shown in Fig. 8-21 is centered over the annulus, only the positive values overlap, yielding a nice central peak. As the decoding function is displaced, both positive and negative values lie on top of the annular shadow. It is easy then to argue that the full width at half-maximum (FWHM) of the central core is equal to the width of the annular shadow, just as the FWHM for the decoded zone-plate PSF is equal to the width of the smallest zone. This has proven to be true experimentally.

The behavior of the PSF as the size of the decoding function is changed is also important to the tomographic performance of the aperture. A series of reconstructions is shown in Fig. 8-22 in which the aperture shadow remains the same size and the size of the decoding function is changed. The parameter "focus" is the ratio of the size of the decoding function relative to the shadow. The perfect aperture would yield nothing if it were out of focus. While the annulus does not achieve this utopian ideal, the behavior of the out-of-focus PSF does not have any particularly bad features.

The tomographic resolution of the annular-coded-aperture system can be calculated with the help of the data in Fig. 8-22. When focus = 0.95, the peak value of the reconstruction has fallen to 50% of the peak value

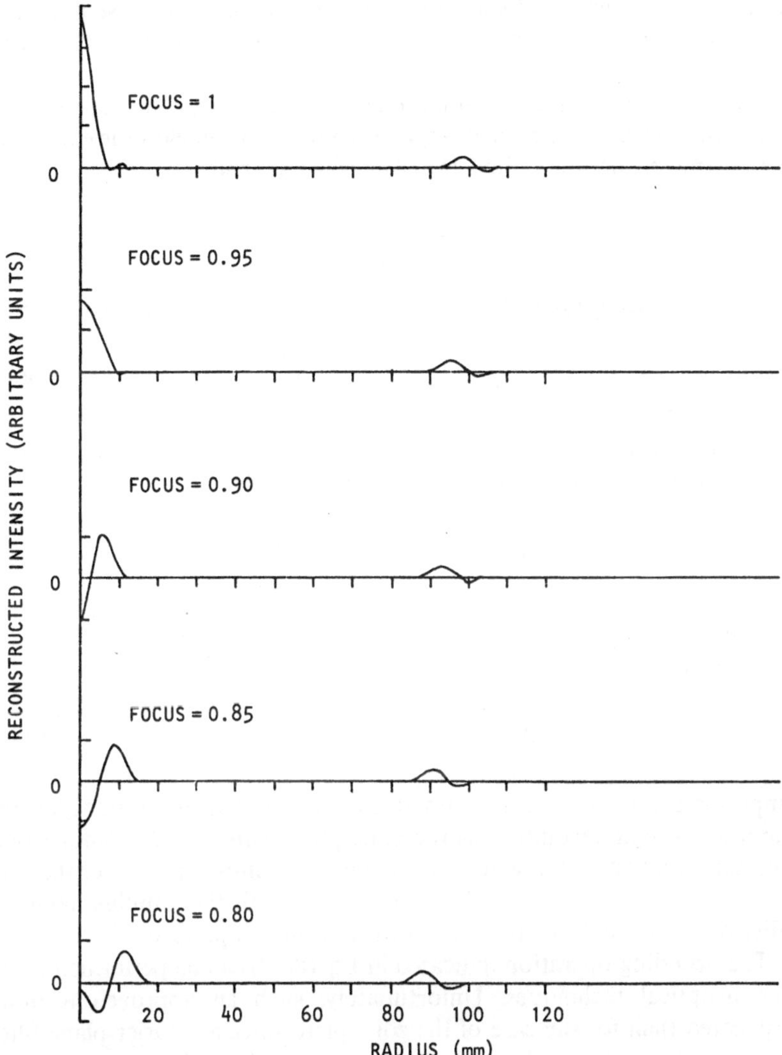

Fig. 8-22. Out-of-focus PSF for an annular-coded-aperture system. "Focus" is the ratio of the scale of the decoding function in Fig. 8-21 to the scale of the annular shadow.

achieved when focus = 1.0. This suggests a depth-of-focus criterion defined as the change in the axial distance s_1 necessary to cause a 5% decrease in the size of the annular shadow. For the annular dimensions used in the formulation of Fig. 8-22, a relative change in the annular radius of 5% decreases the annular radius r by an amount equal to half the annular width Δr. For a general annulus with a mean physical radius of $\bar{r}$ and an annular width of $\Delta\bar{r}$, the depth-of-focus criterion can be expressed in the more general terms as the change in s_1 necessary to change the relative scale of the annulus by $\frac{1}{2}\Delta\bar{r}/\bar{r}$.

In order to calculate the minimum detectable change in s_1 corresponding to a relative annular scale change of $\frac{1}{2}\Delta\bar{r}/\bar{r}$, we begin with the expression for r, the mean shadow radius, in terms of s_1, s_2, and $\bar{r}$:

$$r = \frac{s_1 + s_2}{s_1}\bar{r} \tag{8-60}$$

After differentiating Eq. (8-60) with respect to s_1 and rearranging, we have

$$ds_1 = -\frac{s_1}{s_2}(s_1 + s_2)\frac{dr}{r} \tag{8-61}$$

The minimum detectable change in s_1, designated Δs_1, corresponds to a relative change in shadow radius, dr/r, given by $\frac{1}{2}\Delta\bar{r}/\bar{r}$:

$$\Delta s_1 = -\frac{s_1(s_1 + s_2)}{s_2}\frac{\Delta\bar{r}}{2\bar{r}} \tag{8-62}$$

If the annulus is considered as a zone plate with all but the Nth zone made opaque, we can use Eq. (8-43) to write $\Delta\bar{r}/\bar{r}$ in terms of N so that

$$\Delta s_1 = -\frac{s_1(s_1 + s_2)}{s_2}\frac{1}{4N} \tag{8-63}$$

Comparing this expression with Eq. (8-51), we see that the annulus has the same tomographic resolution as the zone plate with $\beta' = 2$. Tomographic resolution of a zone plate with N zone and an annulus the size of the Nth zone of the zone plate should be very similar, with the annulus having a smaller out-of-focus contribution since it is a dilute aperture.

The decoding operation indicated in Eq. (8-57) can be performed using coherent-optical techniques. Unfortunately, such an approach is more complicated than for the case of the zone plate since a Fourier-plane filter has to be generated in order to realize the required bipolar decoding function. Annular-coded-aperture images have been decoded with digital computers using the decoding function that combines the ρ filter and the matched filter (Simpson *et al.*, 1975). Figure 8-23d is a digital reconstruction of the letter E obtained by correlating the composite decoding function with the data in Fig. 8-23b. Figure 8-23c shows the same data decoded without the inclusion of the ρ filter.

It is also possible to decode the coded image using a combination of digital and optical techniques. The ρ filter can be performed digitally and the ρ-filtered coded image can be made into a transparency. A dc bias level

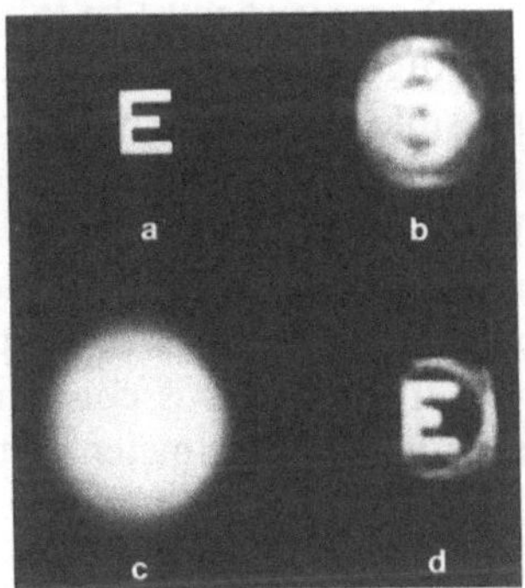

Fig. 8-23. (a) Simulation of the letter E used as the object. The actual E was a radioactive source 10 cm tall with 2-cm bars. (b) Annular-coded image of letter E recorded with an Anger camera detector system. Since the data were digitized into a 64 × 64 array prior to being displayed, the photon noise has been smoothed somewhat. The coded image contained 600K counts. (c) Decoded image obtained by digitally correlating the coded image with an annular template. (d) Decoded image obtained by digitally correlating the coded image with the ρ-filtered decoding function in Fig. 8-21.

is added to the data to eliminate negative values prior to the creation of the transparency. The transparency can then be used in an incoherent-optical correlator to perform the correlation with the annulus (see Fig. 8-24). The distance between the ρ-filtered transparency and the annular mask can be varied, thereby changing the scale of the correlating annulus. In this way, the observer can view the decoded image while scanning through a series of tomographic planes. Improved observer performance has been noted subjectively in other systems which permit an interactive decoding process and it is hoped that such will be the case for the annular aperture.

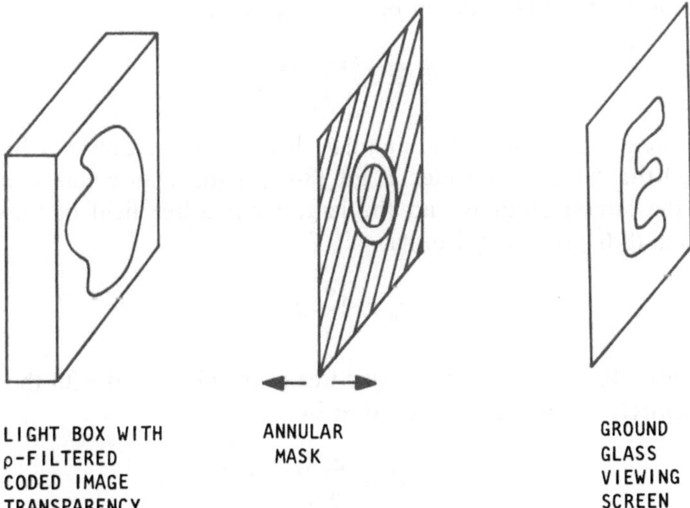

Fig. 8-24. Incoherent optical correlator in which annular-coded-aperture images can be decoded. Continuous adjustment of the depth of the in-focus tomographic plane is possible by moving the annular mask axially. The resulting decoded image is shown instantaneously.

Some care must be taken in designing an annular aperture for use with an Anger camera. The mean radius $\bar{r}$ of the annulus should be as large as possible so as to avoid problems with the glitch at $2\bar{r}$. At the same time, $\bar{r}$ cannot be so large that the coded image is larger than the detector or the lost data will severely degrade the decoded image of object points whose shadows fall partially off the detector. This problem is more serious for the annulus than for the zone plate.

If the object is contained in a circular region of diameter d_o and the annulus has a diameter d_a, the size of the coded image d_c is

$$d_c = \frac{s_2}{s_1} d_o + \frac{s_1 + s_2}{s_1} d_a \qquad \text{(8-64)}$$

where s_2/s_1 is the object magnification and $(s_1 + s_2)/s_1$ is the magnification of the annular shadow. If d_d is the diameter of the detector, we must have

$$d_d \geq d_c = \frac{s_2}{s_1} d_o + \frac{s_1 + s_2}{s_1} d_a \qquad \text{(8-65)}$$

if the coded image is to fit onto the detector.

In order to keep the glitch out of the object field, the diameter of the magnified object should be less than the diameter of the annular shadow:

$$\frac{s_2}{s_1} d_o \leq \frac{s_1 + s_2}{s_1} d_a \qquad \text{(8-66)}$$

Equations (8-65) and (8-66) can be combined to get

$$d_d \geq 2 \frac{s_1 + s_2}{s_1} d_a \qquad \text{(8-67)}$$

The diameter of the magnified annular shadow then should not be larger than half the detector diameter. If Eq. (8-67) is made an equality in order to get the largest annulus and the largest glitch-free field of view, Eqs. (8-65) and (8-67) then require that

$$d_d \geq 2 \frac{s_2}{s_1} d_o \qquad \text{(8-68)}$$

The largest object that can be imaged free of the glitch and with the coded image entirely on the detector is given by

$$d_o = \frac{d_d}{2} \frac{s_1}{s_2} \qquad \text{(8-69)}$$

Just as for the zone plate, the width of the annular zone Δr determines the lateral resolution. Since the Anger camera has an intrinsic resolution with a FWHM of ~8 mm, annuli whose shadows are thinner than 8 mm will only decrease collection efficiency without increasing resolution. A system designed for unit object magnification ($s_1 = s_2$) might then have an annulus with a physical diameter of one-fourth the diameter of the camera face and an annular zone width of 4 mm. An object-field diameter equal to half of the camera-face diameter would be possible with no interference from the glitch.

There is a way to eliminate the bipolar glitch in the PSF, but it involves recording two coded images, each formed with a slightly different-sized annulus. This will be discussed later in the section on multicoding.

8.4.3. Pinhole Arrays

Dicke first proposed the use of a multiple-pinhole aperture in a coded-aperture imaging system (Dicke, 1968). Intended for use in X-ray astronomy, the aperture contains a very large number of randomly located pinholes such that the average transmission of the entire aperture is very close to 50%. Decoding is performed by correlating the coded image with the aperture function, an operation easily performed with an incoherent-optical correlator. When the decoding template is in register with the coded image of a point source, all of the recorded counts from that point source are visible. When the template is shifted a distance larger than the width of a single pinhole, on the average, only 50% of the photons from the point source can be seen, provided that there is a very large number of pinholes. The decoded image will then have a peak value surrounded by a background level equal to half the peak. This same sort of behavior occurred when the Fresnel zone plate was decoded using the matched-filter method. When the object contains more than one point, the background terms add, resulting in diminished contrast in the final image. For isolated astronomical X-ray sources, this is not much of a problem, but it rules out this approach for nuclear-medicine imaging situations.

As with the Fresnel zone plate, the decoding function can be changed so that it has values of +1 and −1 rather than 1 and 0. Brown refers to this sort of processing as mismatched processing (Brown, 1972, 1974). It results in a PSF with a mean background level of zero. However, because of the statistical nature of the aperture, there are fluctuations in the zero-mean background even when the coded image is known perfectly (see Fig. 8-27c). The size of the background fluctuations depends on the number of pinholes in the aperture; the more pinholes, the smaller the background fluctuations. For a finite-sized detector, more pinholes mean smaller pinholes, which must in turn be resolved by the detector. Detector resolution then limits how uniform the background can be. Because of the nonuniform background, this array is not used with the Anger camera detector system.

In the preceding discussion, background fluctuations were considered in the context of the expected behavior of an ensemble of possible realizations of the random pinhole array. In an actual coded-aperture system, only one such realization is employed. The question arises, is there a way to construct a particular two-dimensional, 50%-transparent pinhole array with well-behaved sidelobes? With some help from several theorems from communications theory, it is possible to construct such an aperture (Calabro and Wolf, 1968; MacWilliams and Sloane, 1976). These apertures are referred to in the literature as uniformly redundant arrays, pseudonoise arrays, or maximum-length shift-register codes. A simple one-dimensional example of a uniformly redundant array is shown in Fig. 8-25a. If a decoding function is formed by placing three versions of the basic code end-to-end as in Fig. 8-25b, the decoded PSF will have the form shown in Fig. 8-25c. The flat sidelobe in the region between the correlation peaks results from the uniformly redundant nature of the aperture code. As with the glitch artifact in the annular-coded-aperture system, the two side-peaks will not affect the reconstruction of an object that is confined to a limited region of space. When $s_1 = s_2$, an object area as large as the aperture shadow can be imaged with no interference from the side peaks. Within this allowed object region, the PSF sidelobes introduce a uniform background level

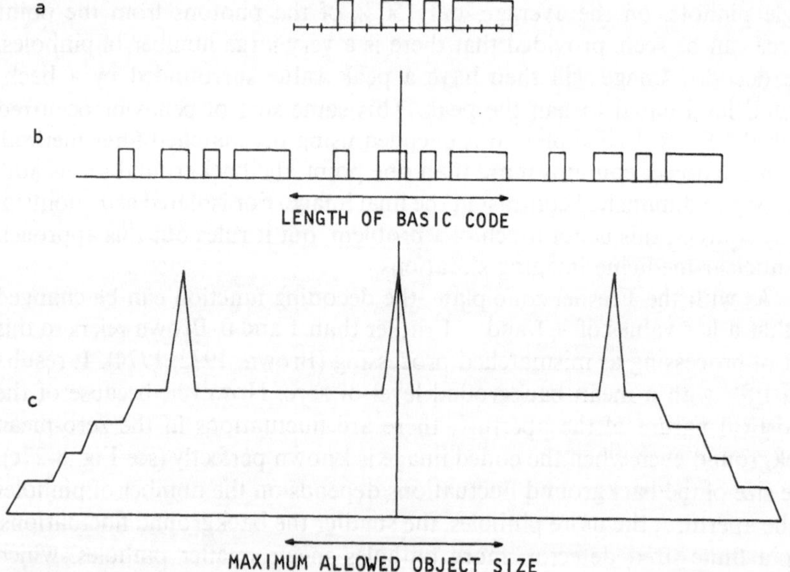

Fig. 8-25. (a) Uniformly redundant pinhole array of length 15. (b) Decoding function obtained by repeating the basic code in (a) three times. (c) Decoded PSF obtained by correlating (a) with (b).

which can be removed by a simple subtraction. In the absence of any noise sources, the background can be removed perfectly, producing no fluctuations in the final background level.

Two-dimensional uniformly redundant pinhole arrays can also be produced, in which case the decoding function is made up of a mosaic of the basic aperture code. Based on the one-dimensional example above, the two-dimensional decoding function should contain nine copies of the basic aperture code. Since reconstructed values outside of the allowed object region are ignored, the size of the decoding array can be reduced without affecting the reconstructed values in the allowed object region (Fenimore and Cannon, 1978). Figure 8-26a shows a reduced two-dimensional decoding function. The central 41 × 43 elements of the 83 × 87 element array form the basic aperture code. Fenimore and Cannon (1978) have used this aperture in some computer simulations and have achieved some very good results. Their test object is shown in Fig. 8-27a. In Fig. 8-27b, the test object has been imaged with the random array in Fig. 8-26b and decoded by simple matched-filter decoding. The large background destroys the contrast in the reconstructed object. The zeros in the decoding function were replaced with unit negative values to produce the decoded image shown in Fig. 8-27c. The background has been greatly reduced, but there are fluctuations in the background even though this was a noiseless simulation. The same object imaged with a uniformly redundant array and decoded with a mosaic of the basic aperture code is shown in Fig. 8-27d with the background subtracted out. The improvement is quite evident.

The uniformly redundant array possesses another nice feature pointed out by Fenimore and Cannon. If the aperture contains a mosaic of uniformly redundant arrays rather than a single array, the coded image need only be detected over a region the size of a single array shadow. This differs from other apertures discussed so far in which the size of the coded image is equal to the size of the object plus the size of the aperture. For a fixed-size detector, a uniformly redundant array can then be larger than other coded apertures, resulting in further improvement in collection efficiency.

Fig. 8-26. (a) Example of a decoding array used with a uniformly redundant array. The basic code is contained in the 41 × 43 element array located in the middle of the 83 × 87 element decoding array. (b) A 40 × 40 element random pinhole array. (From Fenimore and Cannon, 1978; used here with permission.)

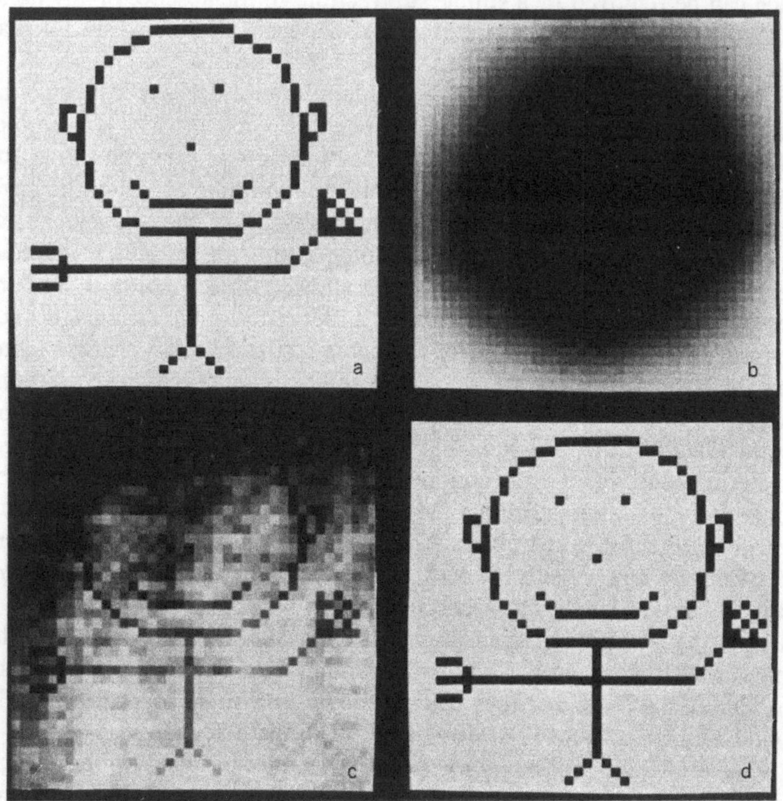

Fig. 8-27. (a) Test object employed in computer simulations of imaging with filled pinhole arrays. (b) Image of (a) obtained by forming a coded image with the random pinhole array in Fig. 8-26b and decoding by matched filtering. (c) Image of (a) obtained by forming a coded image with the random pinhole array in Fig. 8-26b and decoding by correlating with a bipolar version of the aperture function. No statistical noise was added to the data. (d) Image of (a) obtained by forming a coded image with the uniformly redundant array and decoded by correlating with the cyclically repeated uniformly redundant array in Fig. 8-26a. The uniform background has been subtracted. Background variations are due to the inclusion of quantum noise in this simulation. (From Fenimore and Cannon, 1978; used here with permission.)

There are two potential problems with the uniformly redundant arrays. The existence of the uniform background is dependent on the existence of sharp edges in the detected image. If the aperture shadow has blurred edges either from X-rays that penetrate the edge of a pinhole or from too coarse a sampling of the coded image, the background will not be perfectly uniform. Secondly, if the object contains sources in two planes, the out-of-focus plane makes it difficult to determine the amount of background to subtract away. It may be possible to overcome this problem with an iterative, perhaps nonlinear approach, but that remains to be seen.

The problem with background fluctuations in decoded multiple-pinhole images has also been addressed in a second, slightly different manner. In the uniformly redundant arrays discussed above, the peak-to-background ratio in the decoded PSF is 2. For an object consisting of n equal-intensity point sources, the reconstructed peak-to-background ratio (before the background is subtracted away) is $(n + 1)/n$. When there is noise in the coded image, there will be fluctuations in the decoded image background. Because of the small peak-to-background ratio in the PSF, statistical noise in the background, as opposed to inherent aperture-related noise, can become a problem as the object gets large. It might therefore be advantageous to have a pinhole array whose correlation-decoded PSF has well-behaved sidelobes and a large peak-to-background ratio (Lindner, 1975). The largest peak-to-background ratio is achieved with a class of arrays that are known as nonredundant pinhole arrays (Moffat, 1968). A one-dimensional example is shown in Fig. 8-28, along with its autocorrelation. The peak height is equal to the number of pinholes and the background terms are never larger than 1. The array is called nonredundant because no two pairs of pinholes are separated by the same spacing. As the array gets larger, it becomes more difficult to add pinholes without duplicating a previous spacing. As a result, large nonredundant arrays have transmissions much less than 50%.

It is possible to extend this concept of nonredundance to two dimensions by requiring that no two pairs of pinholes be separated by the same vector spacing. Such two-dimensional arrays have been investigated for use in radioastronomy (Golay, 1971). An example of a two-dimensional nonredundant pinhole array that has been used as a coded aperture is shown in Fig. 8-29a (Wouters *et al.*, 1973; Change *et al.*, 1974; Dowdy *et al.*, 1977). Its autocorrelation function is illustrated in Fig. 8-29b. Tipton (Tipton *et al.*, 1976; Dowdy *et al.*, 1977) has performed some computer simulations using this aperture and found that even though the peak-to-back-

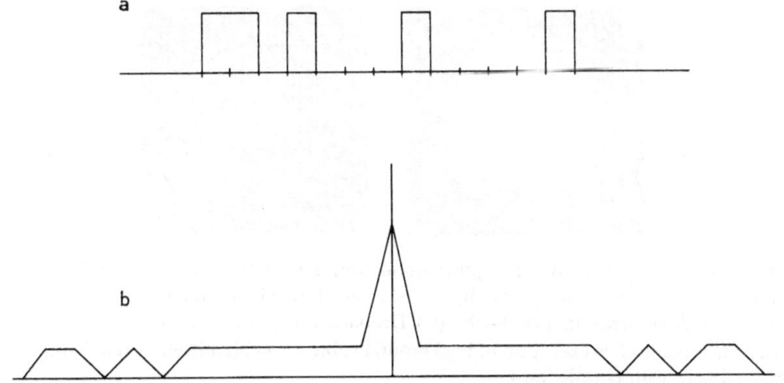

Fig. 8-28. (a) One-dimensional nonredundant pinhole array. (b) Autocorrelation of (a).

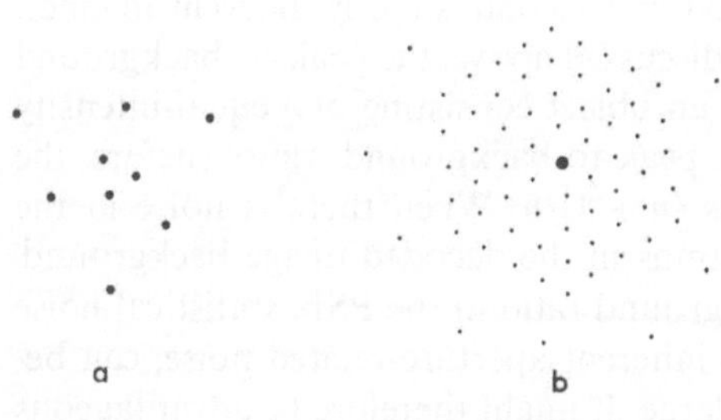

Fig. 8-29. (a) Two-dimensional nonredundant pinhole array. (b) Autocorrelation of (a). All the dots have unit value except for the central spot, which has a value of nine.

ground ratio is large, the background is still a problem (see Fig. 8-30C). While the background cannot be removed by subtracting a uniform bias level from the decoded image, the fact that the background is a deterministic quantity suggests that something might be done to remove it.

If a first estimate of the object can be obtained from the correlation-decoded image, it might be possible to convolve the object estimate with the background portion of the PSF (defined as the PSF minus the central peak) and subtract this "background estimate" from the original decoded image. Such a procedure was suggested by Tipton *et al.* (1976) and Dowdy *et al.* (1977) and striking results have been achieved. Figure 8-30 shows the

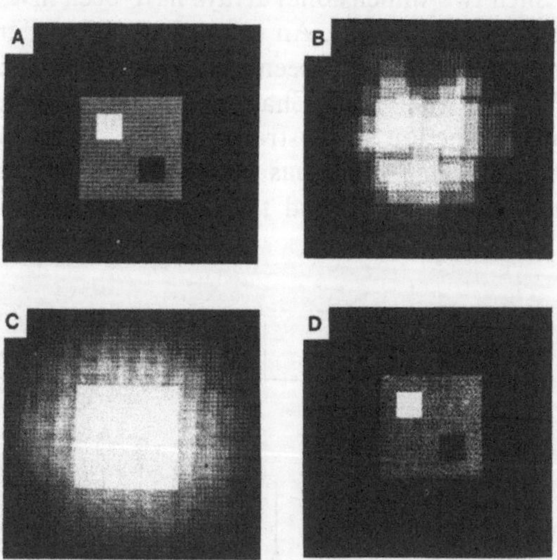

Fig. 8-30. (A) Test object used in computer simulation. The brighter small square has twice the intensity of the darker small square. (B) Coded image formed with the two-dimensional nonredundant pinhole array in Fig. 8-29a. (C) Decoded image obtained by matched filtering. (D) Decoded image after execution of background subtraction algorithm. (From Tipton *et al.*, 1976; used here with permission.)

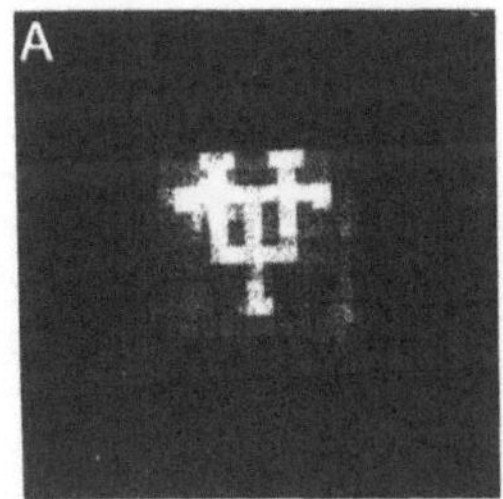

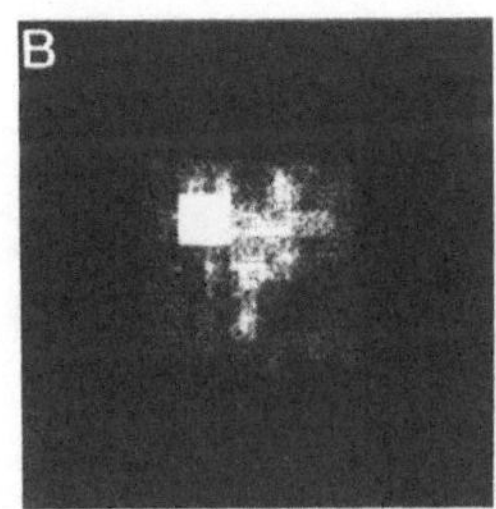

Fig. 8-31. Illustration of tomographic capability. The object contained the UT symbol in one plane and a bright square in another. (A) Tomographic reconstruction of the plane containing the UT symbol. (B) Tomographic reconstruction of the plane containing the bright square. (From Tipton *et al.*, 1976; used here with permission.)

results of a computer simulation of this operation. The original object is shown in Fig. 8-30A. The coded image is shown in Fig. 8-30B. The matched-filter-decoded image with the PSF shown in Fig. 8-29b is displayed in Fig. 8-30C. The initial object estimate is made by discarding reconstructed values below a certain threshold. After convolving the object estimate with the background component of the PSF, the background estimate is subtracted out, leaving the net decoded image shown in Fig. 8-30D. The procedure was also effective in improving the tomographic reconstructions shown in Fig. 8-31.

This same sort of background-subtraction technique has been used by Simpson *et al.* (1977) in a coded-aperture system designed to image fuel pins in a reactor. Because of the long, slender nature of the object and the dependence of the noise in the decoded image on the object distribution (see Section 8.7) a one-dimensional Fresnel-zone-plate aperture was used. As shown in Fig. 8-32, the aperture behaves as a pinhole in one direction and as a coded aperture in the orthogonal direction. Decoding then reduces to a one-dimensional problem. If decoding is performed by one-dimensional correlation with the filter function shown in Fig. 8-33b, the PSF in the coded direction is shown in Fig. 8-33c. Since the background is known, but irregular, Tipton's method should be applicable here. Figure 8-34a shows a ramp object imaged with the one-dimensional zone plate in Fig. 8-33a and decoded with the filter function in Fig. 8-33b. A computer algorithm adjusts a dc bias level until the amount of the decoded image above the bias level is consistent with the number of photons in the coded image. This dc bias level is subtracted from the decoded image and all negative values discarded. This object estimate is then convolved with the PSF with the central peak removed. This background estimate is then subtracted from the original matched-filter-decoded image, resulting in Fig. 8-34c. This result can be used as a new input to the dc bias algorithm and a second object estimate made, leading to a second background estimate which is

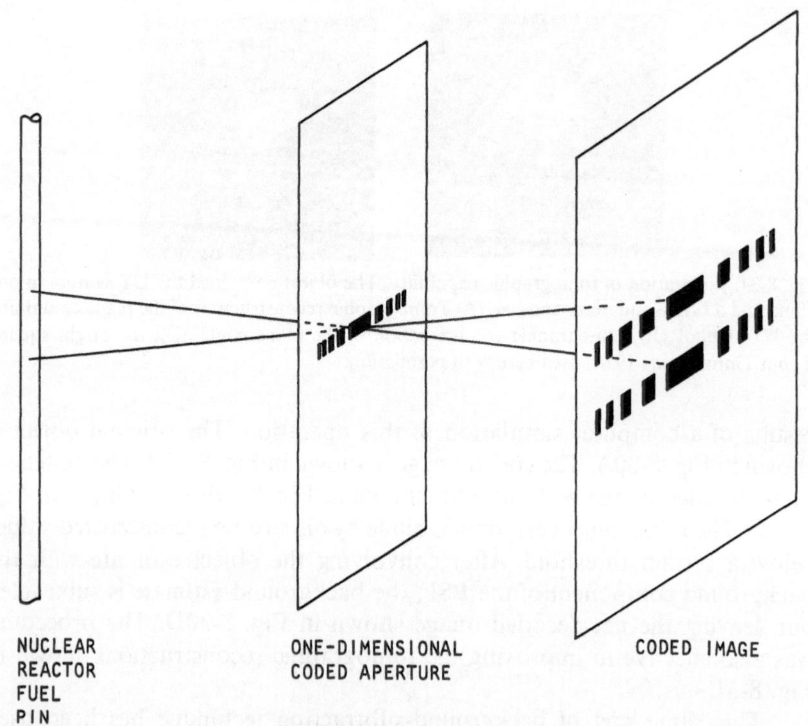

Fig. 8-32. Encoding geometry employed in the one-dimensional Fresnel zone-plate coded-aperture system designed to image nuclear fuel pins.

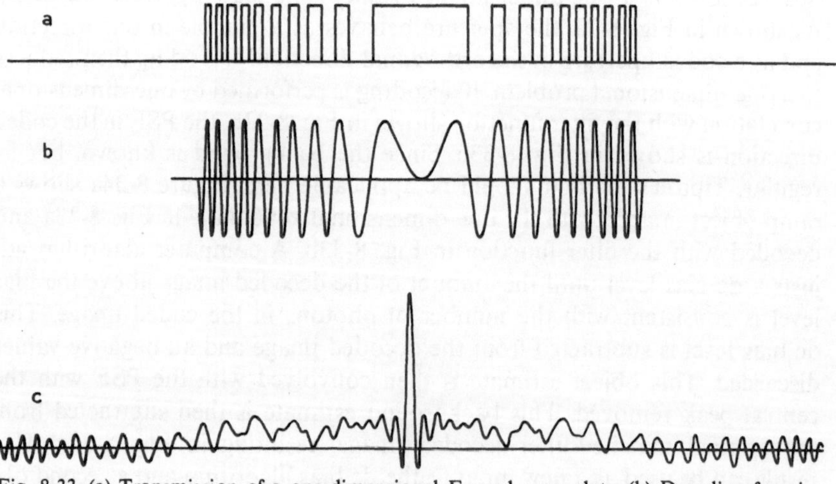

Fig. 8-33. (a) Transmission of a one-dimensional Fresnel zone plate. (b) Decoding function $\sin \alpha x^2$ with α adjusted so that the zeros match with those of the Fresnel zone plate. (c) Decoded PSF obtained by correlating (a) with (b).

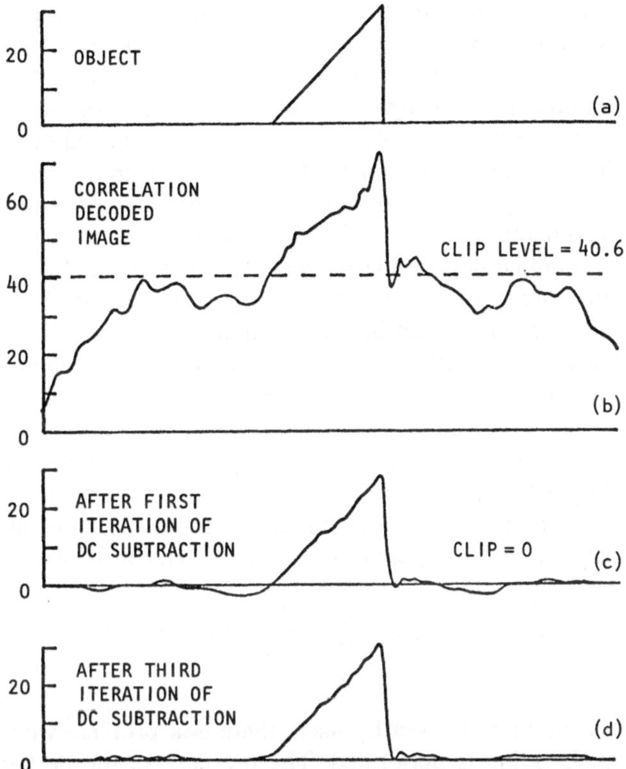

Fig. 8-34. (a) Ramp test object used in computer simulations. (b) Decoded image obtained by correlating the coded image with the decoding function in Fig. 8-33b. (c) Decoded image after one iteration of the background-subtraction algorithm. (d) Decoded image after three iterations of the background-subtraction algorithm.

subtracted from the original decoded image. This process can be repeated as many times as required. The result after three iterations is shown in Fig. 8-34d.

8.5. MULTICODING

While the implementation of the decoding process and the behavior of the decoded PSF varies with each of the apertures discussed so far, they all share the same basic decoding operation. In all cases, some decoding function is correlated with the coded image in order to produce the decoded image. Strict matched filtering of the coded image using a template similar to the coded aperture resulted in PSF's that contained very disturbing, even disastrous, background levels. The background problem was particularly bad for the two apertures that were 50% transparent (the zone plate and the Dicke random pinhole array). In the case of three of the apertures, it was possible to diminish the background level by modifying the decoding function so that it contained negative values. In the case of the nonredundant pinhole array the background was estimated and subtracted out. It is also possible to improve the performance of a coded-aperture system if, instead of a single coded image, several coded images are formed with the same geometry but different apertures. Use of more than one coded aperture is referred to as multicoding. While the way in which the coded images are used may differ depending on the type of apertures involved, the goal is the same: extracting more and better information about the object.

One example of multicoding is the use of complementary on-axis zone-plate apertures (Macdonald *et al.*, 1974; Barrett and DeMeester, 1974; Barrett *et al.*, 1974). A zone plate with a transparent central zone is called a positive zone plate; a zone plate with an opaque central zone is called a negative zone plate. A positive and a negative zone plate make a complementary pair of apertures. The transmission of a positive zone plate $h_+(\mathbf{r})$, and the transmission of a negative zone plate $h_-(\mathbf{r})$, can be written as

$$h_\pm(\mathbf{r}) = \frac{1}{2} \pm \sum_{\substack{m=-\infty \\ m\,\text{odd}}}^{\infty} \frac{1}{i\pi m} \exp(i\pi m r^2/r_1^2) \tag{8-70}$$

When either zone plate is used by itself, there is a problem with dc light when optical decoding is performed. The presence of the dc light is the direct result of the leading constant term of $\frac{1}{2}$ in Eq. (8-70). Suppose two coded images are formed, the first, $g_+(x, y)$, with the positive zone plate and the second, $g_-(x, y)$, with the negative zone plate where

$$g_\pm(x, y) = o(x, y) ** h_\pm(\mathbf{r}) \tag{8-71}$$

If $g_-(x, y)$ is subtracted from $g_+(x, y)$, we get

$$\begin{aligned} g(x, y) &= g_+(x, y) - g_-(x, y) \\ &= o(x, y) ** \left[2 \sum_{\substack{m=-\infty \\ m\,\text{odd}}}^{\infty} \frac{1}{i\pi m} \exp(i\pi m r^2/r_1^2) \right] \\ &= o(x, y) ** h_e(\mathbf{r}) \end{aligned} \tag{8-72}$$

The effective coded aperture $h_e(\mathbf{r})$ no longer has a constant term. With the elimination of the constant, the problem with dc light disappears.

This approach can be implemented easily on a computer (Macdonald *et al.*, 1974). Since the difference coded image $g(x, y)$ will have negative values which have no meaning for an intensity transmission, some ingenuity is required in order to perform the decoding operation optically. In order to realize the subtraction, a method known as grid-coded subtraction can be used (Pennington *et al.*, 1970). The basic arrangement for grid-coded subtraction with positive and negative zone plates is shown in Fig. 8-35. A standard Anger camera is used without any modification except for a grid (Ronchi ruling) which is placed adjacent to the film in the oscilloscope camera. A coded image is first recorded with a positive zone plate in place. Then the negative zone plate is substituted, the grid is shifted by half its period and a second coded image is recorded. Since the film in the oscilloscope camera is not moved between exposures, the two coded images are interleaved on the film. A reduced-scale copy of this film is inserted into the optical system shown in Fig. 8-14. When a single diffraction order (i.e., the -1 beam in Fig. 8-8) is selected with the iris, it can easily be shown that the required subtraction is performed and the dc light is eliminated while the signals add.

An example of an image formed with this technique is shown in Fig. 8-36. An Anger camera detector system was used. The resolution is about 1 cm. The fine lines in the coded image are due to the Ronchi ruling which

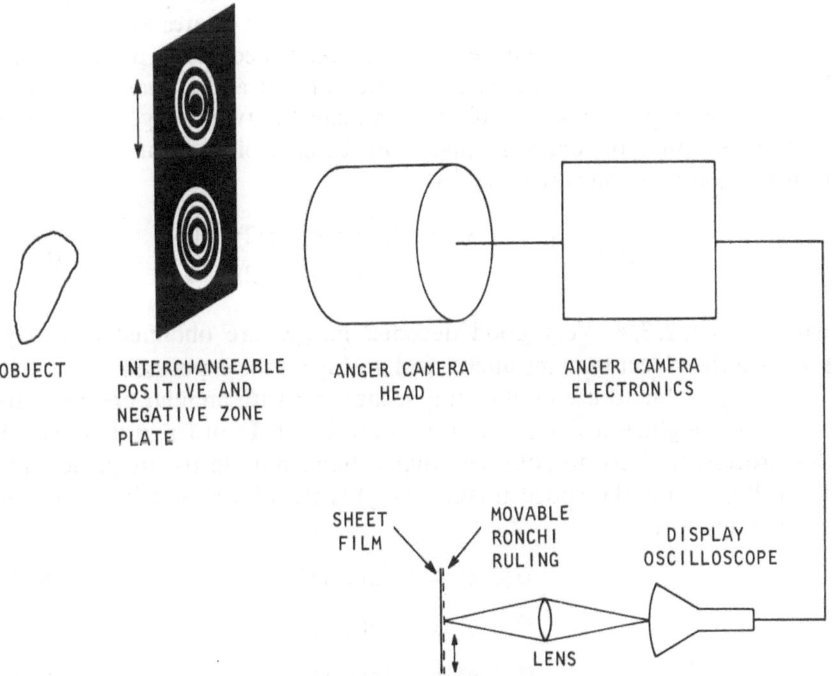

Fig. 8-35. Basic encoding geometry employed in forming a coded image with two complementary zone-plate apertures for later decoding using grid-coded subtraction techniques.

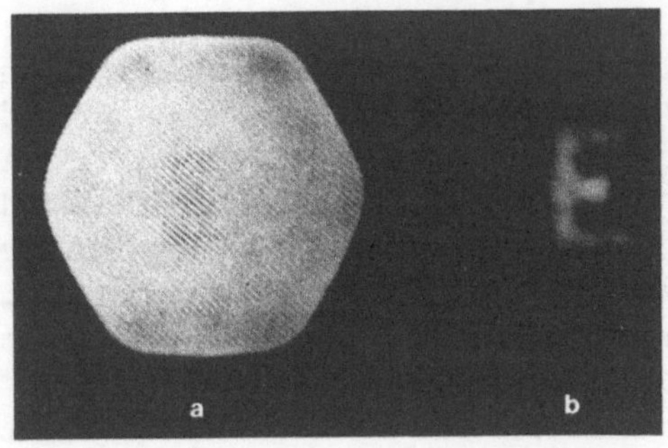

Fig. 8-36. (a) Coded image obtained with apparatus in Fig. 8-35. (b) Decoded image obtained by optical decoding. The object was 12.5 cm tall.

serves the function of the halftone in the off-axis case with one important difference—it is not in the gamma-ray path. Consequently, the extra detector spatial resolution needed with the off-axis zone-plate–halftone combination is no longer required. The Anger camera detector system becomes a practical detector for this system.

After the dc light has been eliminated, there is still a bit of a problem with large objects. Usually either the $+1$ or -1 beam in Fig. 8-8 is used in the reconstruction since they have more energy than the others. Only one of these beams can be used at one time. The other creates what is known in holography as the twin image. The twin image becomes a problem with large objects. Based on an idea due to Burckhardt and Doherty (1968) in optical holography, it is possible to eliminate the twin image by using a sequence of three or four zone plates. In the case of four zone plates, the transmission functions are given by

$$h_n(\mathbf{r}) = \begin{cases} 1 & \text{when } \sin(\alpha r^2 + n\pi/2) \geq 0 \\ 0 & \text{when } \sin(\alpha r^2 + n\pi/2) < 0 \end{cases} \tag{8-73}$$

where $n = 1, 2, 3, 4$. Very good decoded images are obtained this way, provided the object remains unchanged during all the exposures.

It is possible to use multicoding techniques with annular apertures to eliminate the glitch artifact at $2\bar{r}$ (Simpson, 1976). In order to understand this process, we have to consider what is happening in the frequency domain. If $g(x, y)$ is the coded image, $o(x, y)$ is the object, and $h(x, y)$ is the annular aperture, and

$$G(\xi, \eta) = \mathscr{F}\{g(x, y)\} \tag{8-74}$$

$$O(\xi, \eta) = \mathscr{F}\{o(x, y)\} \tag{8-75}$$

$$H(\xi, \eta) = \mathscr{F}\{h(x, y)\} \tag{8-76}$$

where geometric scale factors are neglected for the moment, then the Fourier transform of the coded image is

$$G(\xi, \eta) = O(\xi, \eta)\, H(\xi, \eta) \tag{8-77}$$

[see Eq. (8-15)]. The function $H(\xi, \eta)$ is the transfer function for the encoding system. Let

$$h(\mathbf{r}) = \begin{cases} 1 & \text{when } r_1 \leq r \leq r_2 \\ 0 & \text{otherwise} \end{cases} \tag{8-78}$$

For $\Delta r = r_2 - r_1 \ll r_1$, the Fourier spectrum of the annulus is closely approximated by

$$H(\rho) = kJ_0(2\pi\bar{r}\rho) \tag{8-79}$$

where ρ is the magnitude of the spatial-frequency vector defined as $\rho = (\xi^2 + \eta^2)^{1/2}$, k is a normalization constant, and $\bar{r} = (r_1 + r_2)/2$. The function $H(\rho)$ is shown in Fig. 8-37. Note that the envelope of $H(\rho)$ decays as $1/\sqrt{\rho}$. Since

$$\mathscr{F}\{h(x, y) \star\star\, h(x, y)\} = |H(\rho)|^2 \tag{8-80}$$

matched-filter decoding of the annular-coded image results in a net transfer function with an envelope that decays as $1/\rho$ as shown in Fig. 8-38. The ρ filter serves to eliminate the $1/\rho$ decay in the net transfer function. However, it does nothing to eliminate the zeros in the transfer function. These zeros are responsible for the glitch at $2\bar{r}$. In order to eliminate the glitch, these zeros must be eliminated. With a single annulus, this is not possible without grossly amplifying the noise in the process. One can, however,

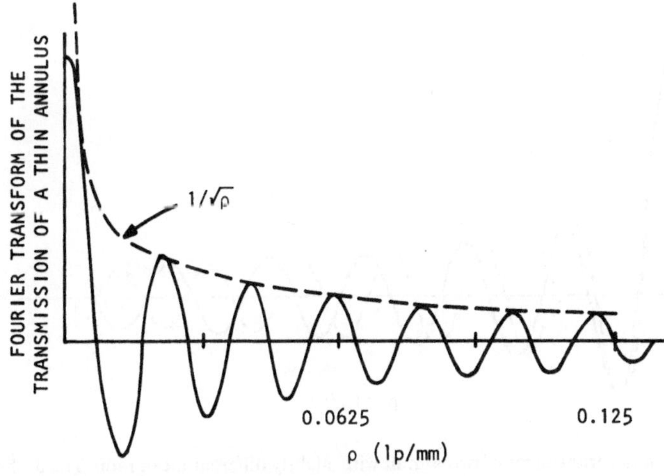

Fig. 8-37. Radial slice through the Fourier transform of a thin annulus.

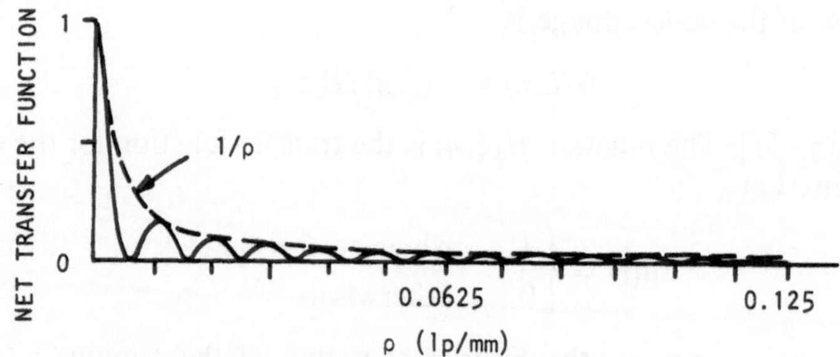

Fig. 8-38. Net transfer function of an annular-coded-aperture system decoded by matched filtering. The transfer function is the square of the function in Fig. 8-37.

think of filling in the gaps in the transfer function if a second coded image made with a slightly larger annulus is available. The transforms of two annuli with mean radii $\bar{r}_1$, and $\bar{r}_2$ are shown in Fig. 8-39. When the spectrum of one annulus is zero, the other may be nonzero. Object frequencies that are lost in one coded image can therefore be recovered by using information from the second coded image.

In order to recover the most information about the object spectrum, the ideal situation would be to have the peaks in the spectrum of one annulus coincide with the zeros in the spectrum of the other annulus. It is not possible to do this merely by using two annuli with different mean radii since changing the mean radius of an annulus only changes the scale of its transform. The best that can be done using two different annuli is to separate the zeros of the two spectra as much as possible. Let us assume

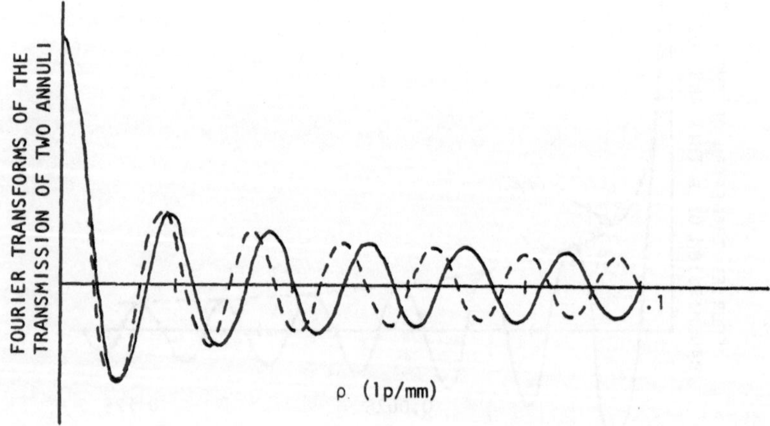

Fig. 8-39. Fourier transforms of two annuli with slightly different mean radii. The dashed curve corresponds to the larger annulus.

that the spectrum of the coded image does not extend beyond some cutoff frequency ρ_c thanks perhaps to limited detector resolution. If the radius of the first annulus is selected based on the considerations in Section 8.4.2, the ratio of the mean radii of the two annuli can be adjusted so that the nth zero of the spectrum of the smaller annulus coincides near ρ_c with the $(n + 1)$st zero of the spectrum of the larger annulus. That ensures that there are no zeros coinciding at frequencies less than ρ_c. Figure 8-39 shows the spectra of two annuli chosen in this way with their 12th and 13th zeros coinciding at $\rho_c = 0.1$ line pairs/mm. The ratio $\bar{r}_2/\bar{r}_1$ is 1.085.

The decoding process is carried out in the spatial-frequency domain. The decoded image spectrum is formed by linearly combining the spectra of the two annular-coded images, frequency by frequency. At each frequency, weighting factors $W_1(\xi, \eta)$ and $W_2(\xi, \eta)$ are calculated such that

$$1 = W_1(\xi, \eta) H_1(\rho) + W_2(\xi, \eta) H_2(\rho) \tag{8-81}$$

where $H_i(\rho)$ is defined in Eq. (8-79) with $\bar{r} = \bar{r}_i$. $H_i(\rho)$ is the effective transfer function for the coded image formed with the ith annulus. When the spectra of the coded images $G_1(\xi, \eta)$ and $G_2(\xi, \eta)$ are then combined using the weights $W_1(\xi, \eta)$ and $W_2(\xi, \eta)$ we have

$$\begin{aligned} W_1(\xi, \eta) G_1(\xi, \eta) + W_2(\xi, \eta) G_2(\xi, \eta) &= W_1(\xi, \eta) O(\xi, \eta) H_1(\xi, \eta) \\ &\quad + W_2(\xi, \eta) O(\xi, \eta) H_2(\xi, \eta) \\ &= O(\xi, \eta) \end{aligned} \tag{8-82}$$

thereby recovering the object spectrum. A second equation is needed to uniquely solve for the weighting factors. Noise considerations suggest that whichever coded image has the larger transfer function at a particular frequency should be weighted more heavily. This leads to the following constraint:

$$\frac{H_1(\rho)}{H_2(\rho)} = \frac{W_1(\rho)}{W_2(\rho)} \tag{8-83}$$

This constraint was used to calculate the set of weights shown in Fig. 8-40; these weights would be used with the spectra of the annuli in Fig. 8-39. Based on experience with inverse filters, the maximum allowed value for a particular weight has to be limited to avoid excessive noise amplification. The weights in Fig. 8-40 were limited to maximum values of ± 10.

The decoded image spectra for a point source is shown in Fig. 8-41b. The dips in the curve are the result of the limit on the magnitude of the weights. The curve has also been apodized (smoothly tapered toward zero rather than sharply truncated at the maximum frequency) to control ringing when the spectrum is inverse transformed. The system PSF is shown in Fig. 8-41a. The glitch at $2\bar{r}$ has been eliminated. Figure 8-42 shows two

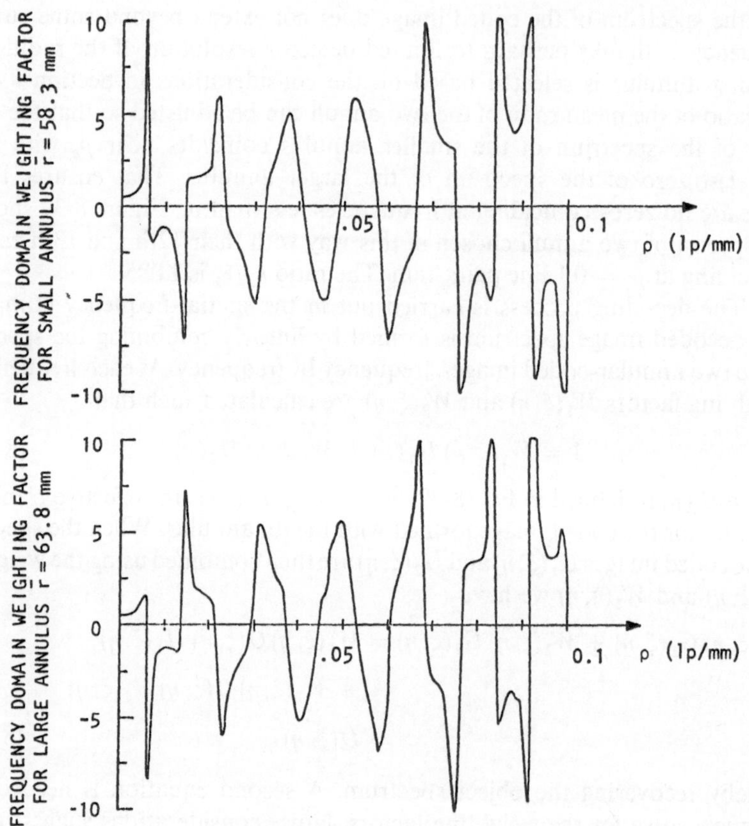

Fig. 8-40. Weighting factors used in combining the Fourier spectra of the coded images formed with the two slightly different annuli whose spectra are shown in Fig. 8-39.

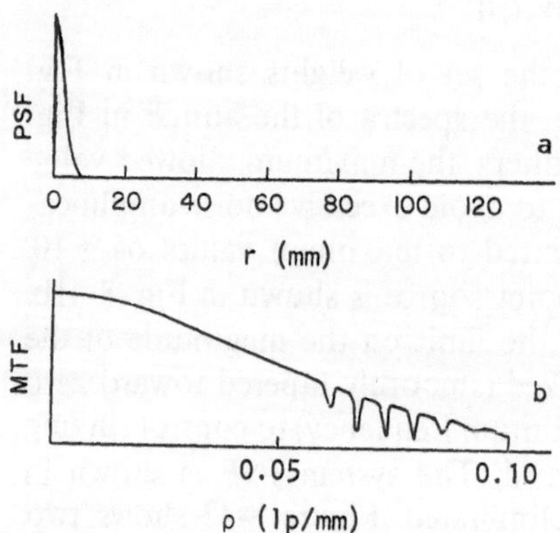

Fig. 8-41. (a) Decoded PSF for the two-annulus system. (b) Effective transfer function for the two-annulus system, obtained by multiplying the annular spectra in Fig. 8-39 by the respective weighting functions in Fig. 8-40 and adding the results together, frequency by frequency. The MTF has been apodized to reduce spurious oscillations in the PSF.

Fig. 8-42. Two phantoms imaged with the two-annulus system. (a) Letter E 10 cm tall imaged at unit magnification ($s_1 = s_2$). (b) Kidney-shaped phantom 20 cm tall with two 3.8-cm-diameter cold regions imaged at a magnification of -0.5. Each coded image contained 600K.

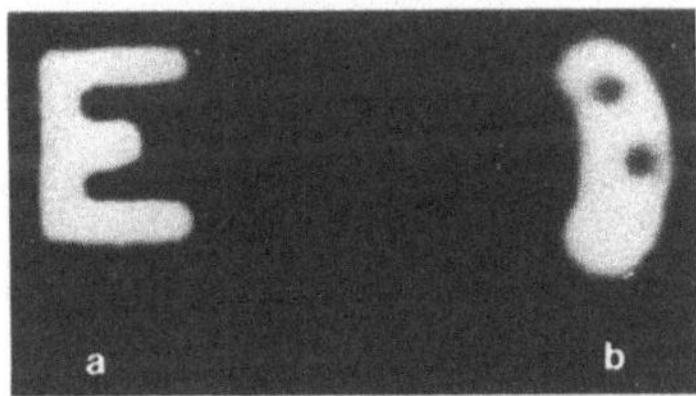

phantoms imaged with the two-annulus system. While out-of-focus behavior has not been discussed much, it should be noted that when the two-annulus system images object points lying outside of the assumed object plane, the glitch is not entirely eliminated.

8.6. TIME-VARYING APERTURES

In the previous section, improved decoded images were achieved by allowing the use of more than one aperture. Although the change occurs in discrete steps, these systems can be considered as time-varying apertures and the improved performance can be attributed to the additional degree of freedom associated with the temporal variable. This additional degree of freedom has been made an integral part of several coded-aperture imaging systems that have been reported in the literature. Very impressive results have been achieved, especially in tomographic performance. It should be remembered, however, that this improvement has been made at the expense of temporal resolution in the decoded image. If there are no dynamic changes occurring in the object, the loss of temporal resolution is unimportant and the improved tomography may be quite important.

One time-varying aperture has been described by Chang and Macdonald (Chang *et al.*, 1974; Macdonald *et al.*, 1975; Chang, 1976). Strictly speaking, their system is not a coded-aperture system but a tomographic system. An outgrowth of their work on nonredundant pinhole arrays, the system uses the array of nine pinholes shown in Fig. 8-43. The object, aperture, and detector are arranged in the usual coded-aperture configuration (see Fig. 8-44). Instead of recording the resulting coded image, all but one of the pinholes are blocked out and the resulting image is recorded.

Fig. 8-43. Nonredundant array of nine pinholes.

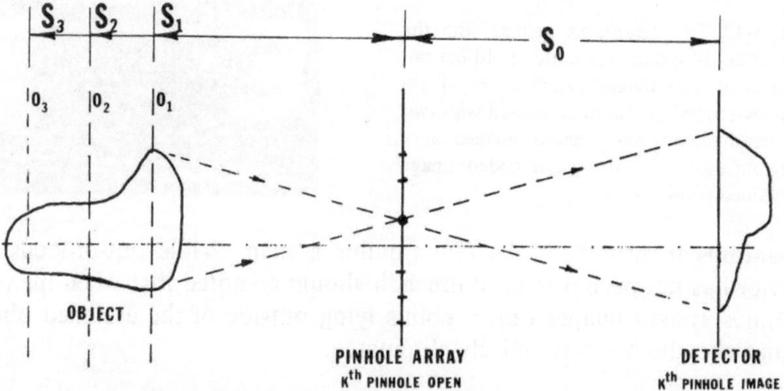

Fig. 8-44. Recording geometry for the sequential-pinhole tomographic system. (From Chang, 1976; used here with permission.)

This process is repeated for each of the nine pinholes, resulting in a set of nine images. Each image is a recognizable representation of the object since it is just a pinhole image. If the object is planar, any one of these images is just as good as the other. However, any single image contains no tomographic information. If the object is not contained in a single plane, the nine images will be different since the object is viewed from slightly different positions. Chang and Macdonald found that it was possible to use these nine images to produce tomographic images that were very free of artifacts from the other object planes.

Figure 8-45 illustrates the recording process and the first step in the reconstruction process. Everything to the left of the detector involves gamma rays. Everything to the right of the detector plane illustrates the mathematical operations that are performed in a computer in order to

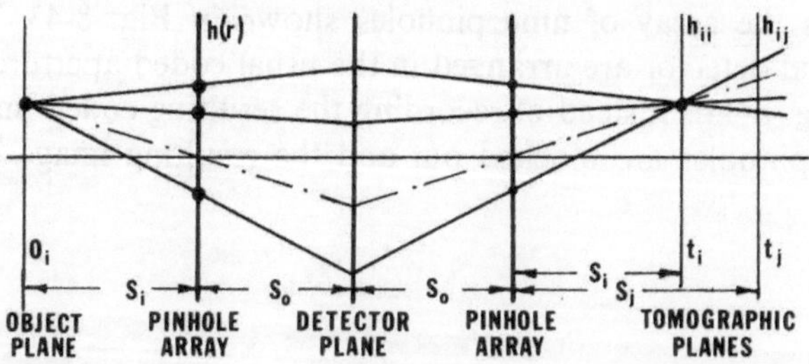

Fig. 8-45. Schematic representation of the data-collection and tomogram-synthesis steps in the sequential-pinhole tomographic system. Everything to the left of the detector plane involves actual gamma rays. Everything to the right represents mathematical operations performed in the computer. (From Chang, 1976; used here with permission.)

reconstruct the object. The object point creates a spot on the detector whose position in that particular image depends on which pinhole is open. This image is then mathematically projected back through a pinhole whose position corresponds to the position of the recording pinhole. This is done for all of the individual pinhole images. In one particular plane, all of the backprojected lines intersect. In other planes, the pattern fans out.

A computer simulation of this backprojection process is shown in Fig. 8-46. The object was assumed to exist in three planes. The distribution in each of the three planes is shown in Fig. 8-46B. The tomographic images that would be formed with the above method are shown in Fig. 8-46C. The out-of-focus artifacts are very evident. In order to understand how these are eliminated, the equations describing the three tomographic images must be considered.

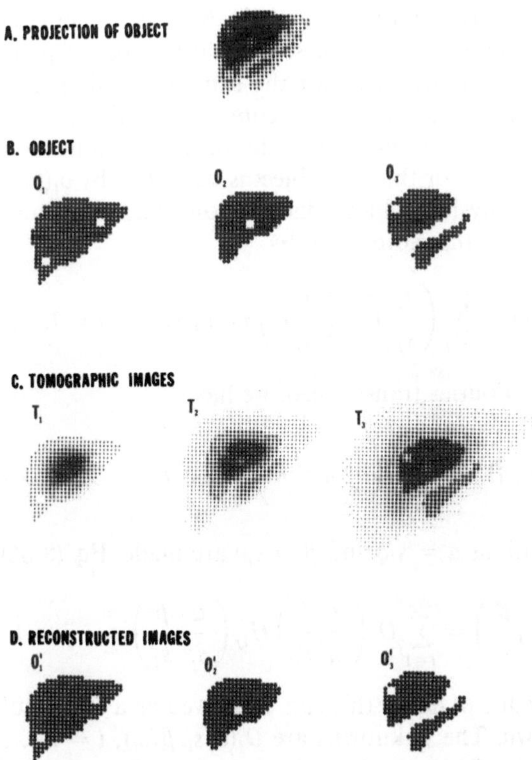

Fig. 8-46. (A) View of the three-plane object in (B) that would be obtained with a parallel-hole collimator. (B) Object distributions in the three planes. Planes are separated by 2 cm. (C) Tomographic images obtained by backprojection. (D) Reconstructed object planes derived from the tomograms in (C). (From Chang, 1976; used here with permission.)

As with all linear systems it is convenient to determine the response to a single point source and use a convolution to describe the output due to more complex objects. Clearly, the response to a point source will depend on both the particular plane that contains the object point and the choice of reconstruction plane. Denoting the object planes by the subscript i and the reconstruction plane by j such that when $i = j$ the ith object plane is in focus, let $h_{ij}(\mathbf{r})$ be the response in the jth reconstruction plane due to a point in the ith object plane, where $\mathbf{r}$ is a two-dimensional position vector in the reconstruction plane. Approximating the pinholes by Dirac delta functions, it is easy to show that

$$h_{ij}(\mathbf{r}) = \sum_{k=1}^{N_h} \delta(\mathbf{r} - m_{ij}\mathbf{r}_k), \qquad i, j = 1, \ldots, N_p \tag{8-84}$$

where $m_{ij} = (s_i - s_j)/s_i$, s_i, and s_j are the axial distances shown in Fig. 8-45, $\mathbf{r}_k$ is the location of the kth pinhole, N_p is the number of object planes, and N_h is the number of pinholes. An odd number of pinholes is used so that the response function is not the same on both sides of the in-focus plane. The object intensity that is convolved with this response function is also dependent on i and j since the object magnification changes with i and j. Accounting for this, the object is described by $o_i(\mathbf{r}s_i/s_j)$, where $o_i(\mathbf{r})$ describes the physical object distribution. The distribution in the jth tomogram $t_j(\mathbf{r})$ is therefore given by

$$t_j(\mathbf{r}) = \sum_{i=1}^{N_p} \left(\frac{s_i}{s_j}\right)^2 o_i\left(\frac{s_i}{s_j}\mathbf{r}\right) ** h_{ij}(\mathbf{r}), \qquad j = 1, \ldots, N_p \tag{8-85}$$

If Eq. (8-85) is Fourier transformed, we have

$$T_j(\xi, \eta) = \sum_{i=1}^{N_p} O_i\left(\frac{s_j}{s_i}\xi, \frac{s_j}{s_i}\eta\right) H_{ij}(\xi, \eta), \qquad j = 1, \ldots, N_p \tag{8-86}$$

If the substitutions $\alpha = s_j\xi$ and $\beta = s_j\eta$ are made, Eq. (8-86) becomes

$$T_j\left(\frac{\alpha}{s_j}, \frac{\beta}{s_j}\right) = \sum_{i=1}^{N_p} O_i\left(\frac{\alpha}{s_i}, \frac{\beta}{s_i}\right) H_{ij}\left(\frac{\alpha}{s_j}, \frac{\beta}{s_j}\right), \qquad j = 1, \ldots, N_p \tag{8-87}$$

For a given value of (α, β), this can be viewed as a system of N_p equations in N_p unknown. The unknowns are $O_i(\alpha/s_i, \beta/s_i)$, $i = 1, \ldots, N_p$, while the values of $T_j(\alpha/s_j, \beta/s_j)$, $j = 1, \ldots, N_p$ are known from the N_p backprojected tomograms and the matrix of values $H_{ij}(\alpha/s_j, \beta/s_j)$ are known from the shape of the pinhole pattern and the position of the tomogram planes. The solution of these equations for the value of O_i at a particular frequency involves the inversion of the $N_p \times N_p$ matrix $[H_{ij}]$. The elements of $[H_{ij}]$

are easily derived from Eq. (8-84):

$$H_{ij}\left(\frac{\alpha}{s_j},\frac{\beta}{s_j}\right) = \sum_{k=1}^{N_h} \exp\{i2\pi(\alpha x_k + \beta y_k)[(s_i - s_j)/s_i s_j^2]\},$$

$$i, j = 1, \ldots, N_p \tag{8-88}$$

The success of this method will depend on whether the matrix $[H_{ij}]$ is singular for any values of (ξ, η). When $\xi = \eta = 0$,

$$H_{ij}(0,0) = N_h \tag{8-89}$$

Since all values of the matrix $[H_{ij}(0,0)]$ are the same, the determinant of the matrix will be identically zero for all values of N_p. Therefore, the dc component of the object is indeterminant. This should come as no surprise since the dc component in each recorded image would look the same regardless of which pinhole is used. It would be quite an accomplishment to tell how the isotope was distributed between the three planes based on this data. While this loss of dc information might inhibit the determination of the actual amount of isotope present in a given plane, a dc bias can be artificially added to the data so that a very reasonable representation of the object results. If the object is known to be spatially limited, the bias can be set to eliminate negative values outside of the known object region. If other spatial frequencies are indeterminant because of a singular matrix, the problem becomes more serious. There is no proof yet that all other spatial frequencies in the object spectrum can be recovered without encountering a singular matrix. However, none have been encountered in any work reported to date. Tomographic reconstructions of simulated data using this method are shown in Fig. 8-46D.

This tomographic reconstruction algorithm can also be used to remove out-of-focus artifacts from tomograms formed with a variety of other systems. A scanner with a focusing collimator will form the same sort of tomogram formed by backprojecting the pinhole images in the system described above. If several scanner images are recorded with different focal planes, they can be used as the tomographic input data $t_j(x, y)$ in the matrix-inversion technique described above. Data from a positron camera or a dynamic-tomography unit can also be used just as the multiple pinhole images are used. It is curious, however, that the process will not work with a coded-aperture system. In a coded-aperture system where decoding is done by matched filtering, the decoding function which produces an in-focus image of the jth object plane is

$$h_j(x, y) = h\left[\frac{x}{(s_j + s_o)/s_j}, \frac{y}{(s_j + s_o)/s_j}\right] \tag{8-90}$$

where h(x, y) is the actual aperture transmission function. The coded image of an object point in the ith object plane is

$$h_i(x, y) = h\left[\frac{x}{(s_i + s_o)/s_i}, \frac{y}{(s_i + s_o)/s_i}\right] \tag{8-91}$$

The response in the jth tomographic plane due to a point in ith object plane is then

$$h_{ij}(x, y) = h_i(x, y) ** h_j(x, y) \tag{8-92}$$

The decoded image $g(x, y)$ is then

$$g(x, y) = \sum_{i=1}^{N_p} \left(\frac{s_o}{s_i}\right)^2 o_i\left(-\frac{s_o}{s_i}x, -\frac{s_o}{s_i}y\right) ** h_{ij}(x, y) \tag{8-93}$$

The scale factors in o_i have no dependence on s_j so there is no need to make a change of variables to α and β. Proceeding as above, the Fourier transform of $h_{ij}(x, y)$ is

$$H_{ij}(\xi, \eta) = H_i(\xi, \eta)\, H_j^*(\xi, \eta) \tag{8-94}$$

For a three-plane object, the matrix $[H_{ij}]$ becomes

$$[H_{ij}(\xi, \eta)] = \begin{bmatrix} H_1(\xi, \eta)\, H_1^*(\xi, \eta) & H_1(\xi, \eta)\, H_2^*(\xi, \eta) & H_1(\xi, \eta)\, H_3^*(\xi, \eta) \\ H_2(\xi, \eta)\, H_1^*(\xi, \eta) & H_2(\xi, \eta)\, H_2^*(\xi, \eta) & H_2(\xi, \eta)\, H_3^*(\xi, \eta) \\ H_3(\xi, \eta)\, H_1^*(\xi, \eta) & H_3(\xi, \eta)\, H_2^*(\xi, \eta) & H_3(\xi, \eta)\, H_3^*(\xi, \eta) \end{bmatrix} \tag{8-95}$$

It is easy to show that the determinant of this matrix is zero for all values of (ξ, η). This result is independent of both the actual and assumed number of object planes. Since the determinant is zero at all frequencies, tomograms produced by changing the scale of the decoding function in a coded-aperture system cannot be used as input data into this algorithm.

The success of the sequential pinhole system depends on the behavior of the decoded PSF as it goes out of focus. In the sequential pinhole arrangement, the decoded PSF keeps the same functional form as it goes out of focus with only the scale of the function changing. If the pinhole array is used as a coded aperture and matched-filter decoding is performed, the PSF has the behavior shown in Fig. 8-47 since only the scale of the decoding function is changed, not the scale of the net PSF. As long as a spatial correlation is performed to decode the coded image, this problem will persist.

The sequential pinhole system just described is more correctly referred to as a tomographic system rather than a coded-aperture system. The

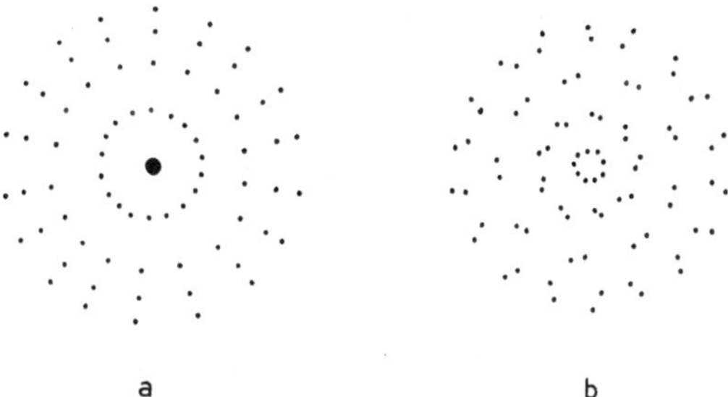

Fig. 8-47. (a) In-focus PSF obtained by correlation decoding of the pinhole array in Fig. 8-43. (b) Slightly out-of-focus PSF for the same pinhole array.

processing that is done provides improved tomographic behavior, but is not essential in order to produce a recognizable image. There is a coded-aperture system that combines features of the sequential pinhole system and coded-aperture systems. Developed by workers at the University of Michigan (Koral *et al.*, 1975; May, 1974; May *et al.*, 1974; Akcasu *et al.*, 1974), the system employs a time-modulated aperture to perform the encoding while the spatial resolution of the detector is used to recover tomographic information in a way analogous to the sequential pinhole system. This system is a true coded-aperture system since the recorded signals must be decoded before a usable image is obtained.

The basic encoding scheme was first proposed by Gottlieb (1968) for use in a television scanning system. The geometry for a one-dimensional time-varying coded-aperture system is shown in Fig. 8-48. The aperture is a pinhole array which moves to the right in discrete steps equal to the width of a pinhole. The output from detector 1 due to object point 1 varies in time in the same way that the transmission of the aperture varies in space. The output from detector 1 due to object point 2 has the same functional form but has a different phase. If the output from detector 1 due to object points 1 and 2 is correlated with the aperture function, two correlation spikes are formed and the distance between the two correlation spikes is related to the separation between object points 1 and 2.

If only the data from a single detector is available, it is not possible to obtain any tomographic resolution in the decoded image. Consider object points 1 and 3 in Fig. 8-48. The signal from detector 1 due to either of these two points will have the same phase. Thus it is impossible to determine where along the line connecting the two points the sources are really located. However, detector 4 *will* see a phase difference between object points 1 and 3. Depth resolution can then be obtained from the parallax information contained in the signals from detectors located at other positions in the detector plane. The situation is identical to that encountered in the sequential pinhole system of Chang and Macdonald. The decoded data from the various detectors can be combined in a manner analogous to the sequential pinhole data to produce a tomogram. A set of tomograms can be

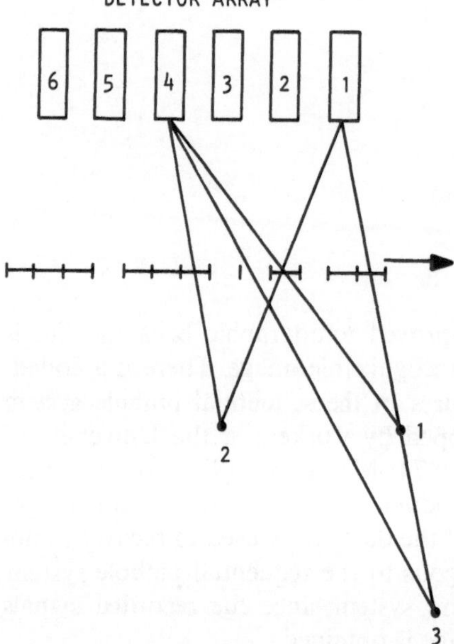

Fig. 8-48. Encoding geometry for a one-dimensional time-varying coded-aperture system. The pinhole array is moved to the right either continuously or in discrete steps while the output of the detectors is recorded for later decoding.

constructed and used as input into the Chang and Macdonald algorithm in order to eliminate out-of-focus contributions. Initially, the Michigan group halted their reconstruction process at the tomogram stage, relying on a large detector array to produce a smooth out-of-focus PSF. Borrowing a technique originally developed for CAT-scanning systems, they have recently used an ART (algorithmic reconstruction technique) algorithm to produce reconstructions in which out-of-focus contributions are almost entirely eliminated. Using the decoded images from all of the detectors, the ART algorithm iteratively seeks a set of reconstructed object planes which is most consistent with the decoded image data. Their results have been quite impressive.

Background contributions to the decoded image due to the sidelobes of the decoded PSF can be eliminated if the sidelobes are uniform. The uniformly redundant arrays and nonredundant arrays discussed earlier are two examples of code functions that can be used to produce uniform sidelobes which can be removed with a simple subtraction. However, as described earlier, in order to produce the flat sidelobes, the decoding function contains a cyclically repeated version of the aperture code. As a result, the largest object that can be successfully imaged with these apertures is determined by the length of the aperture code. Large objects require longer codes, which in the case of a time-varying coded aperture requires that more data be collected.

It is possible to alter the physical arrangement in Fig. 8-48 slightly and circumvent this requirement. An aperture is made which contains two copies of the coded array placed end-to-end. A window whose length is equal to that of a single code sequence is placed in contact with the pinhole array so that only a fundamental length of code can be used at one time (see Fig. 8-49). The window is held fixed while the pinhole array is moved to the right in discrete steps. If a pinhole moves out of the window to the right, a new pinhole moves in from the left. A single detector is then responsible for decoding only those object points that could be seen if only the window were in place. Each detector is therefore responsible for a slightly different portion of the object and there is no longer any constraint on the overall size of the object. This data collection arrangement has an interesting effect on the behavior of the decoded image. Object point 3 in Fig. 8-49 is so far to the right that only the leftmost detector receives any signal from it. In other coded-aperture systems, if an object point produced an aperture shadow that fell that far off the detector, there would be little hope of recovering the object point. However, in the time-varying system, the fact that the aperture shadow falls so far off the detector has no effect on our ability to resolve the point laterally. The only loss is in tomographic resolution since no parallax data is available on that point.

The one-dimensional coded aperture discussed so far could be used to image two-dimensional objects if a two-dimensional array of detectors is used, but the out-of-focus PSF would blur in only one direction. In order to produce a smooth, two-dimensional blur, the aperture must be two-dimensional. A two-dimensional aperture can be made from a one-dimen-

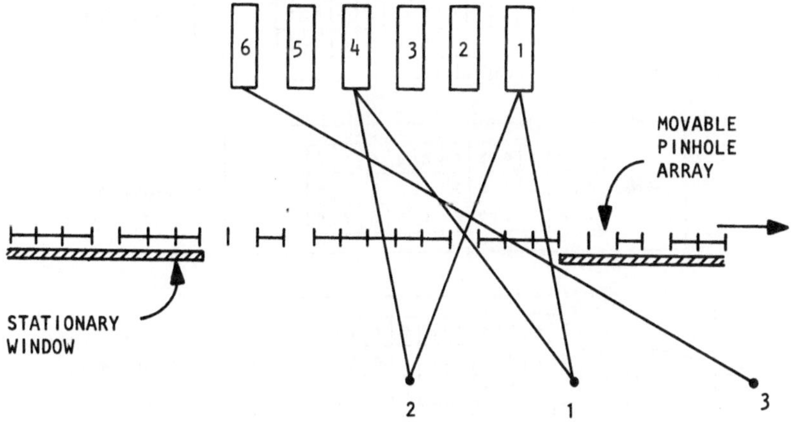

Fig. 8-49. Time-varying coded-aperture system whose aperture code permutes cyclically. Pinhole array contains two lengths of the aperture code placed end-to-end. The stationary window serves to select a fundamental length of the aperture code.

sional code by breaking the one-dimensional code into equal-length segments and stacking up the segments as in Fig. 8-50. If the codes in each row are extended through a complete cycle, it is possible to cyclically permute the two-dimensional code by shifting the coded-aperture plate to the left relative to the window. Data from a single detector will contain information about a square portion of the object.

Experimental results have been obtained at the University of Michigan using a 121-segment sequence arranged in an 11 × 11 square. The aperture segments are 3 × 3 mm resulting in a total aperture that is 3.3 × 3.3 cm. Using the Anger camera scintillation detector, 121 recordings are made, one for each aperture permutation. Figure 8-51 illustrates the tomographic performance of the aperture, using phantoms located in three planes. Figure 8-52 shows a clinical image of a normal thyroid in a human patient. These figures illustrate quite clearly the improved performance that results when the out-of-focus contributions are removed.

Macovski (1974) proposed a time-modulated coded-aperture system in which an array of pinholes is modulated with a set of mechanical shutters. Each pinhole is opened and closed at a characteristic frequency; frequency rather than phase is the encoding parameter in this system. If the arrival

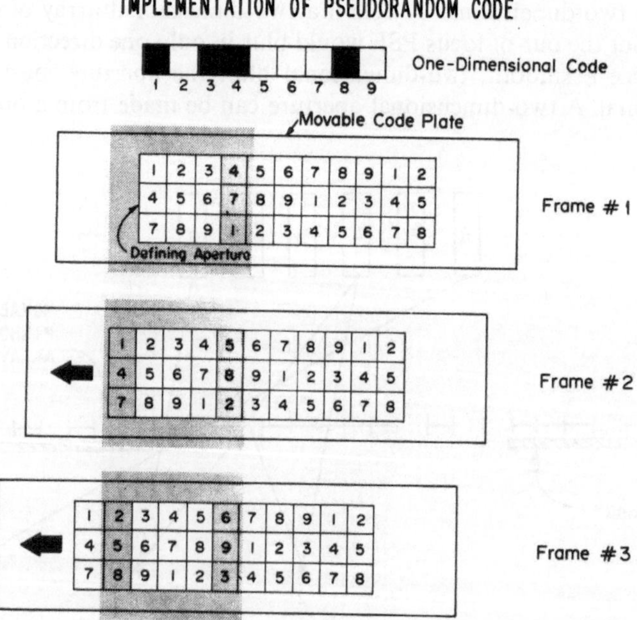

Fig. 8-50. Method for producing a cyclically permutable two-dimensional aperture from a one-dimensional code.

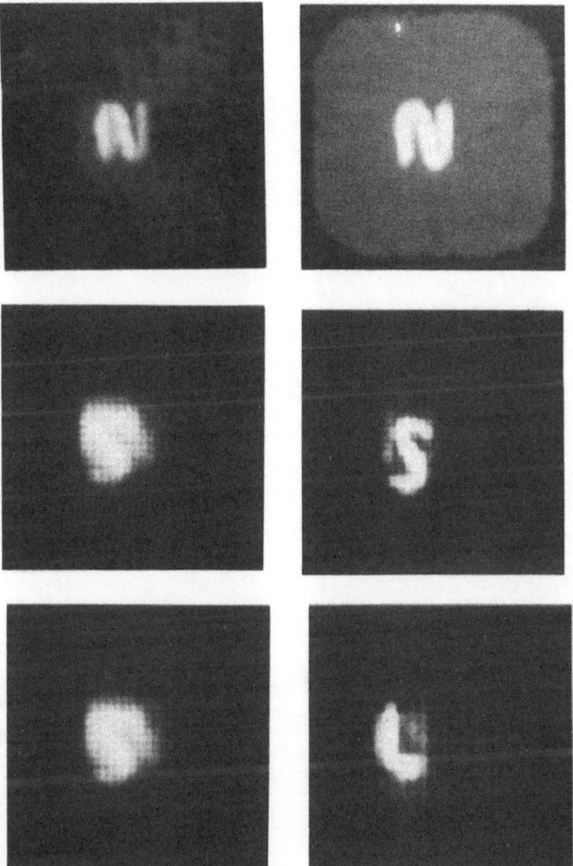

Fig. 8-51. An object consisting of three radioactive letters located in three different planes was imaged with a time-varying, cyclically permuted pinhole array. The simple tomograms are shown on the left, while the results achieved with the use of the ART algorithm are shown on the right. Distance between the aperture and the reconstructed object plane, top to bottom: 2.2 cm, 3.3 cm, 4.4 cm. [Courtesy of W. L. Rogers and K. F. Koral, University of Michigan (Koral *et al.*, 1977).]

time of a photon is recorded as well as the position of the photon, the recorded data can be analyzed temporally and the image from a single pinhole can be separated from the other data. Since each pinhole sees a slightly different view of the object, the resulting parallax information can be used to create a tomographic reconstruction.

Another coded-aperture system which employs an aperture that changes with time is illustrated in Fig. 8-53. First proposed by Tanaka and Iinuma (1975) and also investigated by Miller (1976), the system contains a slit

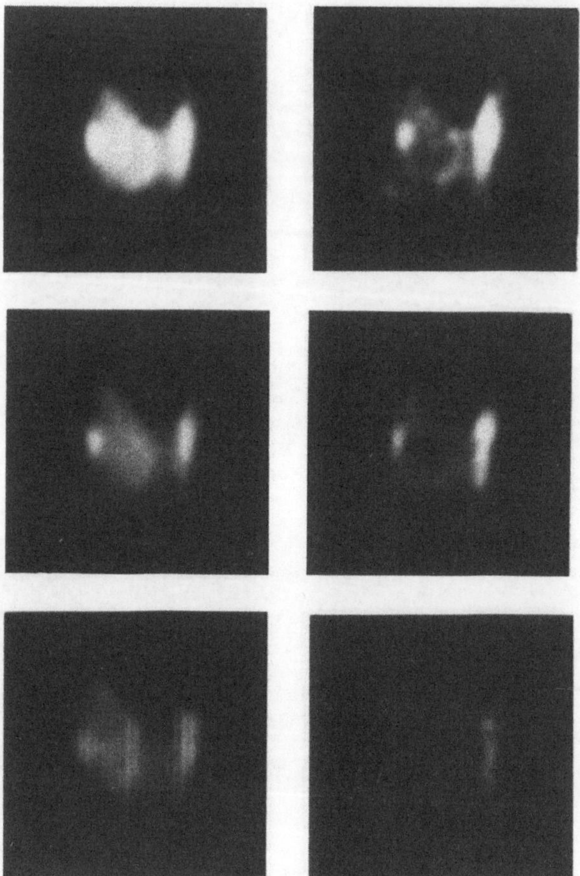

Fig. 8-52. Human thyroid imaged with the time-varying, cyclically permuted pinhole array. The simple tomograms on the left are quite good, but the results with the ART algorithm shown on the right are even more impressive. This patient has a large cystic nodule in the left lobe, producing a cold spot in the left lobe that is evident in the images on the right but is lost in the out-of-focus components in the images on the left. The presence of the nodule was confirmed with ultrasound. Distance between the aperture and the reconstructed object plane, top to bottom: 2.2 cm, 2.6 cm, 3.3 cm. [Courtesy of W. L. Rogers and K. F. Koral, University of Michigan (Koral *et al.*, 1979).]

aperture that rotates about an axis perpendicular to the aperture plane. The operation of this system can be modeled mathematically with a formalism that is analogous to the formalism employed in describing computerized axial tomography; however, there is an important physical difference between the two systems that impacts heavily on the manner in which the data are collected and decoded.

The mathematical similarities are perhaps most obvious if one con-

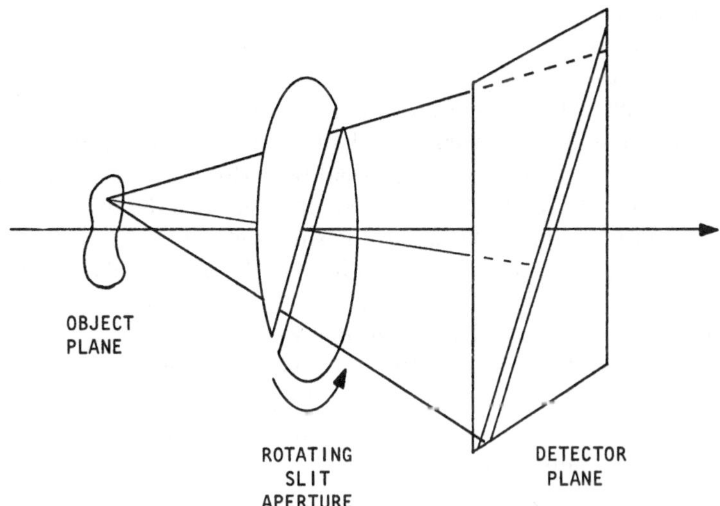

Fig. 8-53. Rotating-slit coded-aperture system. In order to enjoy a SNR advantage, the coded image at each slit orientation must be recorded.

siders a very long narrow slit and a single-point object. At each angular orientation of the slit, a long, thin line is recorded by the detector. If data from a large number of slit orientations are added, a spoke pattern results, just as in computerized axial tomography. In terms of a noise-free image, the comparison is exact. The PSF in both systems, in the limit of a large number of orientation angles, behaves as $1/r$. However, when statistical photon noise is present in the detected image, the two systems differ in an important way. In the computerized axial tomography case in which simple backprojection is performed, all values along a particular backprojected line are the same; in the rotating-slit system, the measured value along any single slit shadow will have statistical fluctuations. If a series of slit images formed with the slit at a variety of orientations are simply added together, the statistical variations along any one slit shadow contribute extra noise to the system. If the composite image is ρ-filtered, the decoded image will have a poorer signal-to-noise ratio (SNR) (see next section for definition of SNR) than if a simple pinhole image had been made with the same total exposure time, even for a single-point object.

The reason for this lackluster performance of a coded-aperture system becomes apparent if the decoding operations are reviewed and compared to other coded-aperture systems. In the rotating-slit system just described, a composite coded image is made and then ρ-filtered. A ρ filter is a sharpening filter; it removes the blurring due to the $1/r$ sidelobes of the PSF. In the other coded-aperture system described in this chapter, decoding is performed by correlating (either spatially or temporally) the coded image with a function that resembles the coded aperture; for simplicity assume that simple template-matching techniques are used. When the template is aligned with the coded image of a point, all of the detected photons from the object point will contribute to the reconstruction of the actual object point, resulting in an improved SNR. Note that at no time in the rotating-slit case was a summation over a slit shadow performed. This suggests that after a sequence of slit images have been recorded with the slit at a discrete set of orientations, the signal along the slit length should be averaged in each coded image *prior* to both the addition of the individual coded images and the ρ-filter operation. Tanaka and Iinuma (1975) calculated the SNR for a slit–aperture system decoded in this way when the object contained a weak point source in a large, uniform background, the situation in which coded apertures usually perform poorly. They found that the SNR of the slit system, normalized to that obtained with a pinhole whose diameter is equal to the slit width W, is given by

$$\frac{\text{SNR}_{\text{slit}}}{\text{SNR}_{\text{pinhole}}} = 1.11(\delta/W)^{1/2} \tag{8-96}$$

where δ is the final resolution after filtering and is constrained to be the same in both systems. If $\delta = W$, the slit has a marginal advantage over a pinhole. If the image is too noisy, it can be reprocessed and smoothed to increase the SNR at the expense of resolution. The final resolution, δ, will then exceed W and the slit will have a larger advantage over a pinhole-aperture image that has been equivalently smoothed, even for the case of a large uniform object. If a high-resolution detector is available, the rotating-slit coded images can therefore be decoded with high resolution and a SNR slightly better than a comparable high-resolution pinhole or it can be decoded with poorer resolution and a much better SNR than would be obtained by smoothing the high-resolution pinhole image.

The PSF obtained with the rotating-slit aperture, both before and after ρ-filtering (with infinite bandwidth) is shown in Fig. 8-54. The finite width of the slit has been included in this calculation but the limited resolution of the detector has not. Note that prior to ρ-filtering, all object points, no matter what their distance from the aperture plane, will be represented by the PSF in Fig. 8-54a; only the size of the central flat region will change. However, the ρ-filter is not sensitive to this difference; the ρ filter only removes the $1/r$ sidelobes. Since the function $h(r) = 1/r$ is a function with no characteristic scale, the ρ filter removes the $1/r$ sidelobes from all object points equally. The final decoded image will have all object planes in focus. This nontomographic nature of the rotating-slit system makes it unique among coded apertures. Depending on the application, this may be a blessing or a curse.

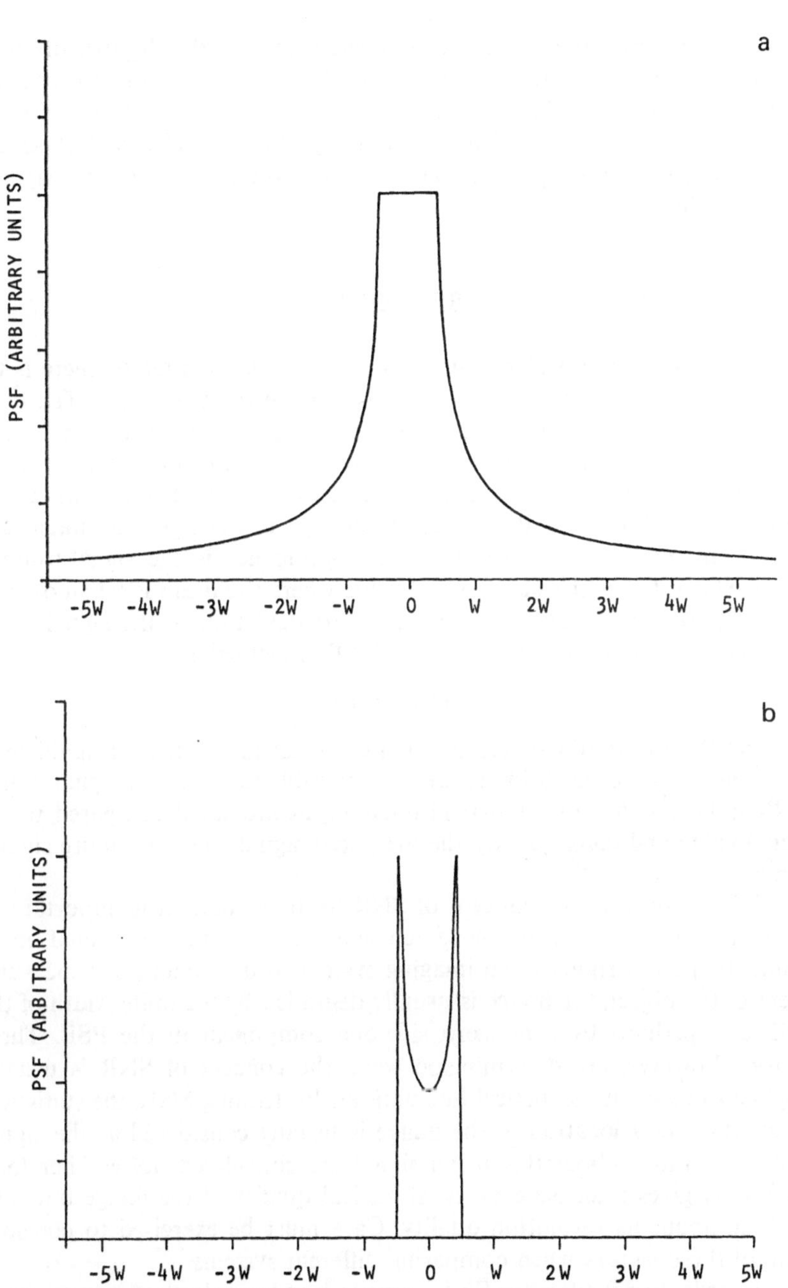

a

PSF (ARBITRARY UNITS)

-5W -4W -3W -2W -W 0 W 2W 3W 4W 5W

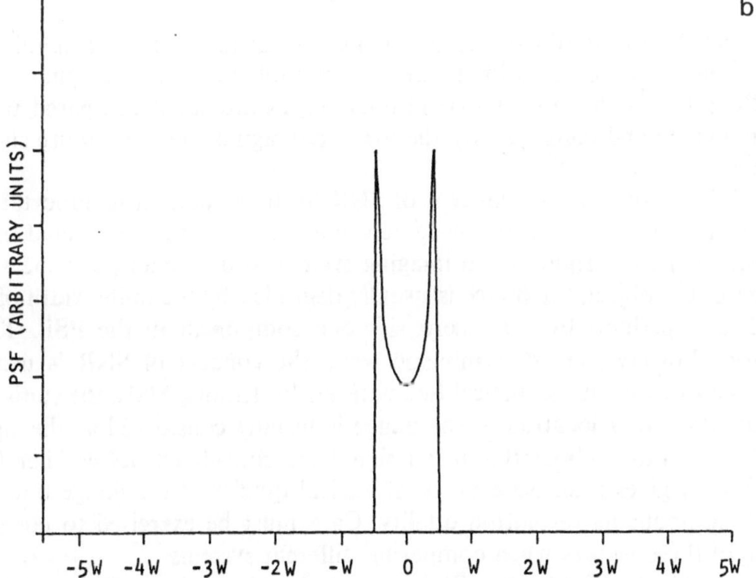

Fig. 8-54. (a) PSF obtained in the limit of an infinite number of slit orientations. W is the width of the slit. (b) PSF obtained after ρ-filtering (a) with infinite bandwidth. The finite width of the slit is included but the limited resolution of the detector is ignored. (From Miller, 1976; used here with permission.)

Tomographic information can be encoded with the slit aperture if the system is changed slightly (Tamura, 1976). If, instead of rotating the aperture plane about an axis that passes through the slit, the aperture is rotated about an axis a distance d away from the slit, the individual slit-coded images can be shifted appropriately to bring a single plane into focus, prior to ρ-filtering.

8.7. NOISE

Any time a physical measurement of some kind is made, there is the possibility that the measured value differs from the true value. The error can be either systematic or random. Since systematic errors can usually be corrected once their presence is known, random errors usually present a bigger problem. When interpreting a measured signal of any kind, it is important to know whether a certain change in the signal is statistically significant. One measure of statistical significance is the signal-to-noise ratio (SNR). If μ is the mean signal value where the mean is taken over an ensemble of signals, and σ is the standard deviation of the signal again averaged over an ensemble of signals, SNR is defined as

$$\mathrm{SNR} = \mu/\sigma \tag{8-97}$$

Low SNR indicates the detected signal value has low statistical significance since the standard deviation is then comparable to the mean signal. Large SNR indicates that the statistical fluctuations are small compared to the signal value and consequently the measured signal value has more significance.

When applying the concept of SNR to image data, it is important to understand clearly what is considered signal and what is considered noise. While the perfect signal in an imaging system would be an exact measurement of the object, the image is usually degraded by the finite width of the PSF and perhaps by a nonzero sidelobe component in the PSF. These factors, however, are deterministic while the concept of SNR is usually applied to data with statistical fluctuations. In defining SNR, the statistical mean value at a location in the image is usually considered as the signal and fluctuations about this mean signal are considered noise. Therefore, SNR only gives a measure of the statistical quality of the image but says nothing about its resolution quality. Care must be exercised to consider both of these factors when comparing different systems.

In order to calculate the SNR, one needs to know both the mean signal and the standard deviation. These two parameters are easily calculated if the statistics of the noise sources are known. Usually, the effect of a single noise source dominates so that other sources of noise can be ignored. In nuclear medicine, the dominant noise source is almost invariably quantum noise. Also known as photon noise, this noise is the result of detecting a finite number of individual photons during a measurement. The arrival of an individual photon at the detector is statistically independent of the arrival of any other photon. In addition, the arrival of an individual photon is equally likely to occur at any time during the measurement. These are the same conditions one encounters in dealing with shot noise in electronics (Davenport and Root, 1958). If $g(x, y)$ is the measured coded image, then $n(x, y) = g(x, y)\,\Delta x\,\Delta y$ will be the number of photons detected in an area element $\Delta x\,\Delta y$ located at (x, y). Using the same argument as for electronic shot noise, $n(x, y)$ can be shown to be a Poisson random variable. If the ensemble mean value of $n(x, y)$ is $\bar{n}(x, y)$ the probability of recording $n(x, y)$ photons is given by

$$p\big(n(x, y)\big) = \frac{e^{-\bar{n}(x,y)}\big(\bar{n}(x, y)\big)^{n(x,y)}}{n(x, y)\,!} \tag{8-98}$$

An important feature of Poisson random variables is the fact that the variance, σ^2, is equal to the mean. Consequently, the standard deviation is equal to the square root of the mean, resulting in a SNR given by

$$\begin{aligned} \mathrm{SNR} &= \mu/\sigma \\ &= \bar{n}(x, y)/[\bar{n}(x, y)]^{1/2} \\ &= [\bar{n}(x, y)]^{1/2} \end{aligned} \tag{8-99}$$

In order to improve the SNR by a factor of 2, the number of detected photons must be increased by a factor of 4.

Since $n(x, y)$ is the number of photons detected in a given area, the size of that area affects how large $n(x, y)$ is and consequently affects the SNR. In the case of a pinhole camera, there is nothing to be gained by dividing the detector into elemental areas larger or smaller than the resolution cell, where the resolution cell is the size of the pinhole shadow. Detector elements larger than the resolution element will degrade the system resolution. Smaller detector elements will merely record a smaller number of photons resulting in a smaller SNR. The SNR can be improved in the latter case by doing some spatial averaging, also referred to as noise smoothing. As long as the averaging is restricted to areas the size of the resolution cell, no resolution will be lost while the resultant SNR approaches the value that would have been achieved if the size of the detector elements had matched the size of the resolution cell initially. The SNR for a pinhole camera in which the detector-element size matches the resolution-cell size is then given by

$$\mathrm{SNR_{ph}} = (\text{number of detected photons per resolution cell})^{1/2} \tag{8-100}$$

For a point source whose coded image is decoded by template matching, the peak value of the reconstruction is just the number of photons that were collected. For a point source, then, the SNR at the peak of the reconstruction is given by

$$\text{SNR}_{ca} = (\text{number of photons collected})^{1/2} \tag{8-101}$$

When the imaging geometry, the object and the exposure time are fixed, the number of collected photons is proportional to the area of the aperture. The ratio of the SNR's in Eqs. (8-100) and (8-101) is then

$$\frac{\text{SNR}_{ca}}{\text{SNR}_{ph}} = \left(\frac{\text{area of coded aperture}}{\text{area of pinhole}}\right)^{1/2} \tag{8-102}$$

This ratio can be quite large, but unfortunately it only holds for a single-point object. When the object contains two resolvable points, Eq. (8-100) is still valid, but Eq. (8-101) has to be modified. In the coded-aperture system, the aperture shadows from each of the two object points may overlap. If they do overlap, portions of the aperture shadow from one point will be visible when the decoding template is centered over the shadow from the other point. Noise fluctuations in the shadow of the first point will act as additional noise in the decoded image of the second point. As the number of points increases, the number of overlapping shadows increases and more noise is introduced. The SNR for the decoded image will then decline as the number of object points increases. This is not a problem with the pinhole since two resolved points produce nonoverlapping pinhole shadows.

In order to determine the dependence of the SNR on object size, one must understand that the Poisson noise is present in the coded image before any processing is done. The decoding operation may alter the behavior of the noise in the decoded image, but it will do so in a deterministic manner. In the cases where decoding consisted of correlating the coded image with a decoding function, the noisy coded image can be thought of as the input to a system whose impulse response is the decoding function. If the noise is stationary such that the variance is independent of position, power-spectral analysis can be used to predict the noise in the output based on the noise in the input. Since the coded image contains Poisson noise, the variance at any location is equal to the mean. The variance will be independent of position (i.e., stationary) only when the mean is the same at all points in the coded image. This will be the case only for a very large, uniform object. Power-spectral analysis is therefore not applicable in almost all coded-aperture situations.

It is possible to calculate the noise in the decoded image by a different technique (Metz, 1969; Metz and Beck, 1974; May, 1974; May *et al.*, 1974;

Akcasu *et al.*, 1974). Let a particular noisy coded image be given by $g(x, y)$. The decoded image $i(x, y)$ is then given by

$$i(x, y) = g(x, y) \star\star h_2(x, y) \tag{8-103}$$

where $h_2(x, y)$ is the decoding function. It will be important to distinguish between the shadow function $h_1(x, y)$ and the decoding function $h_2(x, y)$. The two functions will have the same functional form with equal scales when the decoded point is in focus; the normalization of the two functions may differ, however. The normalization of $h_1(x, y)$ will be important because it determines the number of photons in the coded image and consequently determines the noise. The normalization of $h_2(x, y)$ will not matter, as will become clear shortly.

The mean value of $i(x, y)$ is then

$$\begin{aligned} \langle i(x, y)\rangle &= \langle g(x, y) \star\star h_2(x, y)\rangle \\ &= \langle g(x, y)\rangle \star\star h_2(x, y) \end{aligned} \tag{8-104}$$

since h_2 is a deterministic function. The variance of $i(x, y)$ is defined as

$$\begin{aligned} \sigma_i^2 &= \langle |i(x, y) - \langle i(x, y)\rangle|^2\rangle \\ &= \langle |g(x, y) \star\star h_2(x, y) - \langle g(x, y)\rangle \star\star h_2(x, y)|^2\rangle \\ &= \langle |(g(x, y) - \langle g(x, y)\rangle) \star\star h_2(x, y)|^2\rangle \\ &= \langle |\Delta g(x, y) \star\star h_2(x, y)|^2\rangle \end{aligned} \tag{8-105}$$

where

$$\Delta g(x, y) = g(x, y) - \langle g(x, y)\rangle \tag{8-106}$$

Writing out the integrals, one obtains

$$\begin{aligned} \sigma_i^2 = \Big\langle \iint_{-\infty}^{\infty} \Delta g(\alpha, \beta)\, h_2(\alpha - x, \beta - y)\, d\alpha\, d\beta \iint_{-\infty}^{\infty} \Delta g^*(\gamma, \delta) \\ \times h_2^*(\gamma - x, \delta - y)\, d\gamma\, d\delta \Big\rangle \end{aligned} \tag{8-107}$$

$$\begin{aligned} = \iiiint_{-\infty}^{\infty} \langle \Delta g(\alpha, \beta)\, \Delta g^*(\gamma, \delta)\rangle\, h_2(\alpha - x, \beta - y) \\ \times h_2^*(\gamma - x, \delta - y)\, d\alpha\, d\beta\, d\gamma\, d\delta \end{aligned} \tag{8-108}$$

Since $g(x, y)$ is real, $\Delta g^*(\gamma, \delta) = \Delta g(\gamma, \delta)$. In order to perform the expectation-value operation contained in the integral, it is necessary to again consider $n(x, y) = g(x, y)\,\Delta x\,\Delta y$. In a physical measurement the detector is broken up into area elements with sides of length ε. The available data are then $n(x, y) = g(x, y)\,\varepsilon^2$. The expectation value in Eq. (8-108) can then be written

$$\langle \Delta g(\alpha, \beta)\, \Delta g(\gamma, \delta)\rangle = \frac{1}{\varepsilon^4}\langle \Delta n(\alpha, \beta)\, \Delta n(\gamma, \delta)\rangle \tag{8-109}$$

Provided that the detection of a single photon results in a signal whose spatial extent is much less than ε, any statistical fluctuation at (α, β) will be independent of the fluctuations at (γ, δ) except when $\alpha = \gamma$, $\beta = \delta$ since the arrival of a single photon is independent of the arrival any other photon. Since the fluctuations are independent and since $\Delta n(x, y)$ is a zero-mean random variable, we have

$$\langle \Delta n(\alpha, \beta)\, \Delta n(\gamma, \delta)\rangle = \begin{cases} \langle \Delta n(\alpha, \beta)^2\rangle & \text{for } \alpha = \gamma \text{ and } \beta = \delta \\ \langle \Delta n(\alpha, \beta)\rangle \langle \Delta n(\gamma, \delta)\rangle \equiv 0 & \text{for } \alpha \neq \gamma \text{ or } \beta \neq \delta \end{cases} \tag{8-110}$$

Equation (8-109) then becomes

$$\langle \Delta g(\alpha, \beta)\, \Delta g(\gamma, \delta)\rangle = \frac{1}{\varepsilon^4}\langle (\Delta n(\alpha, \beta))^2\rangle\, \delta_{\alpha,\gamma}\delta_{\beta,\delta} \tag{8-111}$$

where

$$\delta_{a,b} = \begin{cases} 0 & \text{for } a \neq b \\ 1 & \text{for } a = b \end{cases} \tag{8-112}$$

Since $n(x, y)$ is Poisson, we have

$$\begin{aligned} \langle (\Delta n(\alpha, \beta))^2\rangle &= \langle (n(\alpha, \beta) - \langle n(\alpha, \beta)\rangle)^2\rangle \\ &= \sigma_n^2 \\ &= \langle n(\alpha, \beta)\rangle \end{aligned} \tag{8-113}$$

Combining Eqs. (8-111) and (8-113) and associating the ε's differently, we have

$$\langle \Delta g(\alpha, \beta)\, \Delta g(\gamma, \delta)\rangle = \frac{\langle n(\alpha, \beta)\rangle}{\varepsilon^2}\, \frac{\delta_{\alpha,\gamma}\delta_{\beta,\delta}}{\varepsilon^2} \tag{8-114}$$

The first term on the right side of Eq. (8-114) is simply $\langle g(\alpha, \beta)\rangle$ and, for ε small, the second term approximates the two-dimensional Dirac delta function $\delta(\alpha - \gamma, \beta - \delta)$. Equation (8-108) then becomes

$$\begin{aligned} \sigma_i^2 &= \iiiint_{-\infty}^{\infty} \langle g(\alpha, \beta)\rangle\, \delta(\alpha - \gamma, \beta - \delta)\, h_2(\alpha - x, \beta - y) \\ &\quad \times h_2^*(\gamma - x, \delta - y)\, d\alpha\, d\beta\, d\gamma\, d\delta \\ &= \iint_{-\infty}^{\infty} \langle g(\alpha, \beta)\rangle\, |h_2(\alpha - x, \beta - y)|^2\, d\alpha\, d\beta \\ &= \langle g(x, y)\rangle ** |h_2(x, y)|^2 \end{aligned} \tag{8-115}$$

The variance is then given by correlating the mean coded image with the squared magnitude of the decoding function. Note that all dependence on the artificially introduced parameter ε has disappeared. In order to see more clearly the dependence of σ_i^2 on the object, we can write

$$\langle g(x, y)\rangle = \left\langle \frac{1}{m_1^2} o\left(-\frac{x}{m_1}, -\frac{y}{m_1}\right)\right\rangle ** h_1(x, y) \tag{8-116}$$

where $m_1 = s_2/s_1$. Combining Eqs. (8-115) and (8-116), we have

$$\sigma_i^2 = \left\langle \frac{1}{m_1^2} o\left(-\frac{x}{m_1}, -\frac{y}{m_1}\right)\right\rangle ** h_1(x, y) ** |h_2(x, y)|^2$$

$$= \left\langle \frac{1}{m_1^2} o\left(-\frac{x}{m_1}, -\frac{y}{m_1}\right)\right\rangle ** k(x, y) \tag{8-117}$$

where

$$k(x, y) = h_1(x, y) ** |h_2(x, y)|^2 \tag{8-118}$$

and $k(x, y)$ is referred to as the noise kernel. The noise kernel is convolved with the inverted object to yield the variance. The convolution with $k(x, y)$ is a mathematical statement of the shadow-overlap argument that began this discussion. This convolution emphasizes the object dependence of the noise, as well as its nonstationarity. It also shows that points in the decoded image where there is no object to be decoded may still contain noise.

The SNR for the decoded image is therefore

$$\text{SNR} = \langle i(x, y)\rangle / \sigma_i(x, y)$$

$$= \frac{\langle o(-x, -y)\rangle ** h_1(x, y) ** h_2(x, y)}{(\langle o(-x, -y)\rangle ** h_1(x, y) ** |h_2(x, y)|^2)^{1/2}} \tag{8-119}$$

In order to get the correct answer from Eq. (8-119), care must be taken in how the functions are normalized. Clearly the units of $h_2(x, y)$ do not matter, as stated previously. The following set of definitions are self-consistent and yield proper results when used in Eq. (8-119):

$$\langle o_t(x, y)\rangle\, dx\, dy = \text{average number of photons/second emitted by an area element located at } (x, y)$$

$$\equiv N_0(x, y)\, dx\, dy \tag{8-120}$$

and

$$h_1(x, y) = \frac{T}{4\pi(s_1 + s_2)^2} h\left(\frac{x}{m_2}, \frac{y}{m_2}\right) \tag{8-121}$$

where T = exposure time, $h(x, y)$ = transmission of the coded aperture, and $m_2 = [(s_1 + s_2)/s_1]$.

Using this formalism, it is easy to understand the noise properties of many apertures, even the pinhole. Suppose the pinhole is a square of width d such that

$$h_1(x, y) = \frac{T}{4\pi(s_1 + s_2)^2} \operatorname{rect}\left(\frac{x}{m_2 d}, \frac{y}{m_2 d}\right) \tag{8-122}$$

where

$$\operatorname{rect}(x/d, y/d) = \begin{cases} 1 & \text{when } |x| \leq d \text{ and } |y| \leq d \\ 0 & \text{otherwise} \end{cases}$$

Assuming perfect detector resolution, the actual recorded image of a point source imaged with a pinhole aperture would be a set of points corresponding to the detected photons. This set of points would be contained within the bounds of the pinhole shadow. The image of the point would then appear to be grainy and to have high-frequency structure that is known to exceed the resolution capability of the pinhole. This high-frequency structure can be removed and the SNR improved if the pinhole image is correlated with a noise-smoothing filter h_2 given by

$$h_2(x, y) = \operatorname{rect}\left(\frac{x}{m_2 d}, \frac{y}{m_2 d}\right) \tag{8-123}$$

This filter is the same size as the pinhole shadow and serves to average the number of detected photons over a single resolution cell. If the resolution is defined as the full width at half maximum of the PSF, this noise-smoothing filter improves the SNR while leaving the resolution unchanged. Since $|h_2(x, y)|^2 = h_2(x, y)$, Eq. (8-119) simplifies to

$$\mathrm{SNR_{ph}} = \left[\left\langle \frac{1}{m_1^2} o\left(-\frac{x}{m_1}, -\frac{y}{m_1}\right) \right\rangle ** h_1(x, y) ** h_2(x, y) \right]^{1/2} \tag{8-124}$$

If we consider a uniform square object with dimensions $b \gg d$ such that

$$\frac{1}{m_1^2} \left\langle o\left(-\frac{x}{m_1}, -\frac{y}{m_1}\right) \right\rangle = \frac{1}{m_1} N_0\left(\frac{x}{m_1}, \frac{y}{m_1}\right) \operatorname{rect}\left(\frac{x}{m_1 b}, \frac{y}{m_1 b}\right) \tag{8-125}$$

where $N_0(x, y) = N_0$, a constant, Eq. (8-124) becomes

$$\mathrm{SNR_{ph}} = \left[\frac{1}{m_1^2} N_0\left(\frac{x}{m_1}, \frac{y}{m_1}\right) \operatorname{rect}\left(\frac{x}{m_1 b}, \frac{y}{m_1 b}\right) \right.$$

$$\left. ** \frac{T}{4\pi(s_1 + s_2)^2} \operatorname{rect}\left(\frac{x}{m_2 d}, \frac{y}{m_2 d}\right) ** \operatorname{rect}\left(\frac{x}{m_2 d}, \frac{y}{m_2 d}\right) \right]^{1/2} \tag{8-126}$$

For object points more than a distance d from the edge of the object, the implied integral involving the three rectangle functions in Eq. (8-126) reduce to the square of the area of the pinhole shadow, yielding

$$\mathrm{SNR}_{\mathrm{ph}} = \left[\frac{(1/m_1^2)\, N_0(x/m_1, y/m_1)\, T m_2^4 d^4}{4\pi(s_1 + s_2)^2} \right]^{1/2} \tag{8-127}$$

Recognizing that $m_2^2 d^2 / 4\pi(s_1 + s_2)^2$ is the geometric collection efficiency of the aperture and that $N_0 T b^2$ is the total number of counts emitted by the object in a time T, we have

$$\mathrm{SNR}_{\mathrm{ph}} = \left\{ \left[N_0\left(\frac{x}{m_1}, \frac{y}{m_1}\right) T b^2 \right] \left(\frac{m_2^2 d^2}{4\pi(s_1 + s_2)^2} \right) \left(\frac{m_2^2 d^2}{m_1^2 b^2} \right) \right\}^{1/2}$$

$$= \left(\frac{N_c}{M} \right)^{1/2} \tag{8-128}$$

where N_c is the total number of collected photons from the entire object and $M = (m_1 b / m_2 d)^2$ is the number of resolution cells of width $m_2 d$ in the magnified image. Equation (8-128) is then just the mathematical restatement of Eq. (8-100).

As a second example of the use of Eq. (8-119), we can calculate the SNR for optically decoded zone-plate images. For a zone-plate transmission function $h_z(x, y)$ with a central-zone radius of r_1 (see Fig. 8-5), the zone-plate shadow is described by

$$h_1(x, y) = \frac{T}{4\pi(s_1 + s_2)^2} h_z\left(\frac{x}{m_2}, \frac{y}{m_2}\right) \tag{8-129}$$

where $m_2 = (s_1 + s_2)/s_1$. The optical decoding operation can be modeled as a convolution of the coded image with the complex exponential in Eq. (8-33) with the parameter d set equal to the value of f_1 in Eq. (8-37) for the appropriate value of r_1. The effective decoding function is then

$$h_2(x, y) = \exp\{i\pi[(x/m_2 r_1)^2 + (y/m_2 r_1)^2]\} \tag{8-130}$$

Sincc

$$|h_2(x, y)|^2 \equiv 1 \tag{8-131}$$

Eqs. (8-129) and (8-130) can be combined with Eq. (8-118) to obtain the noise kernel,

$$k(x, y) = \frac{T}{4\pi(s_1 + s_2)^2} \frac{1}{2} \pi (m_2 r_N)^2 \tag{8-132}$$

where $m_2 r_N$ is the radius of the zone-plate shadow and the factor of $\frac{1}{2}$ is due to the mean transmission of the zone plate. If we again assume a uniform-intensity rectangular object given by Eq. (8-125), the denominator in the SNR expression in Eq. (8-119) becomes

$$\left[\left\langle\frac{1}{m_1^2}o\left(-\frac{x}{m_1},-\frac{y}{m_1}\right)\right\rangle ** k(x,y)\right]^{1/2}$$
$$=\left[\frac{(1/m_1^2)\,N_0(x/m_1,y/m_1)\,Tb^2}{4\pi(s_1+s_2)^2}\frac{1}{2}\pi(m_2r_N)^2\right]^{1/2} \tag{8-133}$$

Since $h_2(x, y)$ rather than $|h_2(x, y)|^2$ appears in the numerator of the SNR expression, evaluation of the numerator is a bit more involved. The details of the calculation can be found in the Appendix at the end of this chapter. The calculation involves using the series expansion of the zone plate given in Eq. (8-70) and recognizing that it is the $m = -1$ term which produces the sharply focused spot of light (i.e., the $+1$ focus of the zone plate), while the other terms result in the unfocused background light. Considering then only the $m = -1$ term as "signal," we can define an effective coded-aperture function

$$h_{1e}(x,y)=\frac{T}{4\pi(s_1+s_2)^2}\frac{i}{\pi}\exp\left\{-i\pi\left[\left(\frac{x}{m_2r_1}\right)^2+\left(\frac{y}{m_2r_1}\right)^2\right]\right\}$$
$$r \le m_2r_N \tag{8-134}$$

Equations (8-130) and (8-134) can be used to obtain the decoded PSF. After some straightforward but rather tedious recombining of terms, the decoded PSF can be shown to be

$$h_{1e}(x,y) ** h_2(x,y)=\frac{T}{4\pi(s_1+s_2)^2}\exp\left\{i\pi\left[\left(\frac{x}{m_2r_1}\right)^2+\left(\frac{y}{m_2r_1}\right)^2\right]\right\}$$
$$\times\left(\frac{i}{\pi}\right)[\pi(m_2r_N)^2]\,p(x,y) \tag{8-135}$$

with

$$p(x,y)=2J_1(2\pi rN^{1/2}/m_2r_1)/(2\pi rN^{1/2}/m_2r_1)$$

where $J_1(x)$ is the first-order Bessel function of the first kind. The function $p(x, y)$ is well known from optics where the square of $p(x, y)$ describes the intensity distribution in the diffraction-limited image of a point source imaged with a lens with a circular aperture. This function has a sharp central peak and some small, circularly symmetric sidelobes. The first zero of $p(x, y)$, which occurs when the argument of the Bessel function is equal to 1.22, determines the radius of the central core r_c:

$$\frac{2\pi r_cN^{1/2}}{m_2r_1}=1.22$$

or

$$r_c = 1.22 m_2 r_1 / 2N^{1/2} \tag{8-136}$$

$$= 1.22 m_2 \Delta r_N \tag{8-137}$$

where the last expression is obtained with the help of Eq. (8-43). The area of the resolution cell, using the Rayleigh criterion, can then be defined as

$$A_c = \pi (r_c/2)^2 = \pi \left(\frac{1.22 m_2 r_1}{4N^{1/2}} \right)^2 \tag{8-138}$$

With the help of Eq. (8-136), it can be shown that the complex exponential in Eq. (8-135) is essentially constant over the region in which $p(x, y)$ has any appreciable values. Neglecting then the complex exponential, the decoded PSF can be convolved with the uniform-intensity rectangular object in Eq. (8-125) with the result

$$\left\langle \frac{1}{m_1^2} o\left(-\frac{x}{m_1}, -\frac{y}{m_1} \right) \right\rangle ** h_{1e}(x, y) ** h_2(x, y)$$

$$= \frac{i}{\pi} \frac{T N_0(x/m_1, y/m_1)}{4\pi (s_1 + s_2)^2} \pi (m_2 r_N)^2 \left[\frac{1}{m_1^2} \frac{4}{\pi} \left(\frac{m_2 r_1}{2N^{1/2}} \right)^2 \right]$$

$$= \left(\frac{4}{1.22\pi} \right)^2 \frac{2i}{\pi} \frac{T N_0(x/m_1, y/m_1)\, b^2}{4\pi (s_1 + s_2)^2} \frac{1}{2} \pi (m_2 r_N)^2 \frac{A_c}{m_1^2 b^2} \tag{8-139}$$

for points away from the edge of the object.

The SNR in the light amplitude in the output plane is then

$$(\mathrm{SNR}_{\mathrm{zp}})_{\mathrm{A}} = \frac{4}{1.22\pi} \frac{2}{\pi} \frac{A_c}{m_1^2 b_2} \left[\frac{N_0(x/m_1, y/m_1)\, T b^2}{4\pi (s_1 + s_2)^2} \frac{1}{2} \pi (m_2 r_N)^2 \right]^{1/2} \tag{8-140}$$

where the imaginary number i has been dropped. However, since intensity and not amplitude is the measured quantity, this is not yet the final answer. Barrett and DeMeester (1974) have shown that recording the intensity rather than the amplitude results in an additional factor which, for $(\mathrm{SNR}_{\mathrm{zp}})_{\mathrm{A}} \gtrsim 5$, approaches the value of $1/2^{1/2}$. The SNR in the intensity pattern is then

$$(\mathrm{SNR}_{\mathrm{zp}})_{\mathrm{I}} = \left(\frac{4}{1.22\pi} \right)^2 \frac{2^{1/2}}{\pi} \frac{A_c}{m_1^2 b^2} \left[\frac{N_0(x/m_1, y/m_1)\, T b^2}{4\pi (s_1 + s_2)^2} \frac{1}{2} \pi (m_2 r_N)^2 \right]^{1/2} \tag{8-141}$$

Recognizing that $m_1^2 b^2$ is the size of the image and that the expression in parentheses is the total number of counts N_c collected by the zone-plate system, we can write Eq. (8-141) as

$$(\mathrm{SNR}_{zp})_1 = \left(\frac{4}{1.22\pi}\right)^2 \frac{2^{1/2}}{\pi} \frac{N_c^{1/2}}{M} \tag{8-142}$$

where $M = m_1^2 b^2 / A_c$ is the number of resolution cells in the decoded image. The numerical factors in Eq. (8-142) is correct for on-axis-zone-plate images decoded by coherent optical processing. The SNR in other cases can still be calculated using the noise-kernel approach. The exact value of the numerical constant will be affected by the presence of halftone screens, by any limits on the processing bandwidth and by decisions about what is to be considered as the signal component. However, in all cases involving the zone plate, the zone-plate SNR falls off as M^{-1} as compared to $M^{-1/2}$ for the pinhole. Equation (8-142) can be written as

$$(\mathrm{SNR}_{zp})_1 = C(N_c/M)^{1/2}/M^{1/2} \tag{8-143}$$

where N_c/M is the number of photons collected from each resolution cell in the object and $C = (4/1.22\pi)^2 (2^{1/2}/\pi) = 0.490$. As the number of resolvable object points is increased, the SNR_{zp} will decrease if the number of collected photons per resolution cell is not increased.

Before quantitative comparisons of various apertures can be made, the basis for comparison must be adequately defined. When comparing SNR's for different apertures, one must be careful about whether the spatial resolution in the decoded image is the same, whether the same object field of view is involved, whether the object radioactivity is the same, and whether the exposure times are the same. Comparisons are usually made by considering the same imaging geometry with only the aperture changed. This is a little unfair to the pinhole since a much smaller portion of the detector will be utilized with a pinhole than with a coded aperture. Assuming a fixed detector size, the object could be moved closer to the pinhole, resulting in increased image magnification and collection efficiency. It may or may not be possible to move the object closer to the pinhole depending on the physical size and shape of the object. Since it is easier to consider the same imaging geometry, that is what is usually done for comparison purposes.

If the same imaging geometry, the same object and object field of view, the same resolution, and the same imaging time are assumed, the ratio of the SNR for the zone plate and the pinhole is given by

$$\frac{(\mathrm{SNR}_{zp})_1}{\mathrm{SNR}_{ph}} = C\left(\frac{N_{czp}}{N_{cph}} \frac{1}{M}\right)^{1/2} \tag{8-144}$$

The ratio N_{czp}/N_{cph} is simply the ratio of the geometric collection efficiencies η_{zp} and η_{ph} which, for the same imaging geometry, is just the ratio of the transparent area of the zone plate to the area of the pinhole, so that

$$\frac{(\mathrm{SNR}_{\mathrm{zp}})_{\mathrm{I}}}{\mathrm{SNR}_{\mathrm{ph}}} = C\left(\frac{\eta_{\mathrm{zp}}}{\eta_{\mathrm{ph}}}\frac{1}{M}\right)^{1/2}$$

$$= C\left(\frac{\frac{1}{2}\pi r_N^2}{\pi r_{\mathrm{ph}}^2}\frac{1}{M}\right)^{1/2} \quad (8\text{-}145)$$

This ratio is plotted in Fig. 8-55 for the case of the on-axis zone plate. The saturation at the left end of the curve occurs when the object becomes smaller than a resolution cell. If the processing bandwidth is limited such that the decoding function $h_2(x, y)$ is zero for $(x^2 + y^2)^{1/2}$ larger than the outer radius of the zone plate, the curve in Fig. 8-55 saturates on the right when the object becomes larger than the zone-plate shadow. This saturation comes as no surprise since it represents the situation where additional object points are so far away that the shadows do not overlap anymore.

Although the required expressions do not lend themselves to a general, closed-form expression, the SNR at the center of a disk object imaged with an annular-coded aperture and decoded with ρ-filtered correlation decod-

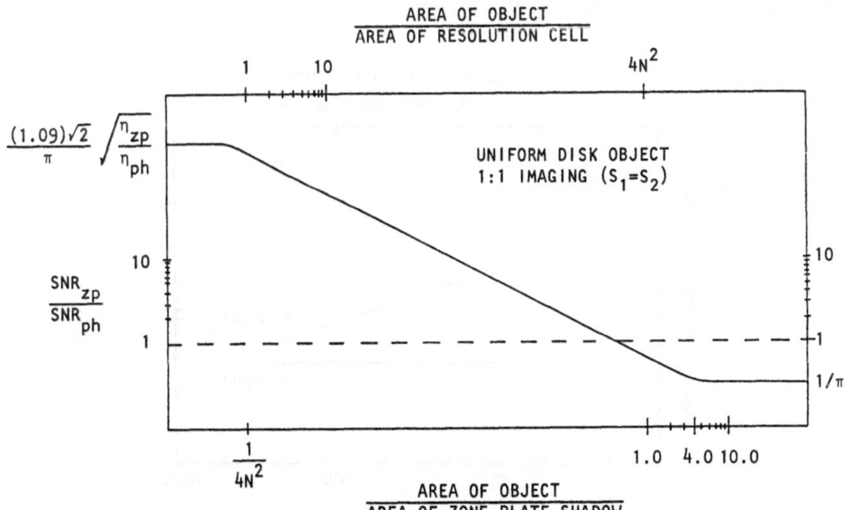

Fig. 8-55. Illustration of the relative SNR advantage of an on-axis Fresnel zone plate compared to a pinhole with the same resolution, exposure time and imaging geometry. Optical decoding is assumed. The log–log plot of SNR advantage vs. number of resolution cells in a variable radius, uniform-intensity disk object is intended to show the qualitative features. The exact curve will depend on N, the number of zones in the zone plate. The slope of $-\frac{1}{2}$ is independent of N. (Note: This illustration appeared in Barrett and DeMeester, 1974, with the slope incorrectly labeled -1.)

ing has been calculated numerically (Simpson 1976). The SNR's for an annulus and a pinhole with the same resolution, object, object field, exposure time, and imaging geometry are shown in Fig. 8-56 as a function of object radius and M. Note that the slope is different than for a zone plate since the amount of overlap is different. The annulus SNR becomes approximately the same as the pinhole just as the glitch begins to interfere with the reconstruction at the center of the disk. The glitch will already have overlapped the rest of the object by then. As long as the object is smaller than the glitch-limited field of view, the SNR will be better for the annulus than for a comparable pinhole.

Different apertures can also be compared in terms of some other important clinical parameters. If SNR is used as a measure of image quality, apertures can be compared based either on the exposure time necessary to collect the required number of photons or on the patient dose needed to produce the required number of photons in a given amount of time. As an example, the data in Fig. 8-56 were used to create the curve shown in Fig. 8-57. This is a plot of relative exposure time for the annulus compared to a pinhole where resolution, object, object field of view, SNR, and imaging geometry are all held fixed. The relative exposure time approaches 1 as the number of resolution cells in the object increases since more counts are needed to maintain the annulus SNR.

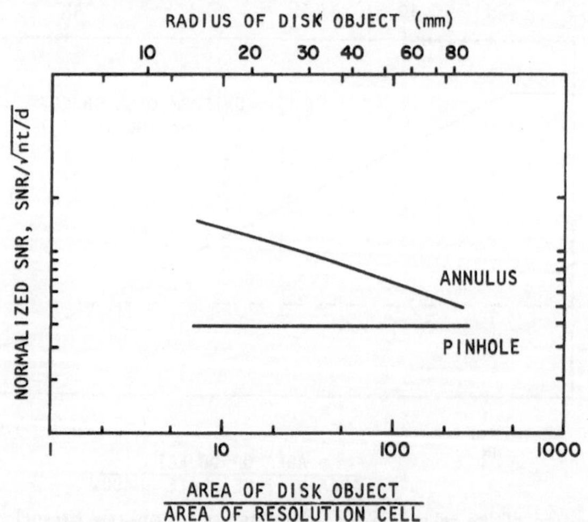

Fig. 8-56. SNR for a pinhole system and an annular-aperture system as a function of object size. The two systems use the same recording geometry and the final images have the same resolution. The annular shadow has a mean radius of 58 mm. The object is a uniform disk of variable radius and the SNR is calculated at the center of the disk. The SNR is normalized by n, the activity per unit area of the object, by t, the exposure time, and by d, the object-to-detector distance.

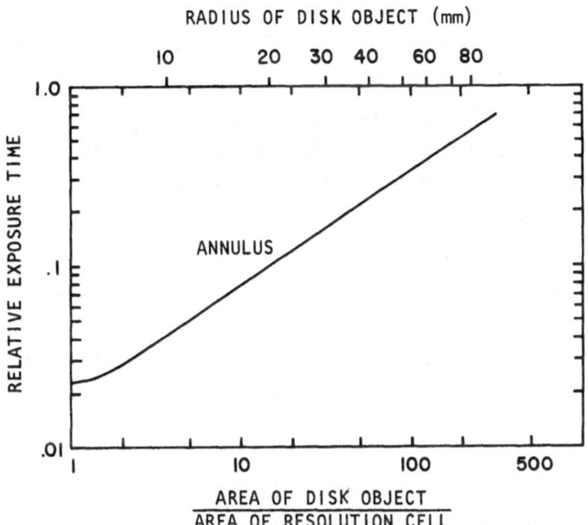

Fig. 8.57. Relative exposure time required for the annular-aperture system to produce the same SNR as the pinhole system, as a function of object size. Same physical constraints as in Fig. 8-56.

One last observation should be made about the SNR expression in Eq. (8-119) before closing this section. Several apertures discussed earlier in this chapter showed better sidelobe or background behavior when $h_2(x, y)$ was a function with values of $+1$ and -1. Changing from a zero–one decoding function to such a bipolar function improves the imaging properties of the system by suppressing sidelobes but it does not increase the peak value of the correlation. The useful image signal therefore remains the same. However, the noise does change since $|h_2(x, y)|^2$ becomes a constant over the aperture, resulting approximately in a $2^{1/2}$ increase in the noise for an aperture that is 50% transparent. In order to achieve the same SNR, the exposure time must be doubled to counteract the increased noise. In the case of the complementary zone plates, this doubled exposure time can be considered to be divided up between the two recorded images. It is also very important that Eq. (8-119) not be used blindly with regard to $h_1(x, y)$. Equation (8-119) is valid only for $h_1(x, y) \geq 0$. If $h_1(x, y)$ is made into a bipolar function by subtracting two coded images, as in the case of the complementary zone plates, $|h_1(x, y)|$ should be used instead.

8.8. SUMMARY

In view of the diversity of encoding and decoding schemes employed in the coded-aperture systems described in this chapter, it seems appropriate to end the chapter with a review of the features that are common to coded-aperture systems in general and a summary of the specific features of the various coded-aperture systems. The common features are important in determining whether a coded-aperture system of any kind is appropriate for a certain application, while system-specific features are important in the selection of an appropriate coded-aperture system.

Coded-aperture systems are shadow-casting imaging devices. They are useful in situations in which conventional refractive or reflective imaging devices are either unavailable or limited in performance—most notably in the X-ray and γ-ray portion of the spectrum. One feature common to all coded-aperture systems is increased collection efficiency compared to a pinhole or collimator with the same resolution as the decoded image. In applications such as nuclear-medicine imagery where the statistical quality of the image improves as more photons are collected, this is an important feature. In order to increase the collection efficiency, the resolution in the recorded image is intentionally degraded in such a way that the recorded image can be processed to recover the lost resolution. All coded-aperture systems therefore involve the detection of a coded image which must be decoded before a recognizable image of the object is obtained. This decoding is an essential part of any coded-aperture system; it is not an optional enhancement process. The decoding generally consists of a correlation operation which is a variant of matched filtering. The decoding operation serves to gather up the detected photons due to a single object point and compact them into the correlation peak. In this way, resolution is recovered and the increased collection efficiency improves the SNR. In order for spatial-correlation decoding (as opposed to temporal-correlation decoding) to work properly, the detection system must be free of geometrical distortions. Correct decoding also requires a linear detector which produces an output directly proportional to the number of arriving photons. This is especially true for large objects where a single detector element may be receiving photons from a large number of object points.

The fact that photons from a single object point are distributed over a large region of the detector results in some behavior not encountered in conventional pinhole or collimator imaging. Since two object points which may be easily resolvable after decoding can have aperture shadows which overlap substantially, one has to be aware of potential sidelobe problems as well as more complicated noise effects. The sidelobe problem is a deterministic feature that is dependent on the particular aperture and decoding method used. While the exact description of the noise in the decoded image is also aperture dependent, a few general comments can be made based on a function called the noise kernel which results from efforts to introduce mathematical precision into the shadow overlap argument. The noise kernel indicates how random fluctuations in the number of photons detected for a particular object point will affect the noise at all locations in the decoded image. Since the noise kernel is defined (see Section 8.7) as the correlation of the aperture shadow with the squared modulus of the decoding function, both positive-valued functions, the noise kernel is a broad, smooth, positive-valued function. If one defines the noise field as the convolution of the object with the broad, positive-valued noise kernel, it is clear that the noise at any location will increase as the object size increases. This general behavior is common to all coded-aperture systems. Because the noise kernel can be quite broad, noise from a particular object point can affect the noise at an image location that is quite distant from the actual object point. Because of this global influence on the noise in the decoded image, photon fluctuations associated with a particular object point can even produce noise in a region of the coded image in which no object points exist. For these reasons, coded-aperture systems work best for small, bright objects rather than dark objects in a large, bright background. The exact noise behavior will depend on the aperture, the decoding function, and the object distribution.

Even though the SNR advantage of a coded-aperture system diminishes as the size of the object increases, the coded-aperture system still possesses a feature not available with a pinhole or collimator. Through sensitivity to the scale of the aperture shadow in systems using spatial encoding or though parallax information in systems employing temporal encoding, coded-aperture systems are capable of producing tomographic views of the object. These tomographic images contain an in-focus image of one object plane and out-of-focus images of other object planes. The depth resolution that results is an important and useful feature. In all cases, the depth resolution becomes better as the angle subtended from an object point by the coded aperture increases. The exact behavior of out-of-focus planes depends on the object as well as the particular aperture and decoding algorithm. One must be aware of possible artifacts due to out-of-focus object planes when viewing a decoded image. Recent work such as that of Chang and Macdonald (Chang, 1976) has raised hopes of recovering images relatively free from out-of-focus contributions. Further advances in this area are anxiously awaited.

The major features of the various coded-aperture systems discussed in this chapter, as well as a few related systems, are summarized in Tables 8-1 and 8-2. The apertures have been divided into two classes: those that are essentially 50% transparent and those that are considerably less than 50% transparent. The first type is referred to as a filled aperture, while the second type is called a dilute aperture. Although dilute apertures have smaller collection efficiencies, they also have less shadow overlap with extended objects. As a result, objects containing more than a few resolvable points can often be imaged as effectively with a dilute aperture as with a filled aperture when noise arguments are considered. The diminished count

Table 8-1. Filled Coded-Aperture Systems

Aperture	Detector	Decoding method	In-focus PSF sidelobes	Limits on object size	Comments	References
On-axis zone plate	Anger camera detector system	Coherent-optical decoding	Sidelobes present due to dc and other diffraction orders	Limited by loss of contrast in image due to PSF sidelobes	Any tomographic plane can be immediately viewed by making a simple mechanical adjustment in the decoding system. Beware of coherent artifacts.	Barrett, 1972b Barrett and Horrigan, 1973 Barrett *et al.*, 1973a,b Rogers *et al.*, 1972 Rogers *et al.*, 1973 Tipton *et al.*, 1973 Tipton *et al.*, 1974
	Anger camera detector system	Coherent-optical matched filtering			A frequency-plane filter must be generated and placed in the Fourier plane of a coherent-optical system.	Gaskill *et al.*, 1972 Whitehead, 1976
	Anger camera detector system or multiwire proportional counters	Digital decoding that imitates optical decoding	Same sort of sidelobes as for optical decoding	Same as coherent optical decoding	Decoding algorithm must be executed for each tomographic plane.	Macdonald *et al.*, 1974 Budinger and Macdonald, 1975 Dance *et al.*, 1975 Wilson *et al.*, 1975
	Anger camera detector system	Digital matched filter	Sidelobes resemble a triangle function; largest sidelobe is approximately one-half of correlation peak	Large sidelobes reduce contrast rapidly as the size of the object increases	Decoding algorithm must be executed for each tomographic plane.	Dance *et al.*, 1975 Wilson *et al.*, 1975

	Anger camera detector system	Digital correlation with bipolar zone plate	Quite small	Limited by size of detector and/or digital-data-handling capabilities	Decoding algorithm must be executed for each tomographic plane. Bipolar decoding function improves sidelobe behavior relative to matched-filter decoding but introduces additional noise in the reconstruction of multiple point objects. Out-of-focus planes are major source of image degradation.	Dance *et al.*, 1975 Wilson *et al.*, 1975
Multiple on-axis zone plates	Anger camera detector system	Grid-coded subtraction	Small	Limited by size of detector	Object must remain unchanged during multiple exposures. Dynamic studies not possible Out-of-focus planes affect final image quality.	Barrett *et al.*, 1974
	Multiwire proportional counters	Digital decoding that imitates optical decoding	Small	Limited by size of detector and/or digital-data-handling capabilities	Object must remain unchanged during multiple exposures. Dynamic studies not possible Out-of-focus planes affect final image quality. Decoding algorithm must be executed for each tomographic plane.	Macdonald *et al.*, 1974 Chang, 1976
Off-axis zone plate	Film	Coherent-optical decoding	Small	Limited by size of detector	Halftone screen necessary. Film must be used to resolve fine structure in coded image Low quantum efficiency of film erodes collection-efficiency advantage. Selection of the in-focus tomographic plane possible with simple mechanical adjustment to the decoding optical system.	Barrett, 1972a,b Barrett *et al.*, 1972 Barrett and Horrigan, 1973 Rogers, 1973 Barrett *et al.*, 1973a, b Jaszczak *et al.*, 1974 Guha, 1976

continued overleaf

Table 8-1. (continued)

Aperture	Detector	Decoding method	In-focus PSF sidelobes	Limits on object size	Comments	References
Random pinhole array	Film	Matched filtering (optical or digital)	Triangular-shaped sidelobes with fluctuations about a mean sidelobe level	Limited by size of detector	Sidelobes produce a signal-dependent background which destroys contrast in large-object reconstructions just as with Fresnel zone plate.	Dicke, 1968 Stroke *et al.*, 1969 Hayat, 1971 Groh *et al.*, 1972 Brown, 1972 Brown, 1974
	Film	Correlation of bipolar pinhole array with coded image	Sidelobes have zero mean but contain fluctuations which depend on the aperture realization	Limited by detector size	Large number of pinholes required to obtain smooth sidelobes. Anger camera incapable of resolving a large number of small pinholes. While bipolar decoding function eliminates sidelobes, it also introduces extra noise. Tomographic performance difficult to predict in general.	Brown, 1972 Brown, 1974 Fenimore and Cannon, 1978
Uniformly redundant pinhole array	Film	Cyclic correlation of aperture code with coded image	Uniform	Number of resolution cells in object must be less than the number of elements in the aperture code	Uniformity of background dependent on sharp edges in recorded pinhole shadow. If decoding is done digitally, sampling rate will also affect the apparent sharpness of the shadow edges. Resolution of Anger camera too poor for use with this aperture. Aperture can be as large as as the detector.	Fenimore and Cannon, 1978

Table 8-2. Dilute Coded-Aperture Systems

Aperture	Detector	Decoding method	In-focus PSF sidelobes	Limits on object size	Comments	References
Single annulus	Anger camera detector system	Analog electronic matched filtering	Sidelobes with $1/r$ behavior	PSF sidelobes severely degrade contrast for non-point objects	Count rates with an annulus are smaller than with a zone plate. The annulus is a better match for the count-rate capabilities of the Anger camera detector system.	Walton, 1973
		Digital matched filter combined with ρ-filter	Glitch at $2\bar{r}$	Object size-limited by glitch. Largest glitch-free field is limited by the size of the detector	Count rates with an annulus are smaller than with a zone plate. The annulus is a better match for the count-rate capabilities of the Anger camera detector system.	Simpson, *et al.*, 1975
Two annuli	Anger camera detector system	Frequency-plane combination of two coded images	None	Limited by size of detector and by out-of-focus glitch	Works very well for planar objects. Glitch reappears as object point goes out of focus	Simpson, 1976 Simpson *et al.*, 1976
Nonredundant pinhole arrays	Anger camera detector system or multiwire proportional counter or film	Matched filtering	Although peak-to-sidelobe ratio is maximum, sidelobes are still present and degrade the contrast	Limited by size of detector and minimum acceptable contrast	Since aperture is dilute it is well suited for use with Anger camera detector system.	Wouters *et al.*, 1973 Chang *et al.*, 1974 Weiss, 1975
		Matched filtering and background subtraction algorithm	Sidelobes well removed by background-subtraction algorithm	Limited by size of detector	Accurate knowledge of the PSF necessary for success of background-subtraction algorithm.	Tipton *et al.*, 1976 Dowdy *et al.*, 1977
One-dimensional zone plate	X-ray image intensifier	Cross-correlation with $\sin \alpha r^2$ and use of background-	Sidelobes well removed by background-subtraction	Limited by size of detector	Accurate knowledge of the PSF necessary for success of background-subtraction.	Simpson *et al.*, 1977

continued overleaf

Table 8-2. (continued)

Aperture	Detector	Decoding method	In-focus PSF sidelobes	Limits on object size	Comments	References
		subtraction algorithm	algorithm		algorithm. Present background-subtraction algorithm has difficulty with objects wider than the central zone of the zone plate. Presence of out-of-focus planes impedes background-subtraction algorithm. Aperture is dilute in one direction, filled in the other. Very good for long, thin objects such as nuclear-reactor fuel pins.	
One-dimensional off-axis zone plate	Anger camera detector system	Electronically filtered with acoustic delay line	Small	Limited by size of detector	System behaves as a coded-aperture system in one direction and as a pinhole in the other. One-dimensional decoding recovers the image.	Barrett 1972a
Sequential pinhole	Multiwire proportional counter	A series of tomograms are produced and used in a frequency-domain algorithm involving matrix inversions	None	Limited by detector size and/or maximum pinhole spacing	Strictly speaking, this system is not a coded-aperture system but a tomographic system. dc component in reconstruction must be introduced artificially.	Macdonald *et al.*, 1975 Chang, 1976

Time-varying, cyclically permuted multiple-pinhole aperture	Anger camera detector system	Temporal correlation with cyclically repeated decoding function. Decoded images from several detector points are combined to provide tomographic information	None	Limited by size of detector	Object point can have a shadow which falls partly off the detector. Only the out-of-focus behavior will be affected. Small objects can be imaged with a filled aperture while large objects are imaged better with a dilute aperture. Smoothness of out-of-focus PSF depends on number and location of detector elements.	Akcasu *et al.*, 1974 May, 1974 May *et al.*, 1974 Koral *et al.*, 1975 Gottlieb, 1968
Frequency-modulated, dilute multiple-pinhole aperture	Anger camera detector system	Temporal-frequency analysis of the detector output as a function of time	None	Limited by size of detector	The arrival time of each photon must be recorded as well as its position and the phase of pinhole-modulating device. Set of nontomographic pinhole images is produced and can be combined to provide tomographic resolution thanks to parallax information.	Macovski, 1974
Rotating slit	Anger camera detector system	Coded images formed at discrete slit orientations. Each coded image is averaged in the slit direction	None	Limited by the size of the detector	If rotation axis passes through through the slit, system is nontomographic. Each of the coded images must be averaged before they are added or SNR will be worse than for a comparable pinhole.	Tanaka and Inuma, 1975 Miller, 1976

rate with dilute apertures may be important when selecting a detector system to record the coded image.

Several features that are common to all coded-aperture systems are listed in separate columns in the tables. The column labeled "Detector" is intended to indicate the detector that has been most commonly used with that particular aperture. Any particular detector requirements will be found in the Comments column. The Comments column also contains notes about special features, performance, or limitations associated with a particular aperture. The References column is intended to indicate sources where a particular aperture and decoding method are discussed. No claims as to the completeness of this list are made or implied.

It should be clear at this point that a large number of coding and decoding schemes have been extensively investigated. In spite of all this effort, no single system has proven itself as *the* system. Acceptable images have been obtained with a number of systems. The best system for any particular application will depend strongly on the actual object distribution. A particularly good example of this is the one-dimensional zone-plate aperture used to image nuclear fuel pins.

Although imaging times for large objects are often as long as the time required with conventional collimators or pinholes, the possibility of recovering accurate three-dimensional information about the object is a very attractive feature of coded-aperture systems. This particular capability alone will probably ensure that coded-apertures will receive further attention and hopefully result in a useful clinical imaging device.

APPENDIX. DERIVATION OF THE POINT SPREAD FUNCTION FOR ZONE–PLATE IMAGING

In this Appendix we present a derivation of Eq. (8-135) in the text. Basically, we must calculate the cross-correlation integral between the effective coded-aperture function $h_{1e}(x, y)$ given by Eq. (8-134) and the decoding function appropriate to coherent optical decoding, viz., $h_2(x, y)$ as given by Eq. (8-130).

The integral is most easily performed in polar coordinates. Let $\mathbf{r}$ be the two-dimensional vector with Cartesian coordinates (x, y) and polar coordinates (r, θ), and let $\mathbf{r}'$ be the vector with coordinates (x', y') or (r', θ'). The desired integral may then be written

$$h_{1e} \star\star h_2 = \int_0^{m_2 r_N} r' dr' \int_0^{2\pi} d\theta' h_{1e}(\mathbf{r}') h_2(\mathbf{r}' + \mathbf{r}) \qquad (8.A\text{-}1)$$

Substituting in the explicit forms for h_{1e} and h_2, we find

$$h_{1e} ** h_2 = \frac{i}{\pi} \frac{T}{4\pi(s_1 + s_2)^2} \int_0^{m_2 r_N} r'\,dr' \int_0^{2\pi} d\theta' \exp[-i\pi r'^2/(m_2 r_1)^2] \times \exp[i\pi|\mathbf{r}' + \mathbf{r}|^2/(m_2 r_1)^2] \tag{8.A-2}$$

But $|\mathbf{r}' + \mathbf{r}|^2$ may be expanded in polar coordinates as

$$|\mathbf{r}' + \mathbf{r}|^2 = r^2 + (r')^2 + 2rr' \cos(\theta - \theta') \tag{8.A-3}$$

Equation (8.A-2) then becomes

$$h_{1_e} ** h_2 = \frac{i}{\pi} \frac{T}{4\pi(s_1 + s_2)^2} \exp[i\pi r^2/(m_2 r_1)^2]\, I \tag{8.A-4}$$

where

$$I \equiv \int_0^{m_2 r_N} r'\,dr' \int_0^{2\pi} d\theta' \exp[i2\pi r r' \cos(\theta - \theta')/(m_2 r_1)^2] \tag{8.A-5}$$

Note that the terms in the exponent proportional to r'^2 have canceled. Had we chosen a different term in the expansion for the zone-plate transmission function, rather than $m = -1$, then this cancellation would not have occurred. The integrand would then have exhibited large oscillations and the resulting integral would have been very small. This argument is the justification for replacing h_1 by h_{1e} at the stage of Eq. (8-134) in the text.

It might seem that the same reasoning could be applied to the integrand in Eq. (8.A-5). It is still an oscillatory function of r', and the integral should still have a small value. This is indeed the case *except* when r is very small. In that case, the exponential is near zero for all values of r', and a large integral is obtained. In other words, the PSF is sharply peaked near $r = 0$.

To make this discussion more precise, we must explicitly evaluate I. The θ' integral may be recognized as an integral representation of the zero-order Bessel function, i.e.,

$$J_0(\alpha) = \frac{1}{2\pi} \int_0^{2\pi} e^{i\alpha \cos\varphi}\, d\varphi \tag{8.A-6}$$

This form jibes with Eq. (8.A-5) if we set $\varphi = \theta - \theta'$ and $\alpha = 2\pi r r'/(m_2 r_1)^2$. We then have

$$I = 2\pi \int_0^{m_2 r_N} r'\,dr' J_0[2\pi r r'/(m_2 r_1)^2] \tag{8.A-7}$$

The r' integral is also a well-known one in the theory of Bessel functions:

$$\int_0^z J_0(t)\, t\, dt = z J_1(z) \tag{8.A-8}$$

Our final result is therefore

$$I = \pi r_N^2 m_2^2 \frac{2J_1(2\pi r r_N/m_2 r_1^2)}{2\pi r r_N/m_2 r_1^2} \tag{8.A-9}$$

which agrees with Eq. (8-135) if we simply recognize that $r_N = r_1 N^{1/2}$.

REFERENCES

Abels, J.G. (1968), Fourier transform photography: A new method for X-ray astronomy, *Proc. Astron. Soc. Austr.* **1**:172.

Akcasu, A.Z., May, R.S., Knoll, G.F., Rogers, W.L., Koral, K.F., and Jones, L.W. (1974), Coded aperture gamma ray imaging with stochastic apertures, *Opt. Eng.* **13**:117.

Barrett, H.H. (1972a), Pulse compression techniques in nuclear medicine, *Proc. IEEE* **60**:723.

Barrett, H.H. (1972b), Fresnel zone plate imaging in nuclear medicine, *J. Nucl. Med.* **13**:382.

Barrett, H.H., and DeMeester, G.D. (1974), Quantum noise in fresnel zone plate imaging, *Appl. Opt.* **13**:1100.

Barrett, H.H., and Horrigan, F.A. (1973), Fresnel zone plate imaging of gamma rays; Theory, *Appl. Opt.* **12**:2686.

Barrett, H.H., and Swindell, W. (1977), Analog reconstruction methods for transaxial tomography, *Proc. IEEE* **65**:89.

Barrett, H.H., Wilson, D.T., and DeMeester, G.D. (1972), The use of half-tone screens in Fresnel zone plate imaging of incoherent sources, *Opt. Commun.* **5**:398.

Barrett, H.H., DeMeester, G.D., Wilson, D.T., and Farmelant, M.H. (1973a), Recent advances in Fresnel zone plate imaging, in *Medical Radioisotope Scintigraphy 1972*, Vol. I, International Atomic Energy Agency, Vienna.

Barrett, H.H., Wilson, D.T., DeMeester, G.H., and Sharfman, H. (1973b), Fresnel zone plate imaging in radiology and nuclear medicine, *Opt. Eng.* **12**:8.

Barrett, H.H., Stoner, W.W., Wilson, D.T., and DeMeester, G.D. (1974), Coded apertures derived from the Fresnel zone plate, *Opt. Eng.* **13**:539.

Born, M., and Wolf, E. (1975), *Principles of Optics*, Pergamon Press, New York.

Bracewell, R. (1965), The Fourier transform and its applications, McGraw-Hill, New York.

Brown, C.M. (1972), Multiplex imaging and random arrays, Ph.D. dissertation, University of Chicago.

Brown, C.M. (1974), Multiplex imaging with multiple-pinhole cameras, *J. Appl. Phys.* **45**:4.

Budinger, T.F., and Macdonald, B. (1975), Reconstruction of Fresnel coded gamma camera images by digital computer, *J. Nucl. Med.* **16**:309.

Burckhardt, C.B., and Doherty, E.T. (1968), Formation of carrier frequency holograms with an on-axis reference beam, *Appl. Opt.* **7**:1191.

Calabro, D., and Wolf, J.K. (1968), On the synthesis of two-dimensional arrays with desirable correlation properties, *Inf. Control* **11**:537.

Chang, L.T. (1976), Radionuclide imaging with coded apertures and three-dimensional image reconstruction from focal-plane tomography, Ph.D. thesis, University of California Berkeley.

Chang, L.T., Kaplan, S.N., Macdonald, B., Perez-Mendez, V., and Shiraishi, L. (1974), A method of tomographic imaging using a multiple pinhole-coded aperture, *J. Nucl. Med.* **15**:1063.

Dance, D.R., Wilson, B.C., and Parker, R.P. (1975), Digital reconstruction of point sources imaged by a zone plate camera, *Phys. Med. Biol.* **20**:747.

Davenport, W.B., Jr., and Root, W.L. (1958), An introduction to the theory of random signals and noise, McGraw-Hill, New York.

Dicke, R.H. (1968), Scatter-hole cameras for X-rays and gamma rays, *Astrophys. J.* **153**:L101.

Dowdy, J.E., Tipton, M.D., Murry, R.C., and Stokely, E.M. (1977), Coded apertures for nuclear medicine imaging, *Appl. Radiol.* **6**(4): 145 (July–Aug.).

Farmelant, M.H., DeMeester, G.D., Wilson, D., and Barrett, H. (1975), Initial clinical experiences with a Fresnel zone plate imager, *J. Nucl. Med.* **16**:183.

Fenimore, E.E., and Cannon, T.M. (1978), Coded aperture imaging with uniformly redundant arrays, *Appl. Opt.* **17**:337.

Gaskill, J.D. (1978), *Linear Systems, Fourier Transforms, and Optics*, Wiley, New York.

Gaskill, J.D., Whitehead, F.R., Gray, J.E., and O'Mara, R.E. (1972), Matched filter restoration of coded gamma and X-ray imagery, *Proceedings of the SPIE*, Vol. 35, November 29–30, *Chicago, 1972, SPIE*, Redondo Beach, Cal., p. 193.

Girard, A. (1963), Spectromètre à Grilles, *Appl. Opt.* **2**:79.

Golay, M.J.E. (1949), Multislit spectrometry, *J. Opt. Soc. Am.* **39**:437.

Golay, M.J.E. (1951), Static multislit spectrometry and its application to the panoramic display of infrared spectra, *J. Opt. Soc. Am.* **41**:468.

Golay, M.J.E. (1971), Point arrays having compact, nonredundant autocorrelations, *J. Opt. Soc. Am.* **61**:272.

Gottlieb, P. (1968), A television scanning scheme for a detector-noise-limited system, *IEEE Trans. Inf. Theory* **IT14**:428.

Groh, G., Hayat, G.S., and Stroke, G.W. (1972), X-ray and gamma-ray imaging with multiple-pinhole cameras using *a posteriori* image synthesis, *Appl. Opt.* **11**:931.

Guha, D.K. (1976), Imaging by shadow casting, Ph.D. dissertation, University of Rhode Island.

Harwitt, M. (1971), Spectrometric imager, *Appl. Opt.* **10**:1415.

Hayat, G.S. (1971), X-Ray and γ-ray imaging with multiple-pinhole cameras, Ph.D. thesis, SUNY Stony Brook, New York.

Jaszczak, R.J., Moore, F.E., and Whitehead, F.R. (1974), Use of an array of three off-axis zone plates for large field of view gamma-ray imaging, in *Proceedings of the SPIE Seminar on Application of Optical Instrumentation in Medicine II, Chicago, 1974.*

Klauder, J.R., Price, A.C., Darlingtin, D., and Ablersheim, W.J. (1960), The theory and design of chirp radars, *Bell Syst. Tech. J.* **39**:745.

Koral, K.F., Rogers, W.L., and Knoll, G.F. (1975), Digital tomographic imaging with a time-modulated pseudorandom coded aperture and an Anger camera, *J. Nucl. Med.* **16**:402.

Koral, K.F., Knoll, G.F., and Rogers, W.L. (1977), Emission tomography with time-coded apertures, in *A Review of Information Processing in Medical Imaging, Proceedings of the Fifth International Conference, Nashville, Tennessee, Vanderbilt University, 1977* (A.B. Brill, P.R. Price, W.J. McClain, and M.W. Lindsay, eds.), pp. 252–265.

Koral, K.F., Freitas, J.E., Rogers, W.L., and Keyes, J.W., Jr. (1979), Thyroid scintigraphy with time-coded aperture, *J. Nucl. Med.* **20**:345–349.

Lindner, J. (1975), Binary sequences up to length 40 with best possible autocorrelation function, *Electron. Lett.* **11**:507.

Macdonald, B., Chang, L.T., Perez-Mendez, V., and Shiraishi, L. (1974), Gamma-ray imaging using a Fresnel zone plate aperture, multiwire proportional chamber detector, and computer reconstruction, *IEEE Trans. Nucl. Sci.* **21**:672.

Macdonald, B., Chang, L.T., and Perez-Mendez, V. (1975), Three dimensional image reconstruction using pinhole arrays, in *International Optical Computing Conference, Washington, D.C., April 23–25, 1975.*

Macovski, A. (1974), Gamma-ray imaging system using modulated apertures, *Phys. Med. Biol.* **19**:523.

MacWilliams, F.J., and Sloane, N.J.A. (1976), Pseudo-random sequences and arrays, *Proc. IEEE* **64**:1715.

May, R.S. (1974), Stochastic aperture techniques in gamma-ray image formation, Ph.D. thesis, University of Michigan.

May, R.S., Akcasu, Z., and Knoll, G.F. (1974), Gamma ray imaging with stochastic apertures, *Appl. Opt.* **13**:2589.

Mertz, L. (1965), *Transformations in Optics*, Wiley, New York.

Mertz, L., and Young, N.O. (1961), Fresnel transformation of images, in *Proceedings of the International Conference on Optical Instruments*, Chapman and Hall, London, p.305.

Metz, C.E. (1969), A mathematical investigation of radioisotope scan image processing, Ph.D. dissertation, University of Pennsylvania.

Metz, C.E., and Beck, R.N. (1974), Quantitative effects of stationary linear image processing on noise and resolution of structure in radionuclide images, *J. Nucl. Med.* **15**:164.

Miller, E. (1976), Aperture coding with a rotating slit, in *Program of the Optical Society of America Annual Meeting, Tucson, Arizona,* October 1976, American Institute of Physics, New York.

Moffat, A.T. (1968), Minimum-redundancy linear arrays, *IEEE Trans. Antennas Propag.* **AP-16**:172.

Papoulis, A. (1962), The Fourier integral and its applications, McGraw-Hill, New York.

Pennington, K.S., Will, P.M., and Shelton, G.L. (1970), Grid coding: A technique for extraction of differences from scenes, *Opt. Commun.* **2**:113.

Rogers, W.L., Han, K.S., Jones, L.W., and Beierwaltes, W.H. (1972), Application of a Fresnel zone plate to gamma-ray imaging, *J. Nucl. Med.* **13**:612.

Rogers, W.L., Jones, L.W., and Beierwaltes, W.H. (1973), Imaging in nuclear medicine with incoherent holography, *Opt. Eng.* **12**:13.

Simpson, R.G. (1976), Decoding of annular coded aperture images, in *Program of the Optical Society of America Annual Meeting, Tucson, Arizona*. October 1976, American Institute of Physics, New York.

Simpson, R.G., Barrett, H.H., Subach, J.A., and Fisher, H.D. (1975), Digital processing of annular coded aperture imagery, *Opt. Eng.* **14**:490.

Simpson, R.G., Barrett, H.H., and Fisher, H.D. (1976). Decoding techniques for use with annular coded apertures, in International Conference on Applications of Holography and Optical Data Processing, Jerusalem, Israel, Aug. 23–26, 1976.

Simpson, R.G., Barrett, H.H., Kelly, J.G., and Stalker, K.T. (1977), Some applications of one-dimensional coded apertures, in *Proceedings of the SPIE, X-Ray Imaging*. Vol. 106, p. 71.

Stroke, G.W., Hayat, G.S., Hoover, R.B., and Underwood, J.H. (1969), X-ray imaging with multiple pinhole cameras using *a posteriori* holographic image synthesis, *Opt. Commun.* **1**:138.

Tamura, P. (1976), private communication.

Tanaka, E., and Iinuma, T.A. (1975), Image processing for coded aperture imaging and an attempt at rotating slit imaging, in *Information Processing in Scintigraphy* (C. Raynaud and A. Todd-Pokropek, eds.), Commissariat à l'Energie Atomique, Orsay, France.

Tipton, M.D., Dowdy, J.E., and Caulfield, H.J. (1973), Coded aperture imaging with on-axis Fresnel zone plates, *Opt. Eng.* **12**:166.

Tipton, M.D., Dowdy, J.E., Bonte, F.J., and Caulfield, H.J. (1974), Coded aperture imaging using on-axis Fresnel zone plates and extended gamma-ray sources, *Radiology* **112**:155.

Tipton, M.D., Dowdy, J.D., and Stokely, E.M. (1976), Background suppression of multiple pinhole-coded aperture scintigrams, in 4th International Conference on Medical Physics, Sponsored by AAPM, Ottawa, Canada, July 1976.

Walton, P.W. (1973), An aperture imaging system with instant decoding and tomographic capabilities, *J. Nucl. Med.* **14**:861.

Weiss, H. (1975), Nonredundant point distribution for coded aperture imaging with application to 3-dimensional online X-ray information retrieving, *IEEE Trans. Comp.* **24:**391–394.

Whitehead, F.R. (1976), A comparison of coded aperture imaging systems containing zone plate and random-phase code functions, Ph.D. dissertation, University of Arizona.

Wilson, D.T., Barrett, H.H., DeMeester, G.D., and Farmelant, M.H. (1973), Point source artifacts in Fresnel zone plate imaging, *Opt. Eng.* **12:**133.

Wilson, B.C., Parker, R.P., and Dance, D.R. (1975), Digital processing of images from a zone plate camera, *Phys. Med. Biol.* **20:**757.

Wouters, A., Simon, K.M., and Hirschberg, J.G. (1973), Direct method of decoding multiple images, *Appl. Opt.* **12:**1871.

Young, N.O. (1963), Photography without lenses or mirrors, *Sky Telescope* **25:**8.

CHAPTER 9

Diagnostic Uses of Ultrasonic Imaging

KAI HABER

9.1. HISTORICAL PERSPECTIVE

Man is a latecomer on the scene of application of ultrasonics to biological problems. This form of energy has been used for millions of years for purposes of orientation within the environment. This process, termed "echolocation", has been adapted to both the aerial and aquatic environments.

The most familiar example of echolocation is that used by the large group of flying mammals, the bats. Bats have developed an extremely sophisticated echo ranging system which can distinguish subtle characteristics of small objects in the environment, allowing them to differentiate between edible and nonedible flying insects. It is of some interest to note that during the course of evolution there have been a number of insects which developed the capability of detecting the ultrasonic waves emitted by nearby bats, thus allowing them to initiate avoidance reactions.

KAI HABER • Department of Radiology, Health Sciences Center, University of Arizona, Tucson, Arizona 85724.

The use of ultrasound for interrogating the environment and deriving meaningful information from it has also been developed to a high degree in certain aquatic mammals. An aquatic environment places serious limitations upon vision. This may have been the driving force in natural selection towards the evolution of the use of ultrasound in orientation within the water. Certain species of dolphin have, in fact, only rudimentary eyes and are essentially blind. Evolution and adaptation have provided certain members of the aquatic mammals with systems of sound production and echolocation for communication, orientation, and food finding. It has recently been demonstrated that sounds covering a broad range of frequencies are produced by many kinds of cetaceans (dolphins, porpoises, and whales). In addition to the use of sound for social communication, underwater sounds are also employed in orientation and food finding. Short bursts of sound are emitted and the animal is able to distinguish the shape, size, and consistency of various objects, even to the point of distinguishing between preferred and nonpreferred food fishes. The sound pulses for echolocation are emitted from concave regions within the skull in the region of the nasal sacs. Some species even have a so-called "melon" of muscular tissue on their foreheads, presumably employed for the purpose of focussing the beam. The shape of this superficial structure on the forehead can be altered voluntarily by the animal to effect a change in the focal characteristics of the ultrasonic beam. The echos which are reflected back to the animal are conducted to the internal portions of the ears, in large part through the lower jaw. The proximal end of the lower jaw terminates next to the auditory apparatus in these animals.

The phenomenon of piezoelectricity was discovered by Pierre and Jacques Curie in 1880. Further development of piezoelectricity and the subsequent apparatus for the generation of directed ultrasonic waves was undertaken in France. The application of ultrasonic waves to echolocation of submarines and other underwater objects, as well as to communication beneath the surface of the sea, took place prior to and during World War I. These applications are first described in the literature in 1928 (Langevin, 1928).

Langevin also described the first effects of ultrasonic radiation upon biological material in an experimental format. Utilizing continuous waves of ultrasonic energy at a frequency of 40,000 cycles per second and a total force of 800 W, he noted that the fish placed within a water bath subjected to this intense radiation were killed. He theorized that intracellular vibrations were set up, leading to local pressures of 5 atm.

Mapping of the sea bottom had advanced significantly by 1928 and an experimental apparatus was mounted on board the ocean liner Ile de France in March of 1928. Another early application of ultrasonic energy to maritime use was that of undersea communication between ships and also between a fixed transmitting station and ships. The direction of an emitting beacon could be detected with a precision of 1° and the distance with a precision of 20 m, at a total distance of 4 km.

The American scientist W. Wood observed the biological experiments of Langevin. Later, he demonstrated independent results showing massive destruction of bacteria subjected to high-intensity ultrasonic waves (Wood, 1927).

Because of the military application of SONAR (*so*und, *n*avigation, *a*nd *r*anging), state-of-the-art instrumentation was not made available to the medical community until after World War II.

Amplitude-mode (A-mode) representations of the brain were obtained in 1947 by Dussik, Dussik, and Wyt in Germany. The data were inconsistent due to the irregular nature of the inner surface of the skull and due to the tremendous attenuation of the ultrasonic beam by bone (Dussik, *et al.*, 1947). Further work on detection of intracranial pathology was reported in 1950 by Ballantine, Bolt, Hueter, and Ludwig from the Acoustic Laboratory at the Massachusetts Institute of Technology (Ballantine *et al.*, 1950). Again, considerable "noise" was imaged and useful clinical information was rarely obtained. Dussik, Dussik, and Wyt as well as Ballantine and his colleagues, utilized the transmission method of recording findings in the human brain. It was later shown that the ventricles could not be consistently outlined by the transmission method due to interposition of the irregular bones in the skull which must be transversed twice (Guttner *et al.*, 1952).

In 1949, Ludwig and Struthers from the Naval Medical Research Institute implanted gallstones into the back muscles of dogs. Following wound healing, the gallstones were localized by the use of ultrasound (Ludwig and Struthers, 1949). In 1950, Dr. J.J. Wild, from the University of Minnesota Medical School, was able to measure bowel wall thickness *in vitro*. He utilized elements from a U.S. Navy Ultrasonic Trainer, device 15-Z-1. He was the first to develop an amplitude-based echo profile of an excised piece of cancerous tissue from a human (Wild, 1950). This work used the echo, or reflection, technique. Since that time, virtually all clinically useful diagnostic ultrasound has been accomplished by the pulse–echo technique.

In 1954, Edler and Hertz described the first time–motion recording (M-mode) of the human heart. They termed this an ultrasonic cardiogram. This work was to lay the foundation of modern echocardiography in the one-dimensional time–motion display (Edler and Hertz, 1954). The first two-dimensional echograms were obtained in 1952 from an apparatus designed by J.J. Wild and J.M. Reid (Wild and Reid, 1952). This technique is now known as brightness mode display (B-mode) and is described in Chapter 10. Working independently, Drs. Holmes and Howry at the University of Colorado developed a sophisticated apparatus for two-dimensional, cross-sectional, ultrasonographic imaging in 1953 (Holmes *et al.*, 1954; Howry, 1965). This instrument was somewhat cumbersone as it used a large water bath system in which the patient was submerged. This early apparatus was termed the "somascope." The brightness mode presentation is obtained by a method called scanning, as described in Chapter 10. In medical technology, the B-mode examination is now referred to simply as the B-scan. The use of B-scanning in obstetrics was pioneered in 1958 (Donald *et al.*, 1958).

As instrumentation became commercially available and more sophisticated, the use of diagnostic ultrasound in medicine expanded rapidly, and continues to expand at the present time. New applications are continually being found (Haber *et al.*, 1975; Pond and Haber, 1976).

The Doppler shift principle has been successfully applied to determination of blood flow in various vessels and organs (Franklin *et al.*, 1961). It is currently in wide, daily clinical use in determining fetal heart tones in obstetrical practice.

9.2. ABDOMINAL ULTRASONOGRAPHY

The most common instrumentation in widespread clinical use today for A-mode, time–motion, and B-mode recording involves direct application of the transducer to the skin of the patient via an acoustic couple such as mineral oil or other specifically designed fluid. When a B-scan is obtained, the entire area to be scanned is coated with the acoustic gel and the resultant scan is termed a compound, contact B-scan. There is no unpleasant sensation. In fact, many patients are quite relaxed by the massagelike motions of the transducer over the body's surface as the information for the scan is gathered. A typical commercial ultrasound unit capable of generating each of the three types of images is pictured in Fig. 9-1.

The abdomen contains a variety of organs belonging to multiple-organ systems. Some organs belong to more than one system.

The abdominal portions of the digestive system include the primary organs of digestion (the hollow tube which reaches from the junction of the esophagus and the stomach to the anus) as well as the secondary organs of digestion (Figs. 9-2a and 9-2b). The hollow tube is divided consecutively into the stomach, the small intestine, and the colon. The small intestine is again divided consecutively into three portions: the duodenum, jejunum, and the ileum. The accessory organs of digestion located within the abdomen are the liver and pancreas. These consist of solid tissue surrounding blood vessels and ducts. In the case of the liver the ductal system is the biliary system. The biliary system transports bile from the liver to the duodenum.

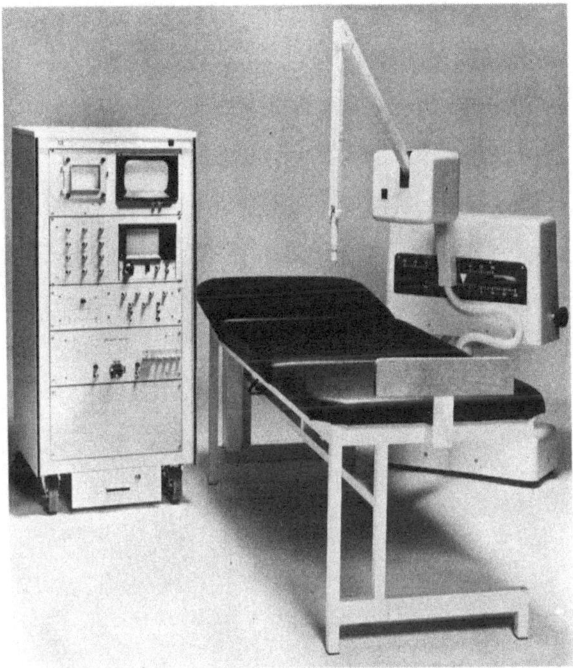

Fig. 9-1. Commercially available diagnostic ultrasound instrument capable of generating A-mode, B-mode, and time–motion images.

A branch of the main biliary duct ends in a storage sac for bile called the gallbladder. The pancreas functions as a hormonal organ (the productions and secretion of insulin and other hormones) as well as an accessory digestive organ. The digestive enzymes that the pancreas produces are carried by a ductal system to the duodenum. These enzymes, together with the bile, act upon the food within the duodenum to further break down the larger molecules to the small molecules, which are then absorbed into the bloodstream and the lymphatic system in the lower portion of the small intestine.

The spleen, liver, lymph nodes, and bone marrow are all part of the reticuloendothelial system (Fig. 9-3). This organ system is involved with the production of blood elements and their removal from the bloodstream, as well as various blood-filtering functions.

The urinary system consists of two kidneys, two ureters, a bladder, and urethra (Fig. 9-4). The kidneys serve both a filtering and regulatory function in the maintenance of homeostasis of the blood. In simplistic terms, the blood is filtered in the kidney, the unwanted products being excreted in the urine and the elements to be retained being reabsorbed into the bloodstream. The urine is then transported via two hollow tubes (the

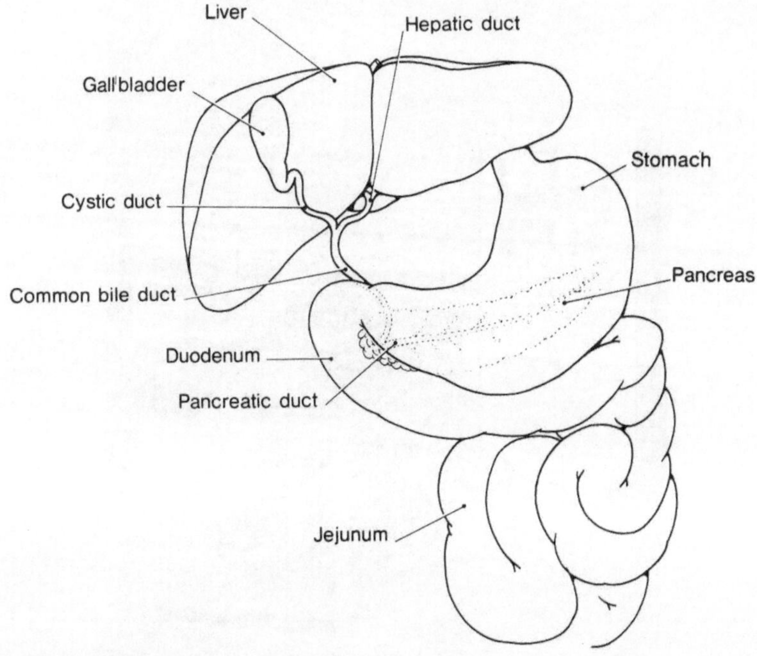

Figure 9-2a. Primary (stomach, duodenum, and jejunum) and secondary (liver, gallbladder, and pancreas) organs of digestion of the upper abdomen.

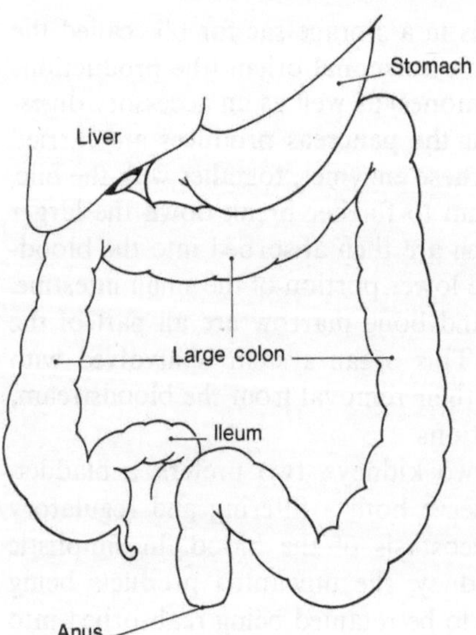

Figure 9-2b. Remaining primary (ileum and large colon) organs of digestion and their relationships to liver and stomach.

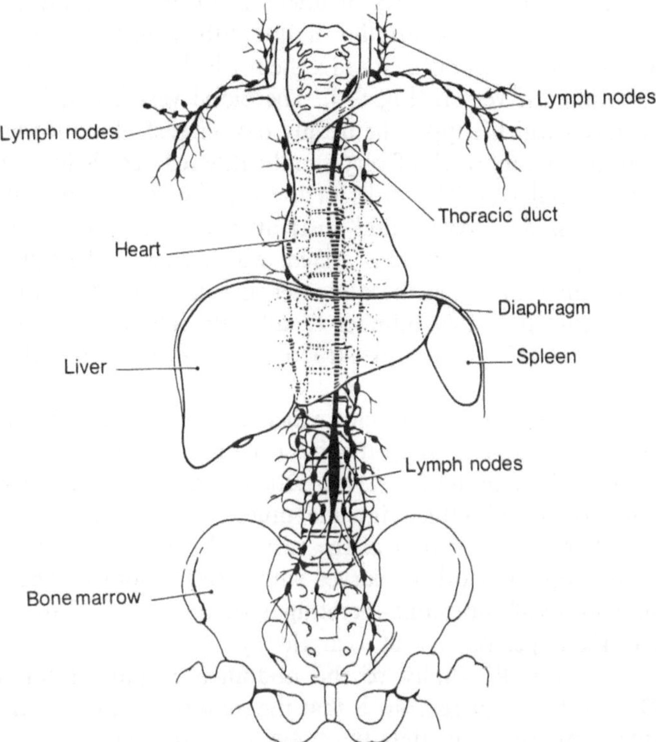

Fig. 9-3. Reticuloendothelial system of the human trunk.

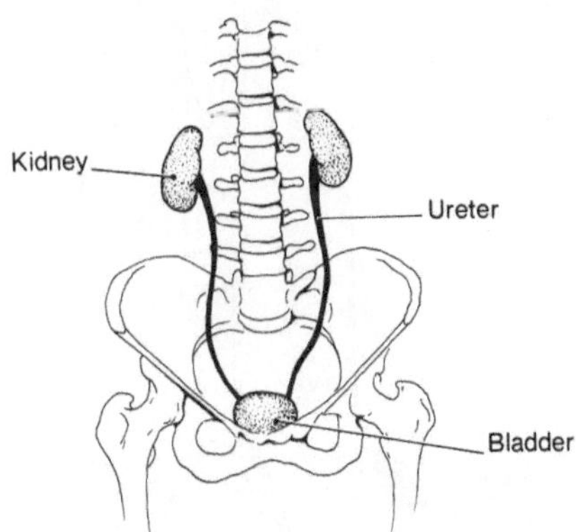

Fig. 9-4. Relationship of urinary system to the axial skeleton.

ureters) to a reservoir (the urinary bladder). From the reservoir, the urine is excreted from the body via another hollow tube called the urethra.

The circulatory system is a closed system which consists of both blood vessels and lymphatic vessels (Fig. 9-5). The blood vessels consist of large-calibered arteries which supply the freshly oxygenated blood from the left side of the heart to a network of very-small-calibered vessels in each of the tissues, called capillaries. The walls of the capillaries are quite thin and allow ready diffusion of oxygen and nutrients across this barrier. The capillaries then empty into the venous system which ends in the right side of the heart. The main artery in the abdomen is called the abdominal aorta and the main vein within the abdomen is called the inferior vena cava. Both of these major vessels have multiple structures supplying each of the above-mentioned organs.

These are the main organ systems which are contained in the abdomen proper. The pelvis contains reproductive organs, as well as blood vessels and elements of the lymphatic system. Other structures which are found in the region of the abdomen include muscles and various connective tissues, as well as the lower part of the vertebral column and spinal cord. There is also a vast network of nerves within the abdomen. The adrenal glands are two small hormone-secreting structures which are in close proximity to the upper portion of each kidney.

Conventional radiography of the abdomen is limited for various reasons. One of the major reasons is that the majority of the organs within the abdomen have approximately the same X-ray tissue density on a conventional radiograph. The outlines of the liver, the kidneys, and the spleen are only visualized because of surrounding fatty tissue. The pancreas, gallbladder, and adrenal glands do not have sufficient fatty tissue around them to be seen routinely on plain radiography. Even if the outlines are delineated, no detail within the organs themselves can be detected without the prior

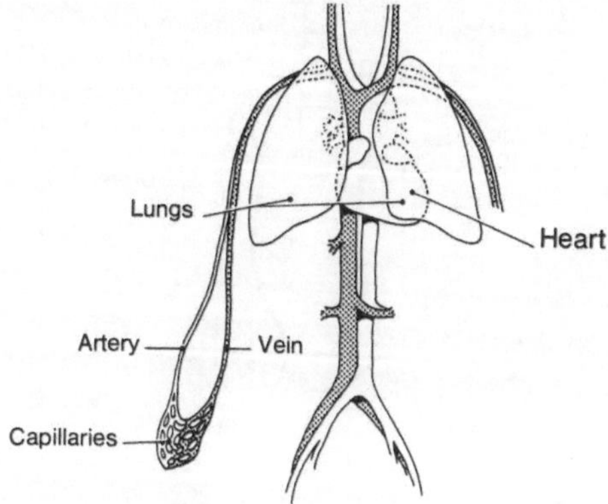

Fig. 9-5. Human circulatory system. The capillaries permeate every portion of the body, including the heart and arteries and veins themselves.

introduction of radiographic contrast material. Ultrasonic B-scanning of the abdomen allows not only ready visualization of the organ outlines but also a sonographic image of the interior of each organ.

Each organ in the abdomen has a typical normal ultrasonic appearance. Thus any significant deviation from the normal is assumed to be a pathologic state.

The discipline of pathology is an extensive, far-reaching field in the medical sciences. There are a vast number of pathologic states which affect various organs and organ systems in a vast number of combinations and permutations. A change in the anatomical structure from the normal will frequently result in a change in function of that organ. It is the anatomic changes involved in many pathologic processes which concern us in ultrasonic imaging.

There are, of course, a large number of anatomical changes which accompany disease processes. Only a few examples will be given, as anything other than a superficial discussion of pathology is beyond the scope of this chapter. This is by no means an exhaustive cataloging of changes to be expected in organs or organ systems which have deviated from the normal.

A common problem occurring in diagnostic medicine is that of a mass within the abdomen. A mass in the abdomen may have been found by the patient himself, or by his physician. Let us assume that the mass was discovered at physical examination and lies deep within the abdomen. Let us further assume that the plain radiograph of the abdomen shows it to be present on the left side and to be associated with the kidney outline. It is possible to inject a radiopaque contrast material into the venous side of the bloodstream and thus visualize the kidney and a portion of the internal architecture of the kidney (intravenous urography). Let us now further assume that the contrast radiographic study showed the mass to be a portion of the kidney. Although, in reality, there are many diseases which can produce a mass in a kidney, let us assume that we have narrowed the choices to a tumor or a cyst. Tumors generally consist of a mass of cancerous cells containing their own blood supply. In general, a tumor, unless it meets significant resistance from surrounding tissue, will grow in a rather spherical manner. Even with the benefit of radiographic contrast material injected into a vein it is not possible to predict with any degree of certainty whether or not a mass in the kidney is a tumor or a cyst. This is, of course, quite important to the patient, as a cyst is a benign condition and generally requires no significant therapy. A tumor, on the other hand, is quite likely to be malignant in this region; and, if surgically excised early enough, the patient can expect to lead a normal life. Therefore, before the advent of ultrasonic scanning, many patients were either taken directly to surgery or were referred for angiographic procedures. One of the areas in which diagnostic ultrasonic B-scanning is highly accurate is in the differentiation between a fluid-filled structure and a solid soft-tissue structure. Thus, in our example, ultrasound is now the next step in the evaluation of an abdominal mass. If the mass is shown to be solid by ultrasound, then angiography can be undertaken. If, however, the mass is shown to be cystic, there is a very high degree of certainty that the patient has a benign condition. One can increase the degree of certainty to almost 100% by inserting a thin needle through the muscles of the patient's back directly into the cyst and aspirating the cyst fluid. The fluid can then be analyzed for malignant cells and certain enzymes which are known to be associated with cancer. The needle can be readily inserted under ultrasonic guidance with a very low risk of complications from the procedure. The entire procedure is done under local skin anesthesia with minimal patient discomfort and takes from 5 to 15 min.

Figures 9-6a and 9-6b show B-mode sonographic images of a normal kidney. A benign cyst is imaged in Fig. 9-7. Contrast the smooth, clear,

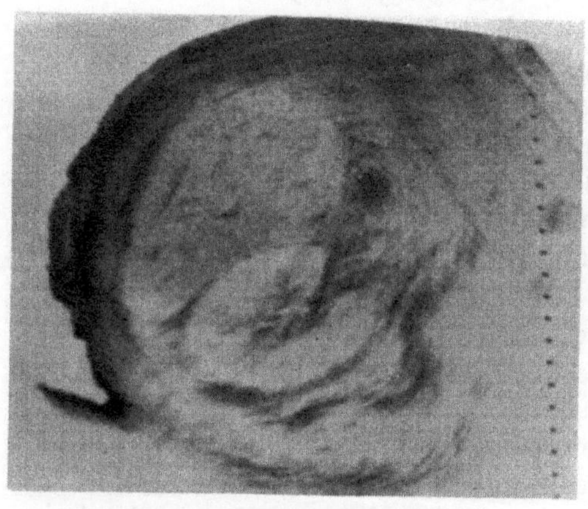

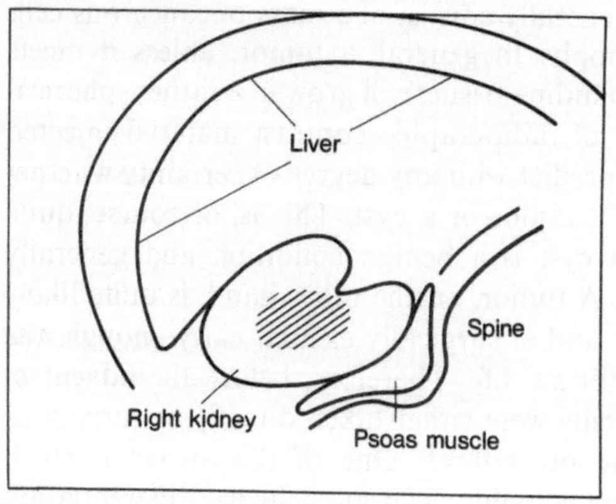

Fig. 9-6a. Transverse B-scan through upper–mid abdomen. Patient is in supine position. Overlying liver serves as excellent sound transmitting medium for imaging of the right kidney.

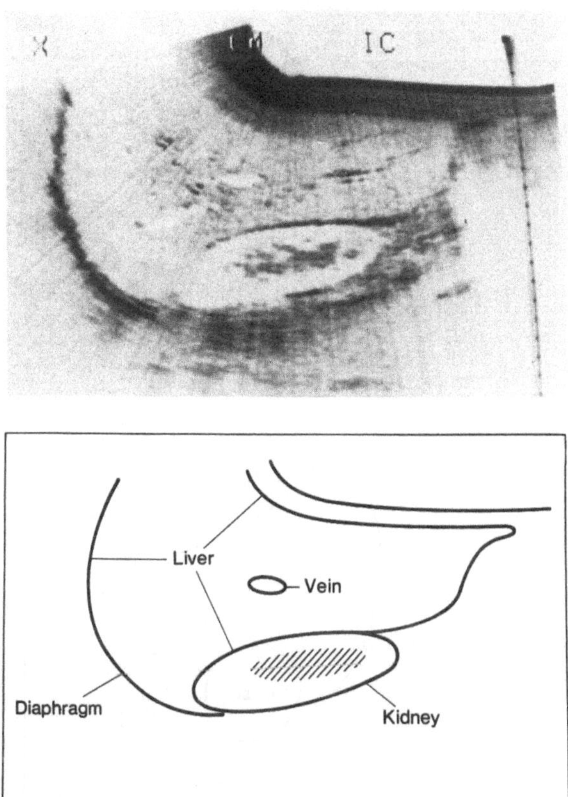

Fig. 9-6b. Longitudinal (parasagittal) B-scan of some patient as in Fig. 6a. Patient is, again, in the supine position. X marks xyphoid and IC marks iliac crest.

echo-free zone with the irregularly shaped mass generating multiple internal echos in Fig. 9-8 (a cancer of the kidney).

Ultrasonography provides an anatomical image of the kidneys. This image is not dependent upon function as are the images obtained with radionuclide scanning of the kidneys or with intravenous urography. A frequent clinical problem arises in patients with very poor renal function. In these cases, intravenous urography often cannot give a reasonable image, and thus not even relative renal sizes can be assessed by this modality. Ultrasonic visualization of the kidneys in this case can be quite helpful in separating the clinical picture of severe renal disease into various distinct pathological categories. This is important in that therapy differs, depending upon the pathological diagnosis. Another area in which ultrasound has become quite useful in diseases of the kidney is in the evaluation of a uni-

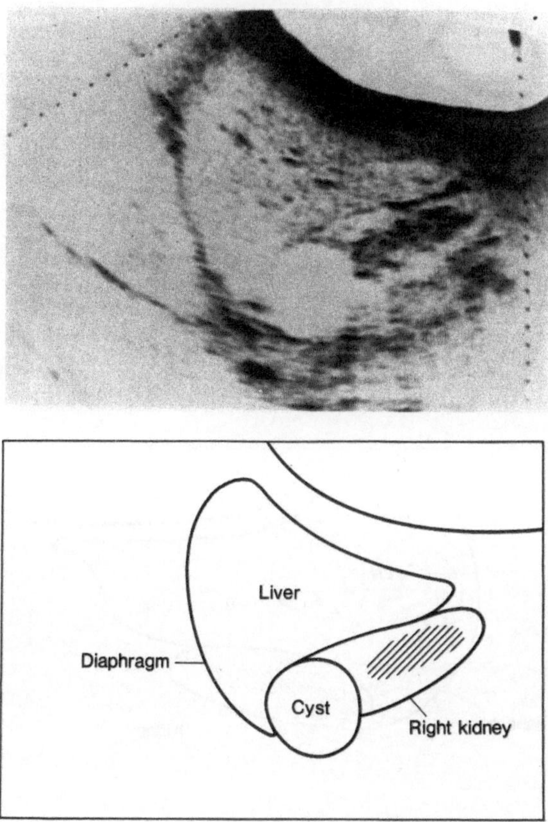

Fig. 9-7. Longitudinal sonogram made 8 cm to the right of the patient's midline in the supine position. Note echo-free nature of the renal cyst.

lateral nonfunctioning kidney at intravenous urography. Again, by various characteristic ultrasonic images, one can arrive at a reasonable pathologic diagnosis and determine the next step in the evaluation of the patient without subjecting him to unnecessary angiographic, surgical, or other diagnostic procedures (Sanders, 1975; Sanders and Conrad, 1975).

The pancreas has classically been an organ which was virtually impossible to image satisfactority before the advent of ultrasound. High-quality B-scan images of the upper abdomen can reveal both the normal and abnormal pancreatic architecture (Haber *et al.*, 1976). Figure 9-9 shows the normal pancreas and its relationship to other structures in the upper abdomen. Ultrasound can distinguish between cancerous and noncancerous enlargement of the pancreas in certain cases. Cancer in the portion of the pancreas adjacent to the termination of the common bile duct into the duodenum can cause obstruction of the bile ducts. This will result in backflow of the bile and subsequent jaundice of the patient. There will be an accompanying dilatation of the entire network of bile ducts both outside and inside of the liver and will of course include the gallbladder, which is connected to the bile duct by a short branch of the bile duct. This will result in a distention of the gallbladder. Ultrasonic scanning of the upper abdomen will show that the gallbladder and the biliary ductal systems are abnormally large. The gallbladder can be readily visualized because it is a fluid(bile)-filled structure (Fig. 9-10). Thus in one ultrasonic examination of the upper abdomen one can visualize the mass within the pancreas as well as the dilated gallbladder and biliary system. This is very specific diagnostic information, given that one is dealing with a patient with jaundice.

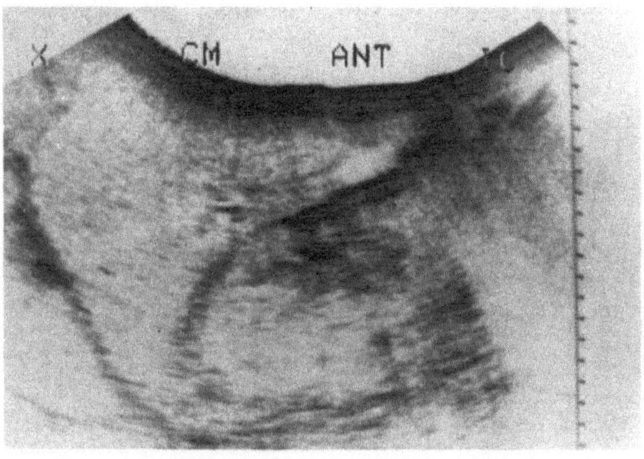

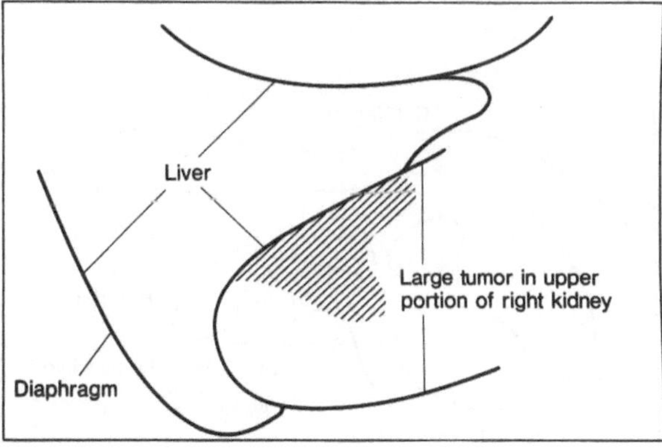

Fig. 9-8. Longitudinal sonogram made 7 cm to the right of the midline, with patient supine. The normal architecture in the upper half of the kidney has been replaced by a tumor. X marks xyphoid and CM marks lower costal margin.

Another example of the complementary role of ultrasound in diagnostic evaluation of a patient with gallbladder disease concerns the diagnosis of gallstones. The gallbladder is visualized by conventional radiography after the patient has taken pills of a radiopaque medium. The radiopaque medium is broken down in the small bowel and absorbed into the bloodstream. From there it is filtered and excreted into the bile. The bile, now containing the radiopaque contrast material, flows passively into the gallbladder. Here, the bile is concentrated. Along with the normal constituents of bile, the radiopaque medium is also concentrated. Radiographs taken at this time will outline the gallbladder. However, in a certain percentage of normal patients and in a large percentage of patients with gallbladder disease (such as gallstones) there is nonvisualization of the gallbladder after the patient has taken the radiopaque tablets. Ultrasonic examination of the gallbladder can readily demonstrate the outlines of the gallbladder and its internal contents. Gallstones frequently cast a characteristic acoustic shadow and

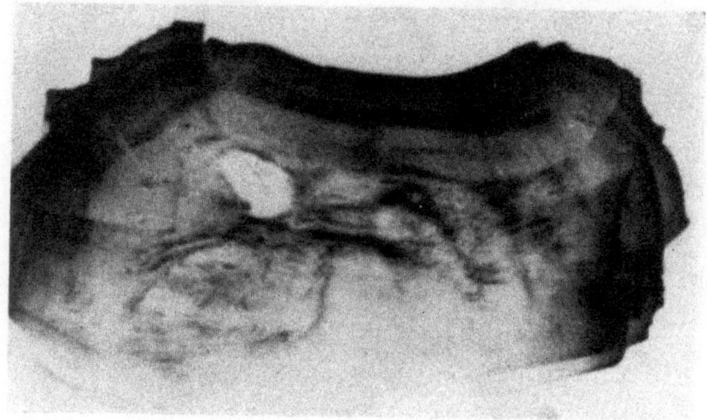

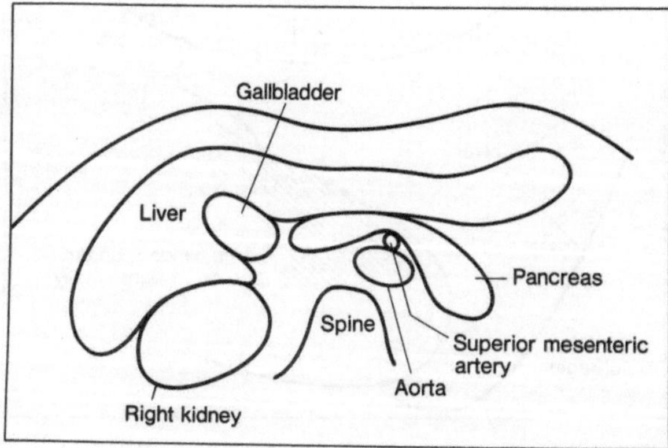

Fig. 9-9. Supine transverse sonogram of the upper abdomen showing relationship of the pancreas to neighboring structures.

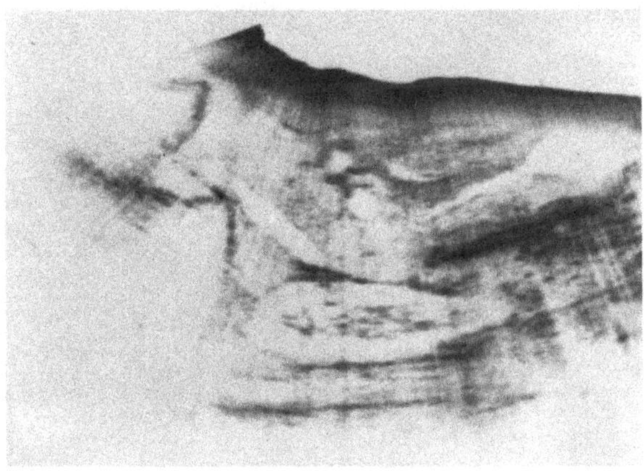

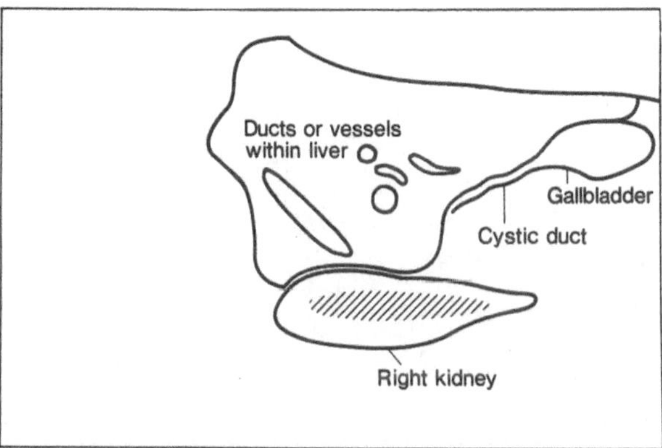

Fig. 9-10. Longitudinal B-scan showing sonolucent gallbladder and an unusually long and straight cystic duct.

can thus be identified (Fig. 9-11). Further confirmation of the diagnosis of gallstones can be made by scanning both in the recumbent and upright positions. The gallstones will, of course, sink to the dependent portion of the gallbladder in each patient position. Thus ultrasonic B-scanning affords a valuable atraumatic adjunct to conventional diagnostic methods in the diagnosis of gallstones (Arnon *et al.*, 1976).

As noted earlier, the aorta is the major artery within the abdomen and from it come various branches to the organs within the abdomen. With good ultrasonic technique, the branches of the abdominal aorta can occasionally be visualized in the normal individual (Fig. 9-12). The abdominal aorta itself frequently undergoes changes of atherosclerosis. This results in a weakening of its walls. The persistent high pressure within the aorta can occasionally result in a ballooning of a portion of the wall of the aorta

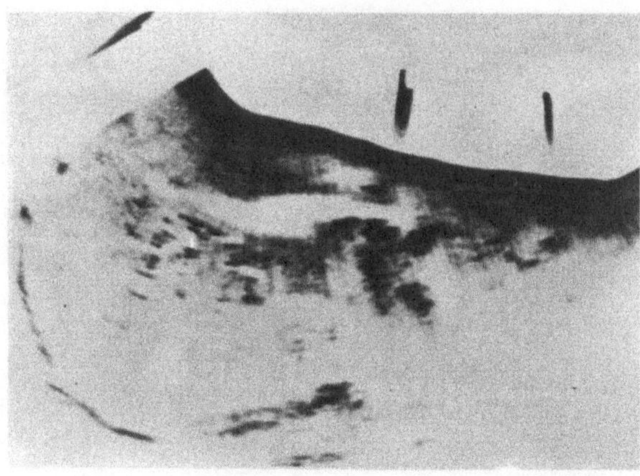

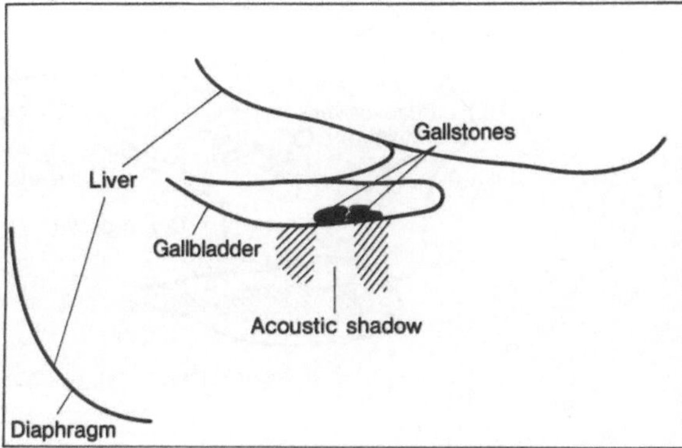

Fig. 9-11. Sonogram of gallbladder with multiple gallstones. Note acoustic shadow cast by the largest gallstone.

(similar to the example of left ventricular aneurysm discussed under "Echocardiography", Section 9.4). The case in the aorta is somewhat different in that the aortic wall is normally much thinner than the wall of the heart. Therefore there is significant danger of rupture of the abdominal aorta, which is fatal in a high percentage of cases. This ballooning-out of the abdominal aorta is called an aneurysm. An aneurysm can be suspected clinically by the presence of a mass in the midabdomen which pulsates due to the blood being pumped through it. The aorta and blood within it cannot be imaged by radiography without the installation of contrast material directly into the lumen by arteriography. This carries a risk in these patients and is frequently difficult to perform because of significant disease in the arteries through which the catheter must pass before it reaches the aneurysmal portion of the aorta. Ultrasonic B-scanning has proven to be highly accurate in the diagnosis of abdominal aortic aneurysms. Very exact measurements of the aorta can be made by this modality. Furthermore, the exact extent of the aneurysmal portion of the aorta can be outlined. Compare the normal aorta in Fig. 9-13 with the abdominal aortic aneurysm in Fig. 9-14.

Ultrasonography of the spleen has proven to be a valuable contribution to diagnostic imaging of the spleen. This examination outlines the anatomical changes within the spleen and changes in the anatomical relationship of the spleen to the rest of the organs in the upper abdomen. Ultrasonic imaging is not dependent upon the function of the organ, as is radionuclide imaging of the spleen. The rapid noninvasive ultrasonic examination has been found to be particularly useful in determination of

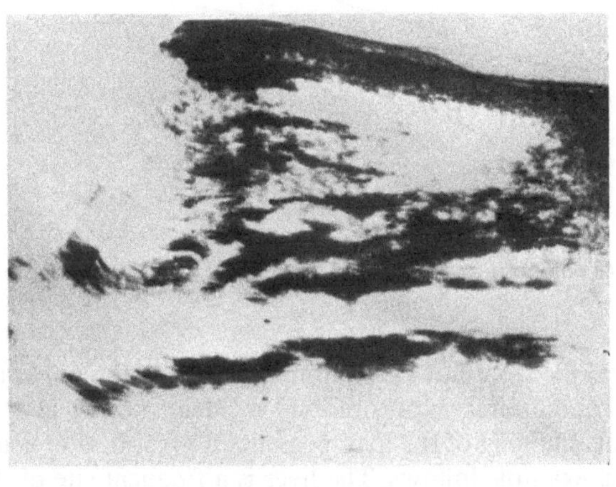

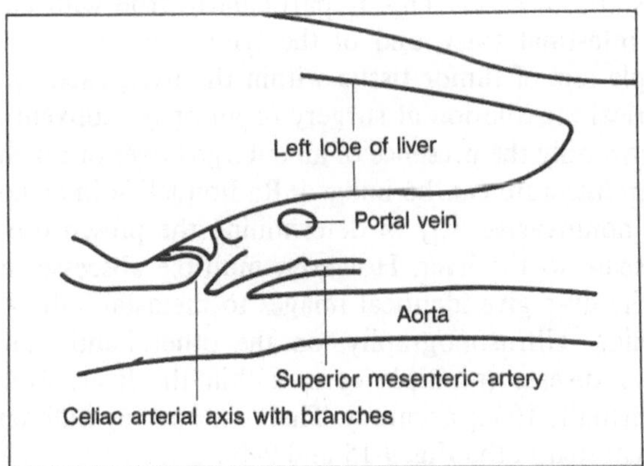

Fig. 9-12. Branches of the upper portion of the abdominal aorta. Note excellent detail, even showing branches of the celiac axis.

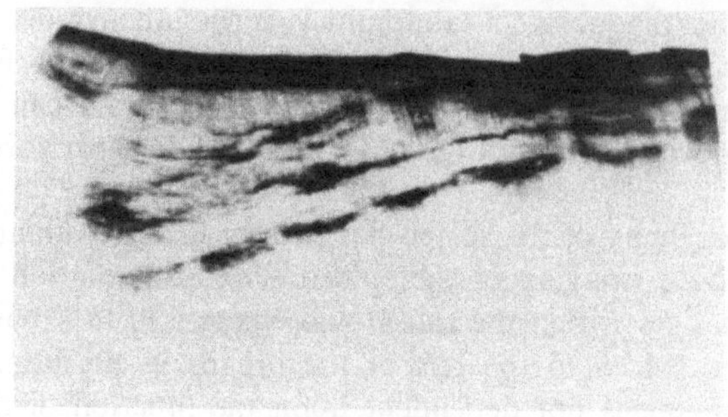

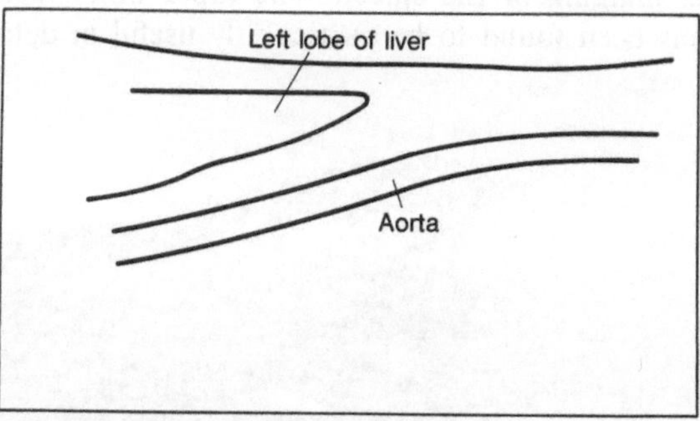

Fig. 9-13. Normal aorta seen in sagittal scan. Note slight taper distally. Scan is at same scale as Fig. 9-14.

damage to the spleen in blunt abdominal trauma to the upper abdomen, as is frequently encountered in automobile accidents (Asher *et al.*, 1976).

Ultrasonic imaging of the liver provides a great deal of useful information. A typical example follows. The liver is a frequent site of the spread of cancer (metastatic disease). This is particularly true with cancers of the breast, lung, intestinal tract, and of the lymph nodes. Frequently, there will be multiple foci of tumor tissue within the liver, each appearing as a roughly spherical mass lesion at surgery or autopsy. Conventional radiography may show only the presence of an enlarged liver or no changes at all. No internal architecture can be imaged. Radionuclide imaging of the liver was the only noninvasive way of determining the presence or absence of metastatic disease to the liver. However, multiple abscesses and multiple cysts within the liver give identical images to metastatic disease by radionuclide scanning. Ultrasonography, on the other hand, can distinguish polycystic liver disease (multiple cysts within the liver) from metastatic disease with virtually 100% accuracy. There are striking differences between the two as illustrated in the Fig. 9-15 and 9-16.

By utilizing the liver as a transmitting medium for the sound beam, one can readily visualize the right side of the diaphragm. The diaphragm separates the abdominal contents from the contents of the thoracic cage. It moves with respiration. One can image the diaphragm by B-scanning. By scanning with the patient holding his breath in deep inspiration and then rescanning the same area on the same scan with the patient holding his breath at full expiration, one can get a graphic representation of diaphragmatic motion (Fig. 9-17). One can accomplish this same task by utilizing M-mode visualization of the diaphragm, obtaining a time–motion representation of a small portion of the hemidiaphragm (Fig. 9-18).

Ultrasonic B-scanning has greatly facilitated nonoperative diagnosis of the female genital system. The ovaries and uterus, being of soft-tissue density for photon purposes, are not ordinarily distinguishable from the surrounding pelvic structure and from each other without installation of contrast material into the uterus. However, the ultrasonic properties are sufficiently different to make routine imaging of these structures possible in both the normal and diseased states. Figure 9-19 shows a full bladder and normal uterus.

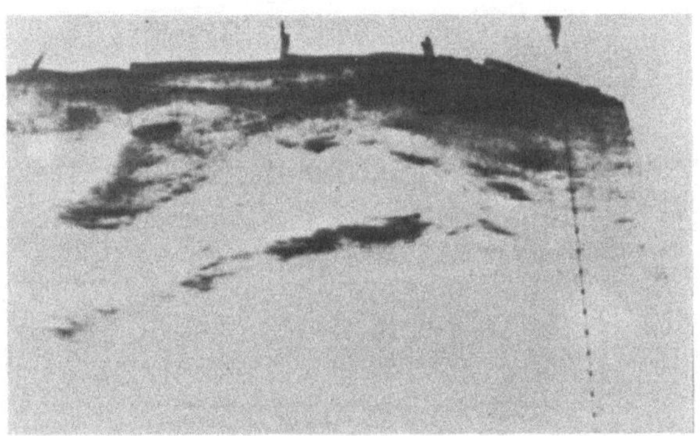

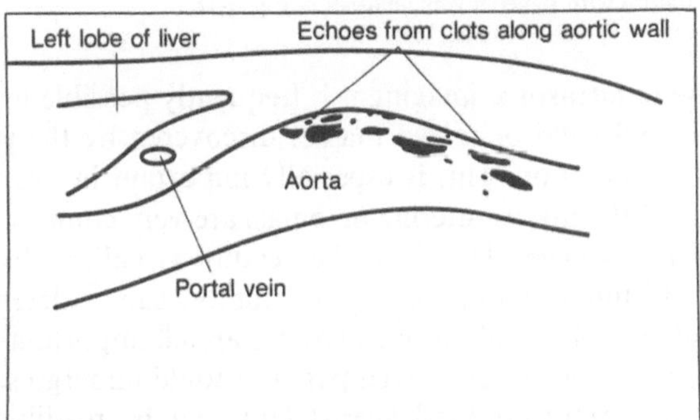

Fig. 9-14. Aneurysm of abdominal aorta. Note echos from blood clots which form in areas of slowed blood flow. The small dots on right-hand side of echogram are 1 cm apart. The aneurysm is 5.2 cm in diameter. The normal aortic lumen is 2 cm or less.

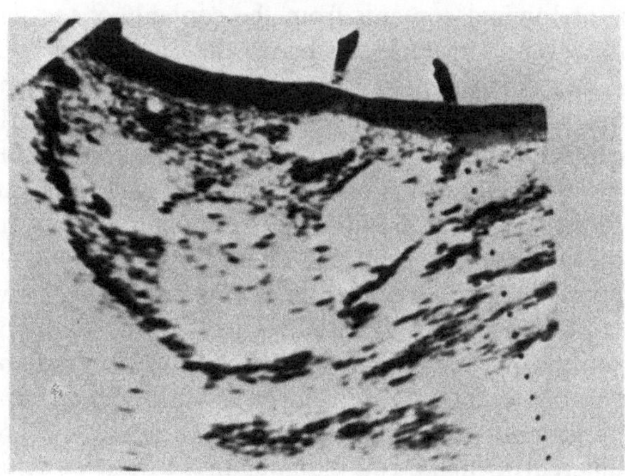

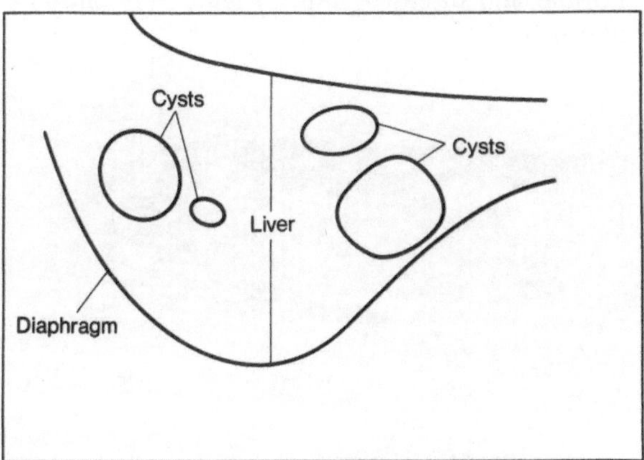

Fig. 9-15. Multiple benign cysts on the liver are shown in this supine longitudinal scan. Contrast their sonolucent nature with the echogenic masses in Fig. 9-16.

By the use of ultrasonic imaging it is frequently possible to distinguish between cystic and solid or mixed masses discovered by the gynecologist during pelvic examination. This is especially important in ovarian masses. Benign tumors of the uterus (uterine myomas) are very common in middle-aged and elderly women. These can be readily visualized by ultrasonic examination. The full extent of these benign tumors can be determined. The presence, number, and size of uterine myomas are all important parameters in determining whether or not a given patient should undergo surgery.

Intrauterine contraceptive devices (IUD) can be readily imaged by ultrasonic B-scanning. A not uncommon problem is the "disappearance" of the string attached to the intrauterine device which normally protrudes from the uterus into the vagina. Usually, it has merely retracted into the uterine cavity or the entire IUD has fallen out of the body unbeknownst to the patient. However, the missing string on vaginal examination occasionally indicates that the IUD has migrated outside the uterus into the pelvic or abdominal cavities. An ultrasonic examination will accurately gauge the presence or absence of the IUD within the uterus without exposing the reproductive organs of the patient to ionizing radiation.

In summary, diagnostic B-scanning of the abdomen (1) is independent of the functional integrity of the organ being examined, (2) allows identification of the organ outline and of its internal anatomical architecture, (3) allows rapid, accurate differentiation between cystic (usually benign) and

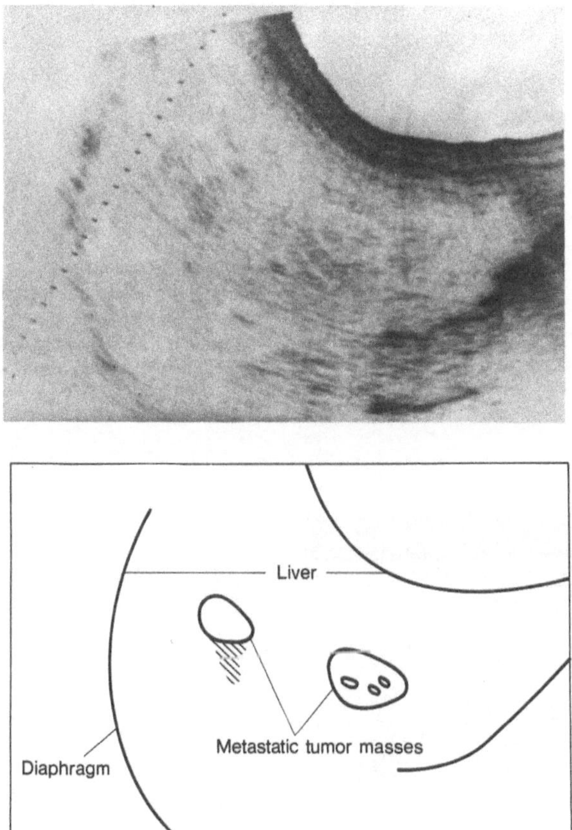

Fig. 9-16. Two foci of metastatic tumor in the liver are shown in this supine longitudinal scan. Note their solid echographic characteristics. Contrast with the liver cysts in Fig. 9-15.

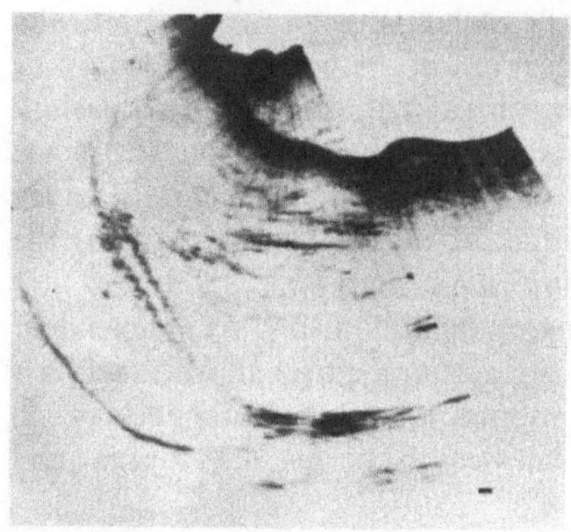

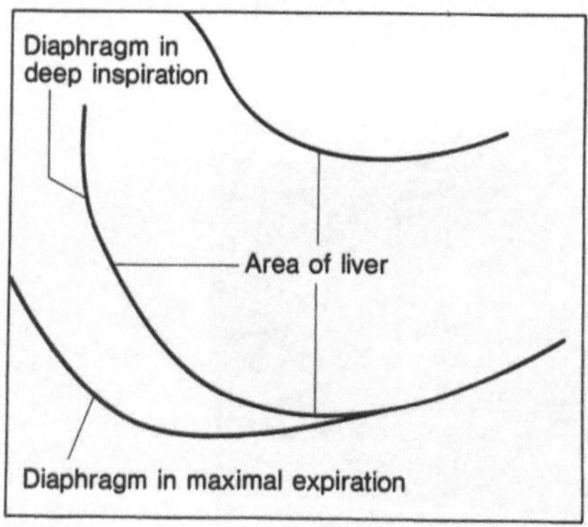

Fig. 9-17. Longitudinal B-scan of the diaphragm showing diaphragmatic position at end of deep inspiration and end of complete expiration. The same area was thus scanned twice, giving a "compound" scan.

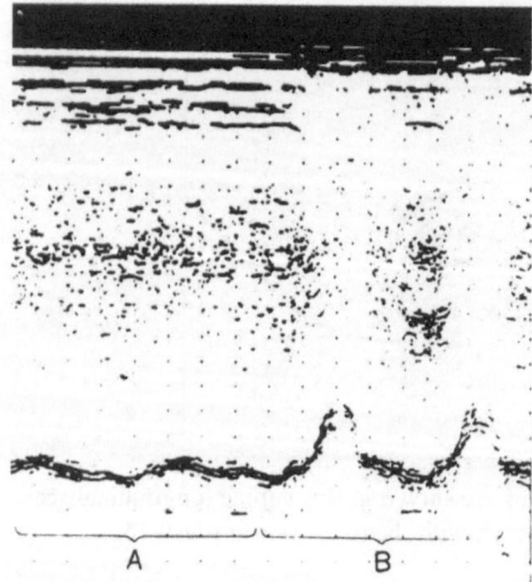

Fig. 9-18. M-mode representation of B-scan in Fig. 9-17. Section A shows two cycles of shallow respiration. Section B demonstrates two cycles of deep inspiration.

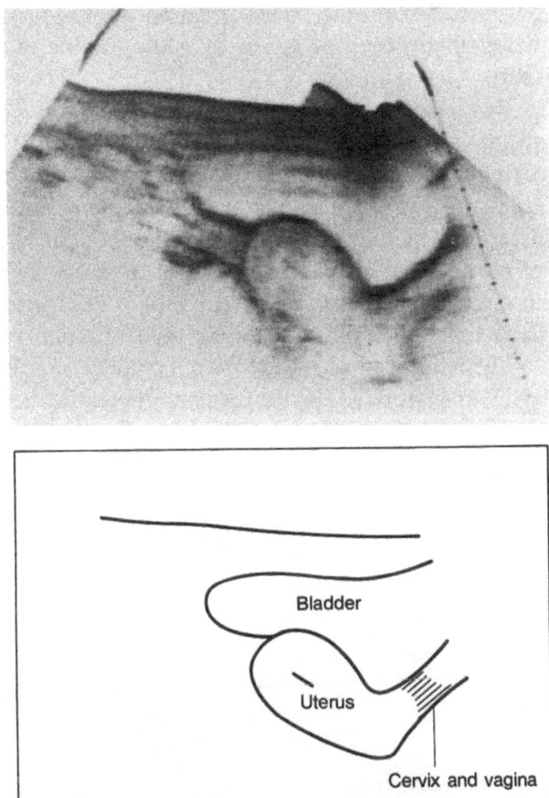

Fig. 9-19. Normal uterus is well imaged in this sagittal scan. Note reverberation artifacts in the anterior portion of the otherwise echo-free bladder.

solid (usually inflammatory or malignant) lesions within the abdomen, and (4) affords a rapid, noninvasive image which occasionally gives information not available by other diagnostic modalities and frequently gives additional information when used as a complementary diagnostic modality.

9.3. OBSTETRICS

It is in the area of obstetrics that diagnostic ultrasonography was an especially welcomed imaging tool (Sanders, 1975). Because of the exquisite sensitivity of the human embryo and fetus to ionizing radiation, the use of conventional radiography (either with or without contrast material) and the use of radionuclide imaging has been severely limited. Not only are there no known harmful effects from ultrasonic imaging at the power levels in use today, but also B-scanning of the pregnant uterus produces images of far greater detail than obtained either by radiographic or radionuclide studies (Fig. 9-20).

Intrauterine measurements of various fetal structures correlate very well with gestational age (Thompson, 1973; Drumm *et al.*, 1976). Of these, the biparietal diameter is the most widely accepted for routine clinical usage (Fig. 9-21). Tables are available giving the normal measurements of the biparietal diameter for different stages of development *in utero*, with appropriate ranges of normal. Serial measurements in time on the same obstetrical patient can give a highly accurate measure of age of the fetus. This has proved to be particularly helpful in planning for Caesarian section. When measurements of the fetal head are made from a standard radiograph, there is a variable degree of distortion of size present, depending on the distance

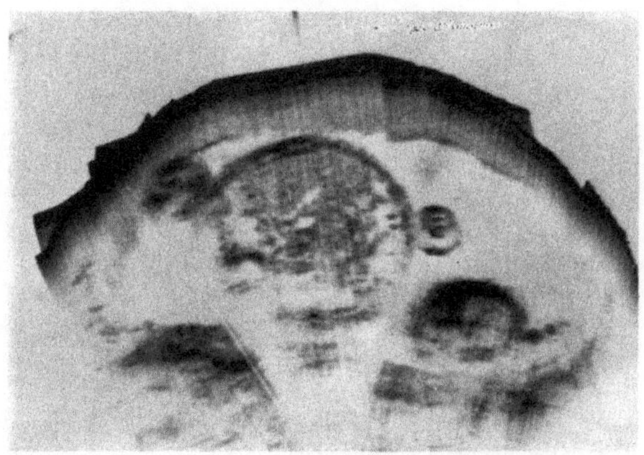

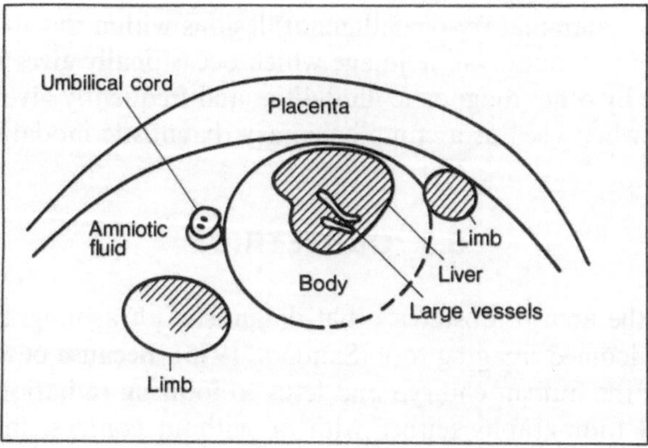

Fig. 9-20. Excellent sonographic fetal detail in normal pregnancy is due to a large degree to the transonic nature of amniotic fluid.

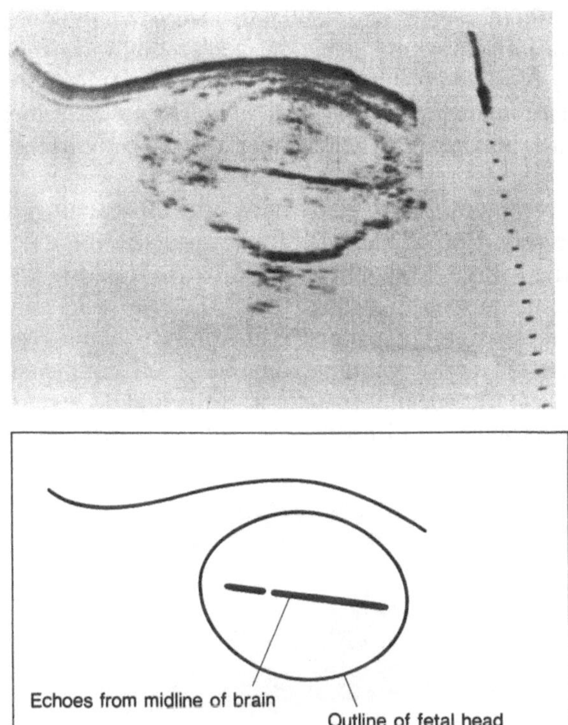

Fig. 9-21. Biparietal diameter of the fetal head can be accurately measured. Gestational age is reliably estimated from correlation with a large data base of normal pregnancies. The dots on the right side of the sonogram are 1 cm apart.

of the head to the film and on the tube-to-film distance. Ultrasonic B-scan systems have range markers which are generally 1 cm apart. These can be superimposed upon the ultrasonic image and a very precise measurement can be obtained directly from the ultrasonogram.

One of the most commonly encountered complications of pregnancy is bleeding in the last three months of pregnancy. Although there are a variety of causes for this symptom, one of the more common underlying conditions is location of the placenta over the cervix of the uterus (so-called placenta previa). Ultrasonic B-scanning is virtually 100% accurate in determining the position of the placenta within the uterus. If a portion of the placenta is covering the outlet of the uterus, this can be readily detected (Fig. 9-22). This condition, of course, makes normal delivery quite hazardous. The patients almost invariably undergo Caesarian section, instead of running the risk of severe, or even fatal, hemmorrhage during delivery. Prior to the use of ultrasonic detection of placental localization, this was carried out by blood-pool imaging with radioactive tracers. Not only was this less accurate in imaging the placenta (with respect to its location within the uterus) but is also resulted in ionizing radiation to both the mother and fetus.

Modern commercially available gray-scale B-scanning devices have made possible very detailed imaging of the fetus itself. If the fetus is a male, the scrotum and penis can often be detected. When these are identified, then one can assure the mother that she is going to deliver a male infant. On the other hand, if these structures cannot be identified, then one is either dealing with a female fetus or the scanning angle has been insufficient for proper imaging of the external genital structures of the male. Therefore, failure to demonstrate a scrotal sac and a penis does not imply that a female fetus will

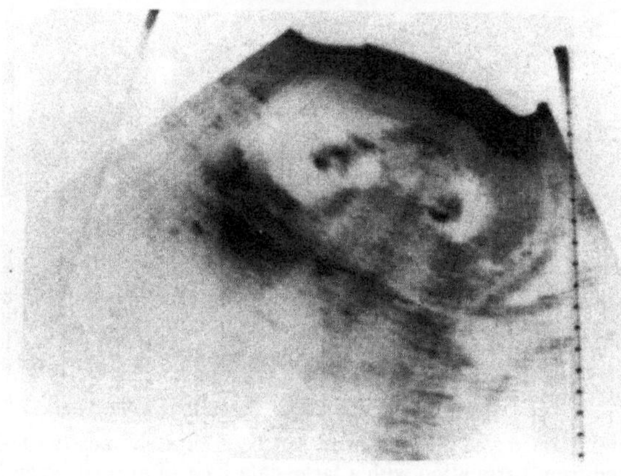

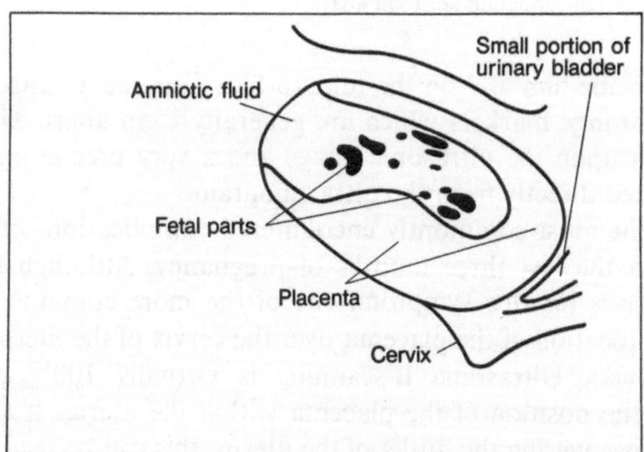

Fig. 9-22. Midline scan in midpregnancy. Placenta completely covers the outlet of the uterus (cervical os).

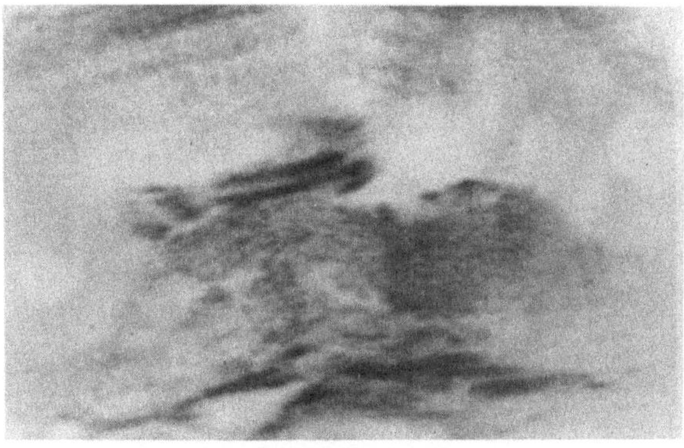

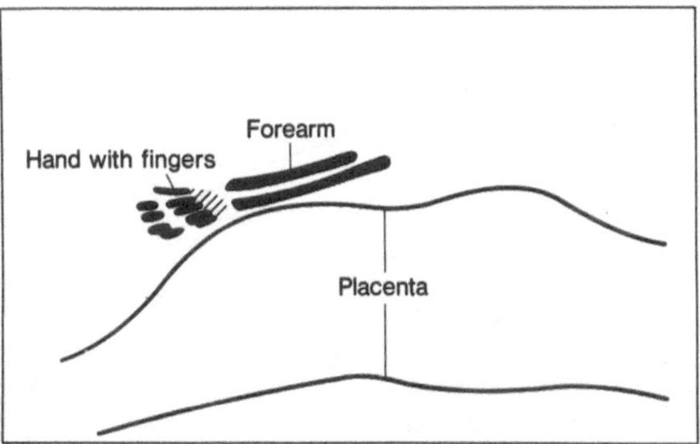

Fig. 9-23. Fetal detail with gray-scale ultrasound has become exquisite.

be delivered. The detail of the normal fetus, as imaged by ultrasonic energy, is such that one can frequently image fingers on a hand *in utero* (Fig. 9-23).

Prenatal diagnoses of multiple congenital abnormalities have been reported. These include deformities of the skull and brain (such as hydrocephalus), cystic disease of the kidneys, obstruction of the urinary tract, and various other developmental or congenital abnormalities (Herzog, 1975) (Figs. 9-24a and 9-24b).

Multiple pregnancy (such as twins) can be diagnosed quite early by ultrasound. To make the diagnosis, one should see two distinct and separate heads.

Pregnancy can be detected quite early by ultrasonic scanning of the uterus in suspected pregnancy. A small gestational sac which shows up as a so-called gestational "ring" can frequently be seen as early as 4 or 5 weeks after conception (Fig. 9-25). It is not uncommon for one to be able to make the ultrasonic diagnosis of pregnancy before chemical determinations of the patient's urine become positive for pregnancy.

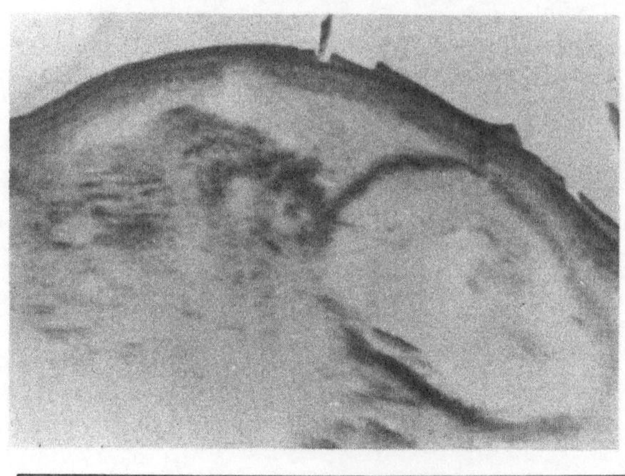

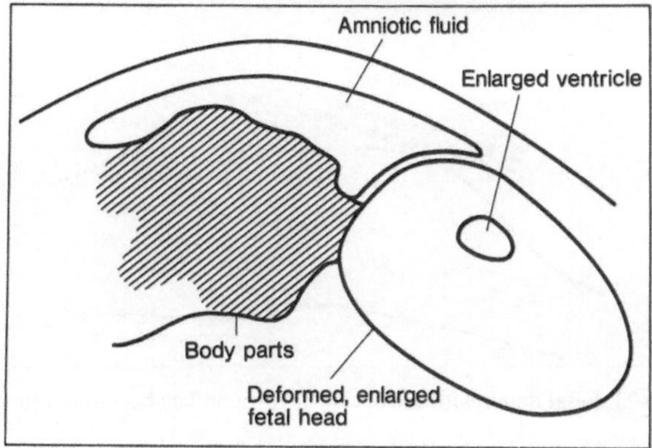

Fig. 9-24a. Longitudinal scan of hydrocephalic fetus in the vertex (head first) position.

The fetal heart tone is detected by Doppler ultrasonic instrumentation. This can take the form of an inexpensive, portable ultrasonic emitter and detector. The Doppler determination of fetal heart rate serves as a valuable adjunct to B-mode scanning in pregnancy.

Occasionally, instead of development of a normal fetus after implantation of the egg into the uterine wall, there is the development of a large cystic growth which is called a hydatidiform mole. Its subsequent growth causes the uterus to continue to enlarge, as if there were a normal pregnancy. Pathologically, the tissue represents multiple small cystic areas which appear similar to clusters of grapes. Clinically, the uterine enlargement may occur more rapidly than in normal pregnancy. This frequently leads to the suspicion of hydatidiform mole, instead of a normal pregnancy. There will not, of course, be any fetal movements present and there will be no fetal heart tones. The diagnosis of hydatidiform mole can be made very reliably

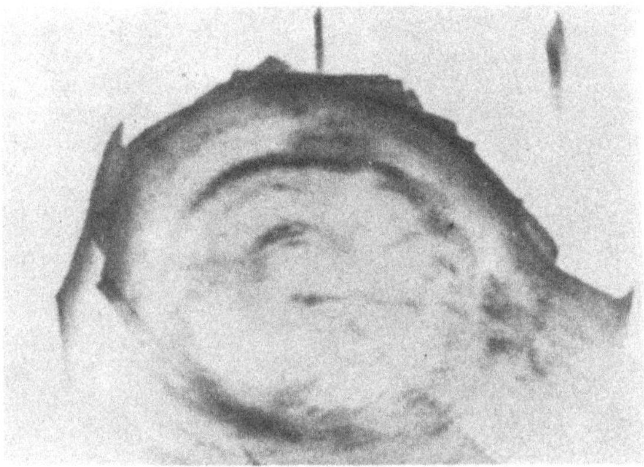

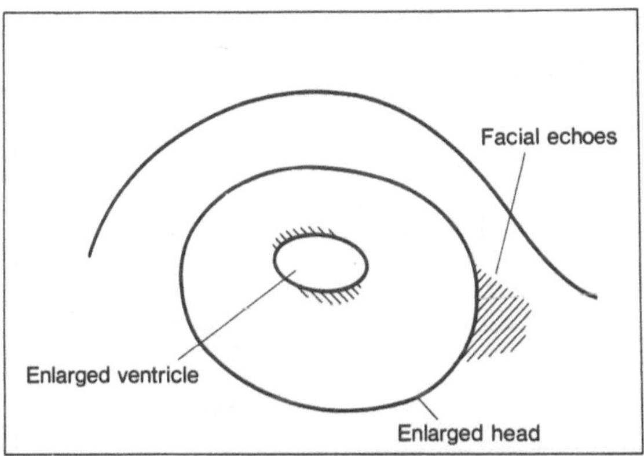

Fig. 9-24b. Transverse scan of same fetus as Fig. 9-24a. Note dilated ventricles causing the very large head.

with diagnostic ultrasonic B-scanning of the uterus since it results in a characteristic complex (cystic and solid) ultrasonic image (Fig. 9-26).

There is a method of detecting some genetic defects in the embryo or fetus before birth. This involves placing a thin-walled needle through the abdominal wall and uterine wall of the mother and into the sac of fluid which surrounds the fetus (amniotic sac). A small amount of fluid is then withdrawn and chromosomal and cytologic studies are performed to detect abnormalities. Before the advent of ultrasonic scanning, this procedure (amniocentesis) was performed in a standard site on each patient. However, occasionally the placenta will lie between the uterine wall and the embryonic fluid and in the path of the needle tract. This is an undesirable situation, as the placenta is quite vascular and there may be a significant amount of bleeding associated with the procedure. In addition, there may be part of the fetus in the path of the needle. Ultrasonic scanning immediately prior

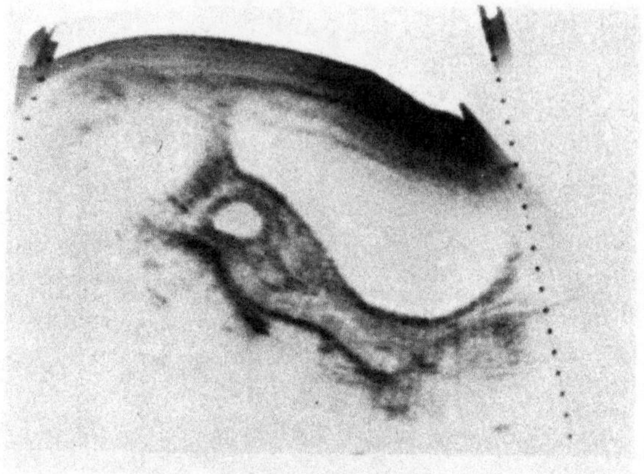

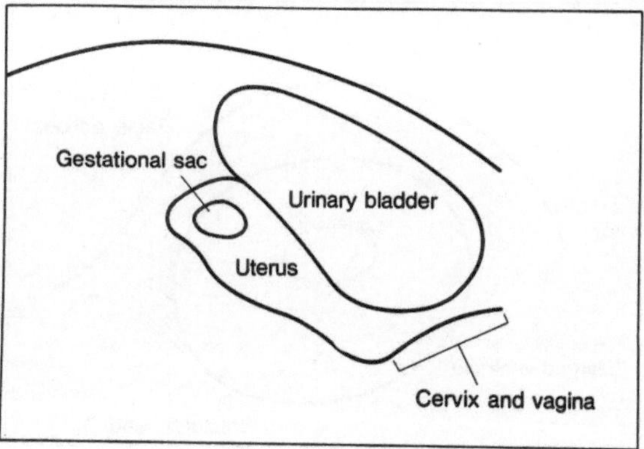

Fig. 9-25. Very early (5 weeks) gestation. Note characteristic ringlike structure at the fundus (top) of the uterus. This represents the gestational sac.

to placement of the needle can direct the obstetrician to the area of embryonic fluid with no part of the fetus or placenta intervening (Gerbie *et al.*, 1975).

9.4. ECHOCARDIOGRAPHY

Since the original time–motion ultrasonic images of the heart by Edler and Hertz in 1954, echocardiography has proven to be a potent noninvasive tool for the physician in the diagnosis of cardiac disorders (Edler and Hertz, 1954). With advances in commercially available instrumentation, echocardiography now has an impact on virtually every category of heart disease (Gramiak *et al.*, 1975; Feigenbaum, 1972).

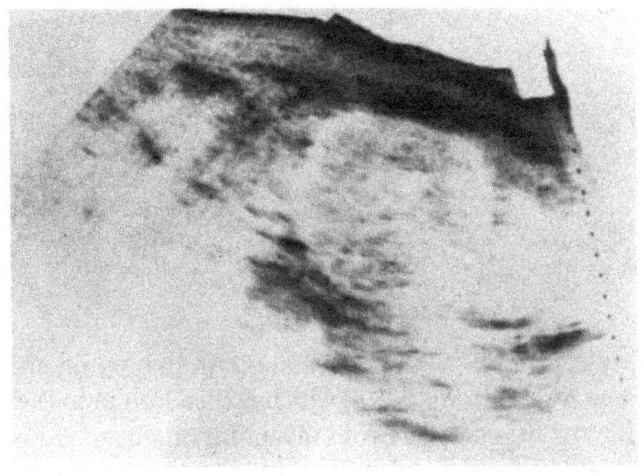

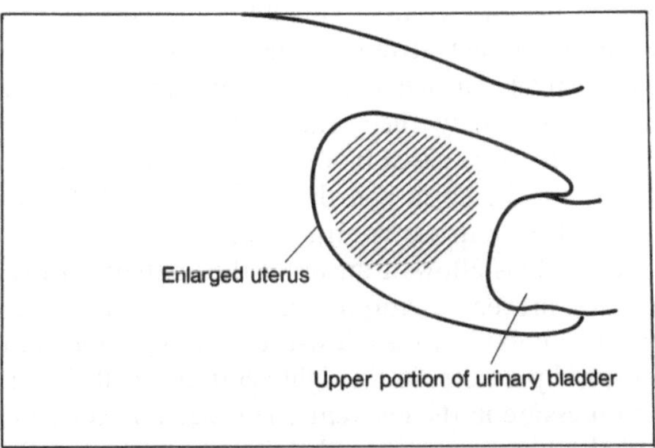

Fig. 9-26. Longitudinal scan of hydatidiform mole. Note the multiple tiny solid and cystic structures within the enlarged uterus.

The heart contains four chambers (Fig. 9-27). These chambers are divided into two sets of atria and two sets of ventricles and can be thought of as separate pumping systems. One is called the right "heart" and the other is called the left "heart." Each side of the heart has an atrium and each side has a ventricle. The right atrium receives the unoxygenated blood returning from the veins of the body. The blood is then pumped through a one-way valve (the tricuspid valve) into the right ventricle. The right ventricle then pumps the blood into the main arteries of the lungs (the pulmonary circulation). As the right ventricle contracts, the valve between the right ventricle and the main pulmonary artery (the pulmonic valve) opens. At the same time, the tricuspid valve closes, thus preventing blood from regurgitating into the right atrium. The blood then flows through the

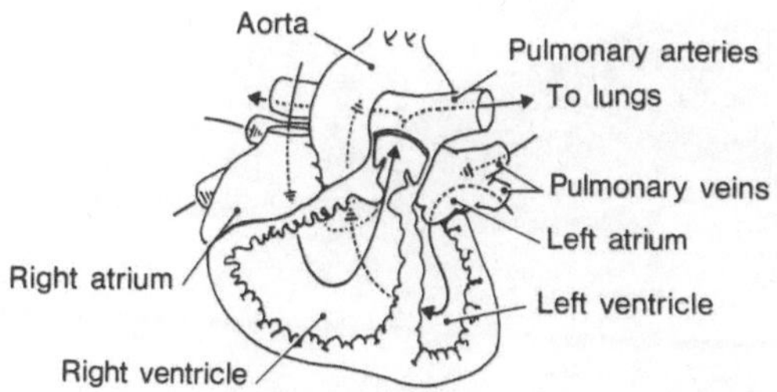

Fig. 9-27. Diagram showing the four chambers of the heart and the major vessels leading into and out of them. Arrows indicate direction of blood flow.

millions of tiny capillaries within the lungs. At this point, there is an exchange of carbon dioxide for oxygen, which is then bound to the hemoglobin molecules in the red blood cells. From this point on, the blood is oxygenated and has a characteristic red color. The blood is then returned to the left side of the heart (the left atrium), via eight pulmonary veins. The blood is next pumped from the left atrium to the left ventricle through an other valve (the mitral valve). The left ventricle pumps the oxygenated blood into the major artery of the body (the aorta), thus supplying all of the tissues of the body with freshly oxygenated blood. There is, of course, a valve between the left ventricle and the aorta and this valve is called the aortic valve. At the time that the left ventricle contracts, the mitral valve closes, and the aortic valve opens. This allows transfer of the contents of the left ventricle into the aorta and prevents regurgitation of the blood into the left atrium.

The right side of the heart is a low-pressure system in comparison with the left side. Typical pressures in the right ventricle are 0–25 mm of mercury. The maximum pressure in the left ventricle is equal to the so-called systolic component of the blood pressure: that is to say, the upper value of the blood pressure figure, typically somewhere around 120–140 mm of mercury. Since the heart is a specialized, highly efficient muscle, it stands to reason that the left ventricular wall is significantly thicker than that of the right ventricle, due to the large differences in pumping pressure.

The average adult human has a cardiac output of approximately 5 l/min. Less than 5% of this cardiac output goes to supply the muscle fibers of the heart itself via the coronary circulation. When an individual suffers occlusion of one of the main coronary arteries or a main branch of a main coronary artery, he may well develop infarction (death) of the portion of the heart muscle which was supplied by that artery. This is the well known heart attack or "coronary." This portion of the heart muscle will then develop a scar. The area of the scar will not contract normally. It may, indeed, be quite weak and actually show dilation while the rest of the heart contracts in a manner similar to ballooning of a structural weakness in a tire inner tube. Echocardiography can readily detect these areas. These areas most frequently occur in the left ventricle and are termed left ventricular aneurysms. If these are large enough, they can significantly affect cardiac function and result in heart failure. Surgical techniques in the last decade have been perfected to the point where a large number of persons suffering from ventricular aneurysms can receive marked benefits as a result of excision of the dead muscle. When the ultrasonic transducer is moved from a position of normal heart function to the area of dead heart muscle, there will be seen either no motion or paradoxical motion of the area of ventricular aneurysm.

When the left ventricle pumps against greater resistance than normal, the muscle of the left ventricular wall will undergo concentric enlargement. This is termed hypertrophy. This is the same phenomenon that takes place when an individual embarks upon a body-building program and increases the size of muscles which are strongly exercised. This condition of cardiac hypertrophy is most frequently encountered in the population at large in patients who have high blood pressure (hypertension). With the increase in peripheral blood resistance (and a subsequent increase in the blood pressure), the heart must work significantly harder. The capillary blood supply to the heart muscle does not increase proportionately to the increase in muscle mass of the heart. Thus a person with long-standing hypertension is much more prone to heart attacks than is an individual with normal blood pressure. Ultrasonography can very accurately image the wall of the left ventricle. Precise measurements of the left ventricular muscle thickness can be obtained. Thus one can separate patients who have the cardiac effects of hypertension from those who have not yet developed them. The severity of the disease process can be better gauged than before this information was available.

Pathologic states not only involve the heart muscle itself, but may involve the valves of the heart. When a valve is structurally damaged its function is impaired to a variable degree. This can be detected in two ways. The first is the direct effect, which will be shown as an actual pathologic change in the structure or function of the valves, or a combination of the two. A common example of this is in patients who have rheumatic valvular heart disease. Different valves are affected to a greater or lesser extent, the most commonly affected being the mitral and aortic valves. In this disease entity the valve leaflets become quite stiff, resulting in either a smaller opening in the valve or an incompetent valve, or both. Another aspect of disordered valve function results in secondary effects. This involves the chambers on either side of the valves and results in alterations in chamber size. Due to scarring and subsequent narrowing of the aortic valve, the left ventricle will have a significantly increased workload. In addition, to maintain cardiac output, the same volume of blood will need to be pumped through a smaller opening. This will cause a jet effect in the aorta beyond the aortic valve, eventually resulting in dilation of the aorta. The left ventricle will undergo hypertrophy as a result of the same process as involved in hypertension.

In the case of narrowing of the aortic valve (aortic stenosis), echocardiography can reveal the limited excursion of the aortic valve as a result of the scarring, the limited opening of the aortic valve, the hypertrophy of the muscle of the left ventricle, and the dilated portion of the aorta. The only other effective way of determining all this data is by introduction of a catheter into the arterial system in a retrograde fashion into the left ventricle and subsequently obtaining radiography after injection of radiopaque material into the left ventricle. This, of course, carries a risk of morbidity and mortality. Ultrasonic investigation, although it does not give images of the same resolution as the radiographic procedure, is, nonetheless, totally noninvasive and without the hazards of ionizing radiation.

Ultrasonography has become the imaging modality of choice in the diagnosis of fluid accumulation around the heart (pericardial effusion).

Echocardiography also plays a major role in "state-of-the-art" diagnostic evaluation of cardiac problems in the pediatric age group (Goldberg *et al.*, 1975). The vast majority of diseases in this patient population are congenital in nature. These congenital cardiac problems run the spectrum from asymptomatic lesions, such as very minor narrowing of a valve orifice, to disorders which are frequently fatal shortly after birth, such as marked underdevelopment of the left-sided cardiac chambers (hypoplastic left heart syndrome). The pressure and volume dynamics of virtually all of the known congenital heart lesions have been well worked out, or can be reasoned out, based on basic physical and physiological principles. These result in anatomical changes of varying degrees in the four chambers of the heart as well as in the aorta and pulmonary arteries. It is these changes in anatomical configuration which are imaged by echocardiography.

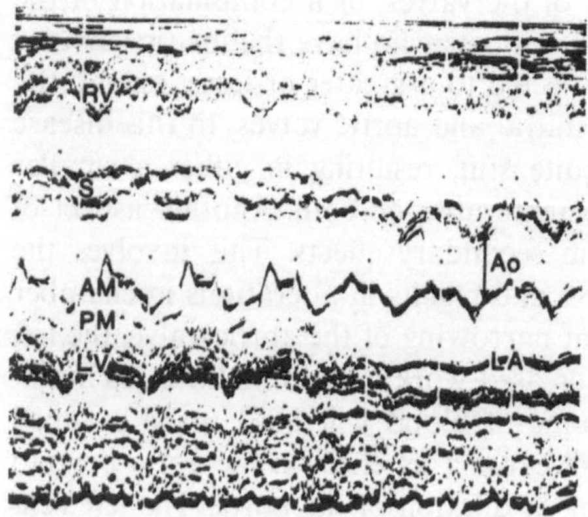

Fig. 9-28. Normal time–motion (M-mode) tracing of the heart. The transducer is stationary. RV is wall of right ventricle. S is interventricular septum. AM and PM are anterior and posterior leaflets of the mitral valve. L.V. is left ventricle wall. AO is aortic lumen. LA is left atrium.

This modality is ideally suited for diagnostic investigations in the pediatric age group because of the fact that there is no ionizing radiation in an ultrasonic examination. Repeated examinations can be obtained without the danger of cumulative tissue damage posed by imaging modalities utilizing photons, since there is no evidence for biological damage at the frequencies and dosages employed in echocardiography (or in other diagnostic examinations for that matter). Furthermore, ultrasonic examination is completely painless and poses no danger to the operator or other persons in close proximity to the child during the examination. Finally, it requires very little, if any, voluntary cooperation on the part of the child (who is frequently a newborn), since the examination is in real time. Because the heart is a structure which is virtually in constant motion, the time–mode method of ultrasonic imaging is the modality of choice.

The most common instrument in use today is the single-crystal, time–motion ultrasonic instrument with a strip-start recorder. An example of this type of tracing in a normal individual is given in Fig. 9-28.

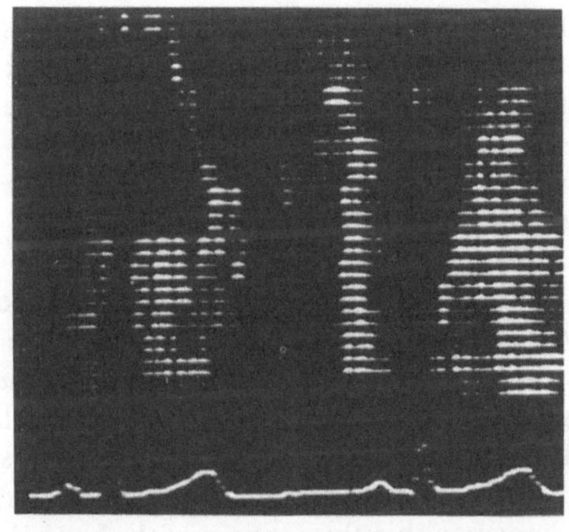

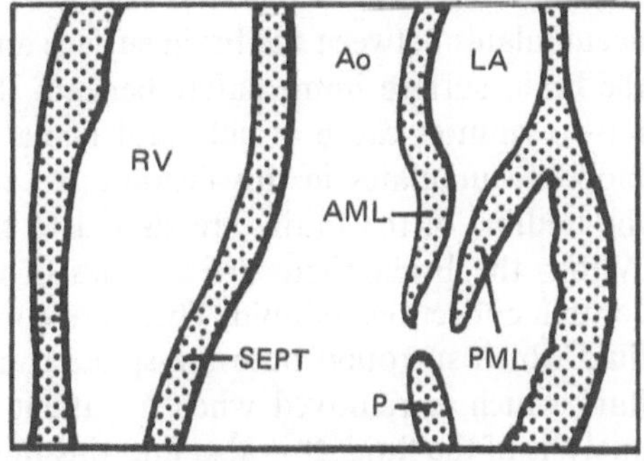

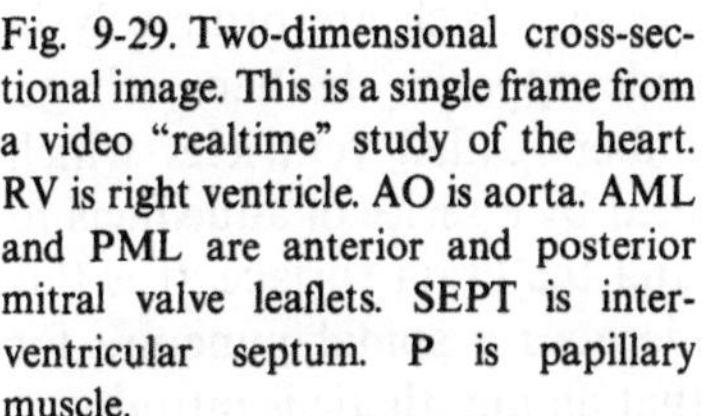
Fig. 9-29. Two-dimensional cross-sectional image. This is a single frame from a video "realtime" study of the heart. RV is right ventricle. AO is aorta. AML and PML are anterior and posterior mitral valve leaflets. SEPT is interventricular septum. P is papillary muscle.

In recent years, there has been a development of real-time imaging in two dimensions. This is accomplished either by rapid sequential firing of multiple crystals in an array or by rapid sector scanning by a single or multiple crystal (Sahn *et al.*, 1976). This allows examinations of a much larger segment of the heart in real time, and results in a much more rapid and thorough examination than the single, nonmoving crystal in the time–motion mode. A single frame from a cardiac study obtained by a multicrystal instrument is shown in Fig. 9-29.

9.5. NEUROLOGY

The use of ultrasound in the detection of neurologic disorders is termed echoencephalography. The vast majority of echoencephalographic examinations are carried out in the amplitude mode (A-mode). This is because of the tremendous attenuation and deformity of the ultrasonic beam as it traverses the thick bone of the skull. The ultrasonic waves must travel through the skull on their way to the reflecting surface and then must traverse the skull once again as the echos return to the transducer. The fact that the echo information that is received is displayed only in the amplitude mode makes the use of ultrasound in the diagnosis of neurologic disorders somewhat limited, both in comparison to the diagnostic capabilities of ultrasound elsewhere in the body and with respect to the newer computerized tomographic techniques utilized in roentgenology (Tenner *et al.*, 1974).

By far the most common use of echoencephalography is in determining the location of midline structures in the brain (White, 1966). This can be achieved with a wide variety of instrumentation. Towards this diagnostic goal of midline localization, several small inexpensive, portable units have been developed and are in widespread use throughout the world.

The human brain is highly malleable and is quite sensitive to pressure changes within the confines of the bony skull. A rather common injury is the so-called subdural hematoma. This is basically a collection of blood which accumulates between the brain surface and the tough membranes overlying the brain surface immediately beneath the inner portion of the skull. The most common cause of subdural hematoma is, of course, trauma. When blood accumulates in this fashion, the structures, which are ordinarily in the midline of the brain, are shifted to the side opposite the hemorrhage. Within the brain there are a series of chambers called ventricles which contain collections of fluid. These are connected by a series of aqueducts to fluid which surround both the spinal canal and the brain surface. It is this fluid which is removed when a patient undergoes a spinal puncture for analysis of the fluid. It is also into this fluid that an anesthetic is introduced in spinal anesthesia. One of the chambers within the brain, the third ventricle, is located in the midline of the brain. It is reflections from a membrane within this chamber that serve as the landmark for the midline of the brain. In the normal state, there will be a large echo reflection from the portion of the skull nearest the transducer. There will be a reflection of somewhat less amplitude from the third ventricle and, finally, there will be a strong reflection from the portion of the skull which is farthest from the transducer (Shkolnik, 1975). When the midline is shifted by a mass such as a subdural hematoma, there will be a shift of the echos of the third ventricle away from the midline position. The examination is carried out both on the right side of the skull and on the left side of the skull in comparable positions near the temples on each side. These positions are standardized and are constant with respect to certain reference points on each patient.

Subdural hematoma is not the only entity which will cause a midline shift. Any disease process which results in the formation of a mass within the brain may cause a midline shift. The more commonly encountered pathologic states are tumors and abcesses. However, the majority of echoencephalographic examinations which are carried out for the detection of midline shift in the United States are for the inclusion or exclusion of hemorrhage as a direct result of trauma.

Another area in which echoencephalography has become quite useful is in determining the presence or absence of hydrocephalus. Hydrocephalus is a term which literally means "water brain." This is an anatomical description of a pathologic state which has many different etiologies. In a patient with hydrocephalus there is dilation of one or more of the cerebral ventricles. This dilation can range from very mild to being so severe that virtually the entire skull is filled with cerebral spinal fluid, with only a small mantle of brain tissue surrounding massively dilated sacs of fluid within the brain.

As mentioned above, the fully ossified adult skull virtually precludes B-scanning of the brain with presently available commercial equipment.

In young children, however, there has been limited success with B-scanning of the brain. This is because full mineralization of the skull does not occur until late childhood. The images are still crude (Shkolnik, 1975; Galicich *et al.*, 1965). It is hoped that there will be further equipment and clinical refinements in ultrasonic diagnosis of brain disorders by ultrasonic B-scanning in the pediatric age group.

9.6. OPHTHALMOLOGY

In recent years, ultrasonic examination of the eye and other soft-tissue structures within the orbits has come into widespread use and become a valuable modality utilized by ophthalmologists.

Historically, A-scans of the eye were the first to be developed. However, the A-scan has given way to virtually complete universal use of two-dimensional B-scanning. Two major types of instruments are in current use. One involves a scanning head which is applied directly to the eyelid with an acoustic gel or other acoustic couple, while the other involves scanning through a waterbath. The waterbath is applied directly to the eye, without an intervening eyelid. This is carried out under local anesthesia to the eye directly and is the so-called immersion B-scan (Coleman *et al.*, 1969).

Ultrasonic imaging of the eye, whether carried out by the contact B-scan method or the waterbath method, utilizes high-frequency ultrasound (8–20 mHz), giving very high axial resolution.

The most dramatic use of ultrasound in ophthalmology is in patients in whom there is opacification of any portion of the eye (McQuown, 1975). The ophthalmologist relies heavily on his visual inspection of the patient's eye. This involves looking not only through his own eye but also through the cornea, the anterior chamber, the lens, and the vitreous of the patient's eye. Thus if a patient has a cataract (opacification of the lens) or other abnormality restricting the ophthalmologist's visual view of the patient's eye, ultrasonography can result in imaging of the area behind the opacity. This can be especially helpful, not only in patients with cataracts, but also in cases of trauma, tumors, or hemorrhaging into the eye from hypertension or other causes.

Ultrasonography can also be used to document disorders which can be readily visualized by the ophthalmoscope. Such disorders would include retinal detachments, tumors within the eye, and localization of foreign bodies.

Echography can give very accurate measurements of the globe. This application has been utilized in biometry prior to implantation of lenses actually within the eye.

A variety of tumors and other space-occupying processes involve the contents behind the globe and in front of the bony orbit. Until the recent advent of computerized X-ray tomography, ultrasonography provided the only method of imaging these structures short of surgical exposure. Sonographic images of these structures are quite helpful in evaluating patients with protrusion of either one or both eyes (exophthalmos). Occasionally, foreign bodies can be found in the space between the globe and the bony orbit. These can be readily identified by ultrasound.

The experience with computerized X-ray tomography of the orbit and eye has been quite limited to date. Therefore the respective places of ultrasonography and computed X-ray tomography in ophthalmology have not been resolved. However, it is likely that the two imaging modalities will be complementary, and not competitive.

9.7. MISCELLANEOUS USES OF B-SCANNING

B-scan ultrasonic imaging has proven to be of clinical value in a variety of miscellaneous anatomical regions. The thyroid gland is located quite superficially in the neck. Therefore high-quality B-scan images can be obtained with 5.0-mHz ultrasonic waves. As in other areas of the body, ultrasonic B-scanning has found a major application in being able to distinguish between cystic (usually benign) and solid (either benign or malignant) nodules in the substance of the thyroid gland itself. A nodule (lump) is usually found either by the patient himself or by the physician during routine physical examination. If ultrasonic examination reveals the nodule to be cystic, a needle can readily be inserted into the nodule after local anesthetic is applied to the skin. The contents of the cyst are then aspirated and analyzed for the presence of malignant cells. As this technique comes into wider clinical use, more and more exploratory operations are obviated (Perlmutter, 1975).

Ultrasonic examination of the testes has been of some value in a variety of disease states (Miskin and Bain, 1974).

The salivary glands, due to their superficial locations, are likely organs for ultrasonic imaging. Unfortunately, current instrumentation does not allow routine visualization of the normal salivary gland. However, when there is enlargement of one or more of the salivary glands, the nature of these enlargements can be determined by ultrasonic B-scanning (Neiman *et al.*, 1976). This is another area in which the primary contribution of ultrasound in overall diagnosis is in determining whether the enlargement is cystic or solid in nature.

Ultrasonography has also found an important place in the management of patients with malignancy. This is especially true in the abdomen. The extent of a malignant mass in the abdomen can be determined by ultrasonic scanning. A projection of the mass can then be drawn on the patient's skin. This serves as a useful guide for the planning of radiation therapy treatment fields. The outlines of vital structures such as the kidneys and liver which are not involved with the malignancy to be irradiated can also be projected onto the patient's skin. These areas can then be protected from radiation by limiting the radiation beam to the malignant tissue. Serial ultrasonic examinations give a record of tumor response to the radiation therapy (Brascho, 1975). Similarly, serial examinations of malignant masses can give an indication to response or lack of response to chemotherapy.

Another expanding area of the use of ultrasound in diagnosis involves percutaneous aspiration of suspected pathologic masses. This is achieved by first localizing the area in question by standard B-mode scanning.

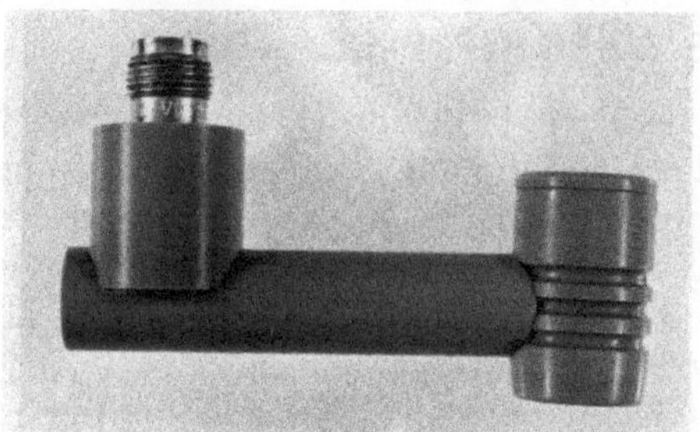

Fig. 9-30. Special biopsy transducer.

Transducers are available which have a central hole through which a needle can be passed (Fig. 9-30). One can then follow the progression of the needle as it is inserted from the skin to the mass (Holm *et al.*, 1975). Generally, the only discomfort the patient feels is the injection of local anesthetic into the skin. The needles are of a very thin caliber. The complication rate for percutaneous aspiration (biopsy) is acceptably low and is certainly much less than surgical morbidity or mortality. This technique has been widely utilized in mass lesions of the kidney, thyroid gland, and pancreas.

9.8. DOPPLER

As we have seen from the foregoing discussions, M-mode imaging results in visualization of structures which show motion during the time frame in which the imaging is carried out. A second method of detecting motions with ultrasound involves utilizing the Doppler shift. Blood velocity can readily be measured by Doppler frequency shift of backscattered ultrasound. The instrument is basically quite simple compared to instrumentation necessary for M-mode and B-mode scanning (Fig. 9-31). Most commercially available instruments utilize a receiving and a transmitting crystal. The signal is emitted continuously, as opposed to the pulsed signal employed in echo imaging systems.

Fortunately, the Doppler shifts which occur are in the audible range (500–6000 cycles/sec). Therefore the signal need only be amplified and processed through a speaker. The most convenient instrumentation is in the form of a light weight, portable stethoscope. The trained observer can determine the directions of blood flow by the change in pitch as the instrument is directed along different portions of the patient's anatomy.

The two main areas of clinical application of continuous wave Doppler are in determining the presence or absence of fetal heart tones and in the area of diagnosis of vascular diseases (Felix *et al.*, 1975).

Ultrasonic Doppler detection of fetal heart tones is highly accurate beginning at 10–12 weeks of gestational age (Johnson *et al.*, 1965). It is much more reliable than electrocardiographic detection of the fetal heart rhythm or standard (nonultrasonic) stethoscopic examination (Bernstein and Callagan, 1966).

The arterial and venous systems in the body are subject to a variety of diseases. Some of these pathologic states result in either a marked diminution in blood flow or a complete absence of blood flow. Ultrasonic evaluation utilizing Doppler can readily determine the presence or absence of flow in major superficial vessels of the body. These include the carotid arteries, the femoral arteries and the major arteries to the arms.

Not only can the presence or absence of flow be detected by Doppler, but the direction of flow can be detected as well. This is particularly important when one is concerned about the presence or absence of collateral circulation. Collateral circulation occurs following the gradual or abrupt occlusion of an artery which normally supplies a given portion of the body. Almost all tissues in the body derive their blood from branches of several major arterial subdivisions. When one of these is completely occluded, the pressure within the artery distal (away from the heart) to this occlusion will have a markedly lowered pressure compared to the remaining, patent arterial system. Thus blood will flow in a reverse direction in the portion of the occluded artery distal to the occlusion. The direction of blood flow in the supraorbital artery is reversed from normal. This reversal of flow is readily detectable by Doppler techniques.

Instrumentation is currently being developed which utilizes elements from both B-scanning and Doppler shift. This is the so-called pulsed-Doppler technique. With this instrumentation an artery or vein can be identified by scanning with the Doppler unit which has built-in devices to determine the position of the vessel in an X, Y plane with respect to a given

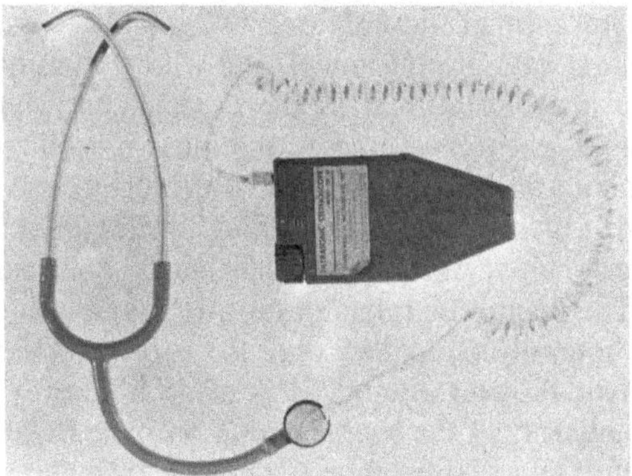

Fig. 9-31. Portable Doppler ultrasonic instrument.

starting point on the patient's anatomy. This allows two-dimensional imaging utilizing the Doppler signal (White, 1975).

The future of Doppler techniques is undoubtedly headed in the direction of more integration with B-scanning equipment. I would envision identification of an artery or vein deep within the body by B-scanning techniques. After the vessel in question is identified, one might switch the instrument to a Doppler mode and determine the direction and velocity of blood flow.

9.9. BIOLOGICAL EFFECTS OF DIAGNOSTIC ULTRASOUND

Diagnostic ultrasound uses low-intensity ultrasonic energy. In the vast majority of diagnostic studies, this ultrasonic energy is emitted in short pulses. In a typical A-, M-, or B-mode diagnostic examination, the piezoelectric element emits ultrasonic waves less than 0.1% of the time. The remainder of the time the piezoelectric element is "listening" for the echo return.

Within the power levels utilized by current ultrasonic instrumentation there has been no evidence to date of any biological effects, either harmful or beneficial.

There is a vast body of literature in both the physical and biological sciences concerning biologic toxicity of ultrasound (Goldstein and Sinskey, 1969; Hill, 1968; Taylor, 1974). There are definite harmful effects to biological tissue which can be imparted by ultrasonic radiation. These biological changes are brought about either by thermal effects or by cavitation within limited cellular loci. To obtain biologically measureable effects, one needs to impart radiation power orders of magnitude greater than is in current diagnostic usage. Many of the experiments which do show biological changes utilize not only tremendous intensities but also apply the ultrasonic energy directly to a small, limited area of biological tissue (such as rat embryos in the first days of pregnancy), and with continuous wave output. The increase in intensity utilized in the experiments which have shown biological damage, when compared to the intensity utilized in diagnostic ultrasonic imaging, can be likened to the difference between a human ear being exposed directly to a cannon (resulting in rupture of the ear drum or destruction of nerve fibers within the cochlea) and a quiet conversation with a good friend. The diagnostic range of ultrasonic beam intensity is several mW/cm^2. This intensity is applied only for very short intervals of time. Experimental data showing biological damage frequently do not give a measure of the intensity of the beam, stating only the frequency employed, the distance from the radiation source, the time of radiation, and the fact that continuous wave irradiation was utilized. In the few well-controlled experiments in which output was measured, or calculated based upon reasonable parameters, the range necessary for biological change was from tens of W/cm^2 to several thousand W/cm^2 (Freimanis, 1970).

Diagnostic ultrasound has been in use for the last 20 years. Over the past several years there has been a marked proliferation in the number of diagnostic ultrasonic examinations. This is especially true in obstetrical patients. If any analogy can be drawn between ultrasonic irradiation and ionizing radiation (such as gamma rays and X-rays), one would expect to find greater sensitivity to harmful effects in rapidly growing tissue, as encountered in embryos, fetuses, and young children. To this date, there is no evidence that irradiation *in utero* causes an increase in any anomalies or other pathologic states subsequently detected after birth. In some cases, the individuals have been observed up to the age of 12 years.

The foregoing does not indicate that diagnostic ultrasound is totally harmless, merely that there have been no effects noted to date. There are many difficulties encountered in obtaining definite "proof" that ultrasound is innocuous at the levels employed in diagnostic usage. One of the main difficulties is that of knowing what biological effect to expect and subsequently seek. Another major problem is that one would need huge volumes of animal data to determine the presence or absence of a threshold for damage while measuring various parameters of the ultrasonic beam such as intensity, frequency, and duration of exposure. This problem can be put into perspective by noting that even though X-rays have been in widespread medical use for over 60 years, there is still active controversy among physicians, physicists, and biological scientists as to whether or not there is a threshold effect present for ionizing radiation. To further complicate the matter, it should be remembered that following Roentgen's discovery of X-rays, it took many years before it was widely recognized that ionizing radiation was directly harmful to biological organisms. It took several more years to recognize the genetic effects of ionizing radiation. Even though our technology has become much more sophisticated, it may not be sensitive enough to give current indications of biological damage from ultrasound, if there is a significantly long lag time between exposure and the biological effects.

In conclusion, it is fair to say that to date there has been no evidence to indicate that ultrasonic irradiation in the diagnostic range is biologically harmful. However, further, long-term data collection is certainly indicated before diagnostic ultrasound can be given an unequivocal clean bill of health.

REFERENCES

Arnon, S., and Rosenquist, C.J. (1976), Gray scale cholecystosonography, an evaluation of accuracy, *Am. J. Roentgenol.* **127**:817–818.

Asher, W.M., Parvin, S., Virgillo, R.W., and Haber, K. (1976), Echographic evaluation of splenic injury after blunt trauma, *Radiology* **118**:411–415.

Ballentine, H.T., Bolt, R.H., Hueter, T.F., and Ludwig, G.D. (1950), On the detection of intracranial pathology by ultrasound, *Science* **112**:525–528.

Bernstein, R.L., and Callagan, D.A. (1966), Ultrasonic Doppler inspection of the fetal heart, *Am. J. Obstet. Gynecol.* **95**:1001–1004.

Brascho, D.J. (1975), Radiation therapy planning with ultrasound, *Radiol. Clin. North Am.* **13**:505–521.

Coleman, D.J., Konig, W.F., and Katz, L. (1969), A hand-operated ultrasound scan system for ophthalmic evaluation, *Am. J. Ophthalmol.* **68**:256–262.

Donald, I., MacVicar, J., and Brown, T.G. (1958), Investigation of abdominal masses by pulsed ultrasound, *Lancet* **1**:1188–1195.

Drumm, J.E., Clinch, J., and MacKenzie, G. (1976), The ultrasonic measurement of fetal crown-rump length as a method of assessing gestational age, *Br. J. Obstet. Gynecol.* **83**:417–419.

Dussik, K.T., Dussik, F., and Wyt, L. (1947), Auf dem Wege zur Hyperphonographie des Gehirnes, *Wien. Med. Wschr.* **97**:425.

Edler, I., and Hertz, C.H. (1954), The use of ultrasonic reflectoscope for the continuous recording of the movements of heart walls, *K. Fysiogr. Saellsk. Lund Foerh.* **24**:40–58.

Feigenbaum, H. (1972), *Echocardiography*, Lea and Febiger, Philadelphia.

Felix, W.R., Sigel, B., and Popky, G.L. (1975), Doppler ultrasound in the diagnosis of peripheral vascular disease, *Sem. Roentgenol.* **10**:315–321.

Franklin, D., Schlegel, W., and Rushmer, R. (1961), Blood flow measured by Doppler frequency shift of back scattered ultrasound, *Science* **132**:564–565.

Freimanis, A.K. (1970), The biological effects of medically applied ultrasound and their causes, *CRC Crit. Rev. Radiol. Sci.* 639–652, December.

Galicich, J.H., Lombrost, D.T., and Matson, D.D. (1965), Ultrasonic B-scanning of the brain, *J. Neurosurg.* **22**:499–510.

Gerbie, A.B., Shkolnik, F., and Shkolnik, A.A. (1975), Ultrasound prior to amniocentesis for genetic counseling, *Obstet. Gynecol.* **46**:716–719.

Goldberg, S.J., Allen, H.D., and Sahn D.J. (1975), *Pediatric and Adolescent Echocardiography*, Year Book Medical Publishers, Chicago.

Goldstein, N., and Sinskey, A.J. (1969), Health hazards from ultrasonic energy, U. S. Department of Commerce PB 185963.

Gramiak, R., Nanda, N.C., and Gross, C.M. (1975), Echocardiography in acquired cardiac and pericardial disease, *Sem. Roentgenol.* **10**:291–297.

Güttner, Von W., Fiedler, G., and Patzold, J. (1952), Über Ultraschallabbildungen am Menschlichen Schädel, *Acustica* **2**:148.

Haber, K., Asher, W.M., and Freimanis, A.K. (1975), Echographic evaluation of diaphragmatic motion in intra-abdominal diseases, *Radiology* **114**:141–144.

Haber, K., Freimanis, A.T., and Asher, W.M. (1976), Demonstration and dimensional analysis of the normal pancreas with gray-scale echography, *Amer. J. Roentgenol. Radium Ther. Nucl. Med.* **126**:624–628.

Herzog, K.A. (1975), The detection of fetal meningocele and meningoencephalocele by B-Scan ultrasound, *J. Clin. Ultrasound* **3**:307–308.

Hill, C.R. (1968), The possibility of hazard in medical and industrial application of ultrasound, *Br. J. Radiol.* **41**:561–569.

Holm, H.H., Pedersen, J.F., Kristensen, J.K., Rasmussen, S.N., Hancke, S., and Jensen, F. (1975), Ultrasonically guided percutaneous puncture, *Radiol. Clin. North Am.* **13**:493–503.

Holmes, J.H., Howry, D.H., Posakony, G.J., and Cushman, C.R. (1954), The ultrasonic visualization of soft tissue structures in the human body, *Am. Clin. Climatol. Ass. Trans.* **66**:208–225.

Howry, D.H. (1965), A brief atlas of diagnostic ultrasonic radiologic results, *Radiol. Clin. North Am.* **3**:433–452.

Johnson, W.L., Stegall, H.F., Lein, J.N., and Rushmer, R.F. (1965), Detection of fetal life in early pregnancy with an ultrasonic Doppler flowmeter, *Obstet. Gynecol.* **26**:305–307.

Langevin, M.P. (1928), Les ondes ultrasonores, *Rev. Gen. Electr.* **23**:626–634.

Ludwig, G.D., and Struthers, F.W. (1949), Consideration underlying the use of ultrasound to detect gallstones and foreign bodies in tissue, U. S. Naval Project NM 004 001, Report No. 4, 16 June 1949.

McQuown, D.S. (1975), Ocular and orbital echography, *Radiol. Clin. North Am.* **13**:523–541.

Miskin, M., and Bain, J. (1974), B-Mode ultrasonic examination of the testes, *J. Clin. Ultrasound* **2**:307–311.

Neiman, H.L., Phillips, J.F., Jaques, D.A., and Brown, T.L. (1976), Ultrasound of the parotid gland, *J. Clin. Ultrasound* **4**:11–13.

Perlmutter, G.S., Goldbery, B.B., and Charkes, N.D. (1975), Ultrasound evaluation of the thyroid, *Sem. Nucl. Med.* **5**:299–305.

Pond, G.P., and Haber, K. (1976), Echography: a new approach to the diagnosis of adrenal hemorrhage of the newborn, *J. Can. Ass. Radiolog.* **27**:40–44.

Sahn, D.J., Allen, H.D., Goldberg, S.J., and Friedman, W.F. (1976), Mitral valve prolapse in children: A problem defined by real-time cross-sectional echocardiography, *Circulation* **53**:651–657.

Sanders, R.C. (1975), The place of diagnostic ultrasound in the examination of kidneys not seen on excretory urography, *J. Urol.* **114**:813–821.

Sanders, R.C., and Conrad, M.R. (1975), Sonography in obstetrics, *Radiol. Clin. North Am.* **13**:435–45.

Shkolnik, A. (1975), B-Mode scanning of the infant brain: A new approach, *J. Clin. Ultrasound* **3**:229–231.

Taylor, K.J.W. (1974), Current status of toxicity investigations, *J. Clin. Ultrasound* **2**:149–156.

Tenner, M.S., Wodraska, G., and Adapon, B.D. (1974), Newer ultrasound techniques in the evaluation of neurologic disorders, *Radiol. Clin. North Am.* **12**:283–295.

Thompson, H.E. (1973), Ultrasonic diagnostic procedures in obstetrics and gynecology, *J. Clin. Ultrasound* **1**:160–171.

White, D. (1975), *Ultrasound in Medicine*, Vol. 1, Plenum Press, New York, p. 355.

White, D.N. (1966), In Grossman, C.C., *et al.* (eds.), *Diagnostic Ultrasound*, Plenum Press, New York, pp. 142–147.

Wild, J.J. (1950), The use of ultrasonic pulses for the measurement of biologic tissues and the detection of tissue density changes, *Surgery* **27**:183–188.

Wild, J.J., and Reid, J.M. (1952), Application of echo-ranging techniques to the determination of structure of biological tissues, *Science* **115**:226–230.

Wood, W. (1927), Extrait congress international des physiciens, *Rev. Gen. Electr.* **22**:614.

CHAPTER 10

Ultrasonic Imaging: Basic Principles

THEODORE BOWEN

10.1. INTRODUCTION

Medical diagnostic imaging with sound waves usually carries the label "ultrasonic" because, as will be shown in the following review, the frequency range useful for diagnostic imaging (1–10 MHz) is well above the hearing range (20–20,000 Hz). The corresponding wavelengths (1.5–0.15 mm) of the imaging waves are much larger than the electromagnetic wavelengths of light or X-rays. In fact, in ultrasonic imaging one must strive to design systems in which the resolution is comparable to the wavelengths of the illuminating radiation; only in the design of optical microscopes does one approach the wavelength limit of resolution in medical-imaging systems using electromagnetic waves. In radar imaging of aircraft and terrain one attempts to approach the wavelength limit of resolution, so there are many similarities between radar and ultrasonic diagnostic techniques.

THEODORE BOWEN • Department of Physics, University of Arizona, Tucson, Arizona 85721.

There is another difference between medical-imaging systems based upon ultrasonic and electromagnetic waves: whereas most electromagnetic wave systems using light or X-rays simultaneously illuminate the entire region of interest, and only a few recently introduced systems (such as the computerized axial tomography with X-rays) scan the illuminating radiation over the subject, most ultrasonic-imaging systems involve scanning a narrow beam of ultrasound through the region to be examined. For this reason, the following review will emphasize physical effects important for scanning-type systems.

Although there are many analogies between the behavior of sound waves and electromagnetic waves, sound waves owe their origin to completely different physical phenomena than electromagnetic waves. Sound waves are the consequence of mechanical motion in regions containing material—gas, liquid, or solid—whereas electromagnetic waves are the consequence of the interaction of electric and magnetic fields in free space.

10.2. FUNDAMENTAL SOUND PROPAGATION EQUATIONS

The propagation of mechanical waves in any material media arises out of combining two fundamental laws of physics: Newton's equation of motion, $F = ma$, and the equation of continuity, which states that motion in a continuous medium, such as a fluid, must take place in such a way that mass is conserved. In a material medium propagating a wave the force arises from pressure differences between nearby regions—the pressure gradient. The accelerated mass in a specified small region is proportional to the density ρ of the material, and the acceleration is the time rate of change of the velocity v of the specified small region. So the only property of the material medium affecting Newton's equation is the density, ρ.

The equation of continuity relates the net flow of material into (or out of) a specified small region to the increase (or decrease) of density which results; hence it relates flow velocity, v, to changes in the density. These changes of density caused by a sound wave are very, very small when expressed as a fraction or percentage of the average density, so these changes can be ignored in the density ρ used in Newton's equation. However, the pressure changes caused by tiny density changes cannot be ignored. The pressure change relative to a fractional change in density is given by the bulk modulus B (or the inverse of the compressibility) for the material medium. Thus the equation of continuity gives a relation between velocity v, and the change of pressure p, which is affected only by the bulk modulus B of the material medium.

An equation for wave propagation emerges from the results of the preceding two paragraphs. Note that Newton's equation of motion relates the rate of change of velocity to the pressure gradient. Also note that the equation of continuity provides an essentially reciprocal relationship between the rate of change of pressure and velocity nonuniformities. Wave motion has the interesting property of satisfying both equations, provided appropriate choices are made for the wave velocity of propagation c and the ratio Z of pressure to particle velocity (where $Z = p/v$).

Sound waves will propagate in any medium characterized by a density ρ and a bulk modulus B. It will be shown in the next sections that the characteristics of the medium are more conveniently summarized in terms of the velocity c of sound propagation, where $c = (B/\rho)^{1/2}$, and the acoustic impedance Z, where $Z = \rho c = (B\rho)^{1/2}$. Other types of mechanical waves exist (for example, shear waves), but only the pressure or compressional wave will propagate appreciable distances in gases, liquids, and soft mammalian tissues.

10.3. WAVE EQUATION FOR SOUND

The equations for propagation of sound waves will be developed for the special case of plane waves propagating in the x direction, since this case will give most of the results of importance for diagnostic ultrasonic imaging. For more detailed discussions, the reader is referred to any standard treatise on acoustics or sound (Morse, 1948, 1968; Malecki, 1969). If one considers the forces on a small element of volume, Newton's equation of motion requires that

$$\rho \frac{\partial v}{\partial t} = - \frac{\partial p}{\partial x} \tag{10-1}$$

where $v(x, t)$ is the particle velocity in the vicinity of the small-volume element at position x and time t, $p(x, t)$ is the pressure, and ρ is the density (considered as constant in this equation). The continuity equation requires that

$$\frac{\partial p}{\partial t} = B \frac{1}{\rho} \frac{\partial \rho}{\partial t} = -B \frac{\partial v}{\partial x} \tag{10-2}$$

where B is the bulk modulus. In order to combine Eqs. (10-1) and (10-2) into an equation for p, differentiate Eq. (10-1) with respect to x and Eq. (10-2) with respect to t, and note that $\partial^2 v/\partial x\, \partial t = \partial^2 v/\partial t\, \partial x$. The result is

$$\frac{1}{\rho} \frac{\partial^2 p}{\partial x^2} = \frac{1}{B} \frac{\partial^2 p}{\partial t^2}$$

or

$$\frac{\partial^2 p}{\partial x^2} - \frac{1}{c^2}\frac{\partial^2 p}{\partial t^2} = 0 \tag{10-3}$$

where $c = (B/\rho)^{1/2}$. If instead Eq. (10-1) is differentiated with respect to t and Eq. (10-2) with respect to x, the result is

$$\frac{\partial^2 v}{\partial x^2} - \frac{1}{c^2}\frac{\partial^2 v}{\partial t^2} = 0 \tag{10-4}$$

where $c = (B/\rho)^{1/2}$ as before with Eq. (10-3). Equations (10-3) and (10-4) show that both the pressure p and particle velocity v obey wave equations with the same wave velocity c. It can be verified by the appropriate differentiations that any function $f(x \pm ct)$ is a solution. Suppose $p(x, t) = f(x - ct)$. This is a wave which at any instant t_1 has the form $p(x, t_1) = f(x - ct_1)$. At a later time t_2 it will have the form $p(x, t_2) = f(x - ct_2)$, where $ct_2 > ct_1$. The x's in the second expression will have to be larger by $ct_2 - ct_1 = c(t_2 - t_1)$ to reproduce the form of the pressure at t_1; hence the wave has moved a distance $c(t_2 - t_1)$ to the right, and the constant c is the velocity of propagation. A solution of the form $f(x + ct)$ represents a wave traveling to the left by analogous reasoning.

If $p(x, t) = f(x \mp ct)$ and $v(x, t) = g(x \mp ct)$, the relationship between the functions f and g can be found by substitution into either Eq. (10-1) or Eq. (10-2). Using Eq. (10-1)

$$\rho g'(x \mp ct)(\mp c) = -f'(x \mp ct)$$

or

$$f(x \mp ct) = \pm \rho c g(x \mp ct) + \text{const} \tag{10-5}$$

If the constant in Eq. (10-5) is set equal to zero by an appropriate choice of the zero of the pressure scale, then the ratio of the pressure to the particle velocity at any point is given by

$$\frac{p}{v} = \frac{f(x \mp ct)}{g(x \mp ct)} = \pm \rho c = \pm Z \tag{10-6}$$

where $Z = \rho c$ is called the acoustic impedance of the medium. Note that p/v is a ratio which is independent of x and t, but its sign depends upon the propagation direction of p. It is also interesting to observe that the information on p/v was not contained in the wave equations for p or v; it was necessary to return to one of the two basic equations from which the wave equation was derived.

Since p/v can have either sign depending upon the direction of travel of the wave, other values for the ratio at a specified x are possible if waves propagating in both directions are present. This is allowed by the wave equations because they are linear in p and v; any linear combination of solutions is also a solution.

10.4. INTERFACES BETWEEN DIFFERENT MEDIA

Suppose there is an interface between two material media at $x = 0$; i.e., two different materials are in contact at the $x = 0$ plane. Let c_A, c_B and Z_A, Z_B be the wave velocity and acoustic impedance in materials A, B, respectively, located to the left and right of $x = 0$. In each material the waves are described by solutions to the wave equations [Eqs. (10-3) and (10-4)]. At the boundary ($x = 0$) the pressure and particle velocity must be the same for a short distance on either side of $x = 0$; i.e., $p(x, t)$ and $v(x, t)$ must be continuous at $x = 0$. If p_A and p_B were not equal at $x = 0$, there would be unbalanced forces; if v_A and v_B were not equal, there would be voids or collapsed material at $x = 0$. So, the boundary conditions at $x = 0$ are

$$p_A(0, t) = p_B(0, t) \tag{10-7}$$

$$v_A(0, t) = v_B(0, t) \tag{10-8}$$

If a wave originating in material A travels to the right from $x = -\infty$ toward $x = 0$ is denoted by pressure $p_A^+(x - c_A t)$ and particle velocity $v_A^+(x - c_A t)$, the ratio p_A^+/v_A^+ must be $+Z_A$. Upon striking the interface at $x = 0$, it will give rise to a wave disturbance in medium B which must also be traveling to the right away from the disturbance at $x = 0$. Therefore, its pressure and velocity are denoted $p_B^+(x - c_B t)$ and $v_B^+(x - c_B t)$, where the $+$ superscript indicates that the wave travels to the right. The ratio p_B^+/v_B^+ must be $+Z_B$, which may be different from Z_A. However, the boundary conditions, Eqs. (10-7) and (10-8), require the same ratio of pressure to particle velocity on either side of the interface at $x = 0$, since Eq. (10-7) divided by Eq. (10-8) gives

$$\frac{p_A(0, t)}{v_A(0, t)} = \frac{p_B(0, t)}{v_B(0, t)} \tag{10-9}$$

Another wave must be added to (p_A^+, v_A^+) and (p_B^+, v_B^+) already mentioned in order to satisfy Eq. (10-9). It must be a wave traveling to the left, and since it must be caused by a mechanical disturbance at its origin, it must be a reflected wave in medium A which can be denoted by pressure $p_A^-(x + c_A t)$ and particle velocity $v_A^-(x + c_A t)$. Since the total wave in medium A is the sum of the two wave solutions for incident and reflected waves, $p_A = p_A^+ +$

p_A^- and $v_A = v_A^+ + v_A^-$ and Eq. (10-9) becomes

$$\frac{p_A^+(-c_A t) + p_A^-(c_A t)}{v_B^+(-c_A t) + v_A^-(c_A t)} = \frac{p_B^+(-c_B t)}{v_B^+(-c_B t)} = Z_B \tag{10-10}$$

A solution for the left-hand side of Eq. (10-10) must be found which is independent of t, since Z_B is a constant determined by the physical properties of medium B. This can be done if the reflected wave is a precise replica of the incident wave except that its amplitude is less by a factor r; i.e., suppose

$$p_A^-(x + c_A t) = r p_A^+(-x - c_A t) \tag{10-11}$$

and

$$v_A^-(x + c_A t) = -r v_A^+(-x - c_A t) \tag{10-12}$$

The minus sign in $-rv_A^+$ of Eq. (10-12) is necessary so that $p_A^-/v_A^- = -Z_A$ as required for waves propagating to the left. Then, setting $x = 0$ in Eqs. (10-11) and (10-12), and substituting into Eq. (10-10), one obtains

$$\frac{p_A^+(-c_A t) + r p_A^+(-c_A t)}{v_A^+(-c_A t) - r v_A^+(-c_A t)} = \frac{(1 + r) p_A^+(-c_A t)}{(1 - r) v_A^+(-c_A t)} = \frac{1 + r}{1 - r} Z_A = Z_B \tag{10-13}$$

Figure 10-1a illustrates the incident, reflected, and transmitted waves; the pressure at a given time is the sum of the pressures due to the incident and reflected waves as is shown in Fig. 10-1b. Solving Eq. (10-13) for r, one obtains

$$r = \frac{Z_B - Z_A}{Z_B + Z_A} \tag{10-14}$$

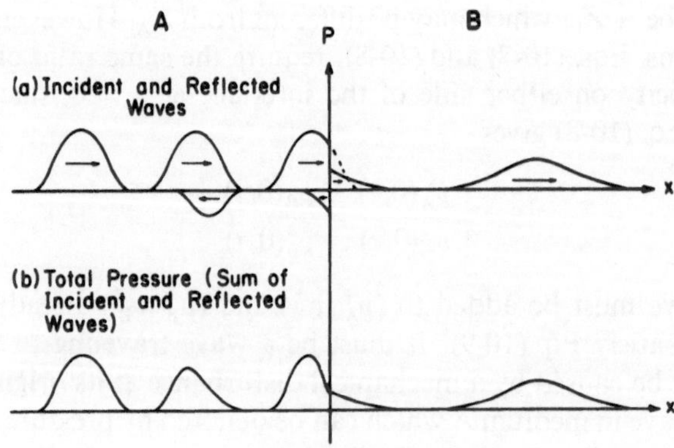

Fig. 10-1. (a) Incident, reflected, and transmitted waves for normal incidence. (b) Total pressure of the incident and reflected waves shown in (a).

Equation (10-14) is fundamental to most applications in diagnostic ultrasonic imaging since it relates the relative amplitudes of reflected and incident waves to the acoustic impedances of the media on either side of the reflecting interface. It is valid only if the plane of the interface is perpendicular to the direction of travel of the incident (and reflected) wave, but this condition is approximately satisfied in most medical applications since only those waves which reflect or backscatter into the transmitting transducer are observed. Note that if $Z_B = Z_A$, $r = 0$; i.e., there is no reflection if impedances perfectly match. It is also interesting to observe that r is positive or negative depending upon whether Z_B is greater or less than Z_A; presently available imaging equipment does not make use of this fact which could in principle detect at each interface whether the impedance increased or decreased.

10.5. ENERGY TRANSPORT BY SONIC WAVES

The energy carried by a sonic wave can be defined as equal to the work it would do if it were completely absorbed. If $Z_B = Z_A$ at an interface at $x = 0$ between media A and B, then a wave from A will be completely absorbed in B, and the energy in the wave can be found by calculating the work done by the forces in A acting on B across the interface. Considering a unit area of the interface, the work per second, W, done by A on B is

$$W(0, t) = \frac{\text{work}}{(\text{unit area})(\text{sec})} = \frac{\text{force}}{\text{unit area}} \cdot \frac{\text{distance moved}}{\text{sec}}$$

$$= p_A(0, t)\, v_A(0, t) \tag{10-15}$$

If MKS units are used with p_A in $\mathrm{N/m^2}$ and v_A in m/sec, then W is in $\mathrm{W/m^2}$. If one is dealing only with a wave traveling from left to right, then $p_A^+ = Z_A v_A^+$ from Eq. (10-6), and

$$W^+ = Z(v^+)^2 = \frac{(p^+)^2}{Z} \tag{10-16}$$

where the subscript A has been dropped since the result applies at any point and the $+$ superscript is a reminder that the wave is traveling in the $+x$ direction. In general, W is a function of time, but often it is useful to define the intensity I of an ultrasonic wave as the power per unit area averaged over a specified time interval:

$$I^+ \equiv \langle W^+ \rangle = Z\langle (v^+)^2 \rangle = \frac{\langle (p^+)^2 \rangle}{Z} \tag{10-17}$$

Note that the energy flow W and the intensity I are both proportional to $(v^+)^2$ or $(p^+)^2$.

It is interesting to compare the reflected intensity I_A^- to the incident intensity I_A^+ for a reflection from an impedance discontinuity with the help of Eqs. (10-11) and (10-14). Assume that the averages for I_A^- and I_A^+ are taken over similar parts of the incident and reflected waves, so

$$\frac{I_A^-}{I_A^+} = \frac{\langle (p_A^-)^2 \rangle}{\langle (p_A^+)^2 \rangle} = r^2 = \left(\frac{Z_B - Z_A}{Z_B + Z_A} \right)^2 \qquad (10\text{-}18)$$

Suppose a wave encountered a 5% impedance change, which would be a large change between typical soft tissues. Equation (10-18) says that only 0.25% of the incident energy would be reflected; the other 99.75% would remain in the wave entering medium B. An ultrasonic wave can pass through many such interfaces with impedance changes of 5% or less, reflecting back a weak but detectable wave or "echo" from each. This provides the basis for most diagnostic ultrasonic imaging.

10.6. REFLECTION AND REFRACTION OF SONIC WAVES

In the case of a sonic wave normally incident to (i.e., direction of propagation perpendicular to) an interface plane, the transmitted wave continues in the same direction in medium B and the reflected wave travels in the exact reverse direction to the incident wave. The relative pressure, particle velocity, and intensity of the reflected wave have been treated in the previous sections.

The problem of a plane wave in medium A obliquely incident at an angle θ_A^+ to the normal on a plane interface between media A and B can be solved by analogous methods. Again there is a reflected wave at angle θ_A^- to normal, and a wave transmitted or refracted into medium B at angle θ_B^+ to the normal (see Fig. 10-2). The relationships among these angles depends only upon the wave propagation velocities c_A and c_B as is also true for reflection and refraction of light. Since the results for light are developed in most introductory physics courses, the reader is referred to any basic physics or introductory optics text for the details; a summary in the notation of this review follows.

(1) The angle of reflection θ_A^- equals the angle of incidence θ_A^+, or

$$\theta_A^- = \theta_A^+ \qquad (10\text{-}19)$$

(2) The angle of refraction θ_B^+ is related to the angle of incidence θ_A^+ by

$$\frac{\sin \theta_B^+}{c_B} = \frac{\sin \theta_A^+}{c_B} \qquad (10\text{-}20)$$

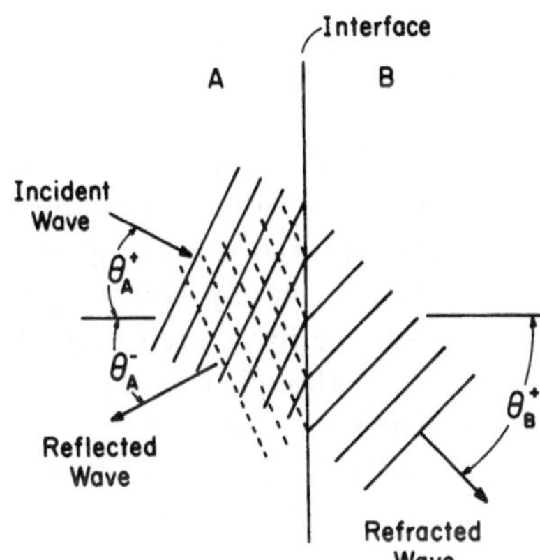

Fig. 10-2. Reflection and refraction from an oblique interface.

Note that the roles of media A and B enter Eq. (10-20) symmetrically; thus a wave incident from B at angle θ_B^+ would emerge in A at angle θ_A^+. This shows that backreflections or echoes retrace the route of the primary wave back through refracting interfaces.

It is useful to put a few numbers into Eq. (10-20) in order to gain an idea of when refraction might seriously deviate a wave from straight-line travel. Suppose a wave encounters a 5% change in sonic velocity across an interface. The resulting change $\theta_B^+ - \theta_A^+$ in the direction of wave propagation is listed in Table 10-1 for several values of the angle of incidence θ_A^+. The table shows that changes of direction remain small except for angles of incidence near 90°.

Table 10-1. Change of Direction of a Wave Encountering a 5% Change of Sound Velocity vs. Angle of Incidence

Angle of incidence, θ_A^+ (deg)	Change of direction, $\theta_B^+ - \theta_A^+$ (deg)
0	0
10	0.5
20	1.0
30	1.6
40	2.4
50	3.3
60	4.6
70	6.8
80	10.7

10.7. SOUND VELOCITIES AND ACOUSTIC IMPEDANCES IN THE BODY

Table 10-2 lists typical results for the velocity of sound and acoustic impedance for various tissues and related substances. The data which would be of greatest interest for diagnostic imaging would concern various living tissues. Unfortunately very few accurate measurements of sound velocity and impedance have been made for living tissue due to the experimental difficulties, although one entry in Table 10-2 shows the range of values obtained from measurements on accessible regions of human soft tissue, such as the calf, thigh, and biceps muscles. The entries in Table 10-2 are meant to give the reader the approximate magnitudes of sound velocity and impedance, and the rough range of variation within a broad group, such as soft tissue.

It is clear from Table 10-2 that tissues or materials found in the body fall into three groups having very different ranges of sound velocity and impedance: gases and inflated lung tissues, fluids and soft tissues, and mineralized tissues. Because of the large impedance differences between these groups, there is very little transmission of sound energy from a region consisting of materials of one group into an adjacent region of another group. These facts effectively limit ultrasonic imaging to regions containing fluids and soft tissues where the viewing is not obstructed by gas (air in the lungs, gas in the intestines) or by bones. (An exception is the head, where some work has been done transmitting the ultrasound through the skull. See Chapter 9, Section 9.5.)

Focusing attention on the fluids and soft tissues group, it is useful to convert the velocity of sound to smaller units: 1500 m/sec = 1.5 mm/μsec —1.5 millimeters per microsecond is a convenient number to memorize for use when needed in "back-of-the-envelope" calculations. Also note from Table 10-2 that 5% is a reasonable estimate of the largest change of velocity or impedance likely to be encountered within a region of fluids and soft tissue. The relatively small range of sound velocities and acoustic impedances in soft tissues provides the basis for diagnostic imaging: (1) sound travels in nearly straight paths to and from the target with little refraction, (2) the time delay in receiving an echo is approximately proportional to the depth of the target, (3) sound waves can "illuminate" any small region with roughly uniform intensity, yet (4) the impedance discontinuities are sufficiently large in magnitude to produce detectable echoes.

10.8. THE ROLE OF ULTRASONIC WAVELENGTH AND FREQUENCY IN IMAGING

Up to this point in the discussion of the propagation of sonic waves no mention has been made of wavelengths or frequency. The waves dis-

Table 10-2. Typical Ultrasound Velocities and Acoustic Impedances in Tissues and Related Substances

	Conditions[a]	Sound velocity (m/sec)	Acoustic impedance[b] (N sec/m)	Reference
		Gases		
Air		353	0.00040×10^6	Beranek, 1963b
Methane		460	0.00024	Beranek, 1963b
Hydrogen		1353	0.00011	Beranek, 1963b
Lung (dog)	Fresh, 35°C	650	0.26	Dunn, 1961
		Fluids and soft mammalian tissues		
Seawater		1558	1.59×10^6	Del Grosso, 1970
Blood	24°C	1556	1.62	Van Venrooij, 1971
Limbs	*In vivo*	1490–1610	1.58–1.70	Ludwig, 1950
Brain (cat)	*In vivo*	1560	1.64	Robinson and Lele, 1972
Nerve (optic)	*In vitro*	1615	1.68	Buschmann *et al.*, 1970
Fat (orbital)	*In vitro*	1462	1.39	Buschmann *et al.*, 1970
Muscle (eye)	*In vitro*	1631	1.73	Buschmann *et al.*, 1970
Muscle (skeletal, dog)	Fresh	1593	1.69	Bowen *et al.*, 1977
Liver (dog)	Fresh	1597	1.68	Bowen *et al.*, 1977
Kidney (dog)	Fresh	1569	1.66	Bowen *et al.*, 1977
Fat (stomach, dog)	Fresh	1412	1.31	Bowen *et al.*, 1977
		Mineralized mammalian tissues		
Bone (skull)	Fresh	3360	5.7×10^6	Theismann and Pfander, 1949
Bone (skeletal, bovine)	Fresh, ~20°C			
	Parallel to bone axis	4030	7.9	Lang, 1970
	Perpendicular to bone axis	3160	6.2	Lang, 1970
Dentine	Fixed, ~20°C	3800	8.3	Barber *et al.*, 1969
Enamel	Fixed, ~20°C	6250	18.1	Barber *et al.*, 1969

[a] Data are for human tissue at body temperature (37°C) unless otherwise indicated.
[b] Acoustic impedance ($Z = \rho c$) estimates in most cases were not obtained from the original data, but by using independent density estimates.

cussed in preceding sections could have arbitrary form—a single unipolar pulse, a bipolar pulse, a periodic oscillatory wave "packet," or a continuous wave (cw) oscillation, to name a few possibilities. These are illustrated in Fig. 10-3. Whatever wave form is initiated, it will propagate through the medium at speed c without a change of shape according to the solutions of the wave equations [Eqs. (10-3) and (10-4)].

Any waveform, even a single pulse, can be mathematically expressed as a superposition of a large or infinite number of continuous waves, each with a different frequency f. If the waveform remains the same as it propagates, each frequency component must propagate at the same speed and without any change in amplitude relative to other frequency components. It can be verified by direct substitution into Eqs. (10-3) and (10-4) that any continuous wave with frequency f and wavelength λ is a solution satisfying these requirements, and that frequency and wavelength are related by

$$\lambda = \frac{c}{f} \tag{10-21}$$

or

$$f = \frac{c}{\lambda} \tag{10-22}$$

It is experimentally observed that there is no measurable change of the sound speed or acoustic impedance of water for frequencies from 0 to more

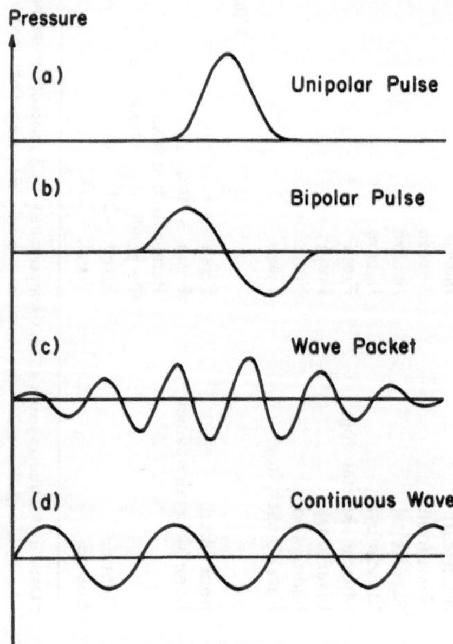

Fig. 10-3. Examples of typical pulse shapes: (a) unipolar pulse, (b) bipolar pulse, (c) wave packet, and (d) continuous wave.

than 100 MHz (i.e., for $\lambda = c/f \gtrsim 10^{-2}$ mm) (Fay, 1957), and that there is only a very small change in the 1–10-MHz range for tissues (Carstensen and Schwan, 1959b). Unfortunately, experiment indicates that waves of differing frequencies in the 1–10-MHz range do not maintain the same relative amplitudes as they propagate through tissue thickness in the 10–300-mm range. In other words, the attenuation of ultrasonic waves in body tissue is a strong function of frequency (or wavelength) (Dunn, 1976).

It can be shown that a single unipolar pressure pulse consists of a broad spectrum of continuous waves where all frequencies from zero to $f_{max} \approx 1/T$ are important, T being a time on the order of the rise or fall time of the pulse, whichever is shorter. On the other extreme, a long wave packet of pressure oscillations, each with period τ, consists of a narrow band of frequencies Δf about a center frequency of $f_0 = 1/\tau$; the order of magnitude of Δf is $1/n\tau$, where n is the number of complete oscillations or cycles in the wave packet. It is clear then that propagation through body tissues may seriously distort the waveforms of pulses, but the distortions become progressively less significant for wave packets of increasing length.

There are further reasons why wave packets consisting of many cycles, rather than lone pulses, are employed in diagnostic ultrasonic-imaging techniques. If a specified finite region initiates the propagation of a wave disturbance and the pressure distribution as a function of position is examined after the wave has traveled some distance, a different pressure distribution will be found for each wavelength component. For example, usually it is desired to produce a narrow beam of ultrasonic radiation; only by restricting emission to a small range of wavelengths can a beam with well-defined profiles be produced.

A practical engineering consideration also favors utilization of a narrow band of frequencies and corresponding wavelengths: the electromechanical devices, called transducers, which provide a convenient means of generating and detecting sonic waves, function most efficiently near frequencies at which they mechanically resonate. Resonant frequencies in the 1–10 MHz region can readily be obtained by appropriate choice of transducer dimensions. Efficient coupling between suitable transducer materials, all of which have much higher acoustic impedance than tissues, and soft tissue can be arranged for a narrow band of frequencies by means of a quarter-wavelength-thickness layer of material with acoustic impedance $Z_c = (Z_1 Z_2)^{1/2}$, where Z_1 and Z_2 are the acoustic impedances of the transducer and tissue, respectively (Goldman, 1962). This coupling technique is exactly analogous to antireflection optical coatings commonly used on lenses.

There are disadvantages of a narrow-band ultrasonic-imaging system: (1) A wave packet consisting of $n(\gg 1)$ oscillatory cycles provides poorer depth resolution than a shorter, wide-band packet or pulse. If echoes are being received from two acoustic impedance discontinuity layers at depths x_1 and x_2, then the echoes will be separated by a time

$$t_{12} = \frac{2(x_2 - x_1)}{c} \tag{10-23}$$

where c is the sound velocity in the layer between discontinuities. For clear resolution of both layers, we must require that

$$t_{12} \gtrsim n\tau = \frac{n}{f} = \frac{n\lambda}{c} \tag{10-24}$$

or

$$x_2 - x_1 \gtrsim \frac{n\lambda}{2} \tag{10-25}$$

(2) The wave packet corresponding to a narrow-band system slowly builds up and dies away (as shown in Fig. 10-3c), resulting in the loss of information concerning the polarity of the received pressure signal. As a result, echoes from increases and decreases of acoustic impedance are indistinguishable, and it is not possible, even in principle, to reconstruct a profile of the impedance as a function of depth from the information in the received signal.

10.9. ATTENUATION OF ULTRASOUND IN TISSUES

If the absorption and scattering of energy in volume dV from an ultrasonic wave is assumed to be proportional to the product of its intensity, $I(x)$, and the volume, then the power dW_{abs} absorbed is

$$dW_{abs} = 2\alpha I(x)\,dV \tag{10-26}$$

where 2α is the constant of proportionality having units of $(\text{length})^{-1}$. We desire to express the effect of this absorption on a plane wave incident on area A. The plane wave delivers power W_{in}, where

$$W_{in} = AI(x) \tag{10-27}$$

In passing through a thickness dx the intensity changes to $I(x + dx)$, and the power passing out through the surface of area A at $x + dx$ is

$$\begin{aligned} W_{out} &= AI(x + dx) \\ &= A\left[I(x) + \frac{dI}{dx}dx\right] \end{aligned} \tag{10-28}$$

The difference $W_{in} - W_{out}$ must equal the power absorbed dW_{abs}:

$$W_{in} - W_{out} = -A\frac{dI}{dx}dx$$

$$= dW_{abs} \qquad (10\text{-}29)$$

Using Eqs. (10-26) and (10-29) and the fact that $dV = A\,dx$, we obtain

$$\frac{dI}{dx} = -2\alpha I(x) \qquad (10\text{-}30)$$

This equation, when integrated, yields the solution

$$I(x) = I_0 e^{-2\alpha x} \qquad (10\text{-}31)$$

where I_0 is the intensity at $x = 0$. Since according to Eq. (10-17) the average pressure amplitude squared is proportional to the intensity, we can also write

$$\langle [p(x)]^2 \rangle^{1/2} \equiv p_{rms}(x) = p_0 e^{-\alpha x} \qquad (10\text{-}32)$$

We have demonstrated that both the intensity and pressure amplitude of an ultrasonic wave of a given frequency can be expected to decrease exponentially with the distance of propagation. Note that the exponential coefficients of the intensity and pressure amplitude differ by a factor of 2. We have defined α as the coefficient of attenuation of the pressure amplitude.

In general α can be a function of the frequency f. In most liquids including water α is proportional to f^2, due in large part to the effects of viscosity (Fay, 1957). In the 1–10-MHz region the attenuation of ultrasound in soft tissues is very much greater than in water, and has a different frequency dependence: α is observed to be proportional to f (see Dunn and O'Brien, 1976, and Hussey, 1975, for surveys of work on absorption of ultrasound in tissue). Thus we can write for frequencies in the 1–10-MHz range

$$\alpha_{mm} = \beta f_{MHz} \qquad (10\text{-}33)$$

where α_{mm} is in mm^{-1}, β is a constant with units of μsec/mm, and f_{MHz} is the frequency expressed in megahertz. Typical values of β for various tissues are given in Table 10-3. If, for example, $\beta = 0.01$ μsec/mm, then at 2.25 MHz $\alpha = 0.0225$ mm^{-1}, and the pressure amplitude would be attenuated by a factor of $e \cong 2.718$ in $1/0.0225 \cong 44$ mm. As the frequency is increased, the attenuation rapidly becomes a serious limitation to observing echoes from interior regions of the body.

Experiments have shown that most of the ultrasonic attenuation in soft tissues, including the linear frequency dependence expressed by Eq. (10.33), is due to the proteins which are present. For example, molecular absorption accounts for about 75% of the attenuation in normal blood for

Table 10-3. Typical Ultrasound Coefficients for Tissue[a]

Tissue	β (μsec/mm)[b,c]
Blood plasma	0.0008
Blood	0.0008 + 0.000031 V[d]
Fat	0.006
Brain	0.008
Liver	0.010
Kidney	0.011
Heart muscle	0.019
Skull bone	0.27

[a] Based upon compilation by D. E. Goldman and T. F. Hueter (Goldman and Hueter, 1957).

[b] β is defined by the attenuation of the pressure amplitude at depth x_{mm} in millimeters according to the relation $p(x_{mm}) = p(0)\exp(-\beta f_{MHz} x_{mm})$, where f_{MHz} is the frequency in megahertz.

[c] The values given for β are approximately valid in the 1–5 MHz region, and are uncertain by roughly ±20%.

[d] V is the volume concentration of cells in percent.

the 1–4-MHz range, the remainder being attributable to viscosity effects arising from motion of the plasma around the more dense red blood cells (Carstensen *et al.*, 1953; Carstensen and Schwann, 1959a). A wide variety of macromolecules in water solution exhibit the same linear dependence of attenuation on frequency. This has led to the hypothesis that the ultrasound attenuation may be due, not to the macromolecules themselves, but to the structure of a hydration layer surrounding the macromolecule when it is in solution in water (Hussey, 1975). It has also been hypothesized that the linear frequency dependence of ultrasonic attenuation is due to a continuous distribution of resonant absorption frequencies (Carstensen and Schwann, 1959b; Edmonds *et al.*, 1970). A fundamental understanding of ultrasonic attenuation by macromolecular solutions awaits further experimental and theoretical investigations.

The attenuation of ultrasound in bone has been included in Table 10-3, even though bone falls outside the general category of soft tissues. This figure has been included for comparison to emphasize that not only does very little acoustic energy cross tissue–bone interfaces, but the attenuation within the bone is great. In spite of these difficulties, methods of transmitting ultrasound through bone continue to receive serious attention because of the immense potential benefits of ultrasonically imaging the brain through the skull (McKinney *et al.*, 1966; Schiefer *et al.*, 1968; Fry *et al.*, 1970; Wells, 1972; Somer *et al.*, 1973).

10.10. GENERATION AND DETECTION OF ULTRASONIC WAVES

The analysis of any wave-imaging system reveals that the wavelength λ of the imaging radiation represents the order of magnitude of a fundamental limit to the resolution of the system. Equation (10-25) shows that the depth resolution of a pulsed-echo system also is proportional to λ. Generally, the best possible resolution is desirable in diagnostic-imaging systems, so the wavelength λ must be chosen as small as possible. By Eq. (10-22) this means that the frequency must be as high as possible. We have seen in the previous section that attenuation becomes more severe as ultrasound frequency is increased; in general shallow depths permit higher frequencies. For example, 2.25 MHz ($\lambda = 0.67$ mm) is most often used for abdominal imaging, whereas 8 MHz ($\lambda = 0.19$ mm) is commonly employed for imaging the eye. Hence, in considering the generation and detection of ultrasound, we are primarily interested in techniques well suited to the 1–10-MHz frequency range. In this range transducers based on the piezoelectric effect are utilized.

In piezoelectric materials an electric field E or displacement D within the material generates a stress T and strain S; conversely, a stress or strain of the material generates an electric field and displacement inside. One of the best known naturally occurring piezoelectric materials is quartz, but a family of ferroelectric ceramics find widest application as they exhibit larger piezoelectric effects, yet are mechanically sturdy, chemically stable, and inexpensive. In piezoelectric materials linear relationships exist between the electrical quantities E and D and the mechanical quantities T and S which are complicated by the presence of four quantities. In diagnostic-imaging applications the transducer is a thin layer whose thickness is varied by application of an electric voltage to generate ultrasonic waves and by received pressure oscillations to generate a signal voltage, so the quantities E, D, T, and S are all parallel to the thickness dimension (commonly denoted the longitudinal or "3" axis) and perpendicular to the surface as shown in Fig. 10-4. The linear relationships are written in the following form for this case:

$$S = \frac{1}{Y_{33}^E} T + d_{33} E \tag{10-34}$$

$$D = d_{33} T + \kappa_{33}^T \kappa_0 E \tag{10-35}$$

where Y_{33}^E is Young's modulus at constant electric field, κ_{33}^T is the dielectric constant at constant stress, $\kappa_0 (= 8.89 \times 10^{-12}\ \text{sec}^2\ \text{m}^{-2})$ is the permittivity of free space, and d_{33} is the piezoelectric constant. If a voltage V is applied across a piezoelectric transducer of thickness l with no external stress, then

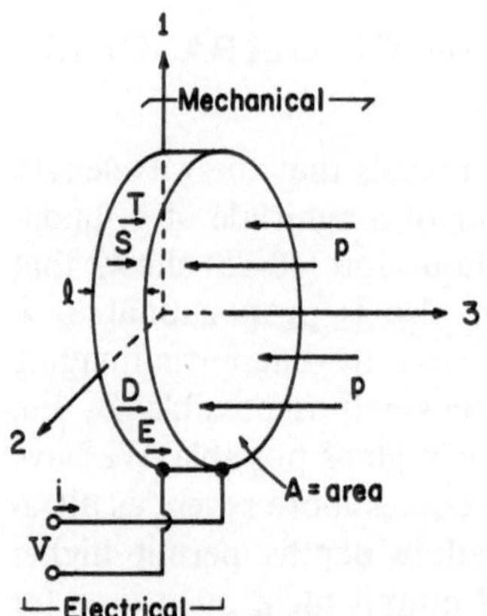

Fig. 10-4. Coordinate system for the definition of transducer characteristics.

$E = V/l$ and $T = 0$. The change of length Δl $(=Sl)$ can be obtained from Eq. (10-34):

$$\Delta l = d_{33}V \tag{10-36}$$

Because d_{33} appears alone in Eq. (10-36), it is often called the transmission coefficient of the piezoelectric material. If instead, the transducer is clamped so the length cannot change ($S = 0$), then the pressure $p(= -T)$ at the surface is from Eq. (10-34):

$$p = (d_{33}Y_{33}^E)\frac{V}{l} \tag{10-37}$$

From Eq. (10-35) for a given applied pressure one finds that the open-circuit voltage ($D = 0$) is

$$V = \frac{d_{33}}{\kappa_{33}^T \kappa_0} lp \tag{10-38a}$$

$$= g_{33}lp \tag{10-38b}$$

where g_{33} $(\equiv d_{33}/\kappa_{33}^T\kappa_0)$ is defined for convenience and is sometimes called the reception coefficient. The charge q for short-circuited electrodes ($E = 0$) is from Eq. (10-35):

$$q = -d_{33}Ap \tag{10-39}$$

where A is the area of the transducer on which the pressure acts. Each of these situations represents an extreme case; equations for the more general situation can be derived and corresponding equivalent circuits can be constructed. However, Eqs. (10-36)–(10-39) can be utilized to obtain good order-of-magnitude estimates, and one or another of the simplifying assumptions is often well satisfied in practice. Table 10-4 lists the constants for quartz, lithium sulfate, and typical ferroelectric ceramics (see Bradfield, 1970, for a review of transducer properties and techniques).

Table 10-4. Properties of Piezoelectric Materials[a]

Physical property	Symbol	Units	Quartz (0° X-cut)	Lithium sulfate (0° Y-cut)	Barium titanate[b]	Lead zirconate-titanate[c] (PZT)	Lead metaniobate
Density	ρ	10^3 kg/m^3	2.65	2.06	5.5	7.5	5.8
Velocity of sound	c_{33}	10^3 m/sec	5.45	5.44	4.49	2.53	2.24
Acoustic impedance	Z_{33}	10^6 kg/m^2 sec	14.4	11.2	24.7	19.0	13.0
Young's modulus	Y_{33}^E	10^{10} N/m^2	7.9	6.1	11.1	4.8	2.9
Dielectric constant	κ_{33}^T	Relative to vacuum	4.57	10.3	1250	3400	225
Piezoelectric constant	d_{33}	10^{-12} m/V	2.25	16	145	593	85
Open-circuit piezoelectric constant	g_{33}	10^{-3} (V/m)/(N/m^2)	55	175	13.1	19.7	42.5
Mechanical quality factor	Q	—	10^6	—	450	65	11
Curie temperature	Θ_C	°C	575	75 (disintegrates)	115	195	550

[a] Based upon compilation by W. P. Mason (Mason, 1963).
[b] Similar to Type 300, Channel Industries, Santa Barbara, California, and to Type EC-31, Edo-Western Corporation, Salt Lake City, Utah.
[c] Similar to Type 5550, Channel Industries, Santa Barbara, California, and to Type PZT-5H, Vernitron Piezoelectric Division, Bedford, Ohio.

The thickness l of the transducer determines the resonant frequencies of the vibrations in the "3" direction. Suppose the back surface of the transducer is cemented to a dense, rigid material of much higher acoustic impedance so the surface can be considered as clamped and motionless. Also assume the front surface is in contact with material of much lower acoustic impedance as would be the case when contacting water or soft tissue; this means the front surface can move almost as if it were free. The resonant frequencies will correspond to the modes of an organ pipe closed at one end as illustrated in Fig. 10-5. Resonances will occur when

$$l = \frac{\lambda_1}{4}, \frac{3\lambda_3}{4}, \ldots, \frac{(2n-1)\,\lambda_{2n-1}}{4} \tag{10-40a}$$

or

$$\lambda_{2n-1} = \frac{4l}{2n-1} \qquad (n = 1, 2, \ldots) \tag{10-40b}$$

The corresponding frequencies are given by

$$f_{2n-1} = \frac{c_{33}}{\lambda_{2n-1}} \tag{10-41a}$$

$$= (2n-1)\frac{c_{33}}{4l} \qquad (n = 1, 2, \ldots) \tag{10-41b}$$

where $c_{33}(\cong (Y_{33}^E/\rho_{\text{transducer}})^{1/2})$ is the velocity of longitudinal elastic waves in the "3" direction in the transducer material. Notice that resonance occurs at a fundamental frequency $f_1 = c_{\text{transducer}}/4l$ and at all the odd harmonics.

If the transducer were to be used in a broadband imaging system—for example, emitting and receiving a single pulse—it would be necessary to avoid the resonant frequencies. This could be done if all the important frequencies in this pulse were below the fundamental frequency f_1, which can always be done by making the thickness l sufficiently small. Equation (10-36), which applies when one surface is free, indicates that the voltage

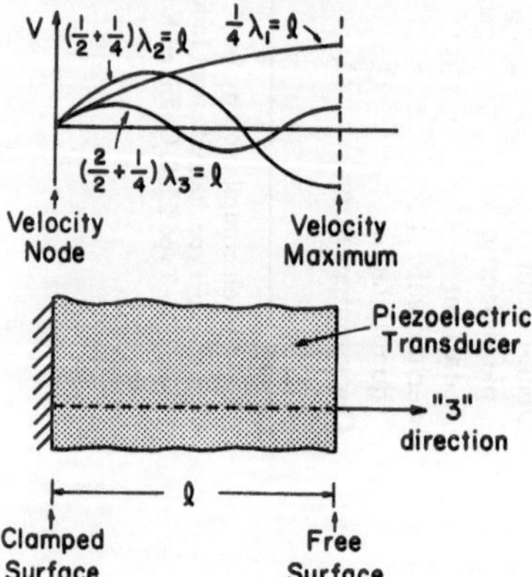

Fig. 10-5. Sketch of resonant velocity modes of a clamped quarter-wave transducer.

required to produce a given displacement is independent of the thickness l. However, as the thickness is decreased, the electrical capacitance across the electrodes will increase, so the current required to charge the transducer to a specified voltage will increase in direct proportion to f_1. Equation (10-38) indicates that the signal voltage when the transducer is used as a detector will decrease as f_1 is increased. Equation (10-39) says that the induced charge which might be measured by a charge-sensitive amplifier is independent of thickness. However, so-called charge-sensitive amplifiers rely on sensing voltage changes caused by the charge and then feeding back a charge which nearly cancels the voltage change; they fail if the voltage as indicated by Eq. (10-38) is below their noise voltage level. In summary, the generation and detection of wide-band pulses brings practical problems with high driving currents and low detector sensitivity.

In narrow-band ultrasonic imaging systems there are many advantages to operating at the fundamental resonant frequency f_1 of the transducer. The drive current requirements are reduced not only by the greater thickness l of the transducer compared to broadband operation, but also because the amplitude of oscillation can be built up over several cycles if necessary. Similarly, the sensitivity as a detector is enhanced both by greater thickness and because there can be a resonant buildup of detector vibration in response to a pressure wave packet. The Q of a resonator—the ratio of total energy stored to the energy lost per cycle—gives a measure of the number of oscillations when left free to "ring" and of the signal enhancement. Assuming that the same or similar transducers are employed for transmitting and receiving, there will be approximately Q cycles in the wave packet and the enhancement of received voltage amplitude relative to a nonresonant system would be roughly by a factor of Q.

As indicated by Eq. (10-24) the depth resolution in an echo-imaging system is proportional to the number of cycles in the wave packet, which in turn is proportional to Q. Therefore, the transducer Q must be kept low —less than about 10—in a pulsed-echo system. This is partially accomplished by virtue of the energy flow from the transducer to the soft tissue under examination. In addition, some piezoelectric materials have intrinsically low Q because of internal damping; chief among these is lead metaniobate. The composition of the high-impedence backing material can also be chosen to reduce the Q—for example, some workers employ a powdered-tungsten-in-epoxy backing (Daly, 1971).

10.11. TRANSMISSION DESIGN PARAMETERS FOR A TYPICAL DIAGNOSTIC ULTRASOUND SYSTEM

Let us examine some typical transducer parameters and circuit voltages for a lead metaniobate transducer operating at a frequency f_1 of 2.25 MHz.

Using Eq. (10-41b) the thickness of the piezoelectric element must be $l = c_{33}/4f_1 = 0.25$ mm if it is backed with a high-acoustic-impedance material. (It would be twice this thickness if unbacked, in analogy to an open organ pipe.) Suppose a voltage $V_0 = 100$ V were imposed across the electrodes—a voltage of this magnitude is near the upper limit for safety from shock hazard without unusual precautions and for transistorized drive circuits of simple design. Using Eq. (10-36) and a sinusoidal representation for the drive voltage, $V(t) = V_0 \sin 2\pi f_1 t$, the velocity v of the front transducer surface would be

$$v \equiv \frac{dl}{dt} = d_{33}\frac{dV}{dt} \qquad \text{(10-42a)}$$

$$= 2\pi f_1 d_{33} V_0 \cos 2\pi f_1 t \qquad \text{(10-42b)}$$

The soft tissue in contact with the transducer face would oscillate with the same amplitude. Since the impedance of the tissue is much lower than for the piezoelectric material, the accompanying sonic pressure will be small compared to the stresses in transducer, thus only perturbing by a small amount the amplitude of motion if it were free, which has been calculated in Eq. (10-42b). If the contact area dimensions are large compared to a wavelength ($A \gg \lambda^2$), then the disturbance in the tissue near the transducer face will propagate like a plane wave, so the average pressure amplitude in tissue can then be calculated from Eq. (10-6):

$$p = Zv \qquad \text{(10-43a)}$$

$$= 2\pi f_1 d_{33} V_0 Z \cos 2\pi f_1 t \qquad \text{(10-43b)}$$

where Z ($\approx 1.6 \times 10^6$ kg/m^2 sec) is the acoustic impedance of soft tissue. Using $d_{33} = 85 \times 10^{-12}$ m/V from Table 10-4, we find that the amplitude p_0 of the pressure wave transmitted into the soft tissue is 1.92×10^5 N/m^2. Since the pressure oscillations are superimposed on a static atmospheric pressure which is approximately 10^5 N/m^2, the negative swings of the $\cos(2\pi f_1 t)$ in Eq. (10-43b) would drive the tissue to a negative absolute pressure of $(1 - 1.92) \times 10^5 = -0.92 \times 10^5$ N/m^2. At high negative pressures ($\sim$100 atm) tissue is damaged by the bubbles formed from cavitation. In order to avoid even a remote possibility of tissue damage we may wish to restrict the piezoelectric transducer drive to not exceed $V_0 = 50$ V amplitude in this example. The corresponding intensity is from Eq. (10-17):

$$I = \frac{\langle p^2 \rangle}{Z} \qquad \text{(10-44a)}$$

$$= \frac{(2\pi f_1 d_{33} V_0 Z)^2 \langle \cos^2 2\pi f_1 t \rangle}{Z} \qquad \text{(10-44b)}$$

$$= 2Z(\pi f_1 d_{33} V_0)^2 \qquad \text{(10-44c)}$$

since $\langle \cos^2 2\pi f_1 t \rangle = 1/2$. If $V_0 = 50$ V, then the intensity $I = 2.9 \times 10^3$ W/m^2 or 0.29 W/cm^2. There appears to be no evidence of biological damage from long exposures at this intensity level and short bursts at much higher intensities appear to be safe when the duty factor (defined as the fractional time with radiation on) is low ($\sim 10^{-3}$) (Hussey, 1975).

The actual drive voltage would be even less than 50 V if it were a 2.25-MHz burst since we have not taken account of resonance enhancement of the amplitude of mechanical oscillations. On the other hand, the modest drive requirements permit an even simpler waveform—a single unipolar pulse with time duration on the order of one-half cycle of the mechanical oscillation. This method is often referred to as "shock excitation" of the transducer; it is analogous to a hammer striking a bell. The voltage pulse amplitude required for shock excitation is on the order of the value of V_0 which is desired.

The driving current required depends also upon one additional parameter, the area A of the transducer. This is determined by the beam profile which is desired for the ultrasonic radiation, and is typically a square centimeter (10^{-4} m^2) or more, which satisfies the assumption in applying Eq. (10-43a) that $\lambda^2 \cong 4.4 \times 10^{-3}$ cm$^2 \ll A$. Since the transducer electrical capacitance C_E is

$$C_E = \frac{\kappa_{33}^T \kappa_0 A}{l} \quad \text{(F)} \tag{10-45}$$

and the current flow into the transducer is given by

$$i = C_E \frac{dV}{dt} \quad \text{(A)} \tag{10-46}$$

we can write, using Eq. (10-41b),

$$i = \frac{8\pi\kappa_0\kappa_{33}^T f_1^2 V_0 A}{c_{33}} \cos 2\pi f_1 t \tag{10-47}$$

For the above example, with $V_0 = 50$ V and $A = 10^{-4}$ m^2, the peak current is 0.57 A, which must be turned on within one-quarter cycle—0.11 μsec. This is well within the range of transistors and silicon-controlled rectifiers.

10.12. RECEPTION DESIGN PARAMETERS FOR A TYPICAL DIAGNOSTIC ULTRASOUND SYSTEM

For the lead metaniobate transducer which we have taken for an example let us estimate its sensitivity as a detector or receiver of ultrasonic waves from soft tissue. The sensitivity of the electronic amplifier attached to the transducer will depend upon the amplifier noise characteristics and the desired bandwidth. If we desire to resolve wave packets which are spaced on the order of 4 cycles apart, then $\Delta f/f \approx 1/4$. Rather than going into an analysis of the best state-of-art amplifiers, we will simply take 5 μV as the order of magnitude of signal which is required for reasonably noise-free amplifier operation for the example which is being considered. The thermal noise always present in the tissue will also have to be considered in estimating the smallest detectable pressure wave.

As above for the case of generating an ultrasonic wave, we will assume that the transducer is in direct contact with the soft tissue without any special impedance-matching layer. The incident wave will encounter an impedance discontinuity at the transducer face, so there will be a reflected wave of amplitude r relative to the incident wave, and the total pressure at the transducer face will be $(1 + r)$ times the incident wave pressure amplitude p_{inc}. Using Eq. (10-14) to find r, we obtain

$$p_{\text{transducer}} = 1 + \frac{Z_{\text{transducer}} - Z_{\text{soft tissue}}}{Z_{\text{transducer}} + Z_{\text{soft tissue}}} p_{\text{inc}} \tag{10-48a}$$

$$= \frac{2Z_{\text{transducer}}}{Z_{\text{transducer}} + Z_{\text{soft tissue}}} p_{\text{inc}} \tag{10-48b}$$

$$\cong 2p_{\text{inc}} \tag{10-48c}$$

where the approximate relation in Eq. (10-48c) is valid if $Z_{\text{transducer}} \gg Z_{\text{soft tissue}}$. It is interesting to note that the pressure in a nonresonant transducer would not be tremendously increased even if there were an impedance-matching layer which allowed all of the incident wave energy, $p_{\text{inc}}^2/Z_{\text{soft tissue}}$, to enter the transducer. In this case,

$$\frac{p_{\text{inc}}^2}{Z_{\text{soft tissue}}} = \frac{p_{\text{transducer}}^2}{Z_{\text{transducer}}} \tag{10-49a}$$

or

$$p_{\text{transducer}} = \left(\frac{Z_{\text{transducer}}}{Z_{\text{soft tissue}}}\right)^{1/2} p_{\text{inc}} \tag{10-49b}$$

For lead metaniobate, the coefficient in Eq. (10-49b) is 2.85, whereas Eq. (10-48b) for the unmatched case gives 1.78.

Using Eqs. (10-38b), (10-41b), and (10-48c), the open-circuit voltage V across the transducer electrodes is given by

$$V \cong 2g_{33}lp_{\text{inc}} \tag{10-50a}$$

$$= \frac{g_{33}c_{33}}{2f_1} p_{\text{inc}} \tag{10-50b}$$

or the incident pressure for a given open-circuit voltage is

$$p_{\text{inc}} = \frac{2f_1}{g_{33}c_{33}} V \tag{10-51}$$

Using the values from Table 10-4 for lead metaniobate, $f_1 = 2.25 \times 10^6$ Hz, and $V = 5 \times 10^{-6}$ V, p_{inc} is 0.24 N/m^2, which is a factor of about 4×10^5 below the maximum safe transmitted pressure of 10^5 N/m^2. Since this estimate does not take account of signal enhancement due to the transducer resonating with the incident wave packet or of the higher intensities which can safely be employed in short bursts, the minimum detectable incident pressure is less than given by Eq. (10-51) by a factor on the order of Q and the maximum transmitted pressure might be as high as 10^6 N/m^2, so there is typically a factor of 10^6–10^7 range between the minimum detectable pressure wave and the maximum safe pressure wave.

The thermal noise pressure can be calculated from a classical physics analysis of the equipartition of energy among all the acoustic modes in an enclosure of arbitrary volume, with each mode having average thermal energy $k\Theta$, where Θ is the absolute temperature and k is Boltzmann's constant ($= 1.38 \times 10^{-23}$ J/°K) (Hunt, 1963). The result for a frequency band Δf ($\ll f$) centered at frequency f is

$$\langle p^2 \rangle_{\text{point}} = \frac{4\pi k\Theta\rho}{c} f^2 \Delta f \tag{10-52}$$

for pressure measured by a detector whose size is small compared to the acoustic wavelength $\lambda (= c/f)$. If the measured pressure is averaged over an area A of the detector, where A cannot be neglected compared to λ^2, then we must divide the result in Eq. (10-52) by the directivity factor (Beranek, 1963a) of the detector and we obtain

$$\langle p^2 \rangle_{\text{detector}} = \frac{k\Theta\rho c \Delta f}{A} \tag{10-53}$$

where the pressure refers to the value which would be measured in the liquid if the transducer were a perfect acoustic match. For $\Delta f = f/Q = 0.56 \times 10^6$ Hz, $A = 10^{-4}$ m^2 (1 cm^2), and $\Theta = 310$°K (body temperature), the root-mean-square thermal noise pressure $(\langle p^2 \rangle_{\text{detector}})^{1/2}$ inferred from the detector is 0.6×10^{-2} N/m^2. We conclude for this example that the fundamental thermal noise limit is only a factor of 10 in pressure amplitude below the level set by the postulated 5-μV amplifier input and a transducer $Q \approx 4$.

10.13. TRANSDUCER EQUIVALENT CIRCUITS

The approximate discussion in the preceding sections of emission and detection of ultrasonic waves was given in considerable detail in an attempt to familiarize the reader with the important physical processes which are involved. An equivalent electrical circuit can be constructed (Mason, 1950) for the low-frequency approximation made in much of the above discussion; this is shown in Fig. 10-6a. All quantities in Fig. 10-6 have been converted to electrical units, regarding voltage as the analog of pressure with conversion factor ϕ defined by

$$\phi \equiv \frac{l}{d_{33} Y_{33}^E} \quad \left(\frac{\mathrm{V}}{\mathrm{N/m^2}}\right) \tag{10-54}$$

and current as the analog of area × velocity with conversion factor $1/\phi$ given by

$$\frac{1}{\phi} = \frac{d_{33} Y_{33}^E}{l} \quad \left(\frac{\mathrm{A}}{(\mathrm{m^2})(\mathrm{m/sec})}\right) \tag{10-55}$$

C_E shown in Fig. 10-6 is the electrical capacitance across the transducer electrodes when clamped, given by Eq. (10-45). The equivalent electrical capacitance C_Y corresponding to the mechanical compliance of the transducer is

$$C_Y = \frac{d_{33}^2 Y_{33}^E A}{l} \quad (\mathrm{F}) \tag{10-56}$$

The equivalent electrical inductance corresponding to the mechanical mass of the transducer is

$$L_\rho = \frac{\rho l^3}{2 d_{33}^2 (Y_{33}^E)^2 A} \quad (\mathrm{H}) \tag{10-57}$$

and the equivalent load resistance Z_L corresponding to the acoustic impedance of the soft tissue is

$$Z_L = \frac{l^2}{d_{33}^2 (Y_{33}^E)^2 A} Z_{\mathrm{acoustic}} \quad (\Omega) \tag{10-58}$$

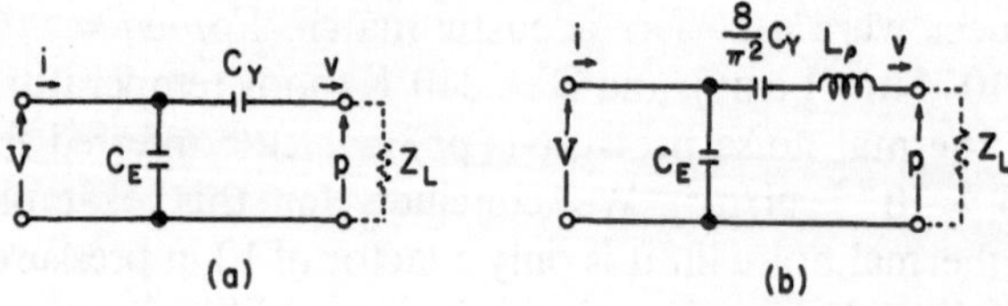

Fig. 10-6. Equivalent electrical circuits of a clamped quarter-wave piezoelectric transducer. (a) For dc and low frequencies ($f \ll f_1$), (b) for frequencies near first resonance ($f \approx f_1$).

provided that all quantities are expressed in MKS units in Eqs. (10-45) and (10-54)–(10-58).

For the lead metaniobate transducer in the above example with $A = 10^{-4}\ \text{m}^2$ (1 cm^2), $Z_L = 163\ \Omega$. In the approximate discussion of ultrasonic wave emission in Section 10.11 we have essentially assumed that the electrical driving impedance is low compared to 163 Ω. If the equivalent electrical circuit of Fig. 10-6 is used for a received ultrasonic pressure wave applied to terminals M_1 and M_2, then it must be regarded as being delivered from the end of a long 163-Ω transmission line; a reflection occurs due to the impedance mismatch. This situation can be taken into account by substituting a generator of voltage $2\phi p_{\text{inc}}$ in series with a resistance Z_L across terminals M_1 and M_2.

For a more accurate analysis at frequencies near the fundamental transducer resonance f_1 the equivalent circuit of Fig. 10-6b may be employed (Mason, 1950). Note that to a good approximation the mechanical portion of the transducer may be regarded as a series-resonant electrical circuit with its capacitor having $8/\pi^2 \cong 0.81$ of the equivalent low-frequency capacitance C_Y.

10.14. DIRECTIONALITY OF ULTRASONIC RADIATION

The development of diagnostic ultrasonic-imaging systems utilizing the detection of echoes from short bursts of emitted radiation depends not only upon favorable physical conditions for the propagation and reflection of ultrasonic waves in soft tissues but upon the possibility of confining emission and reception to a narrow beam. The directional and other properties of ultrasonic beams are most easily discussed with reference to the emission from a flat piston transducer, as described in Section 10-10, which we will assume to have circular cross section.

Referring to Fig. 10-7, suppose we ask for the acoustic pressure at point P due to a piston of infinitesimal area dA set in an infinite rigid (very high acoustic impedance) baffle B–B vibrating with velocity v in the z direction, where

$$v = v_0 \cos 2\pi f t \tag{10-59}$$

Then the pressure dp at point P in the soft tissue is given by

$$dp = -\frac{\rho f v_0 dA}{r} \sin\left[2\pi f\left(t - \frac{r}{c}\right)\right] \tag{10-60}$$

where ρ is the density of the soft tissue, f is the vibration frequency of the piston, r is the distance from the piston element dA to the point P, and $(t - r/c)$ appears in the argument of the sine because the changes at the

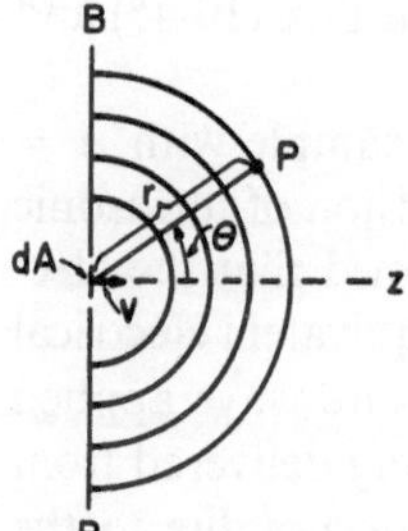

Fig. 10-7. Coordinate system for sound radiation from area dA set in an infinite rigid baffle B–B.

piston are felt a time r/c later at point P. Note that dp is proportional to the frequency f because it is the piston acceleration dv/dt which gives rise to acoustic emission from a small element of area dA. Also observe that the amplitude of dp in Eq. (10-60) depends only upon the distance r to the point P, but not on the angle θ from the z axis to r.

In order to find the pressure p at distance r and polar angle θ relative to a circular piston of radius a as shown in Fig. 10-8, the contributions of all the elements of area dA to the pressure at point P must be summed. The general result takes the form

$$p(r, \theta, t) = -\rho f \int_A \frac{v_0}{q} \sin\left[2\pi f\left(t - \frac{q}{c}\right)\right] dA \tag{10-61}$$

If all points on the surface of the piston vibrate with the same velocity amplitude v_0 and if the point P lies on the z axis, the integration in Eq. (10-61) can be carried out easily, since for this case $dA = 2\pi s\, ds = 2\pi q\, dq$. The simplest and most useful form of the result is obtained if one calculates the intensity, $I = \langle p^2 \rangle / Z$ [see Eq. (10-17) or (10-44a)]:

$$I(r, \theta = 0) = 2Zv_0^2 \sin^2 \pi \left\{ \left[\left(\frac{r}{\lambda}\right)^2 + \left(\frac{a}{\lambda}\right)^2 \right]^{1/2} - \frac{r}{\lambda} \right\} \tag{10-62}$$

where, by comparison of Eq. (10-43b) for a quarter-wave-thickness trans-

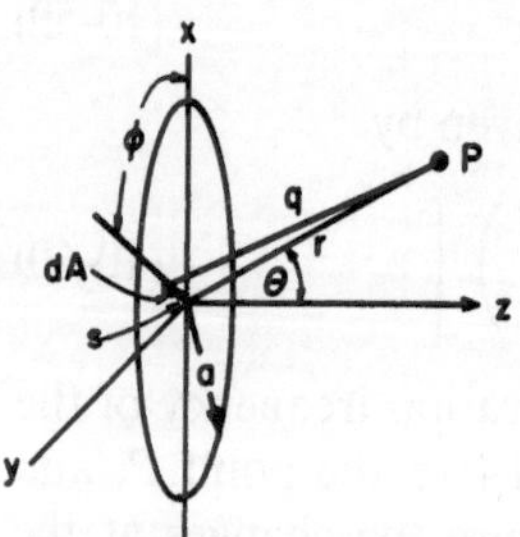

Fig. 10-8. Coordinate system for sound radiation from area dA in a circular piston.

ducer and Eq. (10-59) v_0 is given by

$$v_0 = 2\pi f_1 d_{33} V_0 \tag{10-63}$$

The on-axis intensity given by Eq. (10-62) for $a/\lambda = 10$ is shown in Fig. 10-9 relative to the intensity calculated for emission of a plane wave, Eq. (10-44c); note that the peak intensity reaches four times the plane-wave result. The last maximum occurs at a distance r_1 which corresponds to the argument of the sine in Eq. (10-62) equal to $\pi/2$ rad; r_1/λ is given by

$$\frac{r_1}{\lambda} = \left(\frac{a}{\lambda}\right)^2 - \frac{1}{4} \tag{10-64}$$

The region out to the last intensity maximum at r_1 is known as the *near field* or Fresnel diffraction region. Since the average intensity on axis in the near field remains constant, it is clear that the sound energy is transmitted in an almost parallel beam.

The region beyond r_1 is known as the *far field* or Fraunhofer diffrac-

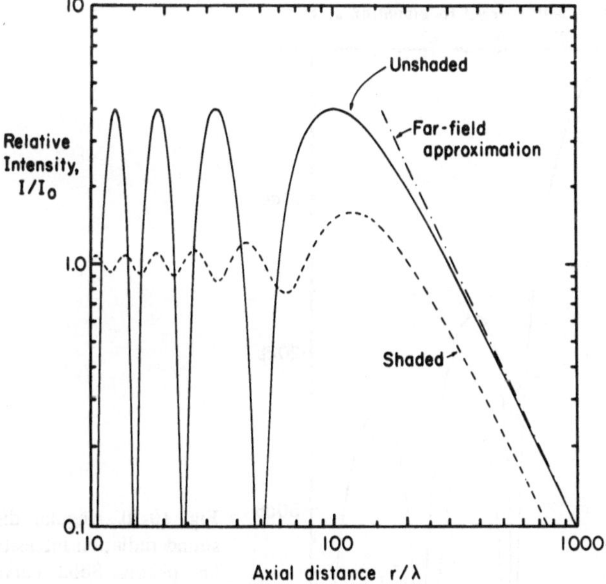

Fig. 10-9. Sound radiation intensity along the axis of a circular piston. Solid curve: unshaded (piston amplitude $= v_0$) and $a/\lambda = 10$; dashed curve: shaded (piston amplitude $= v_0(1 - s^2/a^2)$) and $a/\lambda = 12.4$; dot–dashed line: far-field approximation for unshaded piston. $I_0 = \frac{1}{2}Zv_0^2$, which would be the intensity of a plane wave from a piston of infinite extent vibrating with uniform velocity amplitude v_0.

tion region. If $r \gg r_1$ and $r \gg a$, Eq. (10-62) becomes

$$I_f(r, \theta = 0) \cong (\tfrac{1}{2}Zv_0^2)\left[\pi^2\left(\frac{a}{\lambda}\right)^2\left(\frac{a}{r}\right)^2\right] \tag{10-65}$$

which shows that the intensity is proportional to $1/r^2$ in the far field. In the far field one can return to Eq. (10-61) and obtain an approximate solution valid for all values of the polar angle θ by observing in Fig. 10-8 that $q \cong r - s\sin\theta\cos\phi$, $1/q \cong 1/r$, and $dA = s\,ds\,d\phi$. The final result is (Morse, 1948)

$$I_f(r, \theta) \cong (\tfrac{1}{2}Zv_0^2)\left[\pi^2\left(\frac{a}{\lambda}\right)^2\left(\frac{a}{r}\right)^2\right]\left[\frac{2J_1(ka\sin\theta)}{ka\sin\theta}\right]^2 \tag{10-66}$$

where J_1 is a Bessel function and $k = 2\pi/\lambda$. Note by comparing Eqs. (10-65) and (10-66) that $[2J_1(ka\sin\theta)/ka\sin\theta]^2 = 1$ when $\theta = 0$; this function for $a/\lambda = 10$ is plotted in Fig. 10-10. Most of the radiated far-field intensity is concentrated in the angular region $0 \leq \theta \leq \theta_Q$ where the pressure is, say, one-half or more of its on-axis value ($\theta = 0$), which corresponds to the

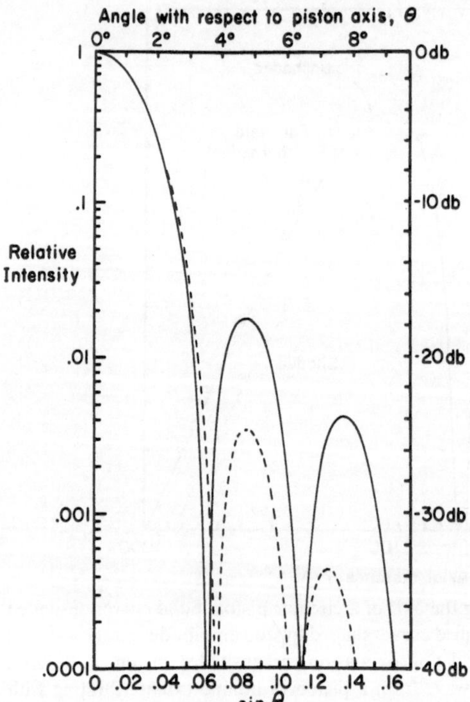

Fig. 10-10. Angular distribution of sound radiation intensity for a circular piston. Solid curve: unshaded (piston amplitude $= v_0$) and $a/\lambda = 10$. Dashed curve: shaded (piston amplitude $= v_0(1 - s^2/a^2)$) and $a/\lambda = 12.4$; the relative intensity for this case is given by $[8J_2(ka\sin\theta)/(ka\sin\theta)^2]^2$.

intensity being one-fourth or more of its maximum value, requiring that

$$ka \sin \theta_Q < 2.2 \tag{10-67a}$$

or, assuming $\theta \ll 1$ rad,

$$\theta_Q \cong \frac{2.2}{ka} = 0.35 \frac{\lambda}{a} \tag{10-67b}$$

Consider the above results in a typical medical-imaging situation. Suppose a frequency of 2.25 MHz, with corresponding wavelength $\lambda = 0.67$ mm, is found to be the highest for which noise-free return echoes can be obtained throughout the 100–300 cm depth of interest. If a transducer diameter of 12.5 mm is chosen, then the radius $a = 6.25$ mm, and $a/\lambda = 9.37$. The beam would remain approximately parallel with roughly a 10-mm diameter out to $r_1 = (0.67)\ [(9.37)^2 - 0.25] = 58.4$ mm. At greater depths, the beam becomes conical with a half-opening angle $\theta_Q \cong (0.35)/9.37 = 0.037$ rad $=$ 2.1°. At a depth of 150 mm the diameter of the beam would still be only about (2)(0.037)(150) = 11 mm, and at 300 mm it would be 22 mm. Since the directivity of the transducer as a receiver also has the form given by Eq. (10-66) and Fig. 10-10, the overall intensity response is proportional to the square of the functions plotted in Figs. 10-9 and 10-10, and the overall received pressure response is directly proportional to the curves in Figs. 10-9 and 10-10. The actual intensity vs. depth curve in tissue requires multiplying the function given in Eqs. (10-62), (10-65), and (10-66) and shown in Fig. 10-9 by the factor $\exp(-2\alpha r)$, where the attenuation coefficient is defined by Eqs. (10-31) and (10-33).

Equation (10-62) and Fig. 10-9 indicate that many nodes can be expected in the spatial distribution of ultrasound intensity in the near field. Along the axis, the number of nodes is the largest integer less than a/λ. It can also be shown that the number of pressure maxima along a diameter of the transducer face is the largest integer less than $2a/\lambda$. In the far field, the number of side lobes, N (not counting the peak at $\theta = 0°$) for θ between 0° and 90° is approximately given by the highest integer less than $a/\lambda + 0.39$.

Since the near-field nodes cause undesirable dead spots and the far-field side lobes cause unwanted responses outside the central beam peak, it is of interest to examine methods of suppressing nodes and side lobes. This can be done by *shading* the velocity amplitude v_0 so that it smoothly decreases to zero as the radius s on the transducer face increases. For example, the dashed curve in Fig. 10-9 shows the on-axis intensity distribution if the velocity amplitude is given by $v_0(s) = v_0(0)(1 - s^2/a^2)$ and Fig. 10-10 shows the corresponding far-field angular distribution of intensity. For comparison with the unshaded piston, the shaded piston was chosen to have $a/\lambda = 12.4$ so that the central peaks in Fig. 10-10 have equal widths at the half-pressure points.

Ultrasonic focusing, in exact analogy to the focusing of light, can be utilized to achieve a beam diameter of a few wavelengths at any specified depth (Eggleton, 1976). However, this is accomplished at the expense of *depth of focus*; i.e., the beam spot will remain small only for a limited range of depths. Thus focusing can improve lateral resolution if information is needed only in a limited region of depth, but a system optimized for imaging a wide range of depths becomes very close to the unfocused arrangement which has been analyzed above.

10.15. THE DOPPLER EFFECT

If ultrasound of frequency f is back-reflected from an acoustic impedance discontinuity which has a velocity component $v_{\|}$ parallel to the direction of the primary beam, then the frequency of the backreflected wave will differ from the original frequency. To calculate the magnitude of the effect, consider the emission of a 1-sec burst containing f cycles of pressure oscillation, each spread over a wavelength λ so that the entire wave packet extends over a distance $c = f\lambda$ = distance traveled by sound in 1 sec. Consider the time t_A when the incident wave packet just reaches the moving reflecting layer and the time t_B 1 sec later as shown in Fig. 10-11. At t_A the reflected wave is just beginning from the position of the reflector; at t_B this first reflected disturbance has propagated back a distance c from the original reflector position, shown dotted in Fig. 10-11B. The number of cycles reach-

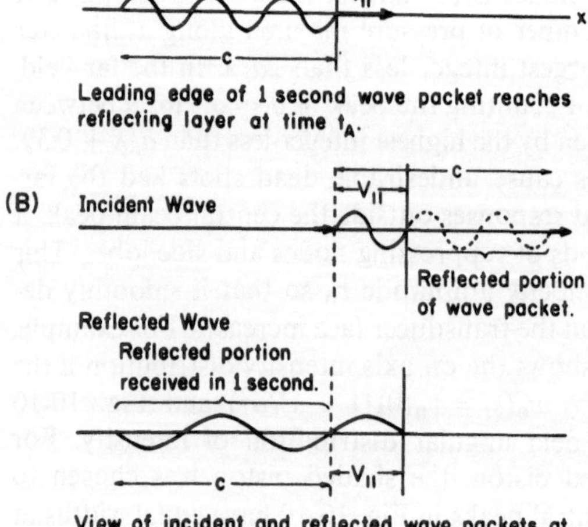

Fig. 10-11. Incident and reflected waves from a moving reflector: (A) at time t_A and (B) 1 sec later.

ing the receiver per second would be exactly the number in a length c of the reflected wave packet, which is a fraction $c/(c + v_{\|})$ of the total number of cycles reflected; the total reflected in turn is $(c - v_{\|})/c$ of the original f cycles. Thus the frequency f_r at the receiver is

$$f_r = \frac{c}{c + v_{\|}} \frac{c - v_{\|}}{c} f \tag{10-68a}$$

$$= \frac{c - v_{\|}}{c + v_{\|}} f \tag{10-68b}$$

$$\cong f\left(1 - \frac{2v_{\|}}{c}\right) \quad \text{if } |v_{\|}| \ll c \tag{10-68c}$$

It is often convenient, using the approximate expression in Eq. (10-68c), to calculate the frequency change or Doppler effect $f_r - f = \Delta f$:

$$\Delta f \cong -\frac{2v_{\|}}{c} f \tag{10-69}$$

where we have taken $v_{\|}$ as positive if the reflecting object is moving away from the transmit-receive transducer, and negative if moving toward the transducer.

Suppose blood or a heart valve moved a millimeter in 0.01 sec; this would correspond to $v_{\|} = 100$ mm/sec if the ultrasound beam could be aligned with the direction of motion and less by a factor of $\cos\theta$ if not aligned. If the primary beam were 3 MHz, then $|\Delta f| \cong (2)(100)(3)(10^6)/(1.5)(10^6) = 400$ Hz, a frequency in the audio range. One type of non-imaging ultrasonic instrument emits a continuous-wave beam and obtains the difference frequency Δf by "beating" the frequencies f and f_r in a non-linear mixer; the audio beat note, whose frequency is directly proportional to valve velocity, is interpreted by the physician's ear (Fieler and Pocock, 1968).

A continuous-wave instrument gives no information on the depth from which the echo originates, nor can signals from several depths be separated. A pulsed ultrasonic wave allows depth discrimination, but the pulse must contain enough cycles of oscillation so that frequency changes can be detected. Thus a trade-off is necessary in pulsed Doppler systems between depth and velocity resolution (Wells, 1969; Barber *et al.*, 1974; White and Brown, 1977).

In a Doppler system reflections are desired not only from blood–wall interfaces, but from the blood itself. This is possible because the random distribution of blood cells in the plasma fluid gives rise to acoustic impedance fluctuations which reflect ultrasound. Since the size of the blood cells and the scale length of the impedance fluctuations are small compared to ultrasound wavelengths in the 1–10 MHz frequency range, the backscattered intensity is proportional to f^4, where f is the ultrasound frequency (Shung, 1975). Usable signals from backscattering in blood and heart valves can be expected at 3 MHz and higher (Reid, 1975).

In the above discussion, we have assumed that the motion of the target reflector could be characterized by a single velocity. An example where this is not valid occurs for turbulent blood flow; in this case the many small eddies or vortices contribute components of varying magnitude and with both algebraic signs. The reflected signal which results is not a single frequency, but rather a broad distribution of frequencies whose spread gives information on the degree of turbulence. The turbulence, in turn, may indicate the presence of an obstruction to the flow of blood in the heart or in an artery or vein. Since regions of turbulent flow are rather small in dimensions—at most a few millimeters—the spectral information must be obtained from a rather short reflected wave train if a pulsed Doppler system is employed. One method which seems to extract considerable information from such a wave train with, say, 10 cycles from the region of interest is to electronically measure, record, and display the time duration of each of the ten cycles of oscillation (Baker and Johnson, 1975). If these ten results agree closely, then there is little or no turbulence; if, on the other hand, there is a large spread among the ten results, this is evidence of turbulent flow.

10.16. DISPLAY OF DIAGNOSTIC ULTRASONIC IMAGES

The principal method of obtaining diagnostic information with ultrasound utilizes short pulses of sound transmitted in a narrow beam, as discussed in previous sections. Reflections or backscattering from successive depths are then separated by the increasing time delay for the arrival of the signal (see Kossoff, 1974, for a general review of display techniques). Perhaps the original and simplest display of this information is the *amplitude* or A-mode display: The horizontal sweep of an oscilloscope moves across the cathode ray tube (CRT) linearly with time, beginning at the moment an acoustic pulse is transmitted. The received echo signals give rise to vertical deflections of the CRT beam. Since time is proportional to depth, the deflections observed on the CRT trace can be directly correlated with depth. If a large acoustic impedance discontinuity is present and is not at too oblique an orientation, a large signal "spike" will be observed on the CRT trace whose position on the trace can be used to infer the depth of the reflecting layer. The raw receiver signal is an alternating-current waveform which would deflect the beam alternately upward and downward. By rectifying the received signal, the deflections can all be in the same direction. If one is primarily concerned with the location of major acoustic discontinuities, an electronic threshold can be provided to display only signals which are greater than some preset amplitude. Also, it is generally desirable to incorporate electronic circuitry to vary the receiver gain as a function of time to compensate the weaker echoes from greater depths.

Let us examine some typical parameters for an A-mode display. Suppose echoes from depths up to 40 cm must be displayed; this corresponds to time delays up to (2)(400 mm)/(1.5 mm/μsec) = 533 μsec = 0.53 msec. Allowing some time between pulses for reverberations to settle, the pulse rate might be as high as 1000 pulses/sec. Traces on the CRT are easily generated with this sweep speed and repetition rate, and the trace appears bright and steady to the eye. If signal spikes are observed on the trace which are echoes from moving interfaces, such as a heart valve leaflet, these spikes will be observed to move back and forth on the trace in what appears to be real time in synchrony with the heart beat.

In *brightness* or B-mode display, the signal is gain compensated and rectified as described above for A-mode display, and the sweep length and repetition rate are the same. However, the rectified signal is used to modulate the intensity or brightness of the trace as it moves in a straight-line path across the screen, with greater signal amplitude corresponding to increased brightness. The position of the ultrasonic transducer is sensed and processed by electronic circuitry which generates each CRT trace with a position and orientation corresponding to the ultrasonic probe position and beam orientation. If the probe position or orientation is gradually changed, the successive traces, each in a slightly different position, correspond to different ultrasonic paths, and a two-dimensional image will appear. However, the human visual system does not average over more than a few successive traces, so some image storage device must be provided if the observer is to be presented with a complete image. Perhaps the simplest means of storage is by means of a camera with fast-developing film which views the CRT screen. Memory-type CRT's are also employed, but suffer from the disadvantage that the memory of a given spot is either *off* or completely *on*; intermediate shades of gray cannot be stored. Other more costly electronic systems are now available for storage and instant replay of two-dimensional images with a gray scale; their application in connection with any B-mode system greatly enhances its diagnostic utility.

In *real-time* display a mechanical or electronic means is provided to rapidly move the ultrasound beam so that a complete image is assembled in a time on the order of 1/30 or 1/25 of a second. Except for the rapidity of scan, a real-time display is identical to a B-mode display. Since a complete image is assembled within the flicker resolving time of human vision, no special storage device is needed for visual observations. However, if the images of a real-time system must be recorded for later replay and analysis, this may be done with a video tape recorder.

It has proved feasible to mechanically rock a single piezoelectronic transducer through a 30°–60° arc 30 times per second; in this case the image appears in a pie-shaped 30°–60° sector region (Somer, 1968; Eggleton, 1976; Shaw *et al.*, 1976). An ultrasound beam can also be shifted in direction by dividing the original transducer into many smaller elements operated as a *phased array* (Thurstone and von Ramm, 1974; Marginness *et al.*, 1976). Electronics must then be provided to independently transmit and receive ultrasonic waves from each element of the array. By appropriate delays between the excitations of successive elements, the beam can be steered in any direction within, for example, an 80° arc (Anderson *et al.*, 1977). Similar delays must be inserted between the received signals before adding so that the receiver sensitivity is also steered. Other real-time diagnostic ultrasound systems have been designed which scan among a succession of side-by-side parallel beams (Pätzold *et al.*, 1970; Bom *et al.*, 1971; Whittingham, 1976).

In *motion* or M-mode display the echo signals modulate the brightness of a linear trace as in a B-mode system. However, the ultrasonic transducer is held in a fixed position while each successive trace is shifted slightly in position so that they appear side by side. This can be done on a CRT screen, but is more often done on a chart recorder where the slow perpendicular motion of the chart paper relative to the traces provides a permanent M-mode recording. If some brightness feature on each trace moves back and forth in synchrony with the heart beat, for example, then the M-mode recording will display the position vs. time waveform of the motion.

Since the same ultrasound signals are utilized in all types of display, the more complicated and costly B-mode and real-time systems usually also provide for selection of A-mode and M-mode display. Computer processing to aid in the interpretation of the information in diagnostic ultrasound images is in its infancy (Gramiak and Waag, 1975; Robinson and Williams, 1975; Willson *et al.*, 1975; White and Brown, 1977). Obvious tasks are to provide more quantitative measures of the signals seen in A-mode scans and to provide M-mode waveforms for the motion of any specified image feature not only for motions along the ultrasonic beam direction, but in any direction lying in the image plane. The optimal combination of Doppler and amplitude information might be achieved through appropriate computer processing. Since the physics of ultrasound propagation in tissues clearly imposes definite limits, the greatest potential for future improvement of diagnostic ultrasonic imaging appears to lie in improved processing and presentation of all the available information.

REFERENCES

Anderson, W.A., Arnold, J.T., Clark, L.D., Davids, W.T., Hillard, W.J., Lehr, W.J., and Zitelli, L.T. (1977), A new real-time phased-array sector scanner for imaging the entire adult human heart, in White, D., and Brown, R.E. (eds.), *Ultrasound in Med.*, Vol. 3B, Plenum Press, New York.

Baker, D.W., and Johnson, S.L. (1975), Doppler echocardiography, in *Cardiac Ultrasound*, Gramiak, R., and Waag, R.C. (eds.), Mosby Press, St. Louis, pp. 264–276.

Barber, F.E., Lees, S., and Lobene, R.R. (1969), Ultrasonic pulse–echo measurements in teeth, *Archs. Oral Biol.* **14:**745.

Barber, F.E., Baker, D.W., Nation, A.W.C., Strandness, D.E., Jr., and Reid, J.M. (1974), Ultrasonic duplex echo-Doppler scanner, *IEEE Trans. Biomed. Eng.* **BME-21:**109.

Beranek, L.L. (1963a), Acoustical definitions, *American Institute of Physics Handbook*, 2nd ed., McGraw-Hill, New York, Sec. 3, p. 2.

Beranek, L.L. (1963b), Acoustic properties of Gases, *American Institute of Physics Handbook*, 2nd ed., McGraw-Hill, New York, Sec. 3, p. 65.

Bom, N., Lancee, C.T., Honkoop, J., and Hugenholtz, P.G. (1971), Ultrasonic viewer for cross-sectional analysis of moving cardiac structures, *Biomed. Eng.* **6:**500.

Bowen, T., Connor, W.G., Nasoni, R.L., Pifer, A.E., and Sholes, R.R. (1977), Measurement of the temperature dependence of the velocity of ultrasonic in soft tissues, in *Proceedings of Second International Symposium on Ultrasonic Tissue Characterization, Gaithersburg, MD,* June 13–15, 1977, Linzer M. (eds.), National Bureau of Standards Special Publication 525, p. 57.

Bradfield, G. (1970), Ultrasonic transducers, *Ultrasonics* **8:**177.

Buschmann, W., Voss, M., and Kemmerling, S. (1970), Acoustic properties of normal human orbit tissues, *Ophthalm. Res. (Basel)* **1:**354.

Carstensen, E.L., Li, K., and Schwan, H.P. (1953), Determination of the acoustic properties of blood and its components, *J. Acoust. Soc. Am.* **25:**286.

Carstensen, E.L., and Schwan, H.P. (1959a), Absorption of sound arising from the presence of intact cells in blood, *J. Acoust. Soc. Am.* **31:**185.

Carstensen, E.L., and Schwan, H.P. (1959b), Acoustic properties of hemoglobin solutions, *J. Acoust. Soc. Am.* **31:**305.

Daly, C.H., and Wheeler, J.B., III (1971), *Int. Dent. J.* **21:**418.

Del Grosso, V.A. (1970), Sound speed in pure water and sea water, *J. Acoust. Soc. Am.* **47:**947.

Dunn, F., and Fry, W.J. (1961), Ultrasonic absorption and reflection by lung tissue, *Phys. Med. Biol.* **5:**401.

Dunn, F., and O'Brien, W.D., Jr. (eds.) (1976), *Ultrasonic Biophysics*, Dowden, Hutchinson & Ross, Stroudsburg, Pennsylvania.

Edmonds, P.D., Bauld, T.J., III, Dyro, J.F., and Hussey, M. (1970), Ultrasonic absorption of aqueous hemoglobin solutions, *Biochim. Biophys. Acta* **200:**174.

Eggleton, R.C. (1976), State-of-the-art of single-transducer ultrasonic imaging technology, *Med. Phys.* **3:**303.

Fay, R.D. (1957), Acoustic properties of liquids, *American Institute of Physics Handbook*, McGraw-Hill, New York, Sec. 3, p. 72.

Fieler, F.D., and Pocock, P. (1968), Foetal blood flow detector, *Ultrasonics* **6:**240.

Fry, F.J., Heimburger, R.F., Gibbons, L.V., and Eggleton, R.C. (1970), Ultrasound for visualization and modification of brain tissue, *IEEE Trans. Sonics Ultrason.* **SU-17:**165.

Goldman, R. (1962), *Ultrasonic Technology*, Reinhold Press, New York.

Goldman, D.E., and Hueter, T.F. (1957), Tabular data of the velocity and Absorption of high-frequency sound in mammalian tissues, *J. Acoust. Soc. Am.* **28:**35, 1956; Errata: **29:**655.

Gramiak, R., and Waag, R.C., (eds.) (1975), *Cardiac Ultrasound*, Mosby Press, St. Louis.

Hunt, F.V. (1963), *Propagation of Sound in Fluids*, American Institute of Physics, Handbook, 2nd ed., McGraw-Hill, New York, Sec. 3, pp. 56–59.

Hussey, M. (1975), *Diagnostic Ultrasound*, Blackie, Glasgow.

Kossoff, G. (1974), Display techniques in ultrasound pulse echo investigations: A review, *J. Clin. Ultrasound* **2**:61.

Lang, S.B. (1970), Ultrasonic method for measuring elastic coefficients of bone and results on fresh and dried bovine bone, *IEEE Trans. Biomedical Eng.* **17**:101.

Ludwig, G.D. (1950), The velocity of sound through tissues and the acoustic impedance of tissues, *J. Acoust. Soc. Am.* **22**:862.

Malecki, I. (1969), *Physical Foundations of Technical Acoustics*, Pergamon/Polish Scientific Publishers, Warsaw.

Marginness, M.G., Plummer, J.D., Beaver, W.L., and Meindl, J.D. (1976), State-of-the-art in two-dimensional ultrasonic transducer array technology, *Med. Phys.* **3**:312.

Mason, W.P. (1950), *Piezoelectric Crystals and Their Application to Ultrasonics*, Van Nostrand, New York.

Mason, W.P. (1963), Properties of transducer materials, *American Institute of Physics Handbook*, 2nd ed., McGraw-Hill, New York, Sec. 3, p. 98.

McKinney, W.M., Kato, M., Pou, B., and Thurstone, F.L. (1966), Echoencephalography, a practical clinical and research tool, *Trans. Am. Neurolog. Assoc.* **91**:297.

Morse, P.M. (1948), *Vibration and Sound*, 2nd ed., McGraw-Hill, New York.

Morse, P.M., and Ingard, K.U. (1968), *Theoretical Acoustics*, McGraw-Hill, New York.

Pätzold, J., Krause, W., Kresse, H., and Solner, R. (1970), *IEEE Trans. Biomed. Eng.* **17**:263.

Reid, J.M. (1976), Challenges and opportunities in ultrasound, in *Proceedings of Seminar on Ultrasonic Tissue Characterization, Gaithersburg, MD*, May 28–30, 1975, National Bureau of Standards Special Publication 453, p. 11.

Robinson, T.C., and Lele, P.P. (1972), An analysis of lesion development in the brain and in plastics by high-intensity focused ultrasound at low-megahertz frequencies, *J. Acoust. Soc. Am.* **51**:1333.

Robinson, D.E., and Williams, B.G. (1975), Computer acquisition and processing of ultrasonic data, in *Ultrasonics in Medicine*, Kazner, E., deVlieger, M., Muller, H.R., and McCready, V.R. (eds.), Excerpta Medica, Amsterdam, p. 96.

Schiefer, W., Kazuer, E., and Kunze, S.T. (1968), *Clinical Echoencephalography*, John Wright & Sons, Bristol.

Shaw, A., Paton, J.S., Gregory, N.L., and Wheatley, D.J. (1976), A real time 2-dimensional ultrasonic scanner for clinical use, *Ultrasonics* **14**:35.

Shung, K.K., Sigelmann, R.A., and Reid, J.M. (1976), The scattering of ultrasound by red blood cells, in *Proceedings of Seminar on Ultrasonic Tissue Characterization, Gaithersburg, MD*, May 28–30, 1975, National Bureau of Standards Special Publication 453, p. 207.

Somer, J.C. (1968), Electronic sector scanning for ultrasonic diagnosis, *Ultrasonics* **6**:153.

Somer, J.C., Oosterbaan, W.A., and Freund, M.J. (1973), Ultrasonic tomographic imaging of the brain with an electronic sector scanning system, in *Proceedings of 1973 IEEE Ultrasonics Symposium*, IEEE, New York, p. 43.

Theismann, H., and Pfander, F. (1949), *Strahlentherapie* **80**:607.

Thurstone, F.L., and von Ramm, O.T. (1974), Electronic beam scanning for ultrasonic imaging, in *Ultrasonics in Medicine*, deVlieger, M., White, D.N., and McCready, V.R. (eds.), Excerpta Medica, Amsterdam, pp. 43–48.

Van Venrooij, G.E.P.M. (1971), Measurement of ultrasound velocity in human tissue, *Ultrasonics* **9**:240.

Wells, P.N.T. (1969), A range-gated ultrasonic Doppler system, *Med. Biol. Eng.* **7**:641.

Wells, P.N. (1972), *Ultrasonics in Clinical Diagnosis*, Williams & Wilkins, Baltimore.

White, D., and Brown, R.E. (eds.) (1977), *Ultrasound in Medicine*, Vol. 3B, Plenum Press, New York.

Whittingham, T.A. (1976), A hand-held electronically switched array for rapid ultrasonic scanning, *Ultrasonics* **14**:29.

Willson, K., Gehrke, J., Gore, J.C., Leeman, S., Oliver, R., and Pridie, R.B. (1975), Digital Processing of ultrasonic cardiac images, in *Ultrasonics in Medicine*, Kazner, E., de-Vlieger, M., Muller, H.R., and McCready, V.R. (eds.), Excerpta Medica, Amsterdam, p. 103.

CHAPTER 11

Medical Aspects of Thermography

IRWIN M. FREUNDLICH

This chapter was written in 1976. Since then a national study has proved that thermography is not sufficiently sensitive as a screening procedure to detect small, particularly nonpalpable, breast carcinomas. Better discrimination among the various causes of venous heat asymmetry is needed. Asymmetry may be secondary to the depth of the vein under the skin or the size of the vein as well as due to a vein carrying blood of increased temperature. The latter group includes increased temperature secondary to inflammatory and neoplastic disease, which two causes might possibly be differentiated by circadian rhythm. Research efforts directed toward better discrimination of the thermographic signal, particularly quantitative discrimination, may well prove to be quite rewarding.

Thermography, however, is still useful in the clinical setting, as an adjunct to mammography, particularly in young patients with extensive benign breast disease for whom routine mammography would not be recommended. In addition, there is some evidence that thermography may be useful in the prognostic sense as a guide for therapy of breast carcinoma.

11.1. HEAT MEASUREMENT IN MEDICINE

Fever, like thunder, lightning, fire, and flood, is accepted by civilized man as a natural phenomenon. As such, it is at least partially understood and

IRWIN M. FREUNDLICH • Department of Radiology, Health Sciences Center, University of Arizona, Tucson, Arizona 85724.

more or less taken for granted. This was not so with our primitive ancestors, who looked upon their world with awe and wonderment. When they burned with fever they attributed their ill health to the wrath of the gods. It was not until about 400 B.C. that Hippocrates, by placing his hand on his patient's brow, recognized and taught that fever was a natural occurrence not due to a divine visitation into the human soul. He was one of the first to attempt a separation of the natural from the theological and the physical from the philosophical. For more than two millennia after Hippocrates, fever was considered a disease in itself, and medical phrases such as scarlet fever and yellow fever lingered well into the 20th century. It was Wunderlich's thousands of temperature measurements in the middle of the 19th century that caused fever to be recognized as a symptom and not the illness itself (van der Star, 1969; Wallace, 1973).

Medicine has been long considered both an art and a science but until the current century was much more of an art, and in light of modern standards, practiced largely in the dark. Immense changes in medical thought followed the application of the scientific method to the investigation of diseases and later, the marriage of clinical medicine to the physical sciences produced the technology we now associate with a modern practice.

Galileo was probably inventor of the first crude thermometer in the latter part of the 16th century. (Strictly speaking, this was a thermoscope since it did not have a scale. A thermometer is a thermoscope with the appropriate calibrated scale.) Whether Galileo himself or one of his students such as Vivani actually fabricated the instrument is uncertain. However, without association with the name of Galileo it would have had little impact as an invention.

In 1612, another Italian, Sanctorius of Padua, devised an air thermometer for measuring the temperature of a person in fever. He was the first to claim to be able to determine the variation of the temperature of the human body during the course of certain fevers. Sanctorius describes a clinical thermometer in the first book of Canon of Avicenna in Venice in 1625 (Garrison, 1963). At the same time two other scientists, Fludd of Ireland and Drebbel of Holland, were developing an air thermometer. These early thermometers are described in detail by S. W. Mitchell (1892).

In 1630, Jean Rey, a French physician, invented the liquid-in-glass thermometer. This open thermometer not only sensed temperatures but was sensitive to barometric pressures also. It therefore could not repeat measurements during calibration. About 1650 the Grand Duke of Tuscany, Ferdinand II, developed a sealed liquid thermometer. In 1660, the physicist Otto Von Guericke, who was then also Burgomeister of Magdeburg, Germany, calibrated his thermometer into seven parts: "freezing hard, freezing, cold, normal, warm, hot, and very hot."

During the seventeenth and early eighteenth centuries, investigators such as Boyle, Hooke, Newton, Roemer, Halley, and Muschembrock tried to define a calibration and standardization of the thermometer scale with no great success (Martine, 1740). One problem these investigators overlooked in making thermometers reliably accurate was the effect of the thermal expansion of the stem, which was made of brass or glass.

Most investigators believed that the freezing and boiling points of water should be used for calibration points, but water thermometers were difficult to calibrate because of the change in state of the expanding liquid at the boiling and freezing point of water. Alcohol thermometers filled with distilled wine spirits could be calibrated nicely at the freezing point of water; they did not freeze when packed in ice, the coldest substance known at that time. However, the alcohol became a gas at the temperature of boiling water.

Other expanding liquids were also tried during these years. Halley and Boyle in 1693 suggested using mercury since no change in state occurs either at freezing or boiling points of water. Newton in 1700 tried linseed oil with no great success. Since calibration and standardization were not established on a firm basis, the thermometer simply existed without achieving a permanent place in medicine or science.

A Danish astronomer, Roemer, the discoverer of the finite speed of light, calibrated his thermometers using snow, ice, and boiling water. In 1708, Gabriel Fahrenheit of Danzig visited Roemer and was impressed by the way Roemer calibrated the scale on his thermometers. Then in 1714, Fahrenheit invented a new method of cleaning mercury by distillation so that it would not stick to the walls of tubes. This enabled him to substitute mercury for alcohol in thermometers. With this mercury thermometer he was able to calibrate both the freezing and boiling points of water without the technical problems of the previous instruments. He gave this mercury thermometer to his friend, Herman Boerhaave, a Dutch clinician, who used it to demonstrate the value of thermometry in the diagnosis of disease among patients at the University of Leiden. These experiments enabled clinicians to record absolute temperature rather than only the subjective feeling of warmth. Fahrenheit chose for his temperature scale the interval between freezing salt water and a healthy person's blood temperature. The zero point was located on the thermometer's stem below the salt water's freezing point at half the interval distance between the two calibration points as shown in Fig. 11-1. He divided the thermometer interval by 12

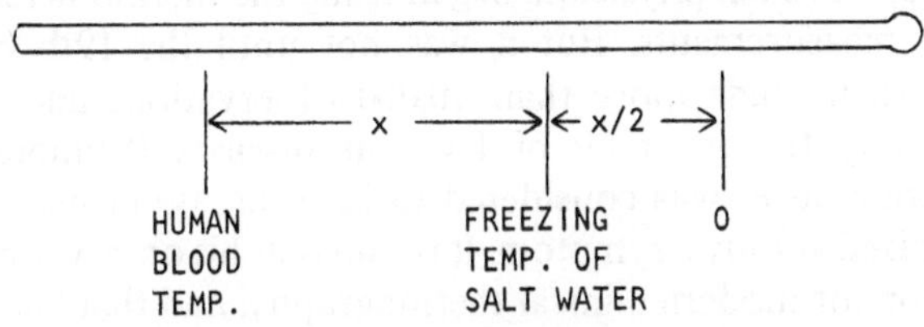

Fig. 11-1. Divisions of Fahrenheit scale.

and then later into 96 divisions; the number 96 being chosen because it had so many divisors.

After Fahrenheit's death in 1736 the freezing point and boiling point were used to calibrate his thermometer. Using this new calibration procedure, the Fahrenheit scale has blood temperatures at 98.6° and the freezing and boiling points of water at 32° and 212°, respectively (Worthington, 1940).

Fahrenheit's success was a result of three developments: (1) establishment of a calibrated scale, (2) establishment of finer subdivisions than previously used, and (3) use of capillary tubes of constant and controlled diameter so that all of the thermometers were identical.

In 1742, a Swedish astronomer, Anders Celsius, recommended that the thermometer be calibrated in 100 parts (centrigrade) between the freezing and boiling points of water (boiling point being zero in the original thermometer). Linnaeus reversed the scale with zero being the freezing point as it is today, although with classic historic irony it is called the Celsius scale (van der Star, 1969).

In the 18th century Hales noted a difference in the temperature between the mouth, the skin, the axilla, and urine in man, while John Hunter, the brilliant English surgeon, also investigated the temperature in various orifices of his own body and in animals. Hunter was evidently fascinated by the ability of certain animals to hibernate and noted body temperature under conditions of hibernation as well.

Very early in the 18th century an acquaintanceship grew between Fahrenheit and Boerhaave, the great Dutch physician, which gave impetus to the use of a thermometer in measuring human fever. One of Boerhaaves' pupils, deHaen, established the use of the thermometer in diagnosis at the Vienna Medical Clinic in the mid-18th century. deHaen realized that subjective sensations of warmth or coolness often did not coincide with objectively recorded body temperature and also noted that in some illnesses a fever persisted after an apparent recovery. Currie, who used one of the earliest mercury thermometers, developed in the latter part of the 18th century, treated fevers with cold water baths. Currie recorded that he used the cold water treatment with his own son, who was critically ill with scarlet fever, and sponged the boy 14 times in 32 hours until he noted a falling temperature, which led to an eventual recovery (Wallace and Cade, 1973). Lorain, a French physician, began using the thermometer for routine temperature measurements. But it was not until the 19th century that Carl Wunderlich made more than 10,000 observations and published a book discussing the meaning of fever in diseases (Wunderlich, 1871). Before his book, fever was considered to be a disease in itself. Thereafter, it was recognized as only a symptom. It is said that his observations provided the foundation for modern clinical thermography, and that "he found fever a disease and left it as a symptom" (Wallace and Cade, 1973). It also led to Albutt's introduction of the clinical thermometer, and attempts to devise meaningful measurements of body surface temperature variations. These efforts failed primarily because of a lack of knowledge about the complex thermodynamic balance of the human body and the fact that contact thermometers modified the temperature structure they were trying to measure.

The discovery of infrared radiation is credited to Sir William Herschel (1800). His discovery made remote sensing of body surface temperatures possible. Herschel discovered that the heating power of the sun's rays increased from the violet to the red end of the spectrum and that the maximum was not reached until the thermometer had been placed beyond the end of the visible red. Herschel found more heating in the infrared spectral region than at the radiation peak of 480 μm predicted by the Wien displacement law because of the prism dispersive character and the finite size (fixed slit width) of the thermometer used. The prism did not disperse the infrared as well as the visible spectrum, thus causing a spatial energy concentration. This pronounced heating effect was attributed to radiation, which he called infrared. The infrared region might well have been discovered by Landriani in 1777, who was the first to examine the energy distribution of the solar spectrum by passing a thermometer through it. Similar experiments were also conducted by Rochon in 1776 and Seniber in 1785 (Barr, 1960). In 1840, Sir John Herschel, son of Sir William, rendered the infrared spectrum visible by means of crude pictures, which he termed "thermographs" (Hershchel, 1840). These were made by coating paper with lamp black and then soaking it in alcohol. When infrared radiation was focused on the prepared paper, the alcohol evaporated more rapidly from parts that received the stronger radiation, causing the paper to appear lighter in those areas. It remained for Seebeck in 1825 to discover the

Table 11-1. Historical Development of Temperature Measurement

Date	Event	Discoverer
400 B.C.	Detected temperature by touch	Hippocrates
1592 A.D.	First thermoscope	Galileo
1608	Discovered thermoscope	Fludd and Drebbel
1630	Liquid thermometer	Jean Rey
1702	Calibrated thermometer	Roemer
1714	Mercury thermometer	Fahrenheit
1742	Centigrade thermometer	Celsius
1800	Discovered infrared	William Herschel
1825	Discovered thermocouple	Seebeck
1840	Imaged infrared	John Herschel
1871	Clinical thermometer	Wunderlich
1881	Discovered bolometer	Langley
1929	Evaporograph	Czerny
1956	Detected breast cancer with thermograph	Lawson

thermocouple, Nobili to refine Seebeck's thermocouple to a sensitive thermopile, and Langley in 1881 to develop the bolometer, before infrared began to be recognized as a quantitative tool.

Nearly a century and a half after the discovery of infrared radiation, Professor Marianus Czerny (1929) developed a method under the name of evaporagraphy that provided the first practical system for "seeing by heat waves." In the 1940's, however, military applications of infrared techniques initiated a technological revolution and extended its practicality. In 1956, a Baird evaporograph was made available and R. N. Lawson (1957), a Canadian surgeon, was able to use it to substantiate his theory that most breast cancers are characterized by a rise in temperature. A synopsis of the historical development is shown in Table 11-1 on page 403.

11.2. HEAT REGULATION AND EMANATION

Maintenance of thermal equilibrium is under central nervous system control, specifically the hypothalamus, which serves as a kind of physiological thermostat (Fulton, 1951). The hypothalamus regulates the rate of heat production and dissipation by its influence upon the somatic and visceral motor neurons of the brain stem and spinal cord. However, the once popular assumption that the hypothalamus is the only location of deep body temperature control is no longer feasible and other temperature sensors are probably distributed throughout the body (Bligh, 1973). The rate of heat production and dissipation is modulated in such a way that the total heat of the body is only slightly altered even in the face of fairly wide variations in environmental temperatures as well as variations in the physiological state of the body (Fulton, 1951). Heat loss by radiation, convection, and conduction consists of sympathetic nervous system influence on peripheral vasomotor tone, especially in the extremities. This influence changes the rate of blood flow through a superficial capillary bed and alters venous motor tone, which controls the route taken by the venous blood. When heat must be conserved, the venous blood returns to the trunk through deep veins lying close to the arteries. A countercurrent heat exchange between the arterial and venous blood lowers the temperature of the arterial blood before it reaches the capillaries and less heat is lost. When heat needs to be dissipated, the venous blood returns preferentially through the superficial veins well removed from the arteries. The opening and closing of arteriovenous shunts probably also influence the non-evaporative heat exchange between the organism and the environment (Bligh, 1973).

The energy derived from food is utilized in humans in one of three ways; the production of heat, work, and storage (Fulton, 1951). Through a series of enzymatic reactions the heat of combustion, upon which mammals depend for the maintenance of their relatively constant body temperature, is gradually released. Heat production is lowest during sleep, higher when the individual is awake but fasting, and shows a further elevation after the ingestion of food or after muscular exercise. Voluntary muscular contractions are accompanied by the liberation of relatively large amounts of heat, an experience most have had in trying to stay warm during cold weather. Shivering is another reaction which accomplishes the same results and is used in maintaining temperature equilibrium. Voluntary exercise, however, may not preserve the equilibrium but actually disturb it, depending upon the environmental conditions at the time (Fulton, 1951).

Heat is not only lost from the skin by radiation, conduction, and convection but also by warming and humidifying the air of respiration, by the evaporation of perspiration, and in the urine and feces (Best and Taylor, 1961). Of the total quantity of heat lost in 24 hours approximately 65% is through radiation, conduction, and convection. Radiation of heat can only be accomplished when a temperature gradient exists between the radiating object and its environment (Fulton, 1951). The reverse may be true under certain circumstances; for example, the body is heated by radiation from the multiple reflecting surfaces of snow while skiing, even though the environmental temperature may be quite low. Conduction includes the transfer of heat to any substance in contact with the body and includes the air which covers the skin under clothing, the clothing itself, the air which is warmed in respiratory passages, in the gastrointestinal tract, and in the urinary system (Fulton, 1951). Heat loss by convection depends upon the movement of warm air from the neighborhood of a heated object and varies with the temperature of the atmosphere. The warm moist air layer in contact with the body is trapped and in the absence of a temperature difference between it and external air, it will remain stagnant and little or no heat will be lost through convection. However when the atmosphere is cooler convection currents are established, which mix the air against the skin with fresh air, and heat is lost (Best and Taylor, 1961).

The evaporation of water from the surface of the skin is an important cooling process and accounts for approximately 30% of heat loss (Best and Taylor, 1961). While heat loss through radiation is only slightly reduced when relative humidity is high, this is not the case when one considers heat loss through evaporation. In the hot dry air of the desert water evaporates almost instantaneously, and the prevention of overheating is easier than in a warm climate with high humidity. Under constant environmental conditions the amount of heat loss depends upon the surface area, temperature, and humidity of the environment as well as the rate of air flow over the skin.

Of the 65% heat loss through radiation, convention, and conduction, approximately 50% is by radiation. The human skin, within the range of the infrared rays to which it is usually exposed, color notwithstanding, is almost a perfect blackbody radiator. It radiates nearly all infrared rays or absorbs to the same extent such rays which fall upon it (Best and Taylor, 1961). The radiation surface of the body is approximately 85% of the total surface. Opposed skin surfaces such as the axillas, medial aspect of the thighs, etc., do not lose heat to the environment by radiation. It is of course, for this reason that one huddles in the cold and spreads out one's limbs in the heat. The subcutaneous layer varies considerably in thickness and is usually thicker in women than in men. This accounts for the greater ability for women to withstand cold temperatures. Generally speaking when the blood vessels are constricted, the skin and subcutaneous tissues are just a little more efficient as an insulating material than a layer of cork of the same thickness (Best and Taylor, 1961).

Although most of the heat loss from the skin is by radiation, this heat reaches the skin predominantly by vascular convection along verticle channels, which either traverse the muscle or connect its vascular system with that of the overlying skin. Cooper *et al.*, whose work established the vascular convection of the heat, also noted that veins were of much greater importance than arteries in this regard, and that the direct nonconvective transfer of heat to the overlying skin is relatively less important than the venous convection (Cooper *et al.*, 1959).

Since veins draining deeper tissues may be carrying blood of increased temperature, it is therefore obvious that the visualization of these veins should be optimized. The same is true for local changes in the temperature of the skin itself. In order to best visualize these temperature changes thermographically the surrounding skin is cooled by reducing the ambient temperature. A room temperature of 68°–70°F for 5–8 min is sufficient to cool the surrounding skin, which improves the signal-to-noise ratio considerably and optimizes visualization of the venous structures.

11.3. DEVELOPMENT OF THERMOGRAPHY

Necessity induced by war is frequently the catalyst which turns the theoretical idea or crude instrument into practical technology. The desire to see in the dark and in the jungle gave tremendous impetus to the development of thermography. The Army recognized its possibilities during World War II and considerable work was carried out at that time and thereafter by the Army Signal Corps engineering laboratories. Theories and crude instrumentation were indeed available in the years before the war. The first working infrared image was developed by Czerny in 1929. It was based on a technique called evaporography and depended upon the differential evaporation of a volatile liquid sprayed on a thin membrane at the time an infrared image is formed on the membrane (Arnquist, 1959). A more advanced instrument based on this principle was developed somewhat later at Baird Associates, with the support of the Air Force and the Army Signal Corps. A few years after Czerny's work the RCA Company was instrumental in producing a device which accepted an infrared image at one end and delivered a visible image at the other (Arnquist, 1959).

In the 1930's Hardy investigated the skin in relation to infrared radiation. He credits Hasselbach with the earliest spectographic observations of ultraviolet and visible radiation from the skin (Hardy and Muschenheim, 1934). Hardy himself found that the skin was essentially a blackbody radiator with the infrared transmission and reflection spectra that would be expected (Hardy and Muschenheim, 1934). In another article Hardy described a radiation instrument for measuring skin temperature, which had the advantages of greater accuracy and simplicity over similar previous radiometers as well as higher sensitivity (Hardy, 1934).

In 1946, Zahl and Golay of the Army Signal Corps described a pneumatic heat detector in which radiant energy was dissipated in a black absorber located in the center of a gas cell (Zahl and Golay, 1946). The resulting heating and expansion of the gas served to distort a collodion film located a few thousandths of an inch from a nearby parallel glass window. The images produced were the first thermograms. The authors noted that the principle could be applied to the design of systems comprising a multitude of these cells and associated detecting film. They acknowledged the superiority of radar to thermography and compared the entities from a military point of view. Golay continued his work with two articles in the following year, the first a mathematical review of the basic factors involved in infrared detection, which included a description of the optical system. The second was a description of the detector in detail. The latter paper included a review of the work which had been done by the Signal Corps from 1932 to 1947 (Golay, 1947 a,b). During the Korean War and thereafter much of the work on infrared technology was accomplished at the Willow Run Laboratories at the University of Michigan. This effort culminated in a fundamental textbook on Infrared Technology published in 1962 (Holter *et al.*, 1962). The military has displayed a continued interest in thermography, and the most sophisticated equipment used today is still classified. For a complete historical review of infrared technology the reader is referred to Arnquist (1959).

11.4. CLINICAL THERMOGRAPHY

Generally speaking, the role of thermography in medical diagnosis is that of a survey instrument, which may detect local excess heat or insufficient heat. Usually a comparison of one side of the body with the other is necessary. When dealing with inflammatory, hyperplastic, or neoplastic diseases, an increase in heat may be a manifestation of illness; while vascular occlusive disease is signaled by a decrease in heat.

In 1956 Dr. Ray Lawson, a Canadian surgeon, acquired a declassified Baird evaporagraph and made the first medical thermograms of increased heat emanating from carcinoma of the breast (Lawson, 1956). Working independently, Lloyd-Williams *et al.*, in England also recognized the medical potential for visualizing infrared radiation emanating from the skin and investigated several diseases (Lloyd-Williams *et al.*, 1960, 1961). These authors noted a rise in skin temperature over a number of different malignancies. They further noted that some benign diseases were also "hot" and indistinguishable from malignancies. Extending their investigation with further observations of breast diseases, they set the stage for detection of carcinoma of the breast by heat emanation, which remains the major interest of clinical thermography today. While the earliest investigators sought the "hot spot" in one breast as the indicator of a neoplasm, it soon became apparent that the venous pattern was of considerable importance. It was noted that a rough symmetry of the venous architecture could be expected and a unilateral increase in venous heat emanation could be an indication of a deeper lesion. Several thousands of patients were gathered by Wallace *et al.*, and the early clinical results were promising (Wallace and Dodd, 1968; Dodd *et al.*, 1969 a,b). Normal breast thermographic patterns were established and considerable variation in the normal was noted (Draper and Jones, 1969; Lapayowker *et al.*, 1971). A review of the two above-mentioned references will demonstrate that both a black-hot and a white-hot polarity are used by various workers. A brief investigation into visual physiology indicates that it is probably easier to detect different shades of gray at the black end of the scale than at the white (Wallace and Cade, 1973). Accordingly, it is recommended that the

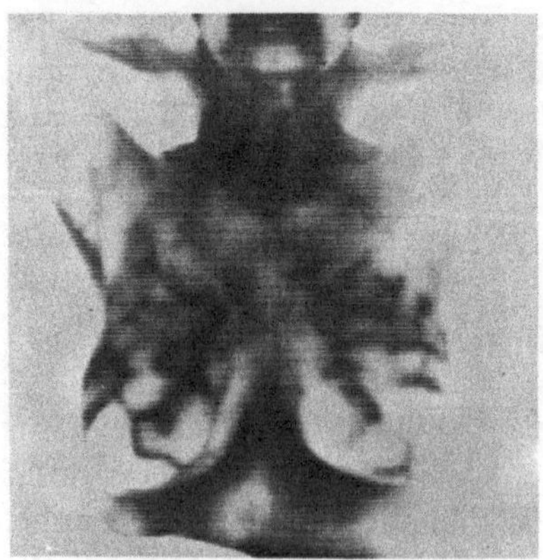

Fig. 11-2. Normal thermogram made in 1968 on facsimile paper by Smith Thermographic Instrument. The polarity is black-hot for this figure and all the remaining figures.

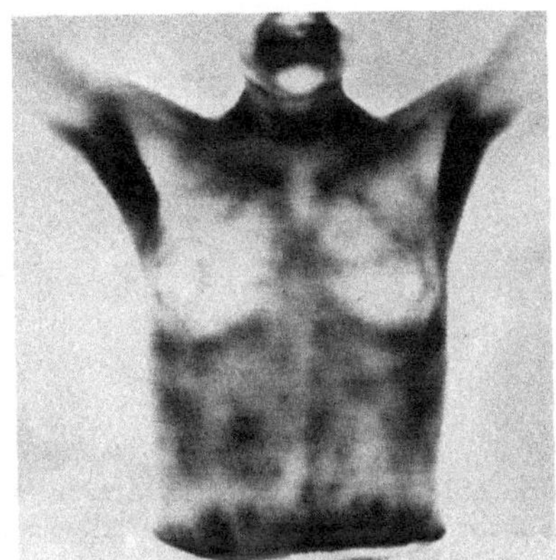

Fig. 11-3. Normal thermogram with relatively "athermal" breasts i.e., there is a lack of superficial venous heat.

black-hot polarity be employed, but a number of thermographers use the opposite polarity. In 1969, Dodd *et al.*, in conjunction with the Texas Instruments Company developed a thermographic instrument with high spatial resolution (Dodd *et al.*, 1969 a,b). The ability to see the details of the thermal pattern was much improved and the stage was set for modern clinical thermography.

Figure 11-2 demonstrates the contrast between an older type of thermogram made on facsimile paper by a Smith Instrument and those made with a modern Texas Instruments thermoscope. Figures 11-3 to 11-6 are various examples of normal thermal patterns of the female breast. The extreme variability from the cold, athermal breast to a marked prominance of venous heat is obvious but of no clinical significance. Abnormal thermograms are recognized by an asymmetry of heat emanating from the

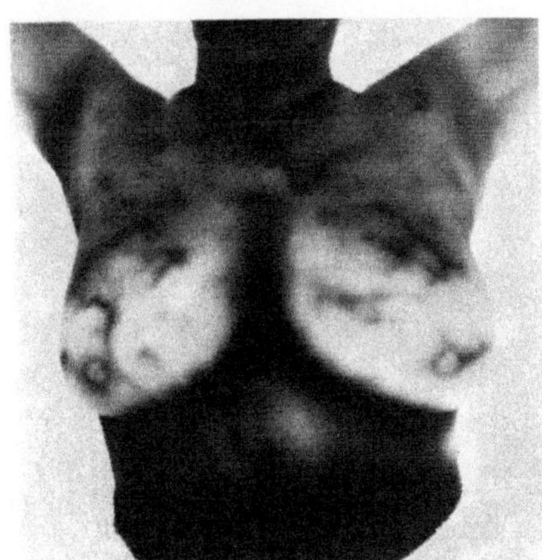

Fig. 11-4. Normal high-resolution thermogram with relatively few superficial veins visible.

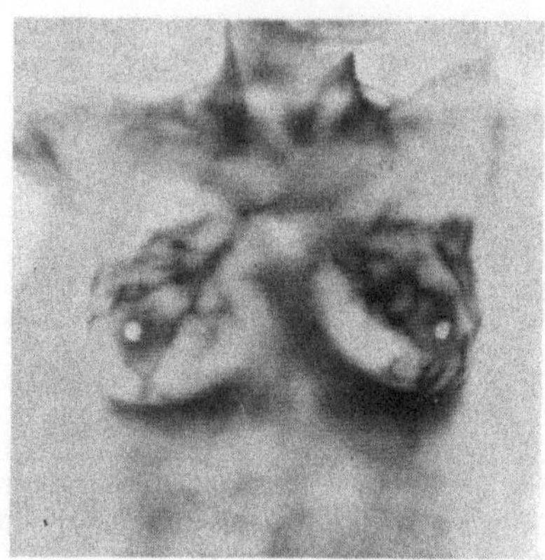

Fig. 11-5. Normal thermogram demonstrating a moderately prominent and roughly symmetrical venous pattern.

breast, which may be manifested by several distinct patterns. A diffuse increase in heat (Fig. 11-7 and 11-8), a localized increase in heat (Fig. 11-9), a unilateral increase in the number and size of veins (Fig. 11-10), and the edge sign (Fig. 11-11) are all indications of thermographic abnormality. The "edge sign" is a distortion of the architecture of the breast, which can be detected by high-quality thermograms as originally described by Isard (1972).

Travis Winsor was one of the earliest pioneers in the investigation of skin temperature in peripheral vascular disease (Winsor, 1954). He described a thermister–thermometer in 1954 prior to Lawson's original thermogram. He has continued his investigations, combining thermography with plethysmography. His work on thermography and cardiovascular disease has been summarized in a recent article (Winsor and Winsor, 1975). Wood initially described the usefullness of thermography in detecting

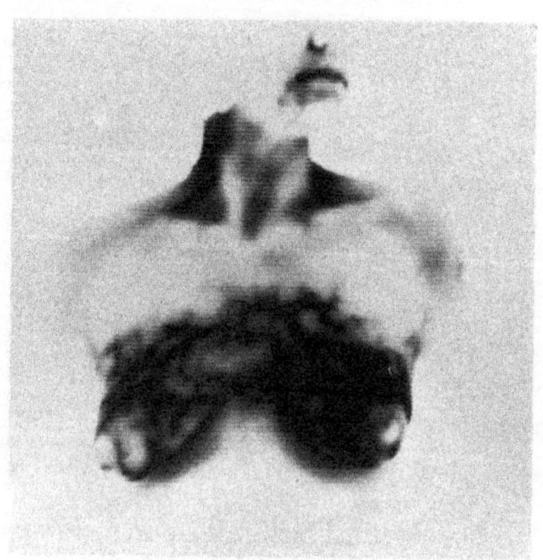

Fig. 11-6. Marked venous engorgement of both breasts in a lactating female.

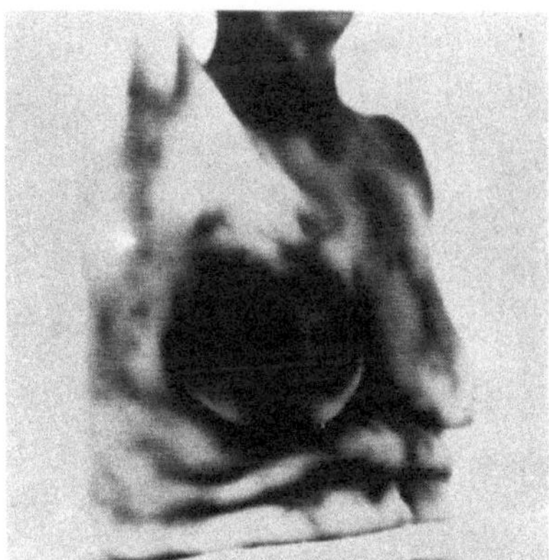

Fig. 11-7. Oblique view of the right breast which demonstrates marked diffuse heat emanating from the breast secondary to a carcinoma.

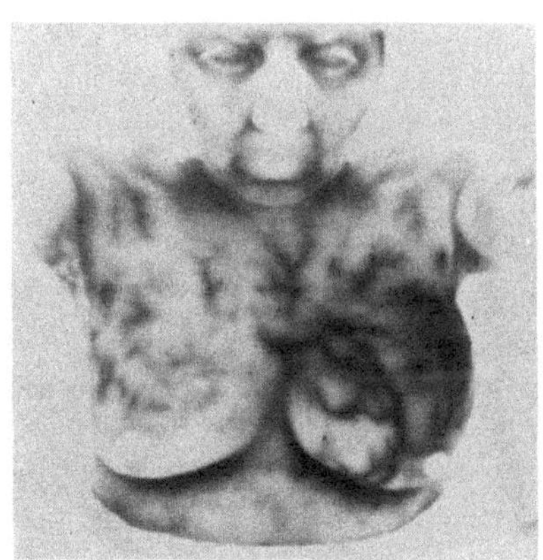

Fig. 11-8. Diffuse heat as well as an increase in the prominance in the veins secondary to a malignancy of the left breast.

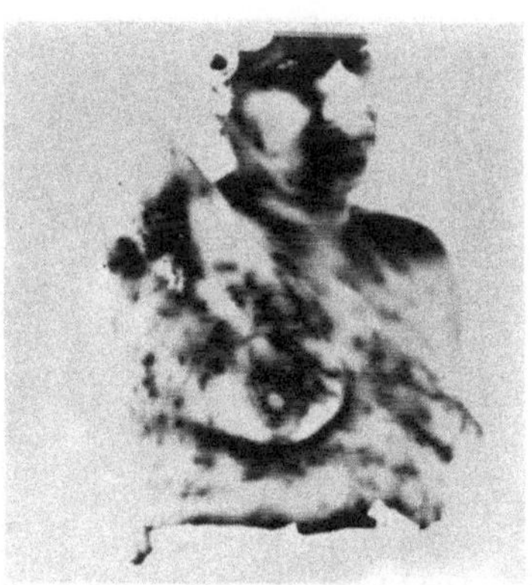

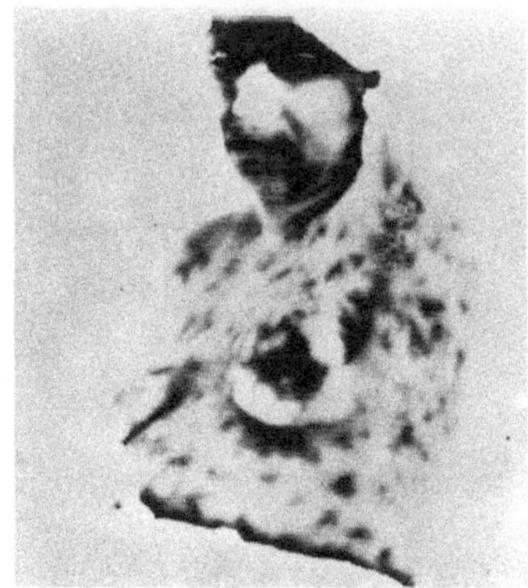

Fig. 11-9. A local increase in pariareolar heat emanating from the left breast. On biopsy only benign disease was found.

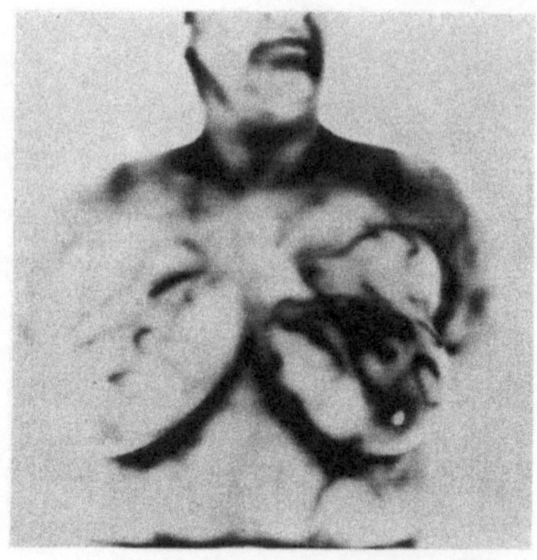

Fig. 11-10. Marked prominance of the venous heat in the left breast secondary to an occult malignancy.

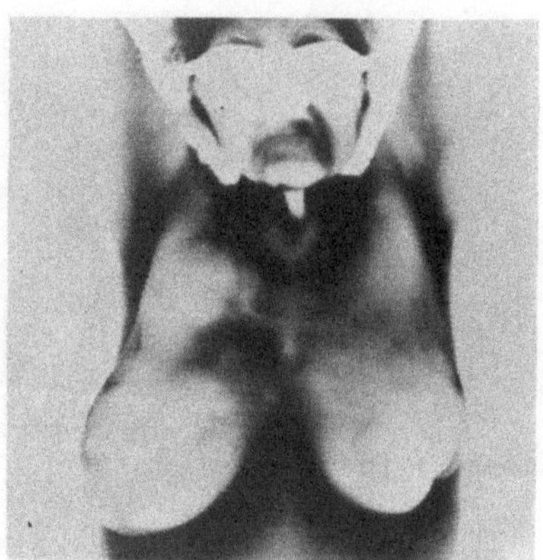

Fig. 11-11. "Edge-sign," a distortion of the contour of the left breast. Note the general absence of heat emanating from both breasts (athermal).

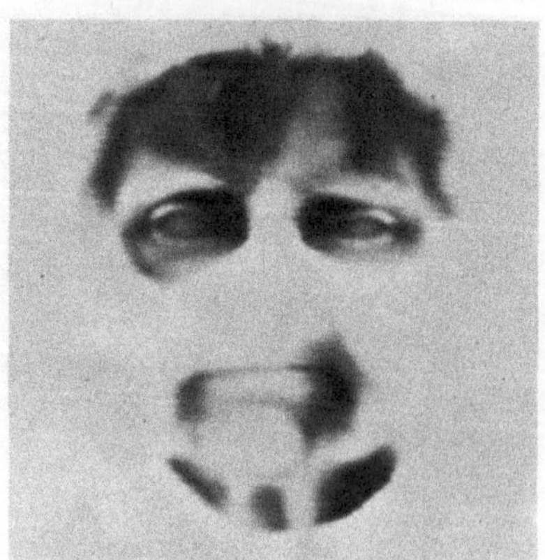

Fig. 11-12. Cool area of brow just to the left of the midline due to significant occlusion of the carotid artery on that side.

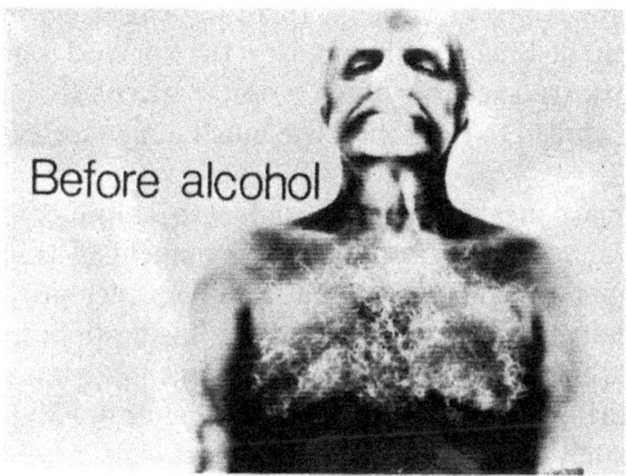

Fig. 11-13. Increase in heat overlying the thyroid and parathyroid glands due to a parathryoid adenoma. (Alcohol cooling is used for thermograms of the neck to enhance the image.)

carotid arterial occlusion in the neck by visualizing the heat of the brow (Fig. 11-12) (Wood and Hill, 1966). Thermography in this area could be very useful as an early detector of potential stroke victims, but unfortunately 60% of the carotid vessel must be occluded before there is thermographic evidence of cooling (Karpman *et al.*, 1972).

The detection of hyperthyroidism and hyperparathyroidism has received considerable attention from Samuels *et al.* (Samuels, 1972, 1975; Samuels *et al.*, 1972). According to these authors, thermography can be employed for detection of parathyroid adenomas but is not as effective in the localization of a hyperplastic gland. However, Dodd has not been able to reproduce the same results and has found the usefulness of the examination for parathyroid adenomas limited (Fig. 11-13) (Dodd, 1975). A thyroid nodule, which is "cold" by radioisotope scanning techniques and could be neoplastic, may well be "hot" by thermographic evaluation. This could be a useful confirmatory clinical parameter, but clinical investigation in this area is needed.

There have been a number of additional reports of medical uses for thermography, which include detection of incompetent perforating veins in the lower extremities, the evaluation of burns, frost bite, wound healing, in the management of the arthritic patient, placental localization, localization of the herniated lumbar disk, and others, but none has found wide clinical acceptance.

11.5. THE PROBLEM OF BREAST SCREENING

Every discussion of breast carcinoma must begin with the knowledge that the mortality rate from carcinoma of the breast has not changed in five decades. This is not to say that there have been no medical advances in the treatment of breast carcinoma as the survival rate has improved. Women with metastatic cancer of the breast, particularly those in whom the malignancy has spread to the bones, live much longer today than in previous years.

The difference in survival rate is due to a limited ability to arrest the disease by altering the hormonal environment of the host, as well as by chemotherapeutic agents, which attack the faster growing tumor cells more readily than normal cells, and by the local application of radiation therapy. Despite this improved survival rate essentially the same percentage of women acquiring breast carcinoma are dying as did 50 years ago.

Approximately 90,000 new cases of breast cancer are found each year in a population of 37 million American women over the age of 35. The vast majority of these malignancies are detected because a mass has grown large enough to be felt by the patient herself or on a routine physical examination. It seems quite clear that the strenuous efforts by the American Cancer Society and other agencies to promote self-examination will not make a significant inroad into the unfortunately constant mortality rate. The limits of palpability in this sense probably have been reached. Although without continued self-examination and physical examination by physicians, the number of women dying of breast carcinoma may actually increase.

It has been clearly demonstrated that smaller neoplasms in the breast have a better prognosis than larger ones. The smaller the lesion found, the less likely that the cancer has spread to the lymph nodes of the axilla. If at the time of surgery these lymph nodes contain no malignant cells, approximately 82% of patients will be free of disease in five years. On the other hand, if the axillary lymph nodes are involved at the time of surgery, this figure drops to about 25%, with an overall figure of 53% being a rather constant one. It is therefore quite clear that detection of smaller lesions will improve the mortality rate. Strax has shown through a mass screening program carried out in New York that breast screening can improve the mortality rate and that X-ray examination of the breast plays a major role. A Breast Cancer Detection Program in 27 centers throughout the United States is now underway, sponsored by the National Cancer Institute and the American Cancer Society. Although it is too early in that program to arrive at definitive conclusions, the trend certainly indicates that a large number of the cancers found are too small to be palpated and are detected only by mammography or xeromammography. These small lesions, very often less than a half a centimeter in size, have an excellent prognosis in that the axillary lymph nodes are seldom involved at the time of surgery. There would be however, several problems associated with an attempt to carry out mammography for the entire American female population over the age of 35. The process is quite time consuming and expensive. Interpretation by a radiologist has been necessary, and the radiation required, although quite small and probably insignificant, must also be listed as a disadvantage. While it may certainly be possible to reduce the cost in a mass program, particularly if lay personnel can be trained to interpret the mammogram, other methods of mass screening must be considered.

It was originally hoped that thermography would be a satisfactory method for screening the American female population. Papers by Stark and Way (1974 a,b), Isard *et al.* (1972) and Jones *et al.* (1975) indicated that, while a significant percentage of false-positive results could be expected, the false-negative rate would be well within acceptable limits. Thermography and physical examination are also included in the NCI/ACS Breast Cancer Detection Program. While the results of these two modalities have been somewhat disappointing in comparison to mammography, a combination of the two should detect approximately 75% of the carcinomas in the population. Thermography can certainly be carried out and interpreted by lay personnel, and nurses can be trained to do an adequate physical examination of the breast.

Certain groups of women fall into a higher risk category for carcinoma of the breast than the general population. Such high-risk groups include those individuals with a strong family history of cancer, particularly breast cancer, those who have had one breast operated upon for breast cancer, those with very extensive benign breast disease, and those with a positive thermogram. Screening of the high risk groups with mammography on an annual basis would seem more feasible than attempting to examine the entire population. However, in order to find those who fall into the high-risk group some type of preliminary screening procedure must be carried out. It is in this realm that thermography and physical examination carried out by lay personnel can play a role.

The "pap" test for cervical carcinoma has shown that mass screening not only is feasible but will improve the mortality rate considerably. Dr. Papanicolaou's original cytological examinations were much more cumbersome, time consuming, and expensive than the test as it is carried out today. This is the hope for breast screening as well. Historical information from the patient, a thermogram, and a physical examination should separate the high risk from the low-risk patients. High-risk individuals can be examined by mammography or xeromammography each year and low-risk individuals every five years. With such a program early detection can be achieved and many lives saved.

11.6. PROBLEMS AND POTENTIAL

Tremendous technological strides have been made in the production of the thermographic image since Lawson's original picture. However, in the diagnosis of breast cancers thermography suffers from a lack of both specificity and sensitivity. A relatively high percentage of false-positives has plagued thermography since the early days of Lloyd-Williams. Two major reasons for this problem have come to light. First, veins of one breast may merely be larger than the other or closer to the skin. Asymmetry due to these congenital variations cannot now be distinguished from asymmetry secondary to veins of one breast actually carrying blood of increased temperature. Second, any benign inflammatory process can also cause increased heat, which cannot be differentiated from heat produced by malignant neoplasms. In addition, trauma as well as alterations in body metabolism can change the pattern of heat convection to the skin and radiation from it. It may be safely said, therefore, that any of the five major categories of human disease—congenital, inflammatory, traumatic, neoplastic, and metabolic—may cause an increase in heat emanation from the body surface. But the problem is not a hopeless one as traumatic and metabolic diseases are usually diagnosed from historical information and will not fall into the differential diagnosis. This would leave only congenital variations and inflammatory diseases with which to contend. Inflammation is usually self-limited and may be differentiated from neoplasm by a serial study over several weeks, which would further reduce the false-positive rate. The major problem therefore in the specificity of thermography is an inability to detect veins carrying blood, the temperature of which is actually increased in comparison with veins of the opposite breast. Experimental work has begun along these lines. The initial step has been the elimination of skin emissivity by measurment of a ratio temperature (Dereniak, 1976). The next step is construction of an instrument to subtract electronically an active infrared image from the passive thermographic image, a step already suggested by Zermeno *et al.* (1975). Success of this project will significantly improve specificity.

Sensitivity is even a greater problem at the present time as the smallest of cancers often do not increase the local production of heat enough to be measured by current instrumentation. Likewise, if one is seeking to detect arterial occlusive disease, severe occlusion must be present before there is sufficient cooling to be detected. However, fundamental changes in technology are now underway. A more sensitive instrument may well result.

Fever is a manifestation, albeit nonspecific, of mammalian ill health. Despite its nonspecificity, the detection of an increase in whole body temperature plays a significant role in the differential diagnosis of a multitude of diseases. Likewise, the detection of a local increase or decrease in heat production may be entirely nonspecific, but nevertheless very useful.

The nonspecificity and lack of sensitivity of current instrumentation should be the impetus for further advances in technology. The concept of a total body thermogram as a routine survey for areas of local increased heat production or deficiency is not without merit; and the thermogram can find its place, as did the thermometer, in the study of human diseases.

REFERENCES

Adams, F. (1849), *The Genuine Works of Hippocrates, Vols. I & II*, London Sydenham Society, London.

Arnquist, W. (1959), Survey of early infrared developments, *Proc. IRE* **47**:1420–1430.

Barr, E. A. (1960), Historical survey of early development of infrared spectral regions, *Am. J. Phys.* **28**:42.

Best, C., and Taylor, N. (1961), The physiological basis of medical practice, 7th ed., Williams and Wilkins Company, Baltimore.

Bligh, J. (1973), *Temperature Regulation in Mammals and Other Vertebrates*, from the North Holland Research Monographs, London.

Bolton, H.C. (1900), *Evaluation of the Thermometer, 1592–1743*, 12° Easton, Pennsylvania.

Cooper, T., Randall, W., and Hertzman, A. (1959), Vascular convection of heat from active muscles to overlying skin, *J. Appl Physiol.* **14**:207–211.

Czerny, M. (1929), Ueber Photographie in Ultraroten, *Z. Phys.* **53**:1.

Dereniak, E. (1976), Ratio temperature measurement, a dissertation submitted to the Committee on Optical Sciences (Ph. D. degree), University of Arizona.

Dodd, G. (1975), Genetics and cancer of the gastro-intestinal system, presented at the Radiological Society of North America Meeting, December.

Dodd, G., Wallace, J., Freundlich, I., Marsh, L., and Zermeno, A. (1969a), Thermography in cancer of the breast, *Cancer* **23**:797–802.

Dodd, G., Zermeno, A., Marsh, L., Boyd, D., and Wallace J. (1969b), New developments in breast thermography, *Cancer* **24**:1212–1221.

Draper, J., and Jones, C. (1969), Thermal patterns of the female breast, *Brit. J. Radiol.* **42**:401–410.

Fulton, J. (1951), *Textbook of Physiology*, 16th ed., W.B. Saunders Company, Philadelphia.

Garrison, F.H. (1963), *History of Medicine*, W. B. Saunders Company, Philadelphia and London.

Golay, M. (1947a), Theoretical considerations in heat and infrared detection with particular reference to the pneumatic detector, *Rev. Sci. Instrum.* **18**:347–356.

Golay, M. (1947b), A pneumatic infrared detector, *Rev. Sci. Instrum.* **18**:357–362.

Hardy, J. (1934), The radiation of heat from the human body: An instrument for measuring the radiation and surface temperatures of the skin, *J. Clin. Invest.* **13**:593–604.

Hardy, J., and Muschenheim, C. (1934), The radiation of heat from the human body. The emission, reflection and transmission of infrared radiation by the human skin, *J. Clin. Invest.* **13**:817–831.

Herschel, J.F.W. (1840), On chemical action of rays of solar spectrum on preparation of silver and other substances both metallic and nonmetallic and on some photographic processes, *Philos. Trans. R. Soc. London* **130**:1–60.

Herschel, W. (1800), Investigation of powers of prismatic colors to heat and illuminate object with remarks that prove different refrangibility of radiant heat, *Philos. Trans. R. Soc. London* **90**:255–283.

Holter, M., Nudelman, S., Suits, G., Wolfe W., and Zissis, G. (1962), *Fundamentals of Infrared Technology*, Macmillan, New York.

Isard, H. (1972), The edge sign in breast carcinoma, *Cancer* **30**:957–963.

Isard, H., Becker, W., Shilo, R., and Ostrum, B. (1972), Breast thermography after four years and 10,000 studies, *Am. J. Roentgenol.* **115**:811–821.

Jones, C., Greening, W., Davey, J., McKinna, J., and Greeves, V. (1975), Thermography of the female breasts: A five year study in relation to the protection and prognosis of cancer, *Brit. J. Radiol.* **48**:532–538.

Karpman, H., Kalb, I., and Sheppard, J. (1972), The use of thermography in a health care system for stroke, *Geriatrics* **27**:96–105.

Lapayowker, M., Kundel, H., and Ziskin, M. (1971), Thermographic patterns of the female breast and their relationship of carcinoma, *Cancer* **27**:819–822.

Lawson, R. (1956), Implications of surface temperatures in the diagnosis of breast cancer, *Can. Med. Assoc. J.* **75**:309–310.

Lawson, R.N. (1956), Implications of surface temperatures in the diagnosis of breast cancer, *Can. Med. Assoc. J.* **75**:309.

Lawson, R.N. (1957), Thermography – new tool in investigation of breast lesions, *Can. Serv. Med. J.* **13**:, 517.

Lloyd-Williams, K., Lloyd-Williams, F., and Handley, R. (1960), Infrared radiation thermometry in clinical practice, *Lancet* **2**:958–959.

Lloyd-Williams, K., Lloyd-Williams, F., and Handley, R. (1961), Infrared thermometry in the diagnosis of breast disease, *Lancet* **2**:1378–1381.

Martine, G. (1740), *Essays, Medical and Philosophical*, A. Millar, London.

Mitchell, S.W. (1892), *The Early History of Instrumental Precision in Medicine*, the President's address to the 2nd meeting of the Congress of American Physicians and Surgeons, pp. 158–198, Washington, D.C.

Samuels, B. (1972), Thermography: A valuable tool in the detection of thyroid disease, *Radiol.* **102**:53–62.

Samuels, B. (1975), The present status of parathyroid thermography, *J. Am. Med. Assoc.* **233**:907–908.

Samuels, B., Dowdy, A., and Lecky, J. (1972), Parathyroid thermography, *Radiology* **104**:575–578.

Stark, A., and Way, S. (1974a), The use of thermovision in the detection of early breast cancer, *Cancer* **33**:1664–1670.

Stark, S., and Way, S. (1974b), The screening of well women for the early detection of breast cancer using clinical examination with thermography and mammography, *Cancer* **33**:1671–1679.

van der Star, P. (1969), The history of thermometry in medicine (medical thermography), *Bibliogr. Radiol.* **5**:1–7.

Wallace, J., and Cade, C. (1973), *Clinical Thermography*, CRC Reviews in Bio-Engineering, CRC Press, Cleveland, Ohio.

Wallace, J., and Dodd, G. (1968), Thermography in the diagnosis of breast cancer, *Radiology* **91**:679–685.

Winsor, T. (1954), Skin temperature in peripheral vascular disease. A description of the thermistor – thermometer, *J. Am. Med. Assoc.* **154**, 1404–1406.

Winsor, T., and Winsor, C. (1975), Thermography in cardiovascular disease, *Appl. Radiol.* **4**:117–126.

Wood, E., and Hill, R. (1966), Thermography in the diagnosis of cerebrovascular occlusive disease, *Acta Radiol.* **5**:961–971.

Worthington, A.G. (1940), The temperature concept, *Am. J. Phys.* **8**, 28.

Wunderlich, C. (1871), *On the Temperature in Disease: A Manual of Medical Thermometry* (translated by W.B. Woodman), Sydenham Society, J.E. Adlard, Bartholomew Close, London.

Zahl, H., and Golay, M. (1946), Pneumatic heat detector, *Rev. Sci. Instrum.* **17**:511–515.

Zermeno, A., Marsh, L., and Dodd, G. (1975), personal communication.

CHAPTER 12

Thermographic Instrumentation

EUSTACE L. DERENIAK

12.1. INTRODUCTION

During the past 25 years there have been many important technical advances in methods of detecting and curing breast cancer. However, it is surprising to note that in spite of these advances the mortality rate due to breast cancer has not decreased during this period. It is hoped that improvements in thermographic studies of breast cancer in the near future will result in better breast cancer treatment and fewer breast cancer deaths. Mammography, which is presently used in most breast cancer screening programs, involves ionizing radiation (X-rays) and may not be an entirely safe diagnostic procedure. Thermography, a method of producing a thermal image of a surface, is based on the principle that the amount of radiation emitted is dependent on the temperature of the surface. The observation by Lawson, in 1956, that a carcinoma increases the temperature of the sur-

EUSTACE L. DERENIAK • Optical Sciences Center, University of Arizona, Tucson, Arizona 85721.

rounding anatomy resulted in the use of thermography as a clinically useful tool in the detection of malignancies. The considerable technical progress in infrared thermography can largely be attributed to the advances infrared detector technology (Leftwich, 1970). Since present systems are background radiation limited with quantum efficiency approaching 1, we probably have reached the limit of passive system capability in the intermediate infrared region. The present trend is toward automated computer image processing and the development of new concepts in original instrument design, i.e., differential thermography. These new techniques involve measuring the thermal patterns below the epidermis by using the near infrared or very far infrared ("Microwave Thermography," Cronin, 1977), where the skin becomes more transparent. A notable exception to the present application is of a military system called the FLIR (forward-looking infrared) system at the University of Oklahoma, for obtaining improved thermograms (Haberman, 1977). This system uses a multielement array of cryogenically cooled detectors, with very high resolution and sensitivity. The Sloan-Kettering Cancer Center uses a method where the temperature of the mammaries is compared to the forehead temperature.

The next section of this chapter (Present Thermographic Implementation) covers first the skin as a temperature regulator and describes some of the theoretical considerations of radiant power transfer. It then describes presently available thermographs and some of their figures of merits, and finally discusses some future instrumentation. The final section (Pattern Recognition Techniques) discusses techniques that are presently used in image processing, and which at this time requires a large computer.

12.2. PRESENT THERMOGRAPHIC IMPLEMENTATION

The most widely explored and clinically applied area of medical thermography is in the early detection of breast cancer (Freundlich, 1972; Wallace and Cade, 1974; Isard *et al.*, 1969; Isard, 1972). It has received much attention most recently due to the risks involved with xeroradiography and mammography. However, thermography can be used in many other anatomical regions where anomalous heating or cooling occurs. Examples of other medical applications are diabetes (Cronin, 1975), neurology, cardiovascular diseases (Winsor and Winsor, 1975), arthritis and pediatric orthopedics (Rosman, 1976; Farrell and O'Hara, 1972; Viitanen and Laaksonen, 1970).

Although thermography is completely safe and does not expose the patient to dangerous ionizing radiation, it has not been successful as an independent detector system of malignancies. Although it is well known that malignant tumors increase the temperature of the surrounding skin, the exact mechanism is not entirely understood. Malignancies are metabolically active and the veins which drain these tumors are warmer than normal. This increase in vein temperature can account for at least part of the increase in skin temperature.

Body heat is produced by a continuous metabolic process consisting of oxidation of carbohydrates and fats, which are the chief sources of energy (Haberman, 1971). Internal body temperatures represent the balance or equilibrium between the heat produced in the tissue and heat lost to the environment. A detailed account of this process is described by Benzinger and Kitzinger (1963), Burton (1941), and Winslow and Pierce (1941). The role of the skin is unquestioned as a significant organ of the body in the thermoregulatory process (Leider and Buncke, 1954; Hardy, 1939). Its outer surface is about 20 ft^2, or 1.9 m^2, and it comprises 6% of the total body weight. Table 12-1 gives some of the significant properties of skin (Stoll, 1960). The temperature of the skin and its spatial and temporal variations are determined by a number of different factors (Draper and Boag, 1971). First, it is subject to environmental processes such as radiation, conduction, convection, and evaporation. For a 22°C room temperature,

Table 12-1. Dimensions of Properties of Skin (Typical Man)

Parameter	Value
Dimension	
Weight	4 kg (8.8 lb)
Surface area	1.8 m^2 (20 ft^2)
Volume	3.6 liter (3.7 qt)
Water content	70–75%
Specific gravity	1.1
Thickness	0.5–5 mm (0.02–0.2 in.)
Property	
Heat production	240 (?) kg cal/day
Conductance	9–30 kg cal/m^2 hr °C
Thermal conductivity	$(1.5 \pm 0.3) \times 10^{-3}$ cal/cm sec °C at 23–25°C ambient
Diffusivity	7×10^{-4} cm^2/sec (surface layer 0.26 mm thick)
Thermal inertia	90 to 400 $\times 10^{-5}$ cal^2/cm^4 sec $°C^2$
Heat capacity	~0.8 cal/g
Emissivity (infrared)	~0.99
Reflectance (wavelength dependent)	Maximum 0.6–1.1 μm Minima <0.3 and >1.2 μm
Transmittance (wavelength dependent)	Maxima 1.2, 1.7, 2.2, 6, 11 μm Minima 0.5, 1.4, 1.9, 3, 7, 12 μm

these processes dissipate about 200 W for an average-sized person. Radiation accounts for 66% of the heat loss (Haberman, 1971; Hardy *et al.*, 1941). Second, there are physiological mechanisms of heat regulation such as constriction of the skin capillaries and sweat secretion. Third, there is conduction of heat from the body interior, through the fat and the dermal layers to the skin surface, and there is transportation of heat from inside the body by means of blood flow. These conditions are described in detail in the literature (Hardy *et al.*, 1941; Sheard *et al.*, 1941). A typical average temperature of the forehead is 34°C, while that of a thumb is around 28°C, and that of a big toe is around 25°C. These values hold for a room temperature of 20°C with uncovered skin exposed to the room temperature for at least 20 min (Wissler, 1963; Mali, 1969). Here the temperature of the breast skin of women is of greatest concern. The average temperature in this case is about 37°C, again for a room temperature of 20°C. Local variations in the conditions affecting the skin temperature, as described above, will result in deviations from this average temperature.

12.2.1. Description of the Radiation Aspects of Thermography

All objects above absolute zero temperature continuously emit and absorb radiation. The amount of energy an object radiates is dependent on its temperature, T, and emissivity, ε. The ratio of actual rate of energy emission to the rate of energy emission of an ideal blackbody at the same temperature is called emissivity. Stefan (1879) found that the total power emitted by a blackbody ($\varepsilon = 1$) is proportional to the fourth power of temperature; actual surfaces emit and absorb less than an ideal black surface.

The emissive power (emittance) of an arbitrary surface at temperature T is (Bramson, 1968)

$$M_e = \varepsilon \sigma_e T^4 \qquad (\text{W/cm}^2\ \text{sr}) \tag{12-1}$$

$$M_q = \varepsilon \sigma_q T^3 \qquad (\text{photon/sec cm}^2\ \text{sr}) \tag{12-2}$$

Max Planck (1901) developed a radiation law that shows how emitted radiation is spectrally distributed as a function of temperature:

$$L_e(\lambda, T)\, d\lambda = \frac{2c^2 h \lambda^{-5}}{e^{hc/k\lambda T} - 1}\, d\lambda \qquad (\text{W/cm}^2\ \text{sr}) \tag{12-3}$$

$$L_q(\lambda, T)\, d\lambda = \frac{2c\lambda^{-4}}{e^{hc/k\lambda T} - 1}\, d\lambda \qquad (\text{photons/sec cm}^2\ \text{sr}) \tag{12-4}$$

If the emissivity is known, then the radiance is a unique measure of the temperature.

One of the basic limitations in using radiance as a measure of the temperature of the emitting body is knowing the emissivity. The characteristics of the human body surface are extremely important to the accuracy of temperature measurement. Although skin appears to be nearly a blackbody in the infrared region, its emissivity is not unity. Studies (Elam *et al.*, 1963; Lloyd-Williams *et al.*, 1963; Watmough and Oliver, 1968a,b; Watmough and Oliver, 1969a,b,c; Patil and Lloyd-Williams, 1969; Steketee, 1973) have indicated that skin emissivity is about 0.95–0.99 in the 3–14-μm spectral region. There is a disturbing amount of disagreement among investigators. For example, Patil and Lloyd-Williams (1969) reported an apparent emissivity greater than 1. While it is desirable and also technically feasible to determine a temperature difference as low as 0.1°K, uncertainties in the emissivity of the human skin usually limit the accuracy to about 0.8°K. Possible variations in emissivity from one area to another and variations due to viewing angle are not thoroughly understood and should be considered before final exact temperature conclusions are made (Lewis *et al.*, 1973; Watmough and Oliver, 1970; Watmough and Oliver, 1969b; Irwin *et al.*, 1973). Otherwise, image structure in a thermogram due to spatial emissivity variations may be ascribed erroneously to temperature variations.

Reflection is another factor that must be considered when the emissivity is less than unity. From Kirchhoff's law, the reflectivity ρ is given by

$$\rho = 1 - \varepsilon \tag{12-5}$$

Therefore a body can reflect a detectable amount of energy from its environment. Reflections of this type normally have an energy peak at wavelengths less than 4 or 5 μm, which makes systems that operate in the 8–14 μm region insensitive to these influences.

A thermographic apparatus reacts to the radiation emitted by the body itself, thus no special radiation source is necessary. Thermography must, therefore, clearly be distinguished from those methods in which one uses auxiliary infrared sources and detects the radiation reflected by the object (e.g., infrared photography, infrared image converters, sniperscopes, etc.) except in the special case of differential thermography.

The heart of the installation is the detector, normally a photodetector. The detector is responsible for the conversion of the incident radiation into an electrical signal, which can be amplified millions of times. The thermal radiation is focused onto the detector using a mirror system having a large aperture. A picture of a part of the body is obtained by means of a mechanical scanning system which collects radiation from the object—point after point and line after line in rapid succession to form a raster. The electrical signal originating from the detector is, after amplification, used to feed the display unit. The point by point construction of the thermal image must be synchronous with the scanning of the patient. All modern systems use a display tube for representing the thermal picture, which can then also be made a permanent record on film.

The pictorial representation of the radiance pattern formed by the thermographic device is interpreted as a temperature pattern. It is a measure of the change in temperature from point to point on the object.

Since present thermographic systems measure a change in temperature, a comparison between systems can be made in determining how small a temperature difference can be detected by a system.

Assuming that the body can be approximated by a graybody, the radiant excitance (M_e) can be expressed as a function of temperature (T) and emissivity ε_e as shown in Eq. (12-1). The change in excitance with respect to temperature can be found by differentiating Eq. (12-1):

$$dM_e = 4\sigma_e T^3 dT \tag{12-6}$$

The change in radiant intensity (dI_e) with temperature can be expressed as

$$dI_e = \frac{4\sigma_e T^3 A_o}{\pi} dT \tag{12-7}$$

where A_o is the area of the object. Here we are assuming the object to be a Lambertian radiator. The amount of power change ($d\Phi_e$) collected by the optical system at its entrance pupil can be given by

$$d\Phi_e = \frac{4\sigma_e T^3 A_o \Omega_o \tau_a \, dT}{\pi} \tag{12-8}$$

where Ω_o is the solid angle subtended by the optical system entrance pupil at the object and τ_a is the atmospheric transmission between object and entrance pupil.

The change in flux at the focal plane (detector) of the optical system is simply $d\Phi_e$ times the transmission of the optical system (τ_o):

$$d\Phi_e = \frac{4\sigma_e T^3 A_o \Omega_o \tau_a \tau_o \, dT}{\pi} \tag{12-9}$$

The detector performance parameter NEP (noise equivalent power) is the signal radiant power sufficient to produce an rms signal-to-noise ratio of 1. Assuming that the system is detector-noise limited, the expression for NEP is

$$\text{NEP} = \frac{(A_d \Delta f)^{1/2}}{D^*(T, f)} \tag{12-10}$$

where A_d is the detector area, Δf is the effective noise-equivalent bandwidth, D^* (T, f) is the blackbody D^*. By equating Eqs. (12-9) and (12-10) and solving for dT one finds the detectable change in temperature for an infrared system (thermograph):

$$dT = \frac{(A_d \Delta f)^{1/2}}{D^*(T, f)} \frac{\pi}{4\sigma_e T^3 A_o \Omega_o \tau_a \tau_o} \tag{12-11}$$

From a system design point of view there are several parameters in (12-11) which we can investigate to maximize performance: $D^*(T, f)$ is one example, but it is specified by choosing the best available detectors and nothing more can be done with it. The parameters which can be manipulated are Δf, A_d, $A_o\Omega_o$, and A_o.

The electrical bandwidth Δf is the noise bandwidth of the system and is related to the 3-dB electrical bandwidth (Δf_e) by $\pi/2$ for a single-pole filter (Ott, 1976), i.e.,

$$\Delta f = \frac{\pi}{2} \Delta f_e \tag{12-12}$$

It determines the amount of information which can be transmitted through an electrical system. Consider the infrared thermogram, which is made up of a side by side series of contiguous scan lines which comprise a scan frame, a single picture. The temporal length of any resolution element is the reciprocal of twice the electric bandwidth ($\Delta f_e = 1/2t_d$). This time is called dwell time, t_d, and is the time exposure from a single resolution element of the thermogram. It also is the time required for the scanning mechanism to stay on a resolution element in order to transmit the information contained within this resolution element. If one assumes that a single scan line is made up of a linear sequence of N_R resolution elements, then the amount of time, t, to scan one line is $N_R t_d = t_1$. The picture time (frame time) would then be the number of lines which make up the picture (N_F) times the single-line time (t_1).

Since optical scanning system must have line-to-line time losses due to the geometry of scanning, a scan efficiency factor must be introduced. The scanning efficiency, η_s, is the ratio of useful scan time in a frame to the total frame time (t_f), i.e.,

$$\eta_s = \frac{N_R N_F t_d}{t_f} \tag{12-13}$$

therefore

$$\eta_s t_f = N_F N_R \frac{\pi}{4\Delta f} \tag{12-14}$$

solving for noise bandwidth

$$\Delta f = \frac{\pi N_F N_R}{4\eta_s t_f} \tag{12-15}$$

Before substituting this expression into Eq. (12-11), the optical magnification for the system can be found to be related to the detector area and the resolution element size by (Jenkins and White, 1957)

$$m = \left(\frac{A_d}{A_o}\right)^{1/2} \tag{12-16}$$

Then from Eq. (12-11),

$$dT = \frac{(\pi N_F N_R)^{1/2}}{D^*(T, f)\, 2(\eta_s t_f)^{1/2}} \frac{m\pi}{4\sigma_e T^3 (A_o)^{1/2}\, \tau_a \tau_o \Omega_o} \tag{12-17}$$

$$dT = \frac{\pi^{3/2}}{8\sigma_e}\left(\frac{N_F N_R}{\eta_s t A_o}\right)^{1/2} \frac{m}{D^*(T, f)\, T^3 \tau_a \tau_o \Omega_o} \tag{12-18}$$

The differential temperature dT under these conditions is interpreted to be the noise-equivalent temperature difference (NETD). In order to have a system which detects small temperature differences the number of resolution elements ($N_F N_R$) can be reduced but this causes a loss in spatial resolution or a change (increase in the area of the object, A_o), and a decrease in m.

The above analysis was for the case where the detector responds to all spectral regions equally, i.e., a bolometer. For the other extreme case, one can solve for a NETD on a monochromatic basis where simply a photodetector and spectral filter would be applicable.

In the spectral-dependent case, the object under consideration is a blackbody radiator with a spectral photon radiance from Eq. (12-4) and emissivity ε, so that

$$L_q(\lambda, T)\, d\lambda = \frac{2c\varepsilon}{\lambda^4[\exp(hc/k\lambda T) - 1]}\, d\lambda \tag{12-19}$$

The change in the object's radiance with respect to temperature can be found by differentiating Eq. (12-19) with respect to temperature:

$$dL_q(\lambda, T)\, d\lambda = \frac{2c^2 h}{kT^2}\frac{1}{\lambda^5}\frac{e^x}{(e^x - 1)^2}\, d\lambda\, dT \tag{12-20}$$

where $x = hc/kT$. The corresponding change in photon flux, $d\phi_q$, at the entrance pupil of the instrument is

$$d\phi_q d\lambda = dL_q(\lambda, T)\, d\lambda A_o \Omega_o \tau_a \tag{12-21}$$

where A_o is the emitting area of the object, Ω_o is the solid angle subtended by the entrance pupil at the source, and τ_a is the atmospheric transmission.

The change in photon flux at the focal plane of the optical system (detector's sensitive surface) is determined by multiplying Eq. (12-21) by the optical transmission τ_o and hc/λ since further analysis requires the change to be in terms of radiant power:

$$d\Phi_e d\lambda = \frac{2\varepsilon c^3 h^2}{kT^2} \frac{1}{\lambda^6} \frac{e^x}{(e^x - 1)^2} A_o \Omega_o \tau_a \tau_o \, dT \, d\lambda \tag{12-22}$$

If this change of radiant power incident on the detector is sufficient to produce a signal change equal to the noise, this radiant power change can be called the noise-equivalent power (NEP) of the detector.

The NEP can be expressed as

$$\text{NEP} = \frac{(A_d \Delta f)^{1/2}}{D^*(T, f)} \tag{12-23}$$

where A_d is the detector area and Δf the system noise bandwidth. Then

$$dT = \frac{kT^2}{2\varepsilon c^3 h^2} \frac{(A_d \Delta f)^{1/2}}{A \tau_a \tau_o D^*} \frac{\lambda^6 (e^x - 1)^2}{e^x (d\lambda)} \tag{12-24}$$

This equation for NETD is in terms of spectral power. In order to determine the NETD, an integration must be performed over each spectral region of interest (i.e., λ_1 to λ_2).

The system electrical bandwidth is determined by scan efficiency, number of lines per frame, and the number of resolution elements per line, as in the previous case.

Substituting into Eq. (12-24) similar to the wide spectral region case yields the NETD expression as a function of wavelength:

$$\text{NETD} = \frac{kT^2}{2\varepsilon c^3 h^2} \frac{m^2}{(A_d)^{1/2} \tau_a \tau_o D^*(T, f)\, \Omega} \left(\frac{\pi N_R N_f}{4 \eta_s t_f} \right)^{1/2} \frac{\lambda^6 (e^x - 1)^2}{e^x d\lambda} \tag{12-25}$$

For both thc total-spectrum case or the monochromatic case the NETD is dependent on frame time and number of resolution elements as indicated by Eqs. (12-18) and (12-25). The longer the frame time and/or the fewer the picture elements, the better the NETD.

12.2.2. Equipment Description

Most presently available commercial thermographs consist of two units, the camera and the recording/display units. The camera consists of the optical subsystems, optomechanical scanner, electronic drives, position sensor pick-offs, and detector/preamplifier assembly (Atsumi, 1973). The recording/display unit is the control panel and includes the power on/off, focusing, signal processing electronics, CRT display, and a photographic means of recording image and patient identification. Figure 12-1 shows the basic components in block diagram form.

The scanning of the object (patient) is a series of contiguous scans similar to a TV raster scan, which forms the image in a line-to-line sequence. The scanning is accomplished by optical elements (normally mirrors) which move in orthogonal directions (two perpendicular axes) to sweep out a raster. In the case of the thermography manufactured by Texas Medical Inc., scanning is accomplished by means of a rapidly rotating multifaceted mirror whose axis of rotation is slowly moved by means of cams to produce a raster pattern.

The optical systems are normally reflective in order to eliminate the material selection problems associated with transmission in the infrared spectrum. These systems are diffraction limited and can focus from about 1 m to infinity.

The heart of the system is the infrared detector, which converts the radiant signal to an electrical output. The present commercial thermographs use either indium antimonide (InSb) or mercury cadmium telluride (HgCdTe) detectors (Hudson, 1968; Wolfe, 1965). The InSb responds to infrared radiation out to 5 μm, whereas the HgCdTe responds to 10 μm. These detectors are used because the scanning speed and frame time requirements force one to have electrically fast (large electrical bandwidth) detectors. The choice of optimum spectral region has long been discussed and analyzed as to which produces better imagery (Leftwich, 1970; Burrer *et al.*, 1975; Bastuscheck, 1970). The 5-μm spectral region is more susceptible

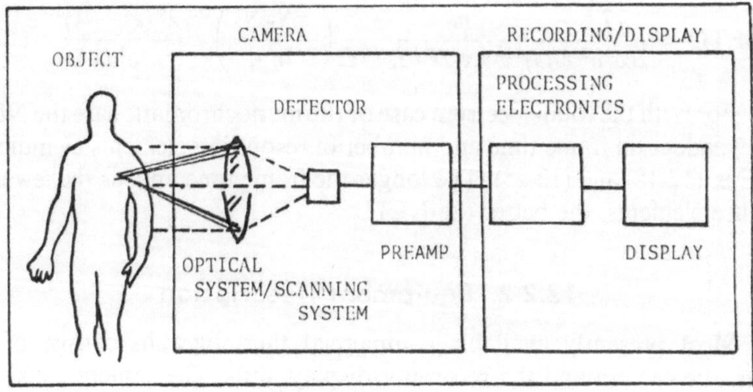

Fig. 12-1. Basic components of a thermograph.

Table 12-2. Performance of Various Thermographic Systems

	Desirable	Thermovision[a]	Model 900[c]	Thermiscope[d]	Model 525[e]	Pyroelectric vidicon[g]	DCATS[h]
Detector		InSb[b]	HgCdTe	HgCdTe	HgCdTe[f]	Triglycine sulfate	HgCdTe
Spectral region		2–5.6 μm	2–14 μm	8–12 μm	8–14 μm	2.2–32 μm (KRS-5)	1–14 μm
Detector temperature		77 K	77 K	77 K	77 K	300 K	77 K
NETD	0.1 K	0.1 K	0.2 K	0.05 K	0.2 K	0.15 K (3 lp/mm)	0.025 K
Resolution							
1. res/line		100 res/line Polaroid/35 mm	512 res/line		150 res/line	252 res/line	256 res/line
2. Instantaneous field of view	1.7 mrad	2.5 mrad	—	0.75 mrad	2 mrad	Not applicable	1 mrad
3. On object	1 mm	Optic dependent	0.25 mm	0.75 mm	0.6 mm	Optic dependent but 8 lines/mm	0.55 mm
Total field of view		40 × 40	30 × 30	33 × 33	14 × 18	18 mm diameter	20 × 20
Optics		Refractive		Reflective		Refractive	
Frametime	1 sec	1/25 sec	1.6/2.0 sec	4.5 sec	1/30 sec	1/30 sec	4 sec
Display	Standard TV hard copy	High-persistance phosphor	Memory storage/ 525 lines; standard TV, Polaroid	High-persistance phosphor; 525 lines Polaroid	Monitor Polaroid	CRT standard TV broadcast	CRT printer
Cost	$ 10,000	$ 40,000	$ 43,000–87,000	$ 45,000	$ 27,500	$ 15,000	$ 125,000

[a] AGA Corporation, 550 County Ave., Secaucaus, N.J. 07094.
[b] Dual systems of HgCdTe and InSb are available at $ 65,000.
[c] UTI, PO Box 519, 325 N. Mathilda, Sunnyvale, CA 94086.
[d] UNICO, 12108 Radium, San Antonia, TX 78216.
[e] Inframetrics, 225 Crescent St., Watham, MA 02154.
[f] Dual systems of HgCdTe and InSb are available at $ 51,000.
[g] ISI Group, 9617 Acoma SE, Albuquerque, NM 87123.
[h] Dorex, Inc., 968 Elm St., Orange, CA 92667.

to temperature contrast changes ($\partial Ep/\partial T$), whereas the 10-μm region has the most energy associated with a 310°K blackbody (human body temperature). Neither system has proven to be superior from a clinical point of view. Both of these detectors require liquid nitrogen cooling (77°K). This adds to the complexity of the system because a Dewar is required to hold the detector/cryogenic liquid (Lloyd-Williams *et al.*, 1963).

A comparison of thermographs is shown in Table 12-2 (Heerma Van Voss, 1969). The NETD sensitivity for these systems is much less than required for clinical application, varying from 0.07 to 0.2°C. As discussed earlier [Eq. (12-18)], the frame time, total number of picture elements, and NETD are interrelated: for longer frame times, the NETD is lower and vice versa. Similarly for fewer picture elements, the NETD is better (lower).

The Inframetrics system works either in the 5-μm region or the 10-μm region by directing the beam either to an InSb detector or a HgCdTe detector. However, the pictures produced in either spectral region are not sufficiently different to make a choice as to optimum spectral region for thermography.

12.2.3. New Instruments

The University of Oklahoma has recently developed a high-resolution thermographic camera modeled after the military's FLIR system (Haberman, 1977). This system has very high thermal sensitivity (NETD, 0.01°C) with standard television frame rates (30/sec), which is accomplished by the use of a multielement detector array. The thermal image is digitized, averaged over several frames, and recorded. The image is then analyzed in a minicomputer and processed using various pattern recognition techniques. The picture also has the advantage of providing quantitative temperature measurements.

The University of Arizona is developing a new method of thermography, differential-ratio temperature thermography (Roehrig *et al.*, 1974; Dereniak and Wolfe, 1970).

The technique applied most commonly today in medical thermography utilizes thermal radiation emitted by the human skin. According to the Stefan–Boltzmann law and the Planck radiation law as stated earlier, the radiance of the skin is a function of the emissivity ε of the skin and its temperature T. As the detector of the thermograph scans across the human body it is exposed sequentially to different radiating elements of the body, each one considered to be of uniform temperature and emissivity. First, the system views a radiating element of temperature T_1 and emissivity ε_1. A short time later it views another element, with temperature T_2 and emissivity ε_2. The differences are ΔT and $\Delta\varepsilon$, which we will assume to be small enough that they can be written dT and $d\varepsilon$. The difference in the radiances of these elements M_q is then from Eq. (12-2):

$$dM_q = 3\varepsilon\sigma_q T^2 dT + \sigma_q T^3 d\varepsilon \tag{12-26}$$

$$dM_q/M_q = 3(dT/T) + d\varepsilon/\varepsilon \tag{12-27}$$

This describes the case for a wide-band detector receiving all the radiation in the spectrum, where the Stefan–Boltzmann law applies. Note that the relative irradiance change is due to a change in temperature and emissivity, unlike Eq. (12-6).

For the case of a narrow-band, or monochromatic, detector, where Planck's law applies, from Eq. (12-4), the relative change in irradiance is

$$dM_q(\lambda, T) = \frac{\varepsilon 2c\pi\lambda^{-4}}{(e^{hc/k\lambda T} - 1)^2} e^{hc/k\lambda T} \frac{hc}{k\lambda T^2} + \frac{2c\pi\lambda^{-4}}{e^{hc/k\lambda T} - 1} d\varepsilon \tag{12-28}$$

and

$$\frac{dM_q(\lambda, T)}{M_q(\lambda, T)} = \frac{e^{hc/k\lambda T}}{e^{hc/k\lambda T} - 1} \frac{hc}{k\lambda T} \frac{dT}{T} + \frac{d\varepsilon}{\varepsilon} \tag{12-29}$$

Some mathematical manipulation gives the case of the narrow-band

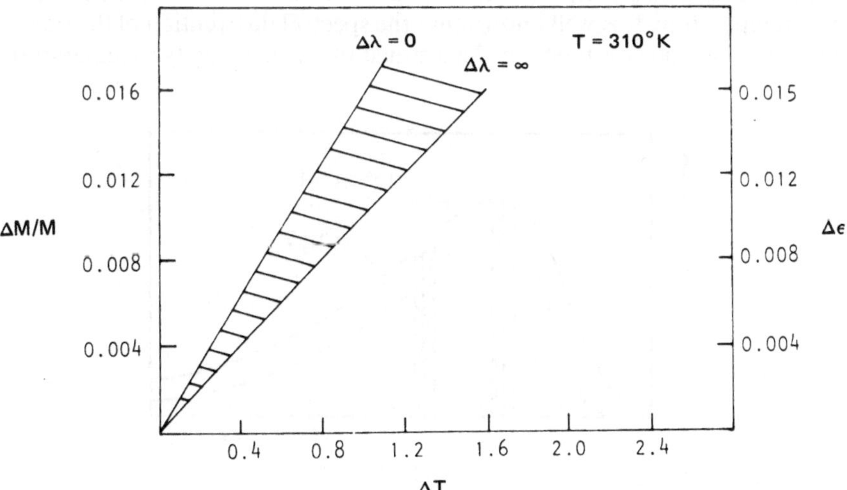

Fig. 12-2. Contrast change vs. relative emissivity and temperature change for monochromatic and total radiation. (From Dereniak, 1976, reproduced with permission from SPIE.)

detector at maximum contrast:

$$\frac{dM_q(\lambda, T)}{M_q(\lambda, T)} = 5\frac{dT}{T} + \frac{d\varepsilon}{\varepsilon} \tag{12-30}$$

Figure 12-2 plots the relative change in irradiance for the two cases.

For a narrow-band detector, for example, a radiance difference dM/M of 0.010 (dashed line) could be due to a $d\varepsilon$ of 0.010 or a dT of 0.6°K (dotted lines), or to some combination of the two.

When a physician interprets the thermograph, he assumes that irradiance changes are due to temperature alone and that the emissivity change from one element to the next is zero ($d\varepsilon = 0$). The signal would then be directly proportional to the temperature difference (dT). However, in reality the emissivity is not constant or is known to only about 1% accuracy. There is sufficient literature to indicate that the emissivity change is on the order of 1% (Steketee, 1973). From the equation one can see that a 1% change in emissivity causes a difference of 0.6°K in the monochromatic case and 1°K in the wide-band case. A temperature difference of 1°K is considered critical by the physician.

12.3. RATIO TEMPERATURE THERMOGRAPHY

A solution to the emissivity problem is ratio temperature thermography, a principle that actually is not new and is widely applied in illumination engineering. This principle relates the spectral distribution of the radiation to a temperature. It is well known that the spectral distribution of the radiation of a blackbody is uniquely determined by the blackbody's temperature

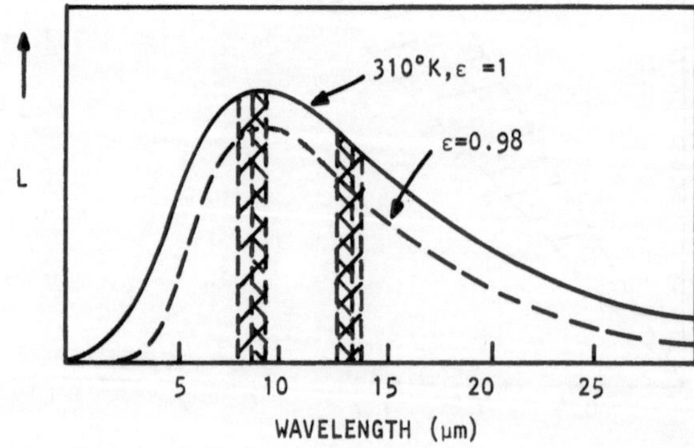

Fig. 12-3. Principle of ratio temperature measurement for graybodies of different emissivity. Note that the ratio of radiance values at λ_1 vs. λ_2 is the same for a body of $\varepsilon = 1$ as for a body of $\varepsilon = 0.98$.

—this is Planck's law. It applies not only for a blackbody but also for a graybody (one that has an emissivity smaller than 1 but that is, however, a constant with respect to wavelength). The spectral distribution can be determined by measuring the radiance at two different wavelengths. Figure 12-3 shows the emission spectra of two 310°K graybodies with emissivities of 1 and 0.98, respectively.

In normal thermography, the detector measures the area under each curve, let us say in the 8–14 μm region. As the detector scans from an element with $\varepsilon = 1$ to one with $\varepsilon = 0.98$, it displays as the signal the difference in radiance.

In ratio thermography, the detector would sample the radiance of any element at two points in the spectrum, say, 9 and 13 μm as indicated in Fig. 12-3, and obtain the ratio of these two values. Mathematically the system output is

$$\frac{E(T, \lambda_1)}{E(T, \lambda_2)} = \frac{\varepsilon_1 c_1 \lambda_1^{-4}[\exp(c_2/\lambda_1 T) - 1]^{-1}}{\varepsilon_2 c_1 \lambda_2^{-4}[\exp(c_2/\lambda_2 T) - 1]^{-1}} \tag{12-31}$$

$$= \frac{c_1 \lambda_2^4[\exp(c_2/\lambda_2 T_c) - 1]}{c_1 \lambda_1^4[\exp(c_2/\lambda_1 T_c) - 1]} \tag{12-32}$$

Solving for ratio temperature,

$$\frac{1}{T_c} = \frac{1}{T} - \frac{\lambda_1 \lambda_2}{c_2(\lambda_2 - \lambda_1)} \ln \frac{\varepsilon_1}{\varepsilon_2} \tag{12-33}$$

The change in ratio temperature is

$$dT_c = \frac{T_c^2}{T^2} dT + \frac{\lambda_1 \lambda_2 T_c^2}{c_2(\lambda_1 - \lambda_2)} \left(\frac{d\varepsilon_1}{\varepsilon_1} - \frac{d\varepsilon_2}{\varepsilon_2} \right) \tag{12-34}$$

It is evident that the ratio of the two radiance values is proportional to the temperature. For the case where the emissivity is constant with respect to wavelength, the ratio is independent of the emissivity, and the temperature measured is the true temperature of the emitter.

If the emissivity is not constant with respect to wavelength, then the temperature determined from the ratio is different from the true temperature and is called the ratio temperature.

The ratio temperature method eliminates the effect of emissivity provided there is a strong correlation between emissivities at wavelengths λ_1 and λ_2. We have found that the correlation need be only 0.366 in order for the ratio temperature measurement to be as good as the present brightness temperature measurement, which measures the radiance at a single wavelength region.

The details of the required emissivity correlation between wavelength regions and an error analysis of ratio temperature thermography is discussed in Chapter 13.

12.4. PATTERN RECOGNITION TECHNIQUES

To eliminate the subjectiveness of thermographic diagnosis and interpretation, computer image processing is beginning to be implemented (Hall *et al.*, 1971; Levine, 1969; Ziskin *et al.*, 1975; Anliker and Friedli, 1976). This technique may relieve trained personnel of the necessity for reading thermograms. However, the physicians' diagnostic capabilities cannot be met with present computer programs. The role of the computer in thermography is to assist the physicians for selected problems where the overwhelming number of thermograms need interpretation. The thermal pattern is either fed directly into a computer via A/D converters or the thermogram is scanned with a microdensitometer and the picture is digitized and computer processed.

The thermogram lends itself to computer processing because its analysis is almost completely dependent on asymmetrical pattern recognition or the "edge sign" (Isard, 1972). The picture production and analysis can best be described in terms of a block diagram such as the one shown in Fig. 12-4. The picture acquisition, data processing, and diagnosis can be divided into three phases: (1) preprocessing, (2) analysis, and (3) diagnosis.

12.4.1. Preprocessing

The preprocessing phase as shown in Fig. 12-4 consists of thermogram acquisition, dividing the picture into an array of picture elements which can be stored digitally, as well as geometrical scaling and gray level setting. In the analysis phase which is done in the computer via command inputs from the operator, the thermogram is analyzed by subroutines which look at pattern asymmetry. The diagnosis is simply the computer's finding based on the pattern asymmetry criterion.

In the preprocessing phase the thermal pattern is taken of the patient,

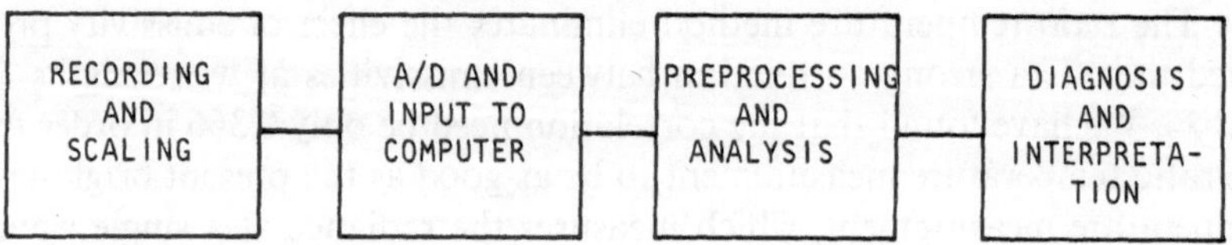

Fig. 12-4. Block diagram of automatic thermograph interpretation.

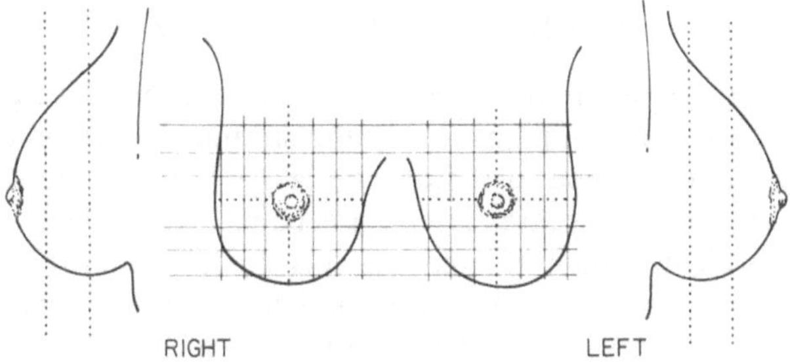

Fig. 12-5. Checkerboard pattern used to subdivide thermograph.

digitized, and computer stored. The thermogram is then divided in half by finding the geometrical center between the nipples of the breast. The nipple is normally used as the center of the matrix or grid which divides each side of the thermogram into a group of picture elements as shown in Fig. 12-5. In this fashion each area of the breast can be assigned a matrix element location. Other housekeeping and auxiliary tasks done in the preprocessing are size scaling, mean gray level setting, and background suppression.

12.4.2. Analysis

The criterion for the evaluation of thermograms as stated earlier was asymmetrical heat patterns. However, there are many variations to this criteria. The absolute temperature is not as important as relative variations (Dodd *et al.*, 1969). The evaluation for cancer detection can be based on one of the following criteria (Winter and Stein, 1973): (1) temperature asymmetry between corresponding regions of each breast, (2) asymmetrical venous patterns, (3) hot spots, (4) local areolar heat, or (5) unilateral elevation of temperature.

Since all can be detected by asymmetrical pattern recognition techniques the analysis in the computer is rather straightforward. This asymmetry can be analyzed on a single picture element by picture element comparison or by groups of picture elements which would cover a region of interest.

The above criteria are partially implemented into the computer diagnosis by the following methods:

(1) geometrical mean vs. thermal mean,
(2) spatial signature analysis,
(3) density distribution,
(4) contour coding, and
(5) Walsh function analysis.

12.4.2.1. Geometrical Mean vs. Thermal Mean

Once the thermogram has been scaled, the location of the geometrical mean, that is, the locus of points along the sternum which produces symmetry, is determined. Then each scan line of the thermogram is evaluated for temperature variations (gray level) for each picture element. The picture elements are weighted and a thermal mean is also determined. The thermal mean may and often does not correspond to the geometrical mean. In addition to this mean value, the variance is also calculated. The mean and variance of the thermal pattern center and compared to the geometrical mean for a diagnosis. This technique requires norms for a baseline analysis to be written into the computer program.

12.4.2.2. Spatial Signature Analysis

Another method of measuring the asymmetry is the use of spatial signature analysis (Hall *et al.*, 1971). As before, the picture is made up of a matrix of picture elements. This analysis consists of summing all the temperature picture elements in each row or column of the picture matrix and plotting the sum either horizontally or vertically. Each point represents a projection of the temperature distribution in two orthogonal directions. The horizontal signature will always show greater symmetry since the sternum will be less vascular than the breasts. The vertical signature, however, gives an asymmetry associated with the cancerous lesion.

12.4.2.3. Density Distribution

This analysis plots a probability density function of the thermal pattern. The plot consists of the number of picture elements which are at a given temperature in the thermogram vs. the temperature (histogram). A variation of this technique is to plot a histogram of each breast individually and compare them. This analysis is important when there is a unilateral temperature increase; however, it discards much of the spatial data.

12.4.2.4. Isothermal Coding

This concept is based on the idea of topography. In this case the areas of equal temperature have been connecting in a series of points of constant brightness producing a contour pattern (Habibi, 1977, and Robinson, 1974; Graham, 1967). Each contour which is formed is a closed loop. This closed contour, called an isotherm, can be analyzed for hot spots and/or asymmetry. By varying the temperature at which the contour is plotted, the areas of highest temperature can be determined rather accurately.

12.4.2.5. Walsh/Hadamard Coding Analysis

The technique of breaking a picture into a set of orthogonal functions has been performed for many years. Due to computational difficulties a new way of analyzing a picture was developed from binary theory where the computation is simply the summing of "ones" or "zeros" to produce a picture. An arbitrary temperature threshold is assigned a value of zero. The total number of ones for a portion of the thermogram representing the right breast is then compared with the total number of ones from a comparable area on the thermogram representing the left breast. In addition, a digitized temperature profile for a single scan line over the right breast is compared with the profile along that same scan line over the left breast. In this analysis the number of ones for each field size is compared for each breast, then the histograms of each breast are compared.

This review of computer analysis of thermographic images is not at all complete and the reader is referred to more extensive discussion and analysis in the text by Andrews and Hunt (1977) and the bibliography by Pratt (1973).

NOTATION

A	Area
A_d	Detector area
A_o	Collector (optic) area
A_s	Area of object
A_x	Area of electrodes
c	Speed of light: 3×10^{10} cm/sec
c_1	$2\pi hc^2$ radiation constant
c_2	hc/k radiation constant
d	Central lens thickness
d	Detector thickness
d	Length of the line joining dA_1 and dA_2
D	Optics diameter
D^*	D "star"—detectivity
D^*_{BLIP}	Background-limited infrared photodetector
D^*_m	D star maximum
D_n	Diffusion constant
$D^*(T, f)$	Blackbody D^* (detectivity)
e	Charge of the electron
E_e	Irradiance (W/cm^2)
E_q	Photon irradiance (photon/sec cm^2)
$E(T, \lambda_1)$	Measured irradiance at λ_1.
$E(T, \lambda_2)$	Measured irradiance at λ_2.
f	Focal length of the optical system
F	Speed or focal ratio of the final optics $F = f/D$
h	Planck's constant
I	Current
I_B	Bias current
I_b	Background current
I_d	Dark current
ifov	Instantaneous field of view
k	Boltzmann's constant: 1.38×10^{-23} J/°K
l	interelectrode spacing
L	Radiance
L_λ^{BB}	Spectral radiance of a blackbody
$L_{q\lambda}^{BB}$	Blackbody photon spectral sterance
$L_e(\lambda, T)$	Radiance (W/cm^2 sr)
$L_q(\lambda, T)$	Photon radiance (photon/sec cm^2 sr) (photon/sec cm^2 sr)
L_{qB}	Photon radiance—background
L_{qs}	Photon radiance—source
L_n	Diffusion length
m	Optical magnification
M_{BB}	Background exitance
M_e	Exitance (W/cm^2)
M_q	Photon exitance (photon/sec cm^2)

n	Density of electrons
n	Refractive index
N	Number of carriers
N	Number of resolution elements
n_b, p_b	Background-generated carrier
N_F	Number of lines in a frame
N_R	Number of resolution elements in a line
n_0, p_0	Equilibrium carrier concentration
NETD	Noise-equivalent temperature difference
P	Density of holes
P_d	Power (watts)
P	Charge of the hole
q	Phase differences
R	Voltage responsivity
R	Resistor
R_L	Load resistor
R_d	Detector resistance
r	Correlation coefficient
r_1	Radius of curvature of first surface
r_2	Radius of curvature of second surface
r_d	Aspect ratio of the detector
r_f	Aspect ratio of the frame
SNR	rms signal voltage or current divided by the rms noise voltage
t	Time constant
t_f	Frame time
t_1	Line time
t_l	Carrier lifetime
T	Kinetic temperature of object
T_c	Ratio temperature of object
t_d	Dwell time
T_s	Scene temperature
T_l	Lens temperature
V	Voltage
v	Velocity
V_B	Bias voltage
V_d	Signal voltage
v_J	Johnson noise
x	$hc/k\lambda T$
x	Distance
z	Object distance
z'	Image distance
α	Prism angle
γ	Correlation coefficient
δ	Deviation angle
Δf	3-dB electrical bandwidth
Δf_e	Effective noise bandwidth
ΔN	Change in number of carriers
$\Delta\theta$	Instantaneous field of view or the size of a detector divided by the focal length
ε	Emissivity
$\varepsilon_1, \varepsilon_2$	Emissivity in wavelength regions 1 and 2
μ	Mobility
η	Detector quantum efficiency
η_{cs}	Efficiency of cold shielding
η_e	Efficiency of the electronics
η_{ab}	Loss in flux due to optical factors
η_s	Scan efficiency
θ	Angular field scanned
λ	Wavelength
ρ	Resistivity $(1/\sigma)$
ρ	Reflectivity
σ	Conductivity
σ_d	Dark conductivity
σ_e	Stefan–Boltzmann's constant: 5.6697×10^{-12} W/°K^4 cm^2
σ_q	Stefan–Boltzmann's constant: 1.5202×10^{11} photons/cm^2 sec° K^3
τ	Carrier lifetime
τ_a	Atmospheric transmission
τ_o	Optical transmission
$\Phi_{e'}$	Radiant power
ϕ_q	Radiant photons
ϕ_1	Angle between the line joining dA_1 to dA_2 and the normal to dA_2
ϕ_2	Angle between the line joining dA_2 to dA_1, and the normal to dA_2
Ω_B	Solid angle of background
Ω_0	Solid angle entrance pupil subtends from source
Ω	Solid angle of the total field of view
ω	Solid angle of one field of view
ω	$2\pi f = 2\pi/t$

Superscripts

a	Atmosphere
B	Background
c	Relates to ratio temperature
d	Relates to detector
e	Relates to electrons
e	Power sterance
l	Relates to lens
h	Relates to holes

o	Optics
p	Relates to holes
p	Photoelectrons
q	Photon sterance
s	Object or scene
t	Total
T	Temperature
1	Related to area (1)
2	Related to area (2)
ε	Emissivity
λ	Spectral response

Subscripts

BB	Blackbody
B	Background

REFERENCES

Andrews, H.C., and Hunt, B.R. (1977), *Digital Image Restoration*, Prentice-Hall Inc., Englewood Cliffs, New Jersey.

Anliker, M., and Friedli, P. (1976), Evaluation of high-resolution thermograms by on-line digital mapping and color coding, *Appl. Radiol.* **5**(3): 114.

Atsumi, K. (ed.) (1973), *Medical Thermography*, University of Tokyo Press, Tokyo.

Bastuscheck, C.P. (1970), Ground temperature and thermal infrared, *Photogramm. Eng.* **XXXVI**: 1064.

Benzinger, T.H., and Kitzinger, C. (1963), The human thermostat, *Temperature, Vol. 3*, Reinhold, New York.

Bramson, M.A. (1968), *Infrared Radiation*, Plenum Press, New York.

Burrer, G.J., Stetson, N.B., and Terrell, M.C. (1975), *Fast Scan Infrared Imaging Devices*, SPIE Seminar Proc., Vol. 62, Mod. Util. of IR Tech., Aug. 19, p. 22.

Burton, A.C. (1941), The operating characteristics of the human thermoregulatory mechanism, *Temperature, Vol. 1*, Reinhold, New York.

Cronin, M.P. (1975), Thermography in the diabetic clinic, *Appl. Radiol.* **4**(4): 31.

Cronin, M.P. (1977), Microwave thermography, *Appl. Radiol.* **6** (3): 139.

Dereniak, E.L. (1976), Preliminary results of ratio temperature thermography, SPIE Proc., Vol. 78, Low Light Level Devices, March 22, p. 126.

Dereniak, E.L., and Wolfe, W.L. (1970), A comparison of the theoretical operations of high impedance and low detectors, *Appl. Opt.* **9**: 2441.

Dodd, G.D., Wallace, J.D., Freundlich, I.M., March, L., and Zermino, A. (1969), Thermography and cancer of the breast, *Cancer* **23**: 797–802.

Draper, J.W., and Boag, J.W. (1971), The calculation of skin temperature distributions in thermography, *Phys. Med. Biol.* **16** (2): 201–211.

Elam, R., Goodwin, D.N., and Lloyd-Williams, K. (1963), Optical properties of the human epidermis, *Nature* **198**: 1001.

Farrell, C., and O'Hara, E. (1972), The use of thermography in the pediatric patient, *Clin. Pediatr.* **II**: 673.

Freundlich, I.M. (1972), Thermography, *New Eng. J. Med.* **287**: 880.

Graham, D.M. (1967), Image transmission by two-dimensional contour coding, *Proc. IEEE* **55** (3): 336.

Habibi, A. (1977), Survey of adaptive image coding technique, *IEEE Trans. Comm.* **25** (11): 1275.

Haberman, J.D. (1971), Image analysis of medical thermograms, *Crit. Rev. Radiol. Sci.* **2**: 427.

Haberman, J.D. (1977), Thermography: A primary consideration in noninvasive testing, in *Breast Carcinoma* (W.W. Logan, ed.). Wiley, New York, p. 265.

Hall, E.L., Kruger, R.P., Dwyer, S.J., III, Hall, D.L., McLaren, R.W., and Lodwick, G.S. (1971), A survey of preprocessing and feature extraction radiographic images, *IEEE Trans. Comput.* **C-20** (9): 1032.

Hardy, J.D. (1939), The radiating power of human skin in the infrared, *Am. J. Physiol.* **127**:454.

Hardy, J.D., Milhort, A.T., and DuBois, E.F. (1941), Heat loss and heat production in women under basal conditions at temperature from 23° to 35°C, *Temperature, Vol. 1*, Reinhold, New York.

Heerma Van Voss, S.F.C. (1969), Currently available thermographic equipment, *Bibliogr. Radiol.* **5**:22.

Hudson, R.D., Jr. (1968), *Infrared System Engineering*, John Wiley and Sons, New York.

Irwin, J.W., Savara, B.S., and Rau, J.A. (1973), Effect of anatomic curvature in real-time intraoral thermography, *Oral Surg.* **36**:616.

Isard, H.J. (1972), Thermographic "edge sign" in breast carcinoma, *Cancer* **30**:957.

Isard, H.J., Becker, W., Shilo, R., and Ostrum, B.J. (1972), Breast thermography after four years and 10,000 studies, *Am. J. Roentgenol. Radium Therm. Nucl. Med.* **115**:811.

Isard, H.J., and Ostrum, B.J. (1974), Breast thermography – the mammatherm, *Radiol. Clin. North Am.* **XII** (1):167.

Isard, H.J., Ostrum, B.J., and Shilo, R. (1969), Thermography in breast carcinoma, *Surg. Gynecol. Obstetr.* **128**:1289.

Jenkins, F.A., and White, H.E. (1957), *Fundamentals of Optics*, McGraw-Hill, New York.

Lawson, R.N. (1956), Implications of surface temperatures in the diagnosis of breast cancer, *Can. Med. Assoc. J.* **75**:309.

Leider, M., and Buncke, C.M. (1954), Physical dimension of the skin, *Am. Med. Assoc. Arch. Dermatol. Syphilol.* **69**:563.

Levine, M.D. (1969), Feature extraction: A survey, *Proc. IEEE* **57** (8):1391.

Leftwich, R.F. (1970), Comparison of InSb and HgCdTe in a real-time scanning infrared camera, *Appl. Opt.* **9**:1941.

Lewis, D.W., Goller, H., and Teates, C.D. (1973), Apparent temperature degradation in thermograms of human anatomy viewed obliquely, *Diagn. Radiol.* **106**:95.

Lloyd, M. (1975), *Thermal Imaging Systems*, Plenum Press, New York.

Lloyd-Williams, K., Cade, C.M., and Goodwin, D.W. (1963), The electronic heat-camera in medical research, *J. Brit. IRE* **25**:241.

Mali, J.W.H. (1969), Some physiological aspects of the temperature of the body surface, *Bibliogr. Radiol.* **5**:8.

Morse, S.P. (1969), Concepts of use in contour map processing, *Assn. Comp. Mach.* **12** (3):147.

Ott, H.W. (1976), *Noise Reduction Techniques in Electronic Systems*, John Wiley and Sons, New York.

Patil, K.D. (1970), Infrared emission from the human skin *in vivo* between 2.0 and 18.0, in Proceedings of the Second International Conference on Medical Physics, *Phys. Med. Biol.* **15**:178.

Patil, K.D., and Lloyd-Williams, K. (1969), Spectral study of human radiation, *Non-Ioniz. Radiat.* **1**:39.

Planck, M. (1901), Ueber das Gesetz der Energieverteilung Normal Spectrum im, *Ann. Phys. Ser. 4* **4**:553.

Pratt, W.K. (1973), Bibliography on digital image processing and related topics, University of Southern California, USCEE, Report No. 453.

Robinson, G.S. (1974), Fourier transforms of Walsh functions, *IEEE Trans. Electromag. Comp.* **16** (3):183.

Roehrig, H., Dereniak, E., Wolfe, W., Nudelman, S., and Freundlich, I. (1974), Reduction of emissivity effects in thermography, in Proceedings of the American Thermography Society Meeting, Chicago, Illinois, June 22, 1974.

Rosman, M.A. (1976), *Thermography in Pediatric Orthopedic Surgery, Appl. Rad.* **5** (1):83.

Sheard, C., Williams, M.D., and Horton, B.T. (1941), Skin temperature of the extremeties under various environmental and physiological conditions, *Temperature, Vol. 1*, Reinhold, New York.

Stefan, J.S. (1879), Uber die Beziehung Zwischen der Wärmestrahlung und der Temperatur, *Widn. Akad. Sitzber.* **79:**391.

Steketee, J. (1973), Spectral emissivity of skin and pericardium, *Phys. Med. Biol.* **18:**686.

Stoll, A.M. (1960), The role of the skin in heat transfer, *J. Heat Transfer* **82,** B-3, 239.

Viitanen, S.M., and Laaksonen, A.L. (1970), Thermography in juvenile rheumatoid arthritis, *Acta Rheum. Scan.* **16:**91.

Wallace, J., and Cade, G. (1974), *Clinical Thermography*, CRC Reviews in Bio-Engineering, CRC Press, Cleveland, Ohio.

Watmough, D.J., and Oliver, R. (1968a), Emissivity of human skin in the wavelength between 2 and 6μ, *Nature (London)* **219:**622.

Watmough, D.J., and Oliver, R. (1968b), Emissivity of human skin *in vivo* between 2.0 and 5.4μ measured at normal incidence, *Nature (London)* **218:**885.

Watmough, D.J., and Oliver, R. (1969a), The emission of infrared radiation from human skin – implications for clinical thermography, *Br. J. Radiol.* **42:**411.

Watmough, D.J., and Oliver, R. (1969b), Variation of effective surface emissivity with angle and implications for clinical thermography, *Nature (London)* **222:**472.

Watmough, D.J., and Oliver, R. (1969c), Wavelength dependence of skin emissivity, *Phys. Med. Biol.* **14:**201.

Watmough, D.J., and Oliver, R. (1970), Some physical factors relevant to infrared thermography, *Phys. Med. Biol.* **15:**178.

Winslow, C.E.A., and Pierce, J.B. (1941), Man's heat exchanges with his thermal environment, *Temperature, Vol. 1*, Reinhold, New York.

Winsor, T., and Winsor, D. (1975), Thermography in cardiovascular disease, *Appl. Radiol.* **4** (6):117.

Winter, J., and Stein, M.A. (1973), Computer image processing techniques for automated breast thermogram interpretation, *Comput. Biomed. Res.* **6:**522–529.

Wissler, E.H. (1963), An analysis of the factors affecting temperature levels in the nude body, *Temperature – Its Measurement and Control in Science and Industry, Vol. III*, Reinhold, New York.

Wolfe, W.L. (1965), *Handbook of Military Infrared Technology*, U. S. Government Printing Office, Washington, D.C.

Ziskin, M.C., Negin, M., Piner, C., and Lapayowker, M.S. (1975), Computer diagnosis of breast thermograms, *Radiology* **115:**341–347.

CHAPTER 13

General Infrared System Analysis

WILLIAM L. WOLFE and EUSTACE L. DERENIAK

13.1. INTRODUCTION

The design and evaluation of infrared image-forming systems for infrared medical radiography (thermography) is based on the interaction of the characteristics of detectors, optics, displays, and the characteristics of the subject and the background. Infrared technology has advanced so much in recent years that systems can be designed and built such that: the optics are limited only by diffraction effects; the detectors are limited only by photon noise; and the system is virtually ideal. Accordingly, this chapter starts with a derivation of an expression for the signal-to-noise ratio of an ideal infrared imaging system and then considers the efficiency factors of each of the components in turn.

WILLIAM L. WOLFE and EUSTACE L. DERENIAK • Optical Sciences Center, University of Arizona, Tucson, Arizona 85721.

13.2. SIGNAL-TO-NOISE RATIO FOR AN IDEAL SYSTEM

Figure 13-1 is a schematic representation of a typical infrared thermograph and its environment. A portion of the scene is imaged by an appropriate optical system onto an image plane. An array of detectors, each element of which transduces the radiant power on it into an electrical signal, is placed in the plane where the image is focused and is usually called a focal-plane array. Each detector element responds to all the flux on its surface in its spectral band of sensitivity. In this manner it behaves as a single grain of silver in a photographic film or an element of the sensitive surface of a television tube. Accordingly, different parts of the scene must be imaged successively on the detectors. The optical mechanical scanning unit performs this function. Each detector is electrically connected to a preamplifier, and this is almost always through a coupling capacitor. The dc or average value of the scene is thereby blocked from the processing system. The individual detector signals may be run in parallel to individual display elements (usually light-emitting diodes in this case), or they may be multiplexed into a single voltage that varies in time like a TV signal. Sometimes various types of linear or nonlinear processing are applied to the electrical signal to enhance the operation of the device, or to improve the final image. Some means must also be accomplished of synchronizing the scan speeds, line positions, frame rates, and start times in the infrared sensor video signal generation with the display.

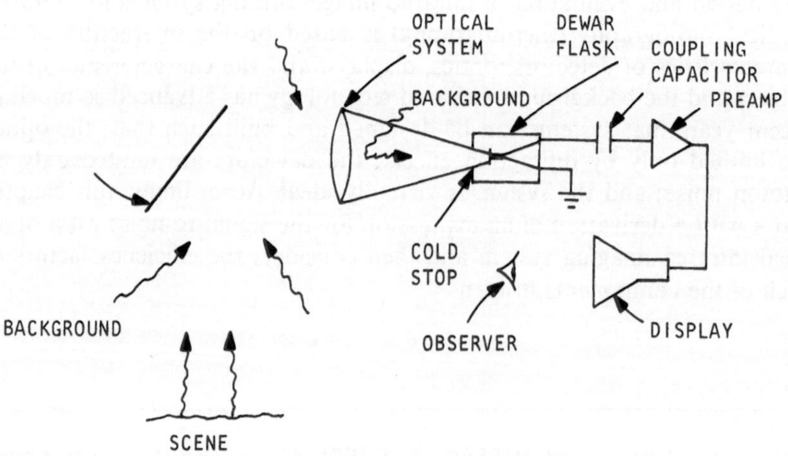

Fig. 13-1. Typical infrared thermograph.

The Signal-to-Noise Equations

The fundamental way to develop an expression for the signal-to-noise ratio is of course to consider the nature of signal generation in a detector and the various possible sources of noise. It has become customary and almost universal in infrared technology to characterize detectors by their D^* values.† We shall do so here. Later it will be appropriate to delve deeper into some of the limitations and nuances of the use of D^* as a summary measure of detector performance. The specific detectivity of D^* is the signal-to-noise ratio per watt on a detector that has a 1-cm^2 area and 1-Hz noise bandwidth:

$$D^* \equiv \frac{(A_\mathrm{d}\Delta_\mathrm{f})^{1/2}}{P_\mathrm{d}} \mathrm{SNR} \qquad (\mathrm{cm\,Hz^{1/2}\,W^{-1}}) \tag{13-1}$$

where A_d is the detector area, Δf the effective noise bandwidth, P_d the power on the detector, and SNR the rms signal voltage or current divided by the rms noise voltage or current, respectively.

The basic equation of radiative transfer can be written

$$d\Phi_\mathrm{e} = L\,dA_1 \cos\phi_1\, dA_2 \cos\phi_2 d^{-2} n^{-2} \tag{13-2}$$

where $d\Phi_\mathrm{e}$ is the flux or power radiating from object differential element dA_1 to image plane differential element dA_2, L is the radiance, dA_1 the differential element of area of object surface, dA_2 the differential element of area of image surface, ϕ_1 the angle between the line joining dA_1 to dA_2 and the normal to dA_1, ϕ_2 the angle between the line joining dA_2 to dA_1 and the normal to dA_2, d the length of the line joining dA_1 and dA_2, and n the refractive index of the medium. For present purposes it will be useful and not very inaccurate to assume that $\phi_1 = \phi_2 = 0$ (or that d is constant over the integration of dA_1 and dA_2). In short,

$$\Phi_\mathrm{e} = \tau_\mathrm{a}\tau_\mathrm{o} L A_1 A_2 d^{-2} n^{-2} \tag{13-3}$$

where τ_a is the atmospheric transmission and τ_o the optical transmission. Next we will assume that the refractive index is 1.0 and the detectors are photon detectors that have constant quantum efficiency, so that

$$D^* = \lambda\lambda_\mathrm{m}^{-1} D_\mathrm{m}^* \tag{13-4}$$

where D_m^* is the maximum value of D^*, λ the radiation wavelength, and λ_m the wavelength at which D_m^* occurs. Finally, we will use the sampling theorem to determine the information bandwidth and the Rayleigh diffraction criterion.

† For definitions of the symbols see the notation list at the end of Chapter 12.

Under these circumstances and assumptions the SNR of the imaging system can be written for a monochromatic radiation signal as

$$\begin{aligned}\mathrm{SNR} &= \Delta\left[\frac{D^{*}\tau_{a}\tau_{o}LA_{o}A_{d}}{(A_{d}\Delta f)^{1/2}f^{2}}\right]\\ &= \Delta\left[\left(\frac{\lambda}{\lambda_{m}}D_{m}^{*}\right)(\tau_{a}\tau_{o}L)\left(\frac{\pi D^{2}}{4f^{2}}\right)\left(\frac{A_{d}}{\Delta f}\right)^{1/2}\right]\\ &= \Delta\frac{D_{m}^{*}}{\lambda_{m}}\frac{\pi}{4}\frac{D\Delta\theta}{F}\left(\frac{1}{\Delta f}\right)^{1/2}\tau_{a}\tau_{o}\lambda L\Big] \end{aligned} \tag{13-5}$$

where A_o is the collector (optics) area, τ_o the optics transmission including obscuration, τ_a the atmospheric transmission, D the optics diameter, f the focal length of the optical system, F the speed or focal ratio of the final optics, $F = f/D$, and $\Delta\theta$ the instantaneous field of view or the size of a detector divided by the focal length. All other symbols have been defined above.

The use of Δ indicates that it is the change in SNR that is important. The image is assumed to be at the focal distance. Figure 13-2 is a schematic representation of the detector output as a detector element scans from one part of the scene to the next. The first part of the scene is at temperature T_1; the second at $T_2 > T_1$. The level of output in both cases needs to be averaged in some way. One simple measure is the average value of the signal plus the noise in each case of $(\overline{S+N})$. If the noise is random, then this can be rewritten as $\bar{S} + \bar{N} \cong \bar{S}$. However, the average value of a random process is zero and the difference in outputs would be just $S_2 - S_1 = \Delta S$. Since recorded noise represents the electrical signal generated from the random arrival of photons (or from internal, electronic sources), it must be evaluated in terms of its rms (root mean square) value, also called the standard devia-

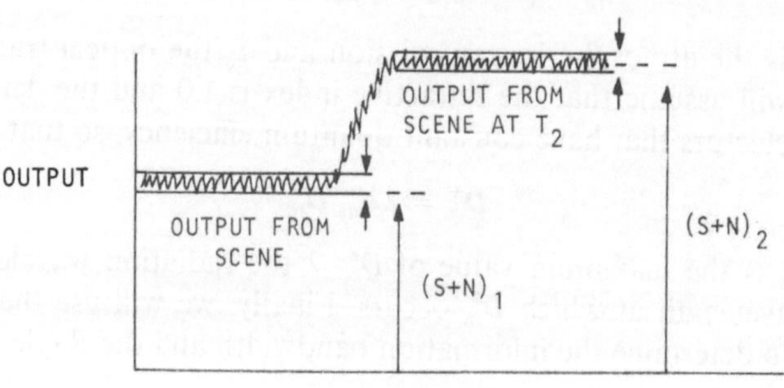

Fig. 13-2. Detector output from two picture elements D^* vs. λ for various detectors.

tion σ. Thus a precise statement is that of the difference in signal-to-noise ratio, i.e., $S_2/\sigma_2 - S_1/\sigma_1$, which can be written without much loss in accuracy by assuming $\sigma_1 = \sigma_2$ and by calling it N. Then $\Delta(S/N)$ is the difference in signal divided by the rms value of the noise. It is customary to write the rms value of signal as well as noise. (For sinusoidal signals the rms SNR is 0.707 times the peak SNR. Values reported for D^* for different detectors are usually for rms SNR's.)

The various parenthetical factors in the final form of the SNR equation will now be considered. Figure 13-3 shows D^* values of many detectors. From this it is clear that the maximum occurs almost at the wavelength at which the detector is no longer sensitive, the cutoff wavelength. It is also true that most of the $D^*_{\rm m}$ values are about 10^{10}–10^{12} for photodetectors.

The second factor in the equation should not cause any conceptual problems; it turns out to be 0.7854.

The third factor involves the diameter of the optics, the instantaneous field of view, and the optical speed denoted by the focal ratio or F/number. It will be considered later what design considerations are necessary to reduce F, increase D, and maintain a specified value for $\Delta\theta$.

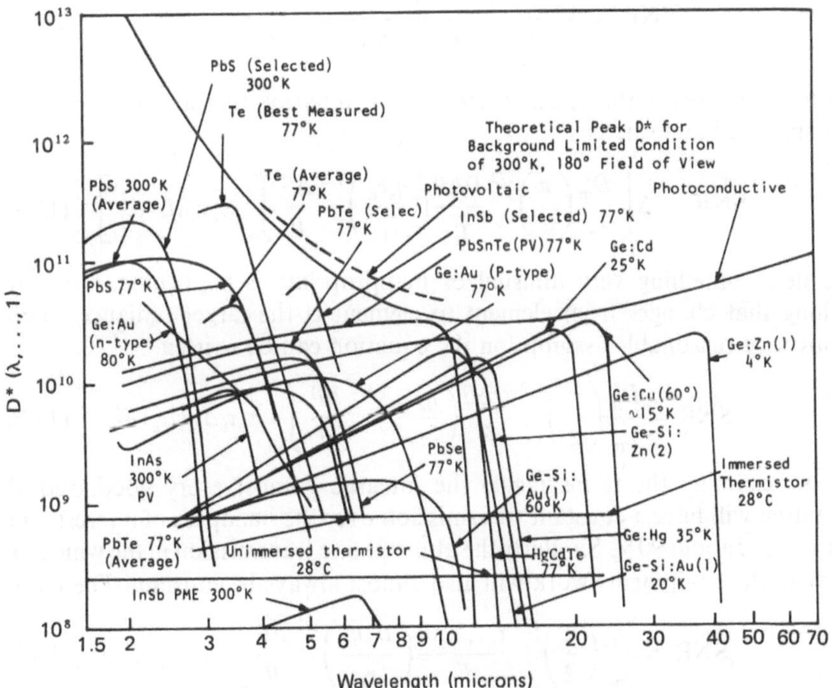

Fig. 13-3. D^* vs. λ for various detectors.

The next factor involves the effective noise bandwidth of the system. By the Whittaker–Shannon sampling theorem the information bandwidth is $(2t_d)^{-1}$, where t_d is the time it takes for the image of a detector to move through the instantaneous field of view (ifov). The dwell time can be calculated in an idealized way by dividing the frame time for a total field of view by the number of resolution elements in the total field of view:

$$t_d = \frac{t}{N} = t\frac{\omega}{\Omega}$$

where ω is the solid angle of one ifov and Ω is the solid angle of the total field:

$$\begin{aligned} \omega &= \Delta\theta\Delta\phi = r_d(\Delta\theta)^2 \\ \Omega &= \theta\phi \quad\;\; = r_f\theta^2 \end{aligned} \tag{13-6}$$

where the aspect ratio of the detector is r_d and that of the frame is r_f. The detector is usually square; the frame usually is not. We can use these substitutions and a scan efficiency factor η_s to obtain

$$\mathrm{SNR} = \Delta\left[\frac{D_m^*}{\lambda_m}\frac{\pi}{4}\frac{D\Delta\theta}{F}\left(\frac{8\eta_s r_d}{\pi r_f}\right)^{1/2}\frac{\Delta\theta}{\theta}\tau_o\tau_a\lambda L\right] \tag{13-7}$$

where the area of the optics is $\pi D^2/4$. For radiation that is integrated over a spectral band one has

$$\mathrm{SNR} = \Delta\left[\frac{D_m^*}{\lambda_m}\left(\frac{\pi}{2}\right)^{1/2}\frac{D\Delta\theta}{F}\left(\frac{\eta_s r_d}{r_f}\right)^{1/2}\frac{\Delta\theta}{\theta}\int_{\Delta\lambda}\tau_o\tau_a\lambda L_\lambda\,d\lambda\right] \tag{13-8}$$

Unless something very unusual or inappropriate is happening, the only thing that changes from element to element is the target radiance. With this very reasonable assumption the equation can be written

$$\mathrm{SNR} = \frac{D_m^*}{\lambda_m}\left(\frac{\pi}{2}\right)^{1/2}\frac{D\Delta\theta}{F}\left(\frac{\eta_s r_d}{r_f}\right)^{1/2}\frac{\Delta\theta}{\theta}\int_{\Delta\lambda}\tau_o\tau_a\Delta(\lambda L_\lambda)\,d\lambda \tag{13-9}$$

Now examine the terms inside the integral. Almost every good optical coating will have a constant transmission over the bandpass of interest and a value of about 90%. Similarly the atmospheric transmission in the windows where the equipments work will also almost always be constant. Therefore

$$\mathrm{SNR} = \frac{D_m^*}{\lambda_m}\left(\frac{\pi}{2}\right)^{1/2}\frac{\tau_o\tau_a D\Delta\theta}{F}\left(\frac{tr_d\eta_s}{r_f}\right)^{1/2}\frac{\Delta\theta}{\theta}\int\Delta(\lambda L_\lambda)\,d\lambda \tag{13-10}$$

the term $\Delta(\lambda L)$ can be written in another form. The equation for the spectral radiance of a blackbody is

$$L_\lambda^{\mathrm{BB}} = c_1\pi^{-1}\lambda^{-5}(e^x - 1)^{-1} \qquad (\mathrm{W\,m^{-1}\,sr^{-1}\,\mu m^{-1}}) \tag{13-11}$$

where $x = c_2/\lambda T$, c_1 is the first radiation constant, c_2 the second radiation constant, λ the wavelength, and T the temperature. The blackbody photon spectral sterance, the number of photons per second per square meter per steradian per micrometer, is given by

$$L_{\mathrm{q}\lambda}^{\mathrm{BB}} = L_\lambda^{\mathrm{BB}}(hc/\lambda)^{-1} \tag{13-12}$$

where the subscript q indicates a photon quantity. It is just the monochromatic power divided by the energy per photon. Therefore

$$\lambda L_\lambda^{\mathrm{BB}} = hcL_{\mathrm{q}\lambda}^{\mathrm{BB}} \tag{13-13}$$

The SNR equation becomes

$$\mathrm{SNR} = \frac{D_{\mathrm{m}}^*}{\lambda_{\mathrm{m}}}\left(\frac{\pi}{2}\right)^{1/2}\frac{\tau_{\mathrm{o}}\tau_{\mathrm{a}}D\Delta\theta}{F}\left(\frac{tr_{\mathrm{d}}\eta_{\mathrm{s}}}{r_{\mathrm{f}}}\right)^{1/2}\frac{\Delta\theta}{\theta}hc\int_{\Delta\lambda}\Delta L_{\mathrm{q}}\,d\lambda \tag{13-14}$$

$\Delta\lambda L_\lambda$ has been simplified to ΔL_{q} since all subsequent analysis relates to blackbody radiation.

The change in radiance ΔL can be written as the combinations of the change due to temperature changes and those due to emissivity change. In differential notation this is

$$dL = \frac{\partial L}{\partial T}dT + \frac{\partial L}{\partial \varepsilon}d\varepsilon \tag{13-15}$$

This expression can be inserted in the integral, but it seems more instructive to write two types of SNR. Since the latter is really measured by the change in signal divided by the noise, one can write

$$\begin{aligned}\mathrm{SNR} &= \frac{\partial\mathrm{SNR}}{\partial T}dT + \frac{\partial\mathrm{SNR}}{\partial\varepsilon}d\varepsilon \\ &= \mathrm{SNR_T}\,dT + \mathrm{SNR}_\varepsilon\,d\varepsilon\end{aligned} \tag{13-16}$$

We note that $\mathrm{SNR_T}$ is the change in the signal-to-noise ratio generated by a 1°K temperature change. A common figure of merit for infrared instruments is the noise-equivalent temperature difference (NETD), i.e., the temperature change required to give a signal-to-noise ratio of 1. Therefore

$$\mathrm{SNR_T} = (\mathrm{NETD})^{-1}$$

$$\mathrm{SNR}_\varepsilon = (\mathrm{NE}\varepsilon\mathrm{D})^{-1}$$

and

$$\mathrm{SNR} = (\mathrm{NETD})^{-1}\, dT + (\mathrm{NE\varepsilon D})^{-1}\, d\varepsilon \tag{13-17}$$

This is a relatively accurate and useful equation as it stands, but there are two other conditions that almost always apply. These are that the detector is limited by photon noise and the optics are diffraction limited. These conditions are certainly true for systems which use narrow fields of view in the 8–14 μm region and which view the earth's environment or people, or any scene that has an average temperature 300°K or above. Under these circumstances, for a photoconductive detector

$$D_{\mathrm{m}}^{*} = D_{\mathrm{BLIP}}^{*} = \frac{\lambda}{2hc}\left(\frac{\eta}{E_{\mathrm{q}}}\right)^{1/2} \tag{13-18}$$

where D_{BLIP}^{*} is the background-limited infrared photodetector, h is Planck's constant, c is the speed of light, η is the detector quantum efficiency, E_{q} is the photon incidance on the detector.

For a photodiode the D_{m}^{*} is $2^{1/2}$ times larger than given by Eq. (13-18). The expression for diffraction-limited resolution is

$$\Delta\theta = 2.44\, \lambda/D \tag{13-19}$$

This is the angle subtended by the Airy disk of an unobscured circular optical system. If λ is taken as the wavelength of the maximum, the calculation will be conservative, that is, $\Delta\theta$ will be a maximum.

The value of E_{q} can be calculated on the assumption that the detector senses radiation from the field of view it sees outside the Dewar flask cold stop. This gives a photon incidance of

$$E_{\mathrm{q}} = \frac{M_{\mathrm{q}}}{4F^2} = \frac{\pi L_{\mathrm{q}}}{4F^2} \tag{13-20}$$

Therefore, for a background-photon-limited infrared sensor system that is also diffraction limited or BLISS one has

$$\mathrm{SNR} = \pi^{1/2}(0.61)(0.84)\, \lambda_{\mathrm{m}}(\Delta f)^{-1/2}\, \tau_{\mathrm{a}}\tau_{\mathrm{o}} \int \Delta L_{\mathrm{q}}\, d\lambda \left(\int L_{\mathrm{q}}\, d\lambda\right)^{-1/2} \tag{13-21}$$

Finally, assume that somehow the designer manages a quantum efficiency of 1 for the detector, and a τ of 1 for both the optics and atmosphere. Then

$$\mathrm{SNR} = 0.91\lambda_{m}(\Delta f)^{-1/2}\left(\int_{\Delta\lambda} L_{\mathrm{q}\lambda}\, d\lambda\right)^{-1/2} \int_{\Delta\lambda} \Delta L_{\mathrm{q}\lambda}\, d\lambda \tag{13-22}$$

This is an interesting result. It is the SNR value for an ideal scanner, using the following simplifying assumptions:

$$\tau_a = 1, \qquad \tau_o = 1$$
$$\eta = 1, \qquad \eta_s = 1$$
$$D^* = D^*_{\mathrm{BLIP}}, \qquad \Delta\theta = 2.44\lambda/D$$

A system can be designed based on this ideal scanner and a set of efficiency factors. One can write the SNR as

$$\mathrm{SNR} = \mathrm{SNR}_{\mathrm{ideal}}\tau_o\tau_a\eta_{cs}\eta\eta_e\eta_{ab} \tag{13-23}$$

where η_{cs} is the efficiency of cold shielding, η the quantum efficiency of the photodetector, η_e the efficiency of the electronics, and η_{ab} the loss in flux due to optical factors. The latter term can usually be forced to be 1 by proper optical design.

In addition solid angles are approximated by areas divided by the square of distance, and the image is at the focal distance, or very close to it.

This result is independent of the field of view, the ifov, the D^*, and everything else except the temporal bandwidth, the spectral bandwidth, and the properties of the target and the background. This situation bears further discussion.

13.3. SUBJECTS

13.3.1. Introduction

The first assumptions we shall make are the ideal ones, i.e., the subjects and the background are blackbodies. Next the assumption will be relaxed to encompass graybodies whose emissivities are independent of wavelength. Finally, the general spectrally varying or colored body will be considered theoretically and some practical examples given.

13.3.2. Theory for Black- and Graybodies

The equation for the signal-to-noise ratio had the following form:

$$\mathrm{SNR} \propto \int_{\Delta\lambda} \Delta L_q \, d\lambda \Bigg/ \left(\int L_q \, d\lambda \right)^{1/2} \tag{13-24}$$

The next step in the analysis is to determine the photon fluxes given by the two integrals. The change in photon sterance can be written

$$dL_q = \frac{\partial L_q}{\partial T} dT + \frac{\partial L_q}{\partial \varepsilon} d\varepsilon \qquad (\mathrm{sec}^{-1}\ \mathrm{m}^{-2}\ \mu\mathrm{m}^{-1}) \tag{13-25}$$

The well-known expression for radiance is

$$L_e = \frac{c_1}{\pi}\lambda^{-5}(e^x - 1)^{-1} \qquad (\mathrm{W\,m^{-2}\,\mu m^{-1}}) \tag{13-26}$$

where c_1 is the first radiation constant, λ the wavelength (μm), x the $c_2/\lambda T$, c_2 the second radiation constant (cm °K), and T the temperature (°K). Then the monochromatic photon sterance is just the monochromatic radiance divided by the energy of the photon

$$L_{q\lambda} = \frac{\lambda L_\lambda}{hc} = \frac{c_1}{\pi hc}\lambda^{-4}(e^x - 1)^{-1} \qquad (\mathrm{sec^{-1}\,m^{-2}\,\mu m^{-1}}) \tag{13-27}$$

The rate of change of this function can be found in a number of ways, which show that

$$\begin{aligned}\frac{\partial L_q}{\partial T}dT &= \frac{xe^x}{e^x - 1}L_q\frac{dT}{T} \qquad (\mathrm{sec^{-1}\,m^{-2}\,m^{-1}})\\ &= \frac{c_1}{hc}\frac{\lambda^{-4}xe^x}{(e^x - 1)^2}\frac{dT}{T}\end{aligned} \tag{13-28}$$

The integral over wavelength then is

$$\int_0^\lambda \frac{\partial L_q}{\partial T}dT\,d\lambda = \frac{c_1}{\pi hc}\frac{dT}{T}\int\frac{\lambda^{-4}xe^x}{(e^x - 1)^2}d\lambda \tag{13-29}$$

The total signal then is (assuming $d\varepsilon$ is not a function of λ)

$$\frac{c_1}{\pi hc}\left(\frac{T}{c_2}\right)^3\left(\frac{dT}{T}\sum_3 + d\varepsilon\sum_2\right) \tag{13-30}$$

where

$$\sum_2 = \sum_{m=1}^{\infty} m^{-3}e^{-mx}\left[(mx)^2 + 2mx + 2\right]$$

$$\sum_3 = \sum_{m=1}^{\infty} m^{-3}e^{-mx}\left[(mx)^3 + 3(mx)^2 + 6mx + 6\right]$$

where m is a running index (see Appendix A). But this is not the whole story for targets which have an emissivity less than 1.

Background effects can be calculated by first writing the irradiation on the aperture in terms of the radiation emitted from the target field and then that which is emitted by the background, reflected by the scene and incident on the aperture. The relative radiance for the entire spectral band can be written as

$$\frac{dL_q}{L_q} = 3\frac{dT}{T} + \frac{d\varepsilon}{\varepsilon} - \frac{\Omega_B}{\pi}\frac{L_{qB}\,d\varepsilon}{L_{qs}}$$

$$= 3\frac{dT}{T} + \frac{d\varepsilon}{\varepsilon}\left(1 - \frac{L_{qB}\Omega_B}{L_{qs}}\right) \tag{13-31}$$

If it can be assumed that the background is black (as a result of emission and many inter-reflections), then

$$\frac{dL_q}{Lq} = 3\frac{dT}{T} + \left(1 - \frac{\sum T_i^3\Omega_i}{T_s^3}\right)\frac{d\varepsilon}{\varepsilon} \tag{13-32}$$

where the summation is over all the different projected solid angles (Nicodemus, 1968) at different uniform temperatures T_i. This can be written for narrow-band radiation as follows:

$$\frac{dL_q}{L_{q\lambda}} = \frac{xe^x}{e^x - 1}dT + \left[1 - \frac{\sum(e^{x_i} - 1)^{-1}\,\Omega_i}{(e^{x_s} - 1)^{-1}}\right]\frac{d\varepsilon}{\varepsilon} \tag{13-33}$$

For values of $x \gg 1$, the following approximation is valid

$$\frac{dL_{q\lambda}}{L_{q\lambda}} \simeq \frac{dT}{T} + 1 - \sum e^{x_s - x_i}\Omega_i\frac{d\varepsilon}{\varepsilon} \tag{13-34}$$

It is reasonable to make the assumption that the system and the scene are at the same temperature. In that case the value of SNR_T in a one cycle bandwidth is given by

$$SNR_T(\Delta f)^{1/2} = 0.296\lambda_m\left(\int_{\Delta\lambda} L_q\right)^{-1/2}\int_{\Delta\lambda}\frac{\partial L_q}{\partial T}\,d\lambda \tag{13-35}$$

The value of SNR_ε in a unit bandwidth is

$$SNR_\varepsilon(\Delta f)^{1/2} = 0.296\lambda_m\left(\int_{\Delta\lambda} L_q\,d\lambda\right)^{-1/2}\int_{\Delta\lambda} L_q\left[1 - \frac{\sum(e^{x_i} - 1)^{-1}\,\Omega_i}{(e^{x_s} - 1)^{-1}}\right]d\lambda \tag{13-36}$$

Therefore if the background term is ignored, for unit bandwidth

$$
\begin{aligned}
\mathrm{SNR} &= \mathrm{SNR}_T\, dT + \mathrm{SNR}_\varepsilon\, d_\varepsilon \\
&= 0.296\lambda_m \left[\frac{\int_{\Delta\lambda} [(\partial L_q/\partial T)\, d\lambda]\, dT}{\int_{\Delta\lambda} (L_q\, d\lambda)^{1/2}} + \left(\int_{\Delta\lambda} L_q\, d\lambda^{1/2} \right) d\varepsilon \right] \\
&= 0.296\lambda_m \left(\int L_q\, d\lambda \right)^{1/2} \left[d\varepsilon + \frac{\int (\partial L_q/\partial T)\, d\lambda}{\int L_q\, d\lambda} dT \right] \\
&= 0.296\lambda_m \left(\int L_q\, d\lambda \right)^{1/2} \left[d\varepsilon + \frac{\sum_3 dT}{T \sum_2} \right] \qquad \text{(13-37)}
\end{aligned}
$$

13.3.3. Assessment of the Background Noise

The total value of E_q on the detector is a result of contributions from scattered light, emission from optical elements, and emission from the scene transmitted (or reflected) by the optical elements. We will give a treatment that is general enough that either transmitting or reflecting elements are included. In both cases the absorption is equal to the emission. For transmitting elements there is no reflection, so $\varepsilon = 1 - \tau$. For reflecting elements, the reflectance is equivalent to the transmittance so that ρ is replaced by τ, $\varepsilon = 1 - \tau$ and no radiation passes through the element. Figure 13-4 shows the geometry of a single optical element and a detector.

The irradiance from the lens on the detector at temperature T is given by

$$E_{qo} = M/4F^2 = (1 - \tau_o)\, M^B/4F^2 \qquad \text{(13-38)}$$

A subscript e will be used for energy hereafter. The radiation that is incident on the lens from the field of view includes those parallel rays in the beam plus that from the ifov. From the far field then the power on the lens in the field is given by

$$
\begin{aligned}
P_{ds} &= \tau_o \varepsilon_s \pi^{-1} M^{BB}(T_s)\, (\mathrm{ifov})^2\, A_o \\
E_{ds} &= \tau_o \varepsilon_s \pi^{-1} M^{BB}(T_s)\, A_o f^{-2} \\
&= \tau_o \varepsilon_s M^{BB}(T_s)/4F^2 \qquad \text{(13-39)}
\end{aligned}
$$

Therefore

$$
\begin{aligned}
E_d &= (2F)^{-2} [\tau_o \varepsilon_s M^{BB}(T_s) + (1 - \tau_o) M^{BB}(T_l)] \\
&= M^B(T_s)(2F)^{-2} [\tau_o \varepsilon_s + (1 - \tau_o)\, M^{BB}(T_l)/M^{BB}(T_s)] \qquad \text{(13-40)}
\end{aligned}
$$

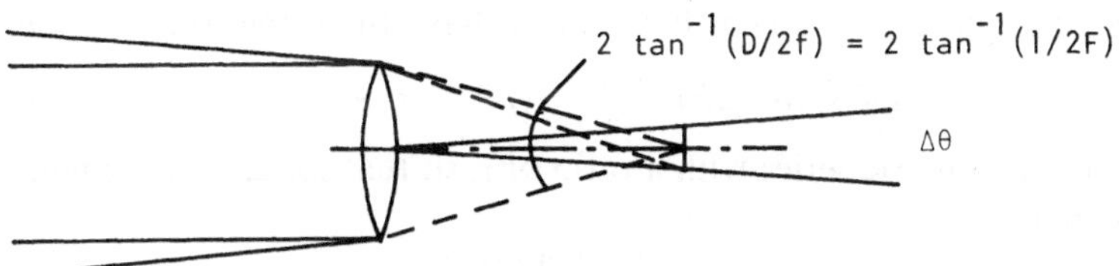

Fig. 13-4. Single optical element and detector.

For situations in which they are the same temperature,

$$E_d = M^{BB}(2F)^{-2}[\tau_o\varepsilon_s + (1 - \tau_o)] \quad (13\text{-}41)$$

Now a second optical element is added increasing the complexity as shown in Fig. 13-5. From this diagram it is easy to see that the first lens subtends the same angle at the detector as does the second. In fact, in a good design both will subtend a slightly greater angle than determined by the (cold) field stop. Therefore, each optical element subtends the same solid angle at the detector in a well-designed optical system. If R_i is the ratio of blackbody emittances of the ith element to that of the scene M^B, then both will subtend a slightly greater angle than determined by the (cold) field stop. Therefore, each optical element subtends the same solid angle at the detector in a well-designed optical system. If R_i is the ratio of blackbody emittances of the ith element to that of the scene M^B, then

$$E_d = M^B(2F)^{-2}(1 - \tau_1)R_1 + \tau_1(1 - \tau_2)R_2 + \tau_1\tau_2(1 - \tau_3)R_3 + \cdots \quad (13\text{-}42)$$

In general, of course, all the optical elements will be at unique temperatures. Often it is useful to assume they are all at the temperature of the scene so that

$$E_d = M^B(2F)^{-2}(1 - \tau_1) + \tau_1(1 - \tau_2) + \tau_1\tau_2(1 - \tau_3) + \cdots \quad (13\text{-}43)$$

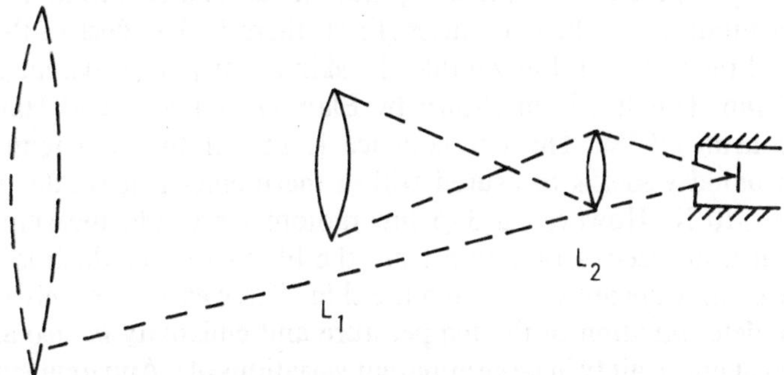

Fig. 13-5. Multielement optical system and detector.

If in addition it is assumed that they all have the same transmission, then

$$E_d = M^B(2F)^{-2}(1-\tau)(1+\tau+\tau^2+\cdots) \tag{13-44}$$

This is a geometric series with a ratio of τ, so that for an infinite number of elements

$$E_d = M^B(2F)^{-2} \tag{13-45}$$

and for a finite number of elements

$$E_d = M^B(2F)^{-2}(1-\tau^n) \tag{13-46}$$

If the system is catadioptric or color corrected with two different kinds of lens materials then the expression can be written as the sum

$$\begin{aligned} E_d &= M^B(2F)^{-2}[(1-\tau_1)+\tau_1(1-\tau_2)+\tau_1\tau_2(1-\tau_1) \\ &\quad + \tau_1^2\tau_2(1-\tau_2)+\cdots] \\ &= M^B(2F)^{-2}\{(1-\tau_1)[1+\tau_1\tau_2+(\tau_1\tau_2)^2+\cdots] \\ &\quad + (1-\tau_2)[\tau_1+\tau_1^2\tau_2+\cdots]\} \\ &= M^B(2F)^{-2}[(1-\tau_1+1-\tau_2)(1+\tau_1\tau_2+\tau_1^2\tau_2^2+\cdots)] \end{aligned} \tag{13-47}$$

The optical elements are counted by starting at the detector.

It seems obvious that the detector field of view should encompass only the optical element, and for practical reasons should be just a little less.

13.3.4. Properties of Thermographic Subjects

It has been fairly well established that in the infrared region of the spectrum at wavelengths beyond about 3 μm, the human skin has an emissivity of 0.95–1.0; it is essentially black. The degree to which the emissivity is not 1.0 is important on a level of about 0.5% to 1% in terms of thermographic diagnosis. Measurements of emissivity with much accuracy in this region of the spectrum are indeed quite difficult. These variations can be due to a number of different causes. First, there is the effect of the transmission of the skin. It is known that the skin is partly transparent between 3 and 5 μm. This has been shown by Elam *et al.* (1963) and Hardy and Muschenheim (1936). The consequence is that if the skin temperature above a blood vessel is measured with a thermometer, it would read, for example, 310°K. However, a 3–5 μm radiometer would measure 313°K because it also receives radiation from the blood vessel (which is warmer than the skin), transmitted through the skin. These effects severely interfere with the determination of the temperature and emissivity *in vivo* and give rise to great uncertainty in large apparent variations of ε. Apparent emissivity values up to $\varepsilon = 1.3$ have been reported and discussed by Steketee (1973a).

There is also the effect of the curvature of the human skin surface. The apparent emissivity depends on the viewing angle. This has been discussed many times, most recently by Lewis *et al.* (1973), Mitchell *et al.* (1967), and Watmough and Oliver (1970). It is pointed out by Lewis *et al.* that a 75° angle of incidence, measured from the normal to the skin, can lead to an apparent 1.5°K temperature differential. Watmough also finds that a 4°K hot spot can be masked or caused by an emissivity change resulting from a 70° viewing angle. Of course, care must be taken with his data as they assume the skin to be a dielectric, which is not really true.

One must conclude from a review of the literature that the emissivity of the skin is not known for a single spot on a human to an accuracy of 1% or better. Further, its variation over the surface of a single person or from person to person are not known in any statistical sense at all.

13.4. THE MTF APPROACH TO A SYSTEM DESCRIPTION

13.4.1. Introduction

In theory, one should be able to describe the imaging performance of a thermograph in terms of its transfer function. Limitations prevail however, due to nonlinearity, shift, and sampling processes that occur. The sophisticated forward-looking infrared scanner (FLIR), for example, is not a linear shift invariant system. But much can still be done and that is the subject of this chapter.

13.4.2. Transfer Functions

Transfer functions describe the ratio of an output spectrum to an input spectrum for a properly defined quantity. The functions can be in the time and frequency domains or in the space and spatial frequency domains. The output $y(t)$ of an electronic system related to the input, $x(t)$ is represented as follows:

$$y(t_2) = \int_{-\infty}^{\infty} h(t_1, t_2)\, x(t_1)\, dt_1 \tag{13-48}$$

In this form the output at time t_2 is related to the input at time t_1. In most applications the function is related only to the time difference; the translation function or weighting function is independent of time. Then

$$y(\tau) = \int_{-\infty}^{\infty} h(t - \tau)\, x(t)\, dt \tag{13-49}$$

By taking the Fourier transform of both sides (see Appendix B for further discussion) one has

$$Y(\omega) = H(\omega)\, X(\omega) \tag{13-50}$$

The spectrum of the output equals the product of the input spectrum and the transfer function. The relationship holds in the spatial domain as well as the temporal domain so that

$$Y(\omega_x) = H(\omega_x)\, X(\omega_x) \tag{13-51}$$

The transfer-function relations can apply to both time and space coordinates and yield no additional conceptual complexity as long as the components are separable (and still shift invariant and linear).

For a scanning system which is scanning at velocity v, the distance will be covered in a time t where

$$t = x/v \tag{13-52}$$

The temporal frequency ω is related to t by

$$\omega = 2\pi/t \tag{13-53}$$

The spatial frequency ω_x is related to x by

$$\omega_x = 2\pi/x \tag{13-54}$$

The two frequencies are related by

$$\omega = 2\pi/t = 2\pi/(x/v) = 2\pi v/(2\pi/\omega_x) = v\omega_x \tag{13-55}$$

This makes sense in that a greater velocity of scan implies a greater required temporal frequency. In electronics one usually deals with the transfer function $H(\omega) = Y(\omega)/X(\omega)$. In optics one usually deals with an MTF, the modulation transfer function that is normalized to a dc value of 1. The next step in the analysis is to determine the MTF for a thermographic system.

13.4.3. Imaging in the Spectral Domain

The scene can be described in terms of the spatial spectrum of variations in radiance. By employing a "hat" notation, the transform of any function f can be written as $\hat{f}$. Thus the spectrum of the photon sterance can be written as $\hat{L}_q(\lambda, T, f_x)$ with dimensions of photons $\text{cm}^{-2}\,\text{sr}^{-1}\,\text{sec}^{-1}$ m.

Then the signal-to-noise ratio as a function of spatial frequency is a function of the (spatial) spectrum of the scene and the transfer function of the infrared instrument. First the scene is imaged by the optical system. The optical system has a transfer function usually labeled the OTF. The detector senses the radiation on its surface and converts any input variations

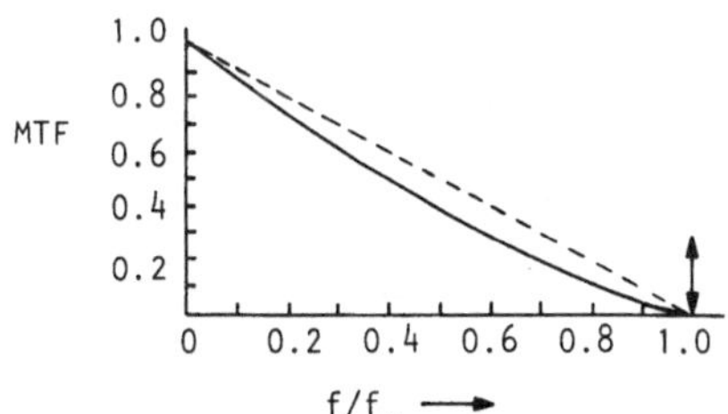

Fig. 13-6. MTF of circular and square aperture (dashed curve for square aperture).

into an electronic signal. Thus the detector has both optical (spatial) transfer and electrical (temporal) transfer functions. The electronics also have a classical temporal transfer function, which is determined by electrical components and by requirements to compensate for the deficiencies of other transfer functions. Finally, of course, the display also has its characteristic spatiotemporal transfer function. The final image should be formed in such a way that the contrast at any spatial frequency is above the threshold contrast of the eye at that frequency.

This procedure is completely equivalent to broadcasting a concert. First, the concert has the full range of frequencies that the instruments can produce. A microphone has both an acoustic and electrical response. (The analogy is a little strained because there is little spatial dependence and a wavelength of sound is larger than the microphone.) The microphone turns the acoustic spectrum into an electrical one. It is processed in that form with some components amplified more than others to account for the deficiencies in the microphone and the speaker of the receiver.

It is therefore of considerable importance to describe in as much detail as a general discussion will permit the appropriate transfer functions for each component. The temporal response of most infrared detectors can be approximated by the response of a single-time constant RC (resistance–capacitance) circuit, i.e., $(1 + j\omega\tau)^{-1}$. The electronics can be described in terms of a combination of different electronic filter functions. The spatial frequency response of the detector can be calculated by assuming the response area is uniform and square with the length of the side given by l. The Fourier transform of such a function is as follows:

$$\begin{aligned} F\{\text{rect}(a, b)\} &= \int_{-a/2}^{a/2} \int_{-b/2}^{b/2} \exp\left[j(\omega_x x + \omega_y y)\right] dx\, dy \\ &= \left[\frac{\exp(j\omega_x x)}{j\omega}\right]_{-a/2}^{a/2} \left[\frac{\exp(j\omega_y y)}{j\omega}\right]_{-b/2}^{b/2} \\ &= \text{ab}\,\text{sinc}(\omega_x a/2)\,\text{sinc}(\omega y b/2) \end{aligned} \tag{13-56}$$

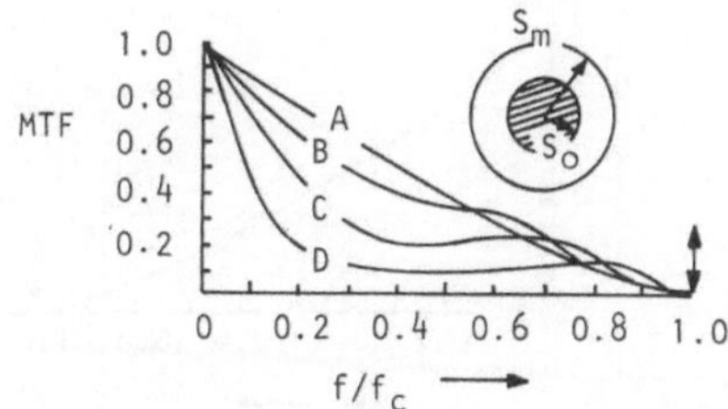

Fig. 13-7. MTF of obscured pupil function.

It can be shown that since the distribution of flux in the image plane is the Fourier transform of the distribution in the entrance pupil, that the MTF is the autocorrelation of the pupil distribution, measured in optical wavelengths, and for a plane wave this gives the MTF. Thus for square optics the MTF is given by $1 - ff_o^{-1}$, where the cutoff frequency f_c is $2a/f\lambda$. For a circularly symmetric system it is

$$(2\pi)^{-1}\left[\arccos(\lambda fy/F) - (\lambda fy/F)\sin\left(\arccos(\lambda fy/F)\right)\right] \qquad (13\text{-}57)$$

where the cutoff frequency is D/f. Figure 13-6 shows these two curves and illustrates the point that the circularly symmetric system is very similar to the square system with just a little sag. A system with obscuration can be calculated in a similar way. There is more sag and additional oscillatory structure, as shown in Fig. 13-7. The cutoff frequencies can be given in linear dimensions as above or in angular dimensions by dividing by the focal length f. Therefore the cutoff frequency in angular dimensions for the obscured, unaberrated circularly symmetric system is $f/2r$ or f/D or F. The cutoff frequency in radians then is $f/F\lambda = D/\lambda$, the same as for the square system.

As a first approximation to the MTF design of a system one need only insure that the aberrations are less than two waves and can then use the straight line $1 - f/f_c$ with $f_c = D/\lambda$, as the MTF of the system. Correction will be 10–20% for final systems. Figure 13-8 shows approximate values of aberrations.

13.5. OPTICAL AND SCANNING SYSTEMS

13.5.1. Introduction

Optical scanning systems for the infrared can conveniently be separated into those which scan in a collimated beam, a convergent beam, and an afocal system. With a few exceptions these require, respectively, high resolution over only the detector or detector array and those which need good resolution over the whole field. The designer needs to consider the combination of the scanning system and the optical system. The scanning should have a high percentage of "on" time with little time used at the beginning

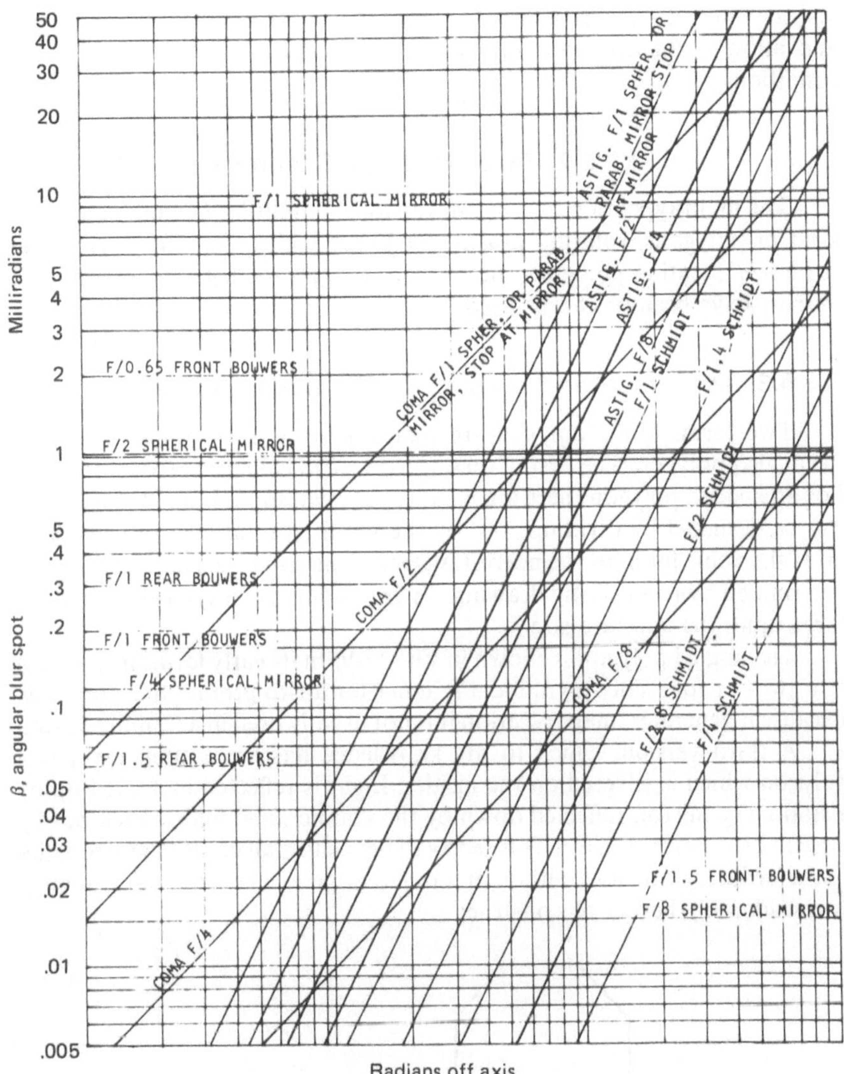

Fig. 13-8. Aberrations of some commonly used optical systems in the infrared.

and end of lines and frames. This helps to keep the bandwidth low and the scan speed slow. This should also be accomplished without introducing obscuration in the optics or increasing the focal ratio unduly. A constant velocity scan is to be preferred because it means (other things being equal) a smaller bandwidth and slower maximum scan speed.

Collimated beam scanners need good resolution over only a narrow field but require a large scanning element. Convergent beam scanners have just the opposite requirements. Afocal systems trade aperture size for angle and allow a smaller scanning element but with more stringent angular conditions.

13.5.2. Parallel-Beam Scanners

The main types of scanners are versions of multifaceted mirrors in the form of polygons, rotating prisms combined with a framing mirror and refractive, rotating polygons. In a few cases galvanometer or tuning fork mirrors have been or can be used.

13.5.3. Multifaceted Mirrors—Reflective Polygon Scanners

Two forms of the polygon are what might be called the straight and the angled polygon. The first of these is very often called a carousel scanner. For an n-sided polygon there are n scans per revolution. Usually the system can be designed by dividing 360° by the required total field of view. This gives the value for n (to the nearest integer). The size of the face can then be determined by engineering drawings or trigonometry; it typically is two or three times the aperture size.

The angled polygon is shown in Fig. 13-9. In its early forms it was used as a two- or four-sided pyramidal scanner for air-to-ground line scanning. Because it generates image rotation it is not usually used in a framing device.

A third version, which to my knowledge has never been used, is a polygon which is silvered on the insides. Light is reflected in, folded up by a stationary mirror, reflected down by the scanner, and folded back out by a second stationary mirror. This seems to have most all of the characteristics of the ordinary carousel, although a different geometry, and unfortunately is considerably harder to construct.

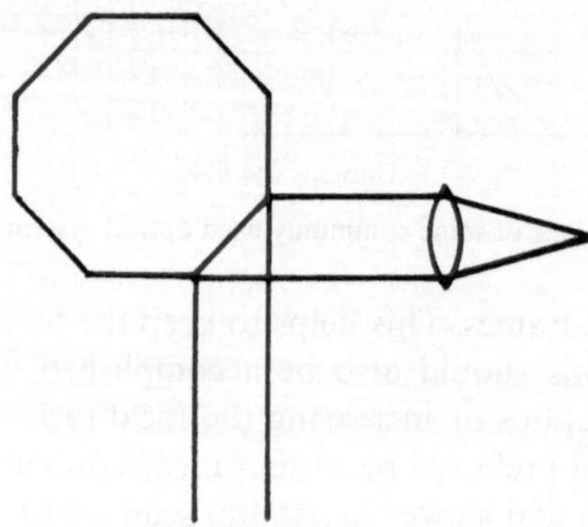

Fig. 13-9. Polygon scanning technique.

With the straight polygon, a framing mirror must be used to generate the scan direction perpendicular to the lines. For a TV-rate scanner 500 lines are generated in 1/30 sec (15,000 lines/sec). Even if there are 100 detectors the scan rate is still $150/n$ per second where n is the number of faces of the polygon. For a 30° field of view the value of n can be 12. In some applications, it might be better to have only six faces and $500/6 = 83$ detectors. Then the exact numbers are determined by design iterations.

13.5.4. Counter-Rotating Prisms and Mirrors

Although this technique uses an identical pair of prisms, other optical elements can be used to generate the angular offset. The prisms can be corotated or counter-rotated at the same speed or different speeds, thereby generating circles, spirals, and rosettes. Exact counterstation of two prisms with equal deviation generates a straight line. This combined with a scanning mirror can generate a frame. The deviation δ in any given direction is given by

$$\delta = (n - 1)\sin\alpha \tag{13-58}$$

where n is the refractive index of the prism and α the prism angle. If we visualize two rotating prisms, each with angle α and index n they will generate a deviation δ in the same angular direction. Any plate perpendicular to the optical axis will be pierced by a given ray at the coordinates (δ_x, δ_y). These are given by

$$\delta_x = \delta_1 \cos(\omega_1 t + q_1) + \delta_2 \cos(\omega_2 t + q_2) \tag{13-59}$$

$$\delta_y = \delta_1 \sin(\omega_1 t + q_1) + \delta_2 \sin(\omega_2 t + q_2) \tag{13-60}$$

where ω_1, ω_2 are the angular rates of the prism rotations for prisms 1 and 2, respectively, q_1, q_2 are the respective phases, and δ_1, δ_2 the respective deviations for counter-rotation at the same rate, $\omega_2 = -\omega_1$. We can start the prisms with the apexes together and wherever desired so that $\delta_1 = \delta_2 = 0$. The deviations are equal so that

$$\begin{aligned} \delta_x &= \delta\left[\cos\omega t + \cos(-\omega t)\right] \\ &= 2\delta \cos t \end{aligned} \tag{13-61}$$

$$\begin{aligned} \delta_y &= \delta[\sin\omega t + \sin(-\omega t)] \\ &= 0 \end{aligned} \tag{13-62}$$

Therefore as time goes by a line is scanned such that the deviation from zero is given by $\delta_x \cos\omega t$ and is only along the x axis. The scan rate is given by

$$v_x = -2\delta\omega \sin\omega t \tag{13-63}$$

The sign shows that the velocity decreases as the deviation increases. The average speed, not velocity, is one-half the maximum or $\delta\omega$. This means of course that the maximum scan efficiency is 50%, which is not very high.

A pair of tilted mirrors can be used in place of the prisms for wide spectral band applications, reduction of chromatic aberration, and maybe a reduction in weight.

The degree of chromatic aberration can be calculated in short order. This can be calculated by the change in deviation with respect to wavelength. The difference in the deviations will just be $(dn/d\lambda)\,\Delta\lambda$, where $dn/d\lambda$ is the dispersion of refractive index and $\Delta\lambda$ is the bandwidth of the systems.

13.5.5. Convergent Beam Scanners

The main forms of convergent beam scanners are refractive polygons, Nipkow scanners, and rotating wheels.

13.5.5.1. Rotating Refracting Polygons

It is noteworthy that with a parallel beam, the use of a refractive polygon in front of the aperture stop in place of a reflective polygon does not work. A plane parallel plate translates but does not deviate a beam, so that the incoming beam would wander over the pupil but continue to be focused in the same place. However, in a convergent beam the image scans an arc. This is the principle used by AGA in the design and construction of their thermographic instrument.

13.5.5.2. Nipkow Scanning Devices

The Nipkow scanning technique was used in the early days of television, before the satisfactory development of scanning electron-beam tubes. It consisted of image-forming optics, a scanning disk, reimaging optics, and a single detector, as shown in Fig. 13-10. The objective optics form an image of the total field of view on the scanning disk. The reimaging optics forms an image of the portion of the disk that comprises the field of view. In theory the only changes which occur are those from the radiation which passes through the hole. This works pretty well in the visible, but in the infrared any temperature or emissivity variations over the surface of the disk will generate a signal output.

The lens which reimages onto the detector is difficult to design because of stringent demagnification requirements. The detector must see the total field of view at all times and cannot be cold shielded very efficiently, and of course, the objective optics must have good resolution over a wide field. One design approach to relieving some of the difficulty of the design re-

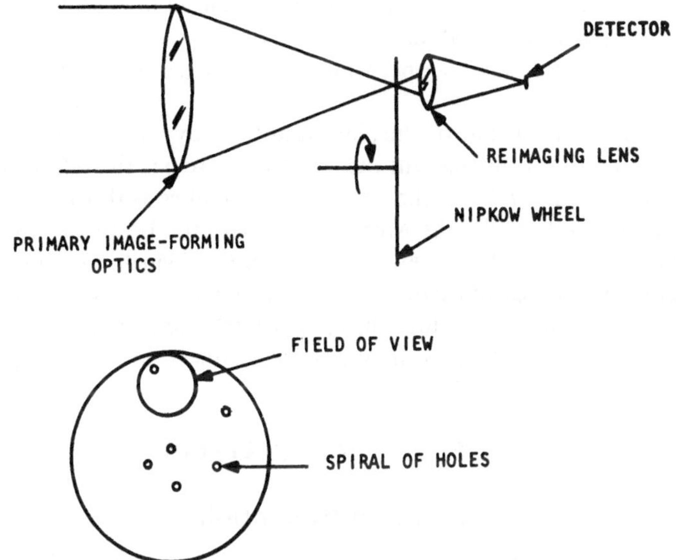

Fig. 13-10. Nipkow scanning technique.

quirements is to insert a small reimaging lens in each hole. There is then one lens for each line of the frame but each is easier to design. One can also use a drum instead of a disk.

13.5.5.3. Rotating-Wheel Scanners

A Schmidt or Bouwers optical system forms an image on a spherical surface—they have curvature-of-field aberration. If one then forms a wheel in which the spokes are optical relay systems, this curved field can be sampled and focused onto a detector array. The major problems here seem to be in the alignment of the various spokes, because the optical and scanning efficiencies are high. A six-spoke system mounted in an airplane was used by Perkin-Elmer and the Air Force in the mid-1950's with considerable success over a period of years, but this design seems to have been abandoned in recent times.

13.5.5.4. Afocal Designs

A recent development in conjunction with the Department of Defense's "Common FLIR" program has been the use of an afocal optical system (such designs are also used as beam expanders and compressors for lasers). An early version of such a system is the Mersenne mirror system. A pair of off-axis parabolas, one larger than the other, is used in a confocal arrangement. The first, large parabola focuses incoming parallel radiation at the focus of the second smaller one, which recollimates the light in a smaller bundle.

The optical invariant or the sine condition says that for good systems $ny \sin\theta$ is a constant throughout the system, where n is the refractive index, y is the ray height, and θ is the angle the ray makes with the optical axis. Therefore if a system like the Mersenne reduces the beam size by a factor m, then the required field of view will be $\arcsin(m^{-1} \sin\theta)$. For small angles, the angular magnification equals the beam demagnification. This usually presents mirror problems for object-space scanners, but can introduce insurmountable difficulties for image-space scanners.

13.6 OPTICAL SYSTEMS

13.6.1. Introduction

We deal here with optical systems that form an image. The relatively special cases of systems which optically enlarge a detector, or which scramble light on it, are not treated. Optical systems can be refractive, reflective, or consist of both refractive and reflective elements. The advantages of refractive (dioptric) systems is that they do not fold the light and therefore do not have large (if any) obscuration. They do suffer from chromatic effects that are almost entirely absent in mirrors and have somewhat lower overall transmission. In fact to bring most infrared materials to the point where they do not reflect over 10% of the incident radiation, one must use multilayer antireflection films. These inherently have an undesirable, nonuniform spectral transmission. Catadioptric systems (the last category), which suffer the afflictions of both the first two, are often the only way to get a truly wide-field, high-resolution system.

13.6.2. Simple Design Equations

The layout and many features of an optical system can be ascertained by use of the first-order ray-tracing equations. The overall resolution performance can be estimated quite well from evaluation of the third-order aberrations. The lens law and lens makers equations give the relationships among the object and image distances, focal length, refractive index, and radii of curvatures of the (spherical) surfaces:

$$\frac{1}{z} + \frac{1}{z'} = \frac{1}{f} = (n-1)\frac{1}{r_1} - \frac{1}{r_2} + \frac{d}{nr_1r_2} \qquad \text{(13-64)}$$

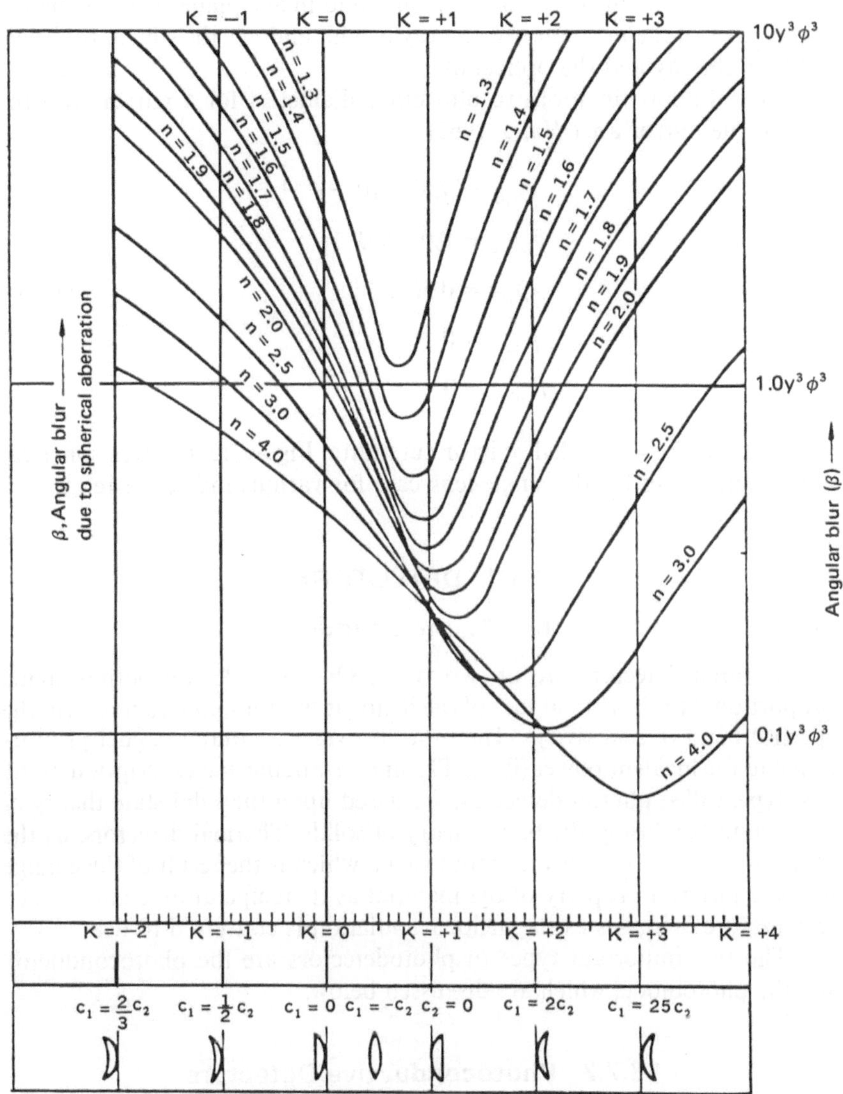

Fig. 13-11. Spherical aberration for single lens of various indices. $K = c_1/(c_1 - c_2)$; $\beta = \{y^3\phi^3/[4(n-1)^2]\}\{n^2 - (2n+1)K + [(n+2)/n]K^2\}$.

where z is the object distance, z' the image distance, f the focal length, n the refractive index, d the central thickness, r_1 the radius of curvature of the first surface, and r_2 the radius of curvature of the second surface. The magnification is given by

$$m = z'/z$$

The optical invariant for aperture planes and image planes is $n\bar{y}u$, where n is the index of the medium, y is the ray height, and u is the sine of the angle between the ray and the optical axis.

Useful approximations to blur circle diameters for a mirror with the stop at the mirror are (Wolfe, 1965)

$$\begin{aligned} \beta_{\text{sph}} &= 7.8 \times 10^{-3}F^{-3} \\ \beta_{\text{coma}} &= 0.0625\theta F^{-2} \\ \beta_{\text{ast}} &= 0.5\theta^2 F^{-1} \\ \beta_{\text{dest}} &= 0 \\ \beta_{\text{color}} &= 0 \end{aligned} \tag{13-65}$$

where curvature = one-half mirror curvature. Figure 13-11 gives spherical aberration values for the single-lens case for various indices of refraction.

13.7. DETECTORS

13.7.1. Introduction

Infrared detectors are of two types. One provides an output signal proportional to the arrival rate of the incident photons on its surface (in the spectral band of sensitivity). The other provides an output signal proportional to the incident power (flux). The understanding and description of the first type, called photon detectors, are based upon the solid state theory of semiconductors using the band theory of solids. Thermal detectors, as the others are called, provide an output signal which is the result of the change in some physical property of the material as its temperature changes. The temperature increases as the incident radiation is converted to heat.

The two important types of photodetectors are the photoconductor and the photodiode, which are discussed below.

13.7.2. Photoconductive Detectors

A typical circuit is shown in Fig. 13-12. The voltage of the battery (or other bias supply) is divided between the load resistance R_L and the detector resistance R_d. Because most arrangements use the blocking capacitor for ac coupling, only the difference in voltage is sensed. The voltage across R_d is

$$V_d = \frac{V_B R_d}{R_L + R_d} \tag{13-66}$$

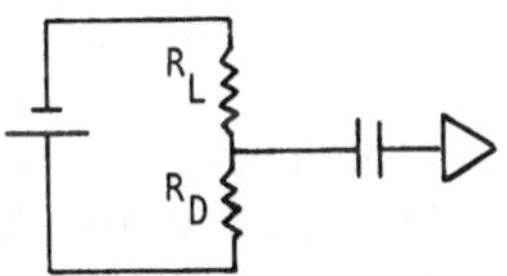

Fig. 13-12. Biasing arrangement for photoconductor.

The voltage change with respect to a change in R_d, written as v_d, is

$$\frac{\partial V_d}{\partial R_d} dR_d = v = \frac{V_B(R_L + R_d) - R_d}{(R_L + R_d)^2} dR = \frac{V_B R_L dR_d}{R_L^2 + 2R_L R + R_d^2}$$

$$= V_B dR_d/(R_L + 2R_d + R_d^2/R_L)$$

$$= \frac{1}{(1 + R_d/R_L)} I_B dR_d \tag{13-67}$$

Without going any further, it is clear that a larger bias current produces a larger detector signal. The signal is in fact proportional to the bias current and detector resistance change. As long as $R_d \leq R_L$ the value of the parenthesis is close to 1, and has little influence on the ac signal voltage.

The conductivity σ of a photoconducting semiconductor is given by

$$\sigma = ne\mu_e + pe\mu_h \tag{13-68}$$

where n is the density of electrons, e the charge of the electron, μ_e the mobility of the electron, μ_h the mobility of the holes, and p the density of holes. The resistance is $\rho l/A_x = l/\sigma A_x$ so that a change in resistance is

$$dR_d = \frac{l}{A_x}\left[d\left(\frac{1}{\sigma}\right)\right] = \frac{l\,d\sigma}{A_x\sigma^2} = \frac{R_d\,d\sigma}{\sigma} \tag{13-69}$$

$$d\sigma = e[\mu_e\,dn + n\,d\mu_e + \mu_h\,dp + p\,d\mu_h]$$

$$= e[n(d\mu_e + a\,d\mu_h) + \mu_e(dn + b\,dp)]$$

$$= e[n\,d\mu_e(1 + ab) + \mu_e\,dn(1 + ab)]$$

$$= e(1 + ab)(n\,d\mu + \mu\,dn)$$

$$a = \frac{p}{n}$$

$$b = \frac{\mu_h}{\mu_e}$$

It can be seen that with no loss of generality the analysis can be completed assuming only a single effective carrier with density n (carriers per cubic meter) and mobility μ (m^2/V sec). The mobility is a velocity per unit field strength.

The change in conductivity results from both a change in mobility and a change in the density of carriers. The question to be asked now is: "What changes the density of carriers and the mobility?" The answer to this question requires a short excursion into solid state theory, which follows. The change in the number of carriers ($N = n_e A_d d$) is given by

$$\frac{d}{dt}(\Delta N) = A_d \eta E_q - \frac{\Delta N}{\tau} \tag{13-70}$$

The first term is the rate of the net change in the total number of carriers. The second term is the detector area times the quantum efficiency times the incident flux rate of photons (the average number of photons per second per area). This term represents the rate of generation of carriers. The next term is the total number of carriers divided by the lifetime and represents the recombination of carriers. The equation can be rewritten as

$$\frac{d\Delta N}{dt} + \frac{1}{\tau}\Delta N = A_d \eta E_q \tag{13-71}$$

The spectrum of the number of carriers is found by solving this equation by Fourier techniques:

$$\begin{aligned} j\omega\tau\Delta N(\omega) + \Delta N(\omega) &= \tau A_d \eta E_q(\omega) \\ \Delta N(\omega) &= \frac{\tau A_d \eta E_q(\omega)}{1 + j\omega\tau} \end{aligned} \tag{13-72}$$

It is a single time constant system with typical low-frequency response. The amplitude is $\tau A_d \eta E_q(\omega)$. Then

$$\begin{aligned} \frac{\Delta N}{N} &= \frac{\tau A_d \eta E_q(\omega)}{(1 + j\omega\tau) n_e A_d} \\ &= \frac{\tau \eta E_q(\omega)}{n_e d(1 + j\omega\tau)} \end{aligned} \tag{13-73}$$

The signal voltage then is given by

$$v_d = \frac{V_B}{R_L} dR_D = \frac{V_B R_d \tau \eta E_q(\omega)}{R_L n_e d(1 + j\omega t_\Omega)} \tag{13-74}$$

and detectors provide a larger signal voltage if the carriers have longer lifetimes, if the detector has better quantum efficiency and low equilibrium density of carriers. Note also the effect of V_B, R_D/R_L, and d. This analysis is applicable to a constant-current mode of detector circuit often used with low impedance detectors. Those which are operated in constant-voltages modes require a different treatment. Full rigor also requires treatment of preamp and load-resistor noises.

The analysis can be carried out as done in Kruse *Elements of Infrared Technology* (Kruse *et al.*, 1962). The quiescent (dc) electrical signal in the absence of a photon signal is V_0, where

$$V_0 = I_0 l / A_d(\sigma_d + \sigma_B) \tag{13-75}$$

The signal voltage is changed by signal radiation to a conductivity $\sigma = \sigma_s + \sigma_B + \sigma_d$. The ac signal voltage can be written

$$v_s = (\sigma_s/\sigma)\, V_0 = \frac{\sigma_s V_0}{\sigma_s + \sigma_B + \sigma_d} \approx \frac{\sigma_s V_0}{\sigma_B + \sigma_d} \tag{13-76}$$

The dark conductivity of an intrinsic photoconductor is

$$\sigma_d = e(n_0 \mu_e + p_0 \mu_h) \tag{13-77}$$

The background conductivity is

$$\sigma_b = e(n_B \mu_e + n_b \mu_h) \tag{13-78}$$

For many cases one can assume $\mu_e \gg \mu_h$, $t_e \approx t_h \approx t$, $n_0 \gg p_0$, and $\sigma_B \ll \sigma_d$ so that the voltage responsivity (V/w) is

$$R_v(\lambda) = \eta \lambda t V_0 / hc A_d n_0 \tag{13-79}$$

$$= \frac{\lambda \eta V_0 t}{dnc A_d n_0} \tag{13-80}$$

This means that (1) responsivity is increased with higher quantum efficiency, bias voltage, and lifetime, and (2) the sample should be as thin as possible and have a small number of equilibrium carriers.

13.7.3. Photodiode Detectors

The current–voltage curve for dark current is given by

$$I_d = I_0(e^{eV/kT} - 1) \tag{13-81}$$

$$= \frac{A D_n n_p}{L_n}(e^{eV/kT} - 1) \tag{13-82}$$

The background-induced current is

$$I_b = Aten/\tau \tag{13-83}$$

The signal current is $I_s = \eta E_q \tau / L_n$. When the diode is open circuited the voltage must be zero so that

$$I_s + I_b = I_d \tag{13-84}$$

The current flowing in a diode detector can be written as the sum of a current generated by photoelectrons I_p and the dark current I_d which flows in the absence of any incident radiation (in the spectral region where the absorption is not zero). A diode detector is usually used with no bias voltage applied or with a small amount of reverse bias. These are called, respectively, photovoltaic and photodiode detectors. The former usually appears in some form of energy conversion, e.g., a solar cell. For the former the total current I_t is zero. Then

$$I_t = I_p + I_d = 0 \tag{13-85}$$

The photocurrent is $\eta e E_q$, where η is the quantum efficiency, e is the charge of one electron, and E_q is the total number of photons on the detector per second (on the average). Then, by using the dynamic resistance of the diode R $(=\partial v/\partial I)_{v=0}$, one can write

$$I_p = I_d = V/R \tag{13-86}$$

and

$$V = RI_p = R\eta e E_q = R\eta e P\lambda/hv \tag{13-87}$$

The monochromatic voltage responsivity, i.e., the output volts per input watts for a monochromatic signal input, is

$$R_\lambda = R\eta e\lambda/hc \tag{13-88}$$

13.7.4. The Seven Deadly Noises

A noise is generally a random fluctuating voltage that is not the voltage variation representing the signal. In all cases the noise is a fluctuation envelope representing a deviation around the signal voltage, and includes the fluctuation around the mean voltage generated by the background flux, that is, the photon-noise-limited condition.

The noises that are covered here are as follows:

1. Johnson–Nyquist, or thermal, noise is caused when, in the normal flow of current, electrons are scattered throughout the crystal "lattice." The random motions thus represent fluctuations in current, a noise.

2. Shot or Schottky noise is also a variation in current flow. The original analysis was applied to the fluctuations in emission times of electrons from the cathode of a vacuum diode. It applies equally well to the flow of carriers from the n to p (or p to n) side of a semiconductor diode.

3. In semiconducting devices the action starts with the generation of a

free carrier. The generation rate has associated with it a statistical variation called generation noise.

4. Recombination noise is the equivalent quantity associated with the recombination time of carriers.

5. Photon noise is related directly to the statistical variation in the arrival rate of photons.

6. Temperature noise is the variation in the heating rate of a thermal detector due to the fluctuation in the rate of arrival of photons.

7. Excess or $1/f$ noise is associated with improperly fabricated contacts, surface states, internal grain boundaries, and other such phenomena. Even after just about everything is done perfectly, there is still some excess noise left. It is still only imperfectly understood.

We will provide an analytical discussion below of Johnson–Nyquist and generation–recombination noise.

13.7.4.1. Thermal Noise

The noise voltage in a resistance due to the Brownian motion of the electrons is given by

$$v_J^2 = 4kTR\Delta f \tag{13-89}$$

For a photoconductive detector in the presence of background radiation this is given by

$$\begin{aligned} v_J &= 4kT\Delta f_l / A_d(\sigma_d + \sigma_b) \\ &= 4kT\Delta f_l / A_d e[(n_0\mu_e + p_0\mu_h) + (n_v\mu_e + P_b\mu_p)] \end{aligned} \tag{13-90}$$

where n_0, p_0 are the equilibrium carrier concentrations and n_b, p_b the background-generated carriers. The detectivity in this case can be written

$$D^*(\lambda) = \frac{\lambda\eta}{}(A_d\Delta f_e)^{1/2}\frac{(\mu_e\tau_e + \mu_h\tau_h)\{Ae[(n_b + n_0)\mu_e + \mu_h(n_b + p_0)]\}^{1/2} V_0}{[(n_0\mu_e + p_0\mu_h) + n_b(\mu_m + \mu_p)]At(4kTBl)^{1/2}} \tag{13-91}$$

$$= \frac{\lambda\eta(\mu_n\tau_n + \mu_p\tau_p)e^{1/2}V_0}{hct[(n_b + n_0)\mu_n + (n_b + p_0)\mu_p]^{1/2}(4kTl)^{1/2}} \tag{13-92}$$

Now we can assume $\mu_e \gg \mu_h$, $\tau_e = \tau_h = \tau$, and $\sigma_b \ll \sigma_d$ so that $n_0 \gg n_b$. Then

$$D^*(\lambda) = \frac{V_0\lambda\eta\tau}{2hct}\left(\frac{\mu_e e}{n_0 kTl}\right)^{1/2} \tag{13-93}$$

This is the interesting result of the D^* for a thermally limited detector, a detector limited by thermal noise. In this case the bias voltage is made as large as Joule heating and the breakdown voltage will allow. The mobility is made large as is the recombination time. The detector should be thin and cold and short.

13.7.4.2. Generation–Recombination (gr) Noise

Long and Schmit (1970) assert that the mean square gr noise voltage is given by

$$v_{gr}^2 = \frac{2V_0(\Delta f + 1)^2}{bn + p} \frac{np\tau \Delta f}{At(bn + p)} \tag{13-94}$$

$$n = n_0 + n_b$$

$$p = p_0 + p_b$$

Burgess (1955 and 1956) and Van Vliet (1958) show that

$$\eta E_{qb} + \eta E_{qt} = \frac{np}{n + p} \frac{t}{\tau} \tag{13-95}$$

In practice it is often true that $n_b \gg p_b \gg p_0$ and $b \gg 1$ so that

$$v_{gr}^2 = \frac{2V_0^2}{n_0} \frac{n_0 \tau \Delta f}{A_d t} \tag{13-96}$$

On the other hand if $n_0 \gg p_0 \gg n_b$, then

$$v_{gr}^2 = \frac{2V_0^2}{n_0} \frac{p_0 \tau \Delta f}{A_d t} \tag{13-97}$$

The important difference is that the noise is related either to the background-generated flux or the *minority*-carrier concentration. The detectivity in the gr case for either of these extremes can now be calculated.

The general calculation is

$$\begin{aligned} D^* &= (A\Delta f)^{1/2} R/v_n \\ &= \frac{\lambda\eta(\mu_e\tau_e\mu_h\tau_h)\, 2V_0(\Delta f + 1)(npB)^{1/2}}{hc[(n_0\mu_e + p_0\mu_h)\, At + n_b(\mu_e + \mu_h)\, At](bn + p)\,[At(bn + p)]^{1/2}} \end{aligned} \tag{13-98}$$

It is hard to do very much with this equation unless or until some simplifying assumptions are made. It would be possible of course to computerize the whole thing and check the sensitivity to the different variables. If

$$\mu_e \gg \mu_h, \quad \tau_e = \tau_h = t, \quad \text{and} \quad n_0, n_b \gg p_0$$

then

$$D^*(\lambda) = \eta_s \lambda t^{1/2} / [2hcd^{1/2}(n_b)^{1/2}] \tag{13-99}$$

However, when $n_b \gg n_0 \gg p_0$, then

$$\begin{aligned} D^*(\lambda) &= \eta_s \lambda / [2hc(\eta_b)^{1/2}(\bar{n}_b)^{1/2}] \\ &= \eta_s \lambda t^{1/2} / hc(2dn_b)^{1/2} \end{aligned} \tag{13-100}$$

However, when $n_b \ll n_0 \ll p_0$, then

$$\begin{aligned} D^*(\lambda) &= \eta_s \lambda t^{1/2} / hc(2dn_b)^{1/2} \\ &= \frac{\eta_s \lambda}{2hc(dp_0)^{1/2}} \end{aligned} \tag{13-101}$$

13.8. REALIZATION OF A THERMOGRAPH DESIGN

13.8.1 Introduction

The realization begins with a set of specifications and an evaluation as to how well each of the terms in the SNR equation can be realized or how large they must be made. The theoretical expression was found in Section 13.3.2 to be

$$\text{SNR} = 0.296(\Delta f)^{-1/2} \lambda_m \left(\int_{\Delta\lambda} L_q \, d\lambda \right)^{1/2} \left(\frac{\int (\partial L_q / \partial \lambda) \, d\lambda \, dT}{\int L_q \, d\lambda} + d\varepsilon \right) \tag{10-102}$$

The efficiency terms which were all set to 1 included η, τ_o, η_s, and τ_a. For thermographic applications $\tau_a = 1$ as long as $\Delta\lambda$ is either the 3–5 μm region or the 8–12 μm region. The quantity η_s, the scanning efficiency, appears in evaluation of the bandwidth.

13.8.2. Specification

Thermographic instruments should resolve about 1 mm on the surface of a patient. Those used for breast screening need to cover about 40 × 40 cm. The field therefore needs to be about 400 × 400 elements (16×10^4 elements). This is very close to that required by TV. The frame rate should also be about 1/30 sec to eliminate perception of flicker. So the data rate can realistically be taken as 6×10^6 elements/sec. Conversely the dwell time on each element can only be 167 nsec, even if scanning is 100% efficient.

It is clear that a TV-rate thermographic system requires about 100 detectors, since HqCdTe and PbSnTe detectors both can have time constants as short as several hundred nanoseconds.

The camera is used about 1 m from a patient so that 1 mm on the surface subtends 1 mrad. For 50% modulation with an ideal system the cutoff would be at 1/2 mrad or 4 cycles/mrad. This means the aperture $D = 400\lambda$, which for a 3–5 μm system is 1.6 cm and for an 8–12 μm system is 4 cm. These are modest apertures.

The total field is 400 × 400 mrad (0.4 × 0.4 rad), which is large for imaging the full field but probably can be accomplished by either an object plane scanner or an image scanner.

The minimum resolvable temperature difference on the subject should be less than 1°K and the smaller the better.

13.8.3. Object-Space Scanner Design

Based on the preliminary concepts discussed in the previous section a scanner with a 10-cm aperture is assumed initially. Spherical aberration is large for the resolution requirements. Since 100 detectors are to be used the resolution must be maintained out to an angle of 50 mrad.

One design approach is the use of aspheric mirrors, singly or in combination.

The coma then is found as follows for a parabola:

$$\beta_C = 0.0625\theta F^{-2} = 3.13F^{-2} \quad \text{(mrad)} \qquad (13\text{-}103)$$

The astigmatism is

$$\beta_A = 0.5\theta^2 F^{-1} = 1.25F^{-1} \quad \text{(mrad)} \qquad (13\text{-}104)$$

These can both be reduced to 1 mrad or less by using an F/ratio larger than 1. Since to a first approximation these aberrations add, we can choose F to be 3 (this also eases manufacture). Thus

$$\beta_c = 0.35$$

$$\beta_A = 0.42 \qquad (13\text{-}105)$$

The choice of F/number leads one to examine the D^* value. For an $F/1$ field of view, the D^*_{BLIP} was found to be 5×10^{10}. This change requires it to be 1.5×10^{11}, which is reasonable. The detector then is placed at about 30 cm from the aperture, so for a 1-mrad resolution element it must be 300 μm (0.3 mm). This is a little large but certainly available with good performance.

An $F/3$ Newtonian system (with a 10-cm parabola) could be made with about 40% obscuration. A Herschellian system could be made with a parent parabola of about 22–25 cm. One probably can get three 10-cm eccentric elements for the parent, but it is still an expensive way to go. The Pfund version of the Newtonian works well for $F/3$ systems like this. There is no need to consider more exotic systems like a Ritchey Chretien or the wide-angle systems like Schmidt's or Bouwer's. For these mirrors one can assume 98% reflectivity for each mirror, which gives a system reflectivity of 96%.

Designs for this system can also be generated with lenses. For a germanium lens with a shape factor of +3 the value of β_s is 1.5×10^{-3}. This is a little large, so an aspheric element or corrections must be used. A silicon element would be about five times worse. Coma for both would be 0.06 mrad, while chromatic aberration for both would be about 0.05 mrad. The main difficulty then is aspherizing the lens and providing it with a good antireflection coating. The singlet lens could be employed so that the system has no obscuration. This would give an optical efficiency over the chosen spectral passband of about 90%.

These design concepts have ignored the fact that the object is a finite distance from the optical system. Thus we need to consider depth of field and depth of focus. To make a reasonable calculation, we assume the convergent cone is $F/3$ to a spot that is 1 mrad. The image spot increases at 1/6 the rate of change of the depth of focus. Thus we assume a system that delivers 0.5 mrad and require that it not be doubled. Such a criterion leads to the fact that the depth of field can be 10 mm. The calculation is shown below. Note that this is not a very large depth of field and can (or could) be one of the main limitations in the imaging performance of thermographs.

For an infrared system the depth of field and focus is mainly concerned with whether all the energy is focused onto a detector or not.

By first-order optics one has

$$\frac{1}{f} = \frac{1}{z} + \frac{1}{z'} \tag{13-106}$$

Therefore, by differentiation and algebraic manipulation,

$$dz = -\left(\frac{z}{z'}\right)^2 dz'$$

$$\frac{dz}{z} = -m\frac{dz'}{z'} \tag{13-107}$$

In the region of focus the beams form a caustic whose minimum waist usually denotes the position of focus. We treat the caustic by constructing asymptotic-type lines and analyzing the linearized situation trigonometrically. The beam in this case is $F/3$ so the image increases one-third as fast as the focus:

$$dz' = 6dy = 3d(2y) \tag{13-108}$$

The angular change is $2dy/f$. Therefore $2dy/f = 0.5$ mrad, $2dy = 0.015$ cm, $dz' = 0.045$ cm, $dz'/z' \approx 1.5$ mrad, and $dz = -m^2 dz' = 0.05$ cm.

13.9. DIFFERENTIAL THERMOGRAPHY

The differential thermography suggested by Dodd *et al.* (1973) at M. D. Anderson hospital is a step in the right direction for improving thermographic techniques. Their system used 0.9 μm as the near-infrared picture (active picture); however, a better wavelength choice may well improve this technique further.

Figure 13-13 shows a simple model of the skin, subcutaneous tissue, and blood vessels. The illuminating radiation is transmitted and reflected at the epidermis and blood vessels. The difference in the reflection of the blood vessels, which is affected by the absorption of the oxyhemoglobin, and the reflection of the subcutaneous tissue is what we want to detect. Optimum imaging will prevail at a wavelength where transmission through the epidermis is maximum, reflection is minimal, absorption of the blood vessels is maximum, and reflection from subcutaneous tissue is optimized. All of these requirements do not fall at one wavelength; therefore, trade-offs and compromises become essential.

The transmission of skin is shown in Fig. 13-14 as measured by Hardy and others (Hardy and Muschenheim, 1936) and in Fig. 13-15 as obtained

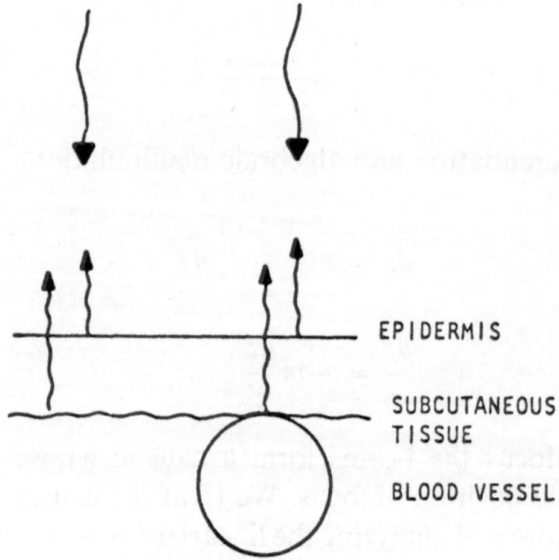

Fig. 13-13. Model of skin.

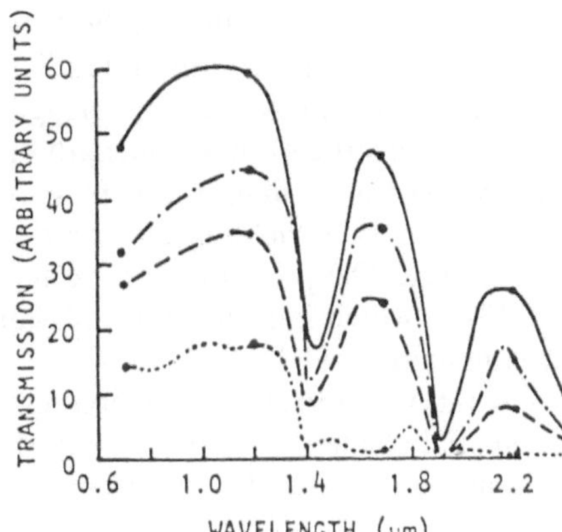

Fig. 13-14. Spectral transmission of excised white human skin. ——, 0.43 mm; —·—, 0.67 mm; ---, 0.84 mm; ···, 1.60 mm (after Hardy *et al.* 1956, reproduced with permission from the American Physiological Society).

in this laboratory. It is obvious that the optimum spectral region is not 0.9 μm. Hardy's data suggest that 1.2 μm may be the optimum region, since this is the maximum of his transmission curve. Figure 13-15 shows that 1.3 or 1.7 μm may be the choice from the transmission viewpoint. The general shape of the two curves is similar; however, Fig. 13-15 does not take into account the diffuse properties of the skin as did Hardy's. The improvement in transmission is about a factor of 2 using 1.7 or 1.2 μm as compared to 0.9 μm.

13.10. RATIO TEMPERATURE TECHNIQUES

Integral temperature thermographs are useful instruments for deriving temperature changes or differences from radiance measurements under certain conditions. The principal requirement for accurate measurements is knowledge of the target's emissivity over the spectral range of the instrument. In addition, all types of thermographs are affected by the absorption in the intervening media between target and sensor. A ratio temperature thermograph substantially reduces these problems.

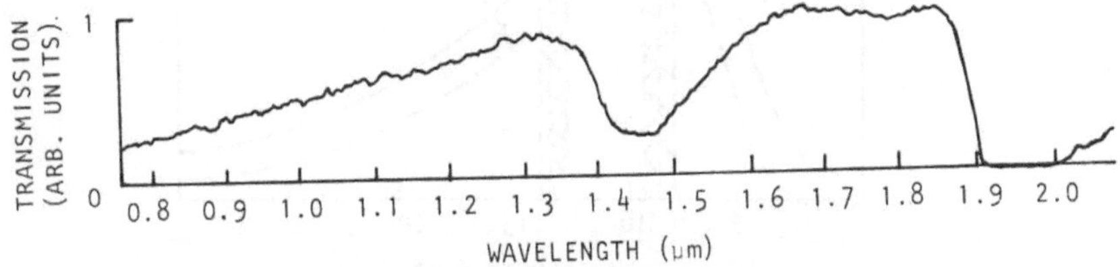

Fig. 13-15. Spectral transmission of human skin.

The ratio temperature of a body is the temperature a blackbody would have in order to emit continuum radiation having the same ratio of spectral radiance at two prescribed wavelengths. At any given temperature, every blackbody has the same wavelength distribution of radiance. This spectral distribution can be determined by measuring the radiance at two different wavelengths, thus yielding an accurate determination of the blackbody's temperature. The principle of ratio temperature measurement is shown in Fig. 13-16, which indicates the emission spectra of 310°K graybodies with the emissivities of 0.98 and 1.00.

A ratio temperature measurement is made by sampling the radiance of a spatial element at two points in the spectrum simultaneously, as indicated in the drawing. The wavelengths of the two passbands are chosen to achieve sensitivity to the change in curvature of the blackbody spectrum with temperature: typical values for the 300°K range are 5 and 13 μm. The ratioing technique eliminates the effect of wavelength-independent spatial and temporal emissivity variations. Mathematically, the system output is

$$\frac{E(T,\lambda_1)}{E(T,\lambda_2)} = \frac{\varepsilon_1 c_1 \lambda_1^{-4}[\exp(c_2/\lambda_1 T) - 1]^{-1}}{\varepsilon_2 c_1 \lambda_2^{-4}[\exp(c_2/\lambda_2 T) - 1]^{-1}} \tag{13-109}$$

where T is the kinetic temperature of the object, $E(T,\lambda_1)$ is the measured irradiance at λ_1, and $E(T,\lambda_2)$ is the measured irradiance at λ_2.

As one can see, the ratio of the two radiance values at given wavelengths is dependent upon temperature except in the Rayleigh–Jeans region ($c_2/\lambda T \ll 1$), which occurs at wavelengths much longer than those used for thermography. For the case in which the emissivity is independent of wavelength ($\varepsilon_1 = \varepsilon_2$), the ratio is independent of the emissivity, and the temperature one measures is the kinetic temperature.

If the emissivity is not constant with respect to wavelength, then the

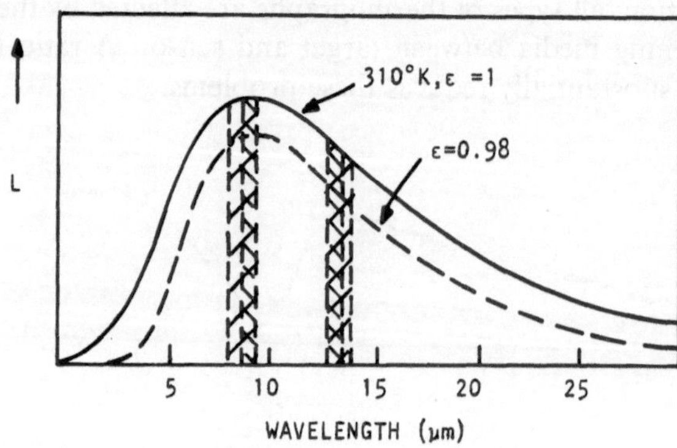

Fig. 13-16. Ratio temperature principles.

ratio temperature will be different from the kinetic temperature of the object. To determine the temperature this way it is not necessary to know the actual emissivity in the two spectral regions, only their ratio. The measurement of the ratio of radiances is less dependent on surface conditions than the measurement of either one of them.

For the same reason, absorption by intervening media will have less effect on color temperature measurements than on brightness temperature measurements, provided the absorption is not highly wavelength dependent since radiance values at two wavelengths are being compared. Over the pathlength used in thermographic applications, the atmosphere will have minimal effect, provided the strong (and possibly time-dependent) absorption bands of H_2O and CO_2 are avoided. For a given instrumental design, the proper choice of λ_1 and λ_2 can almost eliminate ratio temperature errors due to the intervening media.

The ratio temperature is determined by direct measurement of the ratio of the spectral radiances at two wavelengths. In the region for which the Wien law is a good approximation, it can be shown (Bramson, 1968) that the ratio temperature T_c is given by

$$T_c = \frac{c_2[(1/\lambda_2) - (1/\lambda_1)]}{\ln[E(T,\lambda_1)/E(T,\lambda_2)] + 4\ln(\lambda_1/\lambda_2)} \tag{13-110}$$

where $E(T, \lambda_i)$ is a measured value of irradiance. Now let

$$A = 4\ln(\lambda_1/\lambda_2)$$

$$B = c_2[(1/\lambda_1) - (1/\lambda_2)]$$

then

$$T_c = -\frac{B}{A + \ln[E(T,\lambda_1)/E(T,\lambda_2)]} \tag{13-111}$$

For this monochromatic case the relationship between the reciprocal of ratio temperature and the logarithm of the ratio of the spectral radiance can be expressed as a linear equation:

$$\frac{1}{T_c} = -\frac{A}{B} - \frac{1}{B}\ln\frac{E(T,\lambda_1)}{E(T,\lambda_2)} \tag{13-112}$$

For the temperature region of interest, namely, 300–310°K, the equation can be considered linear in the spectral radiance ratio. In a similar fashion, solving for kinetic temperature in terms of ratio temperature from Eq. (13-110), one can show that

$$T = T_c\left[1 - T_c\frac{\ln(\varepsilon_1/\varepsilon_2)}{c_2[(1/\lambda_1) - (1/\lambda_2)]}\right]^{-1} \tag{13-113}$$

Clearly, when $\varepsilon_1 = \varepsilon_2$, the kinetic temperature and ratio temperatures are equal.

As in the case of integral temperature, the important parameter is not the absolute temperature but the difference in temperature measured at two different locations. The expression for ratio temperature, Eq. (13-112), with the appropriate substitution can be shown to be

$$\frac{1}{T_c} = \frac{1}{T} - \frac{\lambda_1\lambda_2}{c_2(\lambda_2 - \lambda_1)} \ln\frac{\varepsilon_1}{\varepsilon_2} \tag{13-114}$$

In order to find the change in temperature and/or emissivity one can take the differential of Eq. (13-114). Since Eq. (13-114) is expressed in reciprocal temperature, the following relationship must be used:

$$d\frac{1}{T} = -\frac{1}{T^2}dT \tag{13-115}$$

or

$$dT = -T^2 d\frac{1}{T} \tag{13-116}$$

Therefore

$$dT_c = \frac{T_c^2}{T^2}dT + \frac{\lambda_1\lambda_2 T_c^2}{c_2(\lambda_1 - \lambda_2)}\left(\frac{d\varepsilon_1}{\varepsilon_1} - \frac{d\varepsilon_2}{\varepsilon_2}\right) \tag{13-117}$$

The ratio temperature difference is made up of two terms: one term is the true kinetic temperature change and a second term causes an error due to emissivity changes. The second term is the one of interest. Equation (13-117) indicates that the emissivity errors subtract, thus making the emissivity uncertainty have less influence on the measurement accuracy. If, for instance, $\varepsilon_1 = 0.99 \pm 0.01$ and $\varepsilon_2 = 0.90 \pm 0.01$, then $d\varepsilon_1/\varepsilon_1 = 0.0101$ and $d\varepsilon_2/\varepsilon_2 = 0.111$. The resulting error in the emissivities would then be $d(\varepsilon_1/\varepsilon_2)/(\varepsilon_1/\varepsilon_2) = 0.001$, which is an order of magnitude better than $d\varepsilon_1/\varepsilon_1$ or $d\varepsilon_2/\varepsilon_2$. This analysis is based on the emissivity uncertainties having a high degree of correlation.

The amount of correlation between ε_1 and ε_2 is a rather subjective argument. An analysis will be carried out in terms of a correlation coefficient, which determines the amount of correlation necessary to have a ratio temperature measurement with the same error as the integral temperature measurement.

If one assumes $d\varepsilon_1/\varepsilon_1$ and $d\varepsilon_2/\varepsilon_2$ are two random variables γ_1 and γ_2 with normal (Gaussian) distribution functions and identical deviations, their joint probability density function is (Papoulis, 1965)

$$f_{\gamma_1\gamma_2}(\gamma_1\gamma_2) = \frac{1}{2\pi\sigma^2(1-r^2)^{1/2}} \exp\left[-\frac{1}{2(1-r^2)\sigma^2}(\gamma_1^2 - 2r\gamma_1\gamma_2 + \gamma_2^2)\right] \tag{13-118}$$

where r is the correlation coefficient between γ_1 and γ_2, and σ is the standard deviation of either ε_1 or ε_2.

If $\gamma_1 - \gamma_2$ is written as γ_c, then the problem is to determine the variance of γ_c as a function of the variances of γ_1 and γ_2 and the correlation coefficient r.

Following Papoulis (1965) one can write

$$\gamma_D = \gamma_1 + \gamma_2 \tag{13-119}$$

Now solving for γ_1 and γ_2,

$$\begin{aligned}\gamma_1 &= \tfrac{1}{2}(\gamma_D + \gamma_c) \\ \gamma_2 &= \tfrac{1}{2}(\gamma_D - \gamma_c)\end{aligned} \tag{13-120}$$

where γ_D is a coordinate transformation variable.

By direct substitution for γ_1 and γ_2 using Eq. (13-120)

$$f_{\gamma_c\gamma}\ (\gamma_c\gamma_D) = \frac{1}{2\pi\sigma^2(1-r^2)} \exp\left\{-\frac{1}{4\sigma^2(1-r^2)}[\gamma_c^2(1+2r) + \gamma_D^2(1-2r)]\right\} \tag{13-121}$$

the density function is Gaussian as expected and is of the general form

$$\exp(-x^2/2\sigma^2) \tag{13-122}$$

where the variance of γ_c is given by

$$\sigma_c^2 = \frac{2(1-r^2)\sigma^2}{1+2r} \tag{13-123}$$

The important result is the value of the correlation when the variance of the ratio temperature is equal to that of the integral temperature or

$$\sigma_c^2 = \sigma^2 = \frac{2(1-r^2)\sigma^2}{1+2r} \tag{13-124}$$

which reduces to a quadratic equation in r with a solution of $r = 0.366$. Therefore, if the correlation is equal to or greater than 0.366, ratio temperature will have less error than integral temperature.

The correlation between the emissivities is strongly related to the choice of the two spectral regions. Spectral emissivity changes should be smooth, so the resulting error in the ratio of the emissivities is expected to be very small. This means that the two spectral bands should be close together, favoring the 8–14 μm region, where no abrupt emissivity changes are reported. Caution is necessary in dealing with the 3–5 μm region because of the apparent emission band reported by Lloyd-Williams *et al.* (1963).

However, one expects the emissivity in both spectral regions to vary in a similar manner, so the ratio is independent over the spatial region being scanned. The situation in which the emissivity of a spatial element in one spectral region increases and in another spectral region decreases is highly unlikely.

13.11. ERROR ANALYSIS, MONOCHROMATIC CASE

The ratio temperature and integral temperature thermographs are compared on the basis of errors involved in the measurements. The changes or difference in temperature can be expressed as follows for either type of system:

$$\Delta T = T_1 - T_2 \tag{13-125}$$

The accuracy of ΔT can be related to how well T_1 and T_2 are measured. Mathematically, the errors can be expressed as

$$\sigma_{\Delta T}^2 = \sigma_{T_1}^2 + \sigma_{T_2}^2 \tag{13-126}$$

If the errors in the measurement of T_1 and T_2 are less for one system, then the total error for that system would also be less for that system. Therefore it remains to be shown that the errors of ratio temperature measurement are smaller than those of integral temperature (Herne, 1953; Pyatt, 1954).

Consider a source having a kinetic temperature T with emissivities ε_b, ε_1, and ε_2 at wavelengths λ_b, λ_1, and λ_2, respectively. Since Wien's law will be used, a small error is introduced as discussed previously; however, both systems will be evaluated with the same approximations so that error should cancel out to the first order. Since temperature appears in the denominator, for mathematical convenience an error in $1/T$ will be found and then translated to an error in T.

For an integral temperature radiometer operating at λ_b, one can call the measured temperature T_B. Equating the measured and predicted radiance one finds from the emittance

$$L_{qb} = c_1\lambda_b^{-4}[\exp(-c_2/\lambda_b T_B)] = \varepsilon_b c_1 \lambda_b^{-4}[\exp(-c_2/\lambda_b T)] \tag{13-127}$$

taking the logarithm of both sides

$$\ln \varepsilon_b = \frac{c_2}{\lambda_b}\left(\frac{1}{T} - \frac{1}{T_B}\right) \tag{13-128}$$

Defining the error

$$E_b = \frac{1}{T} - \frac{1}{T_B}$$
$$E_b = \frac{\lambda_b}{c} \ln \varepsilon_b \tag{13-129}$$

E_b is the systematic error of the integral temperature radiometer. If T_c is the ratio temperature measured between λ_1 and λ_2, by recalling Eq. (13-109) with the appropriate substitutions

$$\frac{\varepsilon_1 c_1 \lambda_1^{-4}[\exp(-c_2/\lambda_1 T)]}{\varepsilon_2 c_1 \lambda_2^{-4}[\exp(-c_2/\lambda_2 T)]} = \frac{c_1 \lambda_1^{-4}[\exp(-c_2/\lambda_1 T_c)]}{c_1 \lambda_2^{-4}[\exp(-c_2/\lambda_2 T_c)]} \tag{13-130}$$

Taking the logarithm of the equation, then

$$\ln \frac{\varepsilon_1}{\varepsilon_2} + \frac{c_2}{T}\left(\frac{1}{\lambda_2} - \frac{1}{\lambda_1}\right) = \frac{c_2}{T_c}\left(\frac{1}{\lambda_2} - \frac{1}{\lambda_1}\right) \tag{13-131}$$

and

$$\ln \frac{\varepsilon_1}{\varepsilon_2} = -c_2\left(\frac{1}{\lambda_2} - \frac{1}{\lambda_1}\right)\left(\frac{1}{T} - \frac{1}{T_c}\right) \tag{13-132}$$

The reciprocal ratio temperature error can be written as

$$E_c = \frac{1}{T} - \frac{1}{T_c}$$
$$E_c = -\frac{\lambda_1 \lambda_2}{c_2(\lambda_1 - \lambda_2)} \ln \frac{\varepsilon_1}{\varepsilon_2} \tag{13-133}$$

As discussed previously, the ratio of the emissivities needs to be equal to 1 for a correct measurement. However, if the ratio is not unity, the error can be plus or minus, unlike the case for integral temperature, where it can only be negative.

E_b and E_c, the systematic errors in the reciprocal temperature, were introduced as a mathematical convenience; the temperature error is of real interest. The corresponding error in the temperature can be expressed as

$$e_b = T_B - T \tag{13-134}$$

and

$$e_c = T_c - T \tag{13-135}$$

With a minor amount of algebra one can obtain e_b and e_c from E_b and E_c.

In order to make a direct comparison between integral and ratio temperature, one can assume that one of the wavelengths, λ_2, is common to both the integral radiometer and the ratio temperature radiometer, ($\lambda_b = \lambda_2$) and ($\varepsilon_b = \varepsilon_2$).

From Eqs. (13-128) and (13-132),

$$\frac{1}{T} - \frac{1}{T_B} = \frac{\lambda_2}{c_2} \ln \varepsilon_2$$
$$\frac{1}{T} - \frac{1}{T_c} = \frac{-\lambda_1 \lambda_2}{c_2(\lambda_1 - \lambda_2)} \ln \frac{\varepsilon_1}{\varepsilon_2} \tag{13-136}$$

The solution of $\ln \varepsilon_1$ in terms of $\ln \varepsilon_2$ can be found to be

$$\ln \varepsilon_1 = \ln \varepsilon_2 \left(1 + \frac{\lambda_1 - \lambda_2}{\lambda_1 \{ (T\lambda_2/c_2) \ln \varepsilon_2 + (e_b/e_c) [1 - (T\lambda_2/c_2) \ln \varepsilon_2] \}} \right) \tag{13-137}$$

The error e_b can be negative only; however, e_c can be positive or negative depending on the selectivity of the surface emissivities vs. wavelength, the worst case being ε_1 with a positive error and ε_2 with a negative error.

There a range of emissivity values can be defined for any given ratio of errors in temperature:

$$\ln \varepsilon_2 \left\{ 1 + \frac{\lambda_2 - \lambda_1}{\lambda_1} \left[\frac{T\lambda_2}{c_2} \ln \varepsilon_2 + \left| \frac{e_b}{e_c} \right| \left(1 - \frac{T\lambda_2}{c_2} \ln \varepsilon_2 \right) \right]^{-1} \right\} < \ln \varepsilon_1$$
$$< \ln \varepsilon_2 \left\{ 1 + \frac{\lambda_2 - \lambda_1}{\lambda_1} \left[\frac{T\lambda_2}{c_2} \ln \varepsilon_2 - \left| \frac{e_b}{e_c} \right| \left(1 - \frac{T\lambda_2}{c_2} \ln \varepsilon_2 \right) \right]^{-1} \right\} \tag{13-138}$$

The ratio of errors in temperature can be less than, equal to, or greater than 1, depending on whether the integral temperature has less error, the same error, or more error than the ratio temperature. A family of curves for ε_1 vs. ε_2 can be plotted as a function of the ratio of the temperature errors for a given system (λ, λ_2, and T defined). The case when the errors are equal ($e_b = e_c$) form a locus of points that defines two regions of minimum temperature error. A plot of ε_1 vs. ε_2 is shown in Fig. 13-17 for $\lambda = 5\ \mu$m and $\lambda = 13.5\ \mu$m and an object temperature of 310°K.

The shaded area is the region in which the ratio temperature has less error than integral temperature ($e_b/e_c > 1$). Shown in the shaded area is a

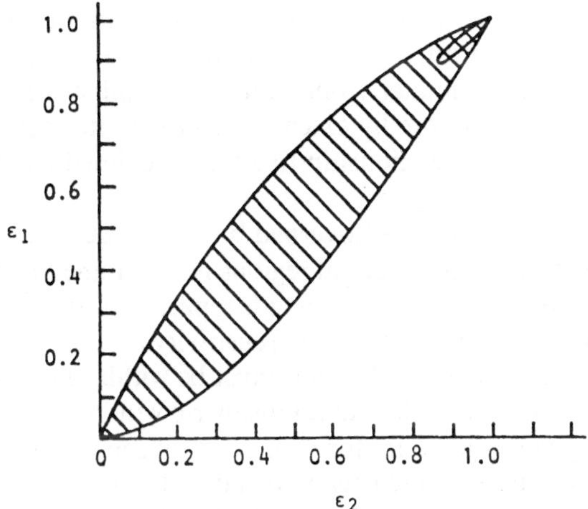

Fig. 13-17. Emissivity plot.

region representing the best guess as to the emissivity of skin (Steketee, 1973a) at 5 and 13.5 μm. Clearly it is in this region that ratio temperature is a more accurate measurement.

13.12. ERROR ANALYSIS, FINITE SPECTRAL BANDWIDTHS

Real radiometers measure irradiances in finite spectral bands, and therefore for a real case the irradiance is integrated over finite spectral regions around λ_1 and λ_2. The monochromatic case treated previously never exists.

Instrumentally the following equation describes color temperature:

$$\frac{\int_{\Delta\lambda} L(T_c, \lambda_1)\,\tau(\lambda_1)\,\tau_f(\lambda_1)\,d\lambda}{\int_{\Delta\lambda_2} L(T_c, \lambda_2)\,\tau(\lambda_2)\,\tau_f(\lambda_2)\,d\lambda} = \frac{E(T, \Delta\lambda_1)}{E(T, \Delta\lambda_2)} \tag{13-139}$$

where $E(T, \Delta\lambda_1)$ is the irradiance measured over a finite bandwidth $\Delta\lambda_1$, $E(T, \Delta\lambda_2)$ is the irradiance measured over a finite bandwidth $\Delta\lambda_2$, $\tau(\lambda)$ is the atmospheric transmission, and $\tau_f(\lambda)$ is the filter transmission.

For a manageable calculation one assumes the emissivity to be nonselective, the atmospheric transmission constant over the spectral regions, and the filters to have equal transmission with rectangular spectral characteristics. Then

$$\frac{\int_{\Delta\lambda_1} \lambda^{-4}[\exp(c_2/\lambda T_c) - 1]^{-1}\,d\lambda}{\int_{\Delta\lambda_2} \lambda^{-4}[\exp(c_2/\lambda T_c) - 1]^{-1}\,d\lambda} = \frac{E(T, \Delta\lambda_1)}{E(T, \Delta\lambda_2)} \tag{13-140}$$

The linearity with temperature is as expected from the monochromatic case. However, of most interest is that the width of the spectral bandwidth is not of great concern; in fact, from an instrumental standpoint the widest bandwidth is best. Therefore by extension to the finite spectral region one still has a pseudolinear relationship like that predicted by the monochromatic analysis.

The choice of λ_1 and λ_2 is governed by several qualitative factors. The slope of the curves for finite spectral regions is determined by the separation of λ_1 and λ_2; the greater the wavelength separation, the greater the slope and, correspondingly, the temperature sensitivity.

In addition, the wavelength bands must be within the spectral response of the detectors and also within an atmospheric window.

Competing with the desire for wide spectral separation is the problem of emissivity variations, which tends to favor the condition that the two wavelengths be close together, and is a factor that favors the 8–14 μm region, where no emissivity changes are reported. Thus it might prove best to pick two wavelengths in this spectral bandwidth. Caution is necessary in dealing with the 3–5 μm region because of the possible emission bands reported by Lloyd-Williams *et al.* (1963).

APPENDIX 13.A. SERIES EVALUATION OF INTEGRALS

The integrals given in the text can be evaluated by a series approach. (There are other ways for evaluating the integral, but I find the series approach satisfying and useful.) First, consider the integral

$$I = \int_0^\lambda \lambda^{-4} x e^x (e^x - 1)^{-2}\, d\lambda$$

$$= \int_x^0 \left(\frac{Tx^{-4}}{c_2}\right) x e^x (e^x - 1)^{-2} \frac{c_2}{Tx^2}\, dx$$

$$= \left(\frac{T}{c_2}\right)^3 \int_x^0 x^3 e^x (e^x - 1)^{-2}\, dx$$

The integrand can be written

$$\frac{x^3 e^x}{e^{2x} - 2e^x + 1} = \frac{x^3}{e^x - 2 + e^{-x}} \times e^x - 2 + e^{-x} \frac{e^{-x} + 2e^{-2x} + 3e^{-3x} + \cdots}{1}$$

$$\times \frac{1 - 2e^{-x} + e^{-2x}}{2e^{-x} + e^{-2x}} \times \frac{2e^{-x} - 4e^{-2x} + 2e^{-3x}}{3e^{-2x} - 2e^{-3x}}$$

Therefore

$$\int_0^\lambda \frac{\partial L_q}{\partial T} dT\, d\lambda = \frac{c_1}{\pi hc} \frac{dT}{T} \left(\frac{T}{c_2} \right)^3 \int_x^0 x^3 \sum_{m=1}^{\infty} me^{-mx}\, dx$$

This integral can be integrated by parts as follows:

$$\int_x^0 x^3 \sum me^{-mx}\, dx = \sum_m m \int_x^0 x^3 e^{-mx}\, dx$$

$$= \sum m \left(-\frac{x^3}{m} e^{-mx} + 3 \int_x^0 \frac{x^2}{m} e^{-mx} \right)$$

$$u = x^3\, dv = e^{-mx}$$

$$du = 3x^2\, dxv = -\frac{1}{m} e^{-mx}$$

$$= \sum m \left[-\frac{x^3}{m} e^{-mx} - \frac{3x^2}{m^2} e^{-mx} - \frac{6x}{m^3} - \frac{6}{m^4} \right]$$

$$= -\sum m^{-3} e^{-mx} [(mx)^3 + 3(mx)^2 + 6mx + 6]$$

$$= \sum m^{-3} e^{-mx} [(mx)^3 + 3(mx)^2 + 6mx + 6]$$

Therefore, if this sum is designated simply as $\sum_3$, then

$$\int_0^\lambda \frac{\partial L_q}{\partial T} dT\, d\lambda = \frac{c_1}{\pi hc} \frac{dT}{T} \left(\frac{T}{c_2} \right)^3 \sum_3$$

The second term in the signal portion of the equation is

$$\int_0^\lambda \frac{\partial L_{q\lambda}}{\partial \varepsilon} d\varepsilon\, d\lambda$$

The quantity $L_{q\lambda}$ can be written as

$$L_{q\lambda} = \varepsilon L_q^{BB}(\lambda, T)$$

Therefore

$$\frac{\partial L_{q\lambda}}{\partial \varepsilon} = L_{q\lambda}^{BB}(\lambda, T) = \frac{c_1 \lambda^{-4} (e^x - 1)^{-1}}{\pi hc}$$

The evaluation of this quantity is as follows:

$$
\begin{aligned}
L_q^{BB} &= \int_0^{\lambda} \frac{c_1}{\pi hc} \lambda^{-4}(e^x - 1)^{-1}\, d\lambda \\
&= \frac{c_1}{\pi hc}\left(\frac{T}{c_2}\right)^4 \int_x^0 x^4(e^x - 1)^{-1} \frac{c_2}{T}\left(-\frac{dx}{x^2}\right) \\
&= \frac{c_1}{\pi hc}\left(\frac{T}{c_2}\right)^3 \int_0^x x^2(e_x - 1)^{-1}\, dx \\
&= \frac{c_1}{\pi hc}\left(\frac{T}{c_2}\right)^3 \sum \int x^2 e^{-mx}\, dx \\
&= \frac{c_1}{\pi hc}\left(\frac{T}{c_2}\right)^3 \sum \left(\frac{x^2 e^{-mx}}{m} + \frac{2x}{m^2} + \frac{2}{m^3}\right) \\
&= \frac{c_1}{\pi hc}\left(\frac{T}{c_2}\right)^3 \sum m^{-3} e^{-mx}[(mx)^2 + 2mx + 2] \\
&= \frac{c_1}{\pi hc}\left(\frac{T}{c_2}\right)^3 \sum_2
\end{aligned}
$$

APPENDIX 13.B. FOURIER AND LAPLACE TRANSFORM RELATIONSHIPS

The Fourier transform is defined as

$$F(\omega) = \mathscr{F}\{f(t)\} = \int_{-\infty}^{\infty} f(t)\, e^{-j\omega t}\, dt$$

In general, $F(\omega)$ is complex so that

$$F(\omega) = R(\omega) + jI(\omega)$$

The inverse transform is

$$f(t) = \mathscr{F}^{-1}\{F(\omega)\} = \int_{-\infty}^{\infty} F(\omega)\, e^{j\omega t}\, dt$$

where $f = \omega/2\pi$.

The Laplace transform in a sense is a stronger transform. The sense is that it has an integrating factor:

$$F(s) = \int_0^{\infty} f(t)\, e^{-st}\, dt$$

where $s = \sigma + j\omega$.

We can also define the two-sided Laplace transform, which is

$$F_{\pm}(s) = \int_{-\infty}^{\infty} f(t)\, e^{-st}\, dt + F_{+}(s) + F_{-}(s)$$

$$F_{\pm}(s) = \int_{-0}^{\infty} f(t)\, e^{-st}\, dt + \int_{-\infty}^{0} f(t)\, e^{-st}\, dt$$

The one-sided Laplace transform requires that $f(t)$ be of exponential order. The Fourier transform function must be such that

$$\int_{-\infty}^{\infty} f(t)\, dt < \infty$$

The region of convergence for the regular Laplace transform is greater than some line $\sigma = \sigma_0$. At all values greater than this $L(s)$ is analytic, that is, it has no poles. The negative one-sided Laplace transform is the reverse of this, so there is a strip of convergence. The Fourier transform is a two-sided Laplace transform with $\sigma = 0$.

Convolution and Multiplication. The convolution of two time functions in the time domain is equivalent to the multiplication of their spectra in the frequency domain, and vice versa:

$$\{f(t)^{*}\, g(t)\} = F(\omega)\, G(\omega)$$

$$\{F(\omega)^{*}\, G(\omega)\} = f(t)\, g(t)$$

$$\{f(t)\, g(t)\} = F(\omega)^{*}\, (\omega)$$

$$\{F(\omega)\, G(\omega)\} = f(t)^{*}\, g(t)$$

The proof of the first of these theorems is given. The remaining ones follow in the same way:

$$f(t)^{*}\, g(t) = \int_{-\infty}^{\infty}\int_{-\infty}^{\infty} f(t)\, g(t-\tau)\, dt e^{-j\omega\tau}\, d\tau$$

$$= \int_{-\infty}^{\infty} f(t)\, e^{-j\omega t}\, dt \int_{-\infty}^{\infty} g(t-\tau)\, e^{-j\omega(\tau - t)}\, d\tau$$

$$= F(\omega)\, G^{*}(\omega)$$

Parseval's Theorem. The basic statement of the theorem is that the integral of the square of a function $f(t)$ over all time is equal to the integral of the square of absolute value of its Fourier transform over all frequencies:

$$F(\omega) = \int_{-\infty}^{\infty} f(t)\, e^{-j\omega t}\, dt$$

$$F(\omega) F(-\omega) = \iint\limits_{-\infty}^{\infty} f(t)\, f(t)\, e^{-j\omega t} e^{j\omega t}\, dt\, dt$$

$$\int_{-\infty}^{\infty} F(\omega)\, F^*(\omega)\, d\omega = \iiint\limits_{-\infty}^{\infty} f(t)\, f(t)\, e^{-j\omega t} e^{j\omega t}\, dt\, dt\, d\omega$$

$$= \int_{-\infty}^{\infty} \left[\iint\limits_{-\infty}^{\infty} f(t)\, e^{-j\omega t} e^{j\omega t}\, d\omega\, dt \right] f(t)\, dt$$

$$= \int_{-\infty}^{\infty} \left[\int_{-\infty}^{\infty} F(\omega)\, e^{j\omega t}\, d\omega \right] f(t)\, dt$$

$$= 2\pi \int_{-\infty}^{\infty} f(t)\, f(t)\, dt$$

Therefore

$$\int_{-\infty}^{\infty} f(t)\, f(t)\, dt = \frac{1}{2\pi} \int_{-\infty}^{\infty} F(\omega)\, F^*(\omega)\, d\omega = \int_{-\infty}^{\infty} F(\omega)\, F^*(\omega)\, d\nu$$

The quantity $F(\omega)\, F^*(\omega) = |F(\omega)|^2$ is a symmetric function so that

$$\int_{\infty}^{\infty} f^2(t)\, dt = 2 \int_{0}^{\infty} |F(\omega)|^2\, d\nu$$

Correlation and Wiener Spectra. The autocorrelation function of a random variable $f(t)$ can be written

$$R_{ff}(\tau) \equiv \overline{f(t)\, f(t+\tau)}$$

$$= \lim_{T \to \infty} \left[\frac{1}{2T} \int_{-T}^{T} f_T(t)\, f_T(t+\tau)\, dt \right]$$

The random variable $f_T(t)$ is just $f(t)$ truncated after time T (in order to keep the total energy of the function finite). The bar above means average with respect to time. It is assumed that the system is shift invariant. Otherwise the time separation parameter τ must be replaced with two variables, the two times of measurement t_1 and t_2.

The power spectrum, or more generally the Wiener spectrum $W(\omega)$, is defined in terms of the spectra of the random variables:

$$W(\omega) = \lim_{T\to\infty}\left[\frac{1}{2T}F_T(\omega)\,F_T^*(\omega)\right]$$

It is called a power spectrum because when $f(t)$ is either a current or voltage, then $W(\omega)$ is the spectrum of the power through a 1-Ω resistor. Since we have other uses for the mathematical forms, we shall be more general and use the term "Wiener spectrum."

The Wiener–Khinchine theorem states that the correlation function of a random variable and the power spectrum of the same random variable are Fourier transforms of each other. We shall prove this now:

$$R_{\mathrm{ff}}(\tau) = \lim_{T\to\infty}\frac{1}{2T}\int_{-\infty}^{\infty} f(t)\,f(t+\tau)\,dt$$

$$\mathscr{F}\{R_{\mathrm{ff}}(\tau)\} = \int_{-\infty}^{\infty}\lim_{T\to\infty}\frac{1}{2T}\int_{-T}^{T} f_T(t)\,f_T(t+\tau)\,dt e^{-j\omega t'}\,dt'$$

The prime is used to keep track of the different time differentials and integrals. With impunity we move the limit operation inside the integral and manipulate on the exponent:

$$\mathscr{F}\{R_{\mathrm{ff}}(\tau)\} = \int_{-\infty}^{\infty}\lim_{T\to\infty}\frac{1}{2T}\int_{-T}^{T} f_T(t)\,f_T(t+\tau)\,e^{-j\omega(t+\tau)}e^{j\omega\tau}\,dt\,dt$$

$$= \lim_{T\to\infty}\frac{1}{2T}\int_{-T}^{T}\int_{-\infty}^{\infty} f_T(t)\,e^{j\omega\tau}f_T(t+\tau)\,e^{-j\omega(t+\tau)}\,dt\,dt$$

$$= \lim_{T\to\infty}\left(\frac{F_T F_T^*}{2T}\right) = W(\omega)$$

The only questions left are the legitimacy of changing the integration variables and moving the limits through the integral sign. Both are all right because integration is from $-\infty$ to $+\infty$.

This relationship holds for cross correlations as well as autocorrelations. The special case for which $\tau = 0$ shows the relationship for the variance and the variance spectrum is

$$\{\sigma_{\mathrm{ff}}\} = \{R_{\mathrm{ff}}(0)\} = W(\omega)$$

REFERENCES

Bramson, M.A. (1968), *Infrared Radiation*, Plenum Press, New York.

Burgess, R.E. (1955), *Proc. Phys. Soc. (London)* **B68**:661.

Burgess, R.E. (1956), *Proc. Phys. Soc. (London)* **B69**:1020.

Dodd, G.D., Zermeno, A., Wallace, J.D., and Marsh, L.M. (1973), Breast thermography: The state of the art, *Curr. Probl. Radiol.* **3**:6.

Elam, R., Goodwin, D.N., and Lloyd-Williams, K. (1963), Optical properties of the human epidermis, *Nature* **198**:1001.

Hardy, J.D., and Muschenheim, C. (1936), Radiation of heat from the human body, V. The transmission of infrared radiation through skin, *J. Clin. Invest.* **15**:1.

Hardy, J.D., Hammel, H.T., and Murgatroyd, D. (1956), Spectral transmittance and reflectances of excised human skin, *J. Appl. Physiol.* **9**:257.

Herne, C.D. (1953), Theoretical considerations of bichromatic pyrometers, *Br. J. Appl. Phys.* **4**:374.

Kruse, P.W., McGlauchlin, L.D., and McQuistan, R.B. (1962), *Elements of Infrared Technology, Generation Transmission and Detection*, John Wiley and Sons, New York.

Lewis, D.W., Goller, H., and Teates, C.D. (1973), Apparent temperature degradation in thermograms of human anatomy viewed obliquely, *Diagn. Radiol.* **106**:95.

Lloyd-Williams, K., Case, C.M., and Goodwin, D.W. (1963), The electronic heat-camera in medical research, *J. Br. IRE* **25**:241.

Long, D., and Schmit, J.L. (1970), in Willardson, R.K., and Beer, A.C. (eds.), *Semiconductors and Semimetals*, Academic Press New York, Chapter 5, p. 222.

Mitchell, D., Wyndham, C.H., and Hodgson, T. (1967), Measurement of the total normal emissivity of skin without the need for measuring skin temperature, *Phys. Med. Biol.* **12**:359.

Nicodemus, F.E. (1968), Emissivity of isothermal spherical cavity with gray lambertian wall, *Appl. Opt.* **7**:7, 1359.

Papoulis, A. (1965), *Probability, Random Variables and Stochastic Processes*, McGraw-Hill Book Co., New York.

Pyatt, E.C. (1954), Some considerations of the errors of brightness and two color types of spectral radiation pyrometers, *Br. J. Appl. Phys.* **5**:264.

Steketee, J. (1973a), The effect of transmission on temperature measurements of human skin, *Phys. Med. Biol.* **18**:726.

Steketee, J. (1973b), Spectral emissivity of skin and pericardium, *Phys. Med. Biol.* **18**:686.

Van Vliet, K.M. (1958), *Proc. IRE* **46**:1004.

Watmough, D.J., and Oliver, R. (1970), Some physical factors relevant to infrared thermography, *Phys. Med. Biol.* **15**:178.

Wolfe, W.L. (1965), *Handbook of Military Infrared Technology*, U. S. Government Printing Office, Washington, D.C.

Index